ACU

your guide to complete knowledge

康

DAVID J. KUOCH

Acumedwest Inc.
PO BOX 14068
San Francisco, CA 94114
www.acupuncturedeskreference.com

ISBN 978-0-615-15463-3
$44.95

Acupuncture Desk Reference™
by David J. Kuoch, L.Ac.

Acumedwest Inc.

Disclaimer: This book is intended as a quick-reference volume for educational purposes only and not as medical information. It is designed to help students and professionals in the acupuncture field make informed decisions about health based on the assumption that the reader has thorough training in acupuncture and herbal procedures and treatment. It is best treated as a supplemental source for information used in daily practice and as a reminder of knowledge gained elsewhere. The information in this book is compiled from reliable sources, and exhaustive efforts have been put forth to make the book as accurate as possible.

The ideas, procedures, and suggestions contained in this book are not intended as a substitute for consulting with your physician. Health care professionals should use sound judgment and individualized therapy for each specific patient care situation. If you suspect that you have a medical problem, seek competent medical help. Neither the author nor the publisher shall have any liability to any person or entity with regard to claims, loss, injury, or damage caused, or alleged to be caused, directly or indirectly by the use of information contained herein, or damage arising from any information or suggestion in this book.

Although great care has been taken to maintain the accuracy of the information contained in this book, the information as presented in this book is for educational purposes only. I cannot anticipate all conditions under which this information might be used. In view of ongoing research, changes in governmental regulation, and the constant flow of information relating to Chinese and Western medicine, as well as herbal therapy, the reader is urged to check with other sources for all up-to-date information.

The staff and authors of Acumedwest Inc. recognize that practitioners accessing this content will have varying levels of training and expertise; therefore, we accept no responsibility for the results obtained by the application of the material within this book. Neither Acumedwest Inc. nor the authors of Acupuncture Desk Reference can be held responsible for human, electronic or mechanical errors of fact or omission, nor for any consequences arising from the use or misuse of the information herein.

The statements in this book have not been evaluated by the Food and Drug Administration. These products are not intended to diagnose, treat, cure or prevent any disease and they are not intended to replace the diagnosis, treatments, prescriptions and services of a trained practitioner or physician.

Published by Acumedwest Inc.
PO Box 14068
San Francisco, CA 94114
Tel: 310-395-9573
www.acupuncturedeskreference.com

Library of Congress Control Number: 2007906092
ISBN 978-0-615-15463-3

Printed in China

"A wise man should consider that health is the greatest of human blessings, and learn how by his own thought to derive benefit from his illnesses." ~ Hippocrates

Purpose of the Book

Acupuncture Desk Reference™ is a quick reference book for Traditional Chinese Medicine practitioners. This is not a medical book; rather, it is designed for educational purposes to help acupuncture professionals make informed decisions on patient care. This book is a collection of information assembled to help the practitioner become effective and successful in TCM practice. The authors assume the reader has familiarity with acupuncture, herbal procedure, treatment, as well as cautions and contraindications of TCM. This text is best used as a supplemental source for information used in daily practice and as a reminder of knowledge and information learned elsewhere. As an acupuncturist, Chinese herbalist, and health care provider, I wrote this book primarily for the licensed practitioner.

To the practitioner who wants to discriminate between formulas, herbs, clinical practice, food as medicine, Western medicine, office procedure, and alternative remedies, Acupuncture Desk Reference is "user friendly." After three years of compiling the information from multiple sources and organizing it in a database, I am able to offer a reference book with easily accessible tables that has integrated both the classics of TCM and Western methodology.

How the Book Came About

I started working on Acupuncture Desk Reference in my third year of acupuncture school at Emperor's College of Traditional Chinese Medicine. I found it cumbersome to need different texts for the variety of different subjects that acupuncture encompasses. It became an exhaustive task to seek out information on a particular herb, formula, or acupuncture treatment. As a student, I quickly became overwhelmed by the amount of information we needed to know in each area. I started compiling the information into a database to help organize what I thought would be pertinent in my practice at a later date.

As my computer database grew, so did the sources of information and volumes of books that I had begun to collect. By the time I graduated, the volumes of information grew to nearly 150 TCM and Western books. In both English and Chinese, some of these books represent the core of TCM and Western medicine, while others are more obscure in content but still contain invaluable information. As you can imagine, in clinical practice, looking up the information while treating patients at the same time became a difficult task. I needed a way to refresh my memory on the options for formulas, herbs and treatment. Eventually, I created one cohesive resource from which I could access both TCM and Western medical theory without pulling several books off the shelf every time.

By the time I graduated, the information from my class notes and textbooks could fit into the palm of my hand thanks to technology and databases. In school I was one of those students who felt that integrative medicine should include a stronger foundation in Western medicine and began assimilating this information. Our approach was integrative in theory, but in clinical practice the Western medicine was used sparingly and strictly adhered to TCM principles. As health care providers, I felt that we had an obligation to treat our patients using every tool possible, whether TCM, Western, or alternative, offering our patients healthcare options. If we needed to do orthopaedic tests, recall a cranial nerve test, look for signs of cancer, or identify a vitamin for a common ailment, this information could be integrated with the appropriate herbs, formulas, zang fu, and treatment procedures.

After graduating from acupuncture school, I consulted my former roommate, who is now an orthopaedic surgeon and professor at NYU. His comment was that the best books he found for reference were books packed with information and tables to refresh his memory. Most physicians hate reading anything too lengthy and prefer content that provides information as quickly as possible. If a patient comes through the door with something the practitioner has never seen before, he could treat the condition with confidence, step out of the room for a moment, and then double check the information in his medical text with his diagnosis. This is when you need your medical text.

INTRODUCTION

Format of Acupuncture Desk Reference

In practice, a TCM practitioner already knows the information. He/she needs something to refresh his/her memory. I mentioned my project idea to Linda Morse, LAc, recognized for her work in national and state board licensing examination review training. She commented that there are many books for students, but so few for licensed practitioners that can be used in everyday practice. Many TCM practitioners have books in their offices but rarely open them unless they need to confirm what they have already read in their medical text. Another colleague, Mick Brackle, LAc, commented that most physicians use their PDR everyday; however, our profession lacks a strong clinical reference book that is easy to use. We have many great reference books but need to condense the information and develop a practitioners guide that can fit in the palm of the hand or the pocket of a medical coat, which a practitioner could reference with ease: a comprehensive and usable handbook that includes herbs, formulas, acupuncture, clinical practice, zang fu, food as medicine as well as Western methodology. Thus began the development of Acupuncture Desk Reference™.

The comments I have received from my colleagues during the peer review are invaluable. I realize that this book could have been organized in a different manner: the formulas and herbs arranged by categories, the exclusion of certain techniques and divergent treatments, the omission of certain formulas and herbs, dosages that were not included or a book that was printed too small.

This is by no means a book lengthy in explanation, but instead, a handbook with material that can be easily referenced. Tables and brevity of content seem the most logical way of disseminating the information without overwhelming the reader. Some readers may enjoy the format and some may find the text too brief or requiring further explanation. It assumes that most of the information is common knowledge to the practitioner. For those who require more information, I have included a section towards the back of the book, "Resources," which will direct the reader to a detailed explanation of the subject at hand. I encourage you to build your library for those times when you need to reference what you already know and treat your patients with confidence.

Please be advised: if you are an unlicensed practitioner or anyone without the proper training in acupuncture and herbology, the ideas, procedures, and suggestions contained in this book are not intended as a substitute for consulting with your TCM practioner or health-care professional.

Table of Abbreviations

Meridians	Channels	(Optional)
Lu	Lung	LU
LI	Large Intestine	LI
St	Stomach	ST
Sp	Spleen	SP
Ht	Heart	HT
SI	Small Intestine	SI
Sj	San Jiao	SJ
Pc	Pericardium	PC
Ub	Urinary Bladder	UB
K	Kidney	Kid or KD
Liv	Liver	LIV
Gb	Gallbladder	GB
Ren	Ren / Conception	REN
Du	Du / Governor	DU
E	Extraordinary	.
g	Gram	
C/I	Contraindicated	

cknowledgement

vould like to express my gratitude to my friends and family, colleagues, and associates for
e support and encouragement. A special thank you to Amy Gayheart Kuoch, for your love,
ht, patience and wisdom to guide me through the process. Without her encouragement, this
ook would not have been available. Thank you to Senika Hatfield, my co-editor extraordinaire
r the many generous hours, eagle eyes, and organization skills. Thank you to Linda Morse
r her contributions with the peer reviews and tremendous input on the chapters. Thank you
Mick Brackle for the marathon brainstorming sessions and creative insight and to Andrew
oulton for your enormous contribution to ADR. Thank you to Butch Hagmoff for his hard work
organizing the information and for the layout design. Thank you to Emily Burt for not making
n of my line drawings and designing the beautiful illustrations. Thank you to my mom, Lily for
owing me how smart work pays off.

e would also like to thank all teachers, students, patients, and associates for their
iluable suggestions with this book. To everyone who continues to support and promote
aditional Oriental Medicine and Acupuncture in this world, we are most grateful to all of you.
cupuncture Desk Reference is dedicated to the promotion of professionalism and clinical
cellence in Traditional Chinese Medicine.

1ank you for your contribution

Amy Gayheart	Emily Burt	Marilyn Allen
Amy Sowecke	Erica Docimo, LAc	Maria Taverne
Andrew Moulton, MD	George Munger	Martin Buitrago, MD
Asha Randall, LAc	Gustaf LaValle, MD	Marston St. John, LAc
Brandie Armijo	Heather Bree	Mick Brackle, LAc
Brandon Leahy	Higgins Gayheart	Mikio Sankey, LAc
Carol Block, MD	Jill Dedera	Richard Tan, OMD, LAc
Cindy Black	John Chen, PhD, PharmD, OMD	Robert Berger, MD
Cory Bilicko	Joy Bainbridge	Senika Hatfield, LAc
Daniel Reid, MD	Jordon Hoffman, LAc	Shelby VanCleve
Dave Halford	Joshua Graner	Shelly Dainty, LAc
David Murray, MD	Justin Curly	Tina Chen, MS, LAc
Don Lee, LAc, QME	Kennedy Sharp	Vladi Starkov
Douglas Andersen, DC	Leigh Gilkey	William Roberts, LAc
Fred Lerner, DC	Linda Morse, LAc	Will Maclean

his book belongs to: ....

found please call: ....

✻ＡＤЯ

TABLE OF CONTENTS

HOW TO USE THE BOOK

How to use the book. The sections include three main categories with Traditional Formulas, Single Herbs, and Acupuncture Points.

Traditional Formulas

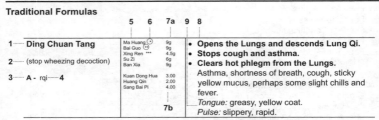

		5	6	7a	9	8

		5 6 7a	9 8
1 — Ding Chuan Tang		Ma Huang ☺ 9g Bai Guo ☺ 9g Xing Ren *** 4.5g Su Zi 6g Ban Xia 9g	• **Opens the Lungs and descends Lung Qi.** • **Stops cough and asthma.** • **Clears hot phlegm from the Lungs.**
2 — (stop wheezing decoction)			Asthma, shortness of breath, cough, sticky
3 — A - rqi — 4		Kuan Dong Hua 3.00 Huang Qin 2.00 Sang Bai Pi 4.00	yellow mucus, perhaps some slight chills and fever. *Tongue:* greasy, yellow coat.
		7b	*Pulse:* slippery, rapid.

1. Traditional Chinese Formulas **2.** Translations **3.** Categories according to importance, **A** = California State Board Formulas, **B** = More commonly used formulas, **C** = Less commonly used formulas **4.** Formula category key (see page 10 for reference) **5.** Herb ingredients **6.** Indicates hierachy of the herb * = chief, ** = deputies, *** = assistants **7a.** Dosage according to (Bensky's *Formulas & Strategies* or Him-che Yeung's *Handbook fo Chinese Formulas*) **7b.** Dosage according to parts per formula **8.** Actions and Indications **9** Tongue and Pulse

Single Herbs

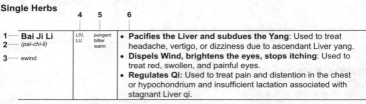

	4	5	6

	4	5	6
1 — **Bai Ji Li** 2 — *(pai-chi-li)* 3 — ewind	LIV, LU	pungent bitter warm	• **Pacifies the Liver and subdues the Yang:** Used to treat headache, vertigo, or dizziness due to ascendant Liver yang. • **Dispels Wind, brightens the eyes, stops itching:** Used to treat red, swollen, and painful eyes. • **Regulates Qi:** Used to treat pain and distention in the chest or hypochondrium and insufficient lactation associated with stagnant Liver qi.

1. Single Herbs **2.** Pinyin proununcications **3.** Single herb category key (see page 104 for reference) **4.** Channels **5.** Taste and Properties **6.** Actions and Indications

Acupuncture Points

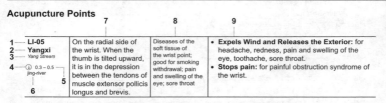

	7	8	9

	7	8	9
1 — **LI-05** 2 — **Yangxi** 3 — *Yang Stream* 4 — ⊥ 0.3 – 0.5 *jing-river* 5 6	On the radial side of the wrist. When the thumb is tilted upward, it is in the depression between the tendons of muscle extensor pollicis longus and brevis.	Diseases of the soft tissue of the wrist point; good for smoking withdrawal; pain and swelling of the eye; sore throat	• **Expels Wind and Releases the Exterior:** for headache, redness, pain and swelling of the eye, toothache, sore throat. • **Stops pain:** for painful obstruction syndrome of the wrist.

1. Acupuncture point **2.** Pinyin name **3.** Translations **4.** Needling directions **5.** Depths **6.** Special points if any **7.** Locations **8.** Use for points **9.** Actions and Indications

Sources

Formulas. Dan Bensky and Randall Barolet, *Chinese Herbal Medicine, Formula & Strategies*, Eastland Press,1990. Yeung, Him-Che, *Handbook of Chinese Herbal Formulas*. Rosemead, CA: Institute of Chinese Medicine, 1983. Jiao Shu De, *Ten Lectures on the Use of Formulas*, Paradigm Publications, 2005. Chongyun Liu & Angela Tseng, *Chinese Herbal Medicine*, CRC Press, 2005. Yi Qiao, *The Traditional Chinese Medicine, Formula Study Guide*, Snow Lotus Press, 2000. Will Maclean & Kathryn Taylor, *The Clinic Manual of Chinese Herbal Patent Medicines*, Redwing, 2003.

Herbs. Dan Bensky and Randall Barolet, *Chinese Herbal Medicine, Materia Medica*, Eastland Press, 1990. John Chen, *Chinese Medical Herbology and Pharmacology*, Art of Medicine, 2001. Yeung, Him-Che, *Handbook of Chinese Herbs*. Rosemead, CA: Institute of Chinese Medicine, 1983. Charles Belanger, *The Chinese Herb Selection Guide*. Phytotech Publishing, 1997.

Acupuncture. Xinnong Cheng & Liangyue Deng, *Chinese Acupuncture and Moxibustion*, Foreign Language Press, 1987. Peter Deadman & Mazin Al-Khafaji, *A Manual of Acupuncture*, Journal of Chinese Medicine, 2001. Gao Lualing, *The Atlas of Layered Anatomy of Acupoints*. Foreign Language Press, 1999. Yu-Lin Lian, *The Seirin Pictorial Atlas of Acupuncture*, Hans Ogal & Wofram Stor, 1999. Arnie Lade, *Acupuncture Points, Images & Functions*, Seventh Printing, 1998. Ellis A, Wiseman & Boss K, *Fundamentals of Chinese Acupuncture*, Paradigm Publications,1988. Qiu Maoliang, *Chinese Acupuncture and Moxibustion*, Churchill Livingstone 1993.

Table of Abbreviations

+ve	Positive
-ve	Negative
1/12	1 month. Similarly 2/12 means 2 months, 3/12 means 3 months, etc
1/24	1 hour. Similarly 2/24 means 2 hours, 3/24 means 3 hours, etc
1/52	1 week. Similarly 2/52 means 2 weeks, 3/52 means 3 weeks, etc
1/7	1 day. Similarly 2/7 means 2 days, 3/7 means 3 days, etc
a c	Before meals
A M A	Advanced maternal age
ad.	Freely as wanted
alt. die	Every other day
alt. h.	Every other hour
aq.	Water
aurist.	Ear drops
B M E	Bi-Manual Examination, i.e. A vaginal examination
B N O	Bowels not open - will be followed by a time span, e.g. B N O 4 days
B P	Blood pressure
b.d. or bd	Twice a day
b.i.d. or bid	Twice a day
c	A lower case c, especially with a line above it, in a medical text means "with"
	A lower case c, without a line above it, in a medical text means about or approximately
	An upper case C usually means century
C N S	Central nervous system
C O or C/O	Complains of
C V S	Cardio vascular system
Ca	Cancer
D R E	Digital rectal examination
Dx	Diagnosis
Dxx	Differential diagnosis
ext.	External
F H	Family history
G or gtt.	Drop or drops
G (number)	This is used in relation to childbirth and pregnancy. A woman described as G2 is in her second pregnancy. G stands for Gravida and is often used with P (see P below)
H O	History of
H P C	History of Presenting Complaint
h.	Hour
h.s.	At bedtime
Hx	History
i.d.	During the day or the same
I D.	Infectious disease
i.d.	Intradermal, between layers of the skin
int.	Internal
Ix	Investigations
mg	Milligram or milligram - a measure of weight
mmHg	Millimeters of mercury, a measure of pressure, usually blood pressure
N A D	No Abnormality Detected (cynics version is Not Actually Done)
N B I	No bone injury
nocte	At night
O E	On examination
o m	Every morning
o n	Every night
O T C	Over The Counter, i.e. A remedy available without prescription
o.c. or occ	Eye ointment
o.d. or od	Daily (or once a day)
O/E	On examination
P (number)	This is used in relation to childbirth and pregnancy. A woman described as P2 has given birth to two live children
P C	Presenting complaint
p c	After meals (on a prescription)
P H	Personal history
P M H	Past medical history
p.m.	Afternoon
p.o. or po	Orally
p.r. or pr	Rectally
p.r.n. or p r n	As required
p.v.	Vaginally
q.	Every
q.2.h.	Every two hours
q.4.h.	Every four hours
q.6.h.	Every six hours
q.8.h.	Every eight hours
q.d. or qd	Every day
q.d.s. or q d s	Four times a day
q.h.	Every hour, hourly
q.i.d. or qid	Four times a day
q.q.h.	Every four hours
q.s.	A sufficient quantity
R O S	Review of Systems or Removal of Sutures (stitches)
R S	Respiratory system
Rx	Prescription
S H	Social history
s.i.d. or sid	Once a day
Sig. or S.	Write on the label
SL.	Sublingual, under the tongue
spec	Short for speculum and will usually mean a visual examination of the vagina and cervix
Stat.	Immediately, with no delay
T	The capital letter T, when followed by an anatomical location, can occasionally stand for tuberculosis
T P R	Temperature, Pulse and Respiratory rate
t.d.s.	Three times a day
t.i.d. or tid	Three times a day
top.	Topically, applied to the skin
Ung.	Ointment
ut dict. or u.d.	As directed
V E	Vaginal examination

FORMULA

Formulas   Formula Category

Release the Exterior - rext
Bai Du San
Cang Er Zi San
Chai Ge Jie Ji Tang
Chuan Xiong Cha Tiao San
Cong Chi Tang
Da Qing Long Tang
Fang Feng Tong Sheng San
Ge Gen Huang Lian Huang Qin Tang
Ge Gen Tang
Gui Zhi Tang
Jia Jian Wei Rui Tang
Jing Fang Bai Du San
Jiu Wei Qiang Huo Tang
Liu Shen Wan
Ma Huang Tang
Ma Huang Xi Xin Fu Zi Tang
Ma Xin Yi Gan Tang
Mai Men Dong Tang
Ren Shen Bai Du San
San Ao Tang
San Huang Shi Gao Tang
Sang Ju Yin
She Gan Ma Huang Tang
Shen Su Yin
Sheng Ma Ge Gen Tang
Shi Shen Tang
Shi Wei Xiang Ru Yin
Wu Ji San
Xiang Ru San
Xiang Su San
Xiao Qing Long Tang
Xin Jia Xiang Ru Yin
Yin Qiao San
Zai Zao San

Reduce Food Stagnation - rfood
Bao He Wan
Jian Pi Wan
Mu Xiang Bing Lang Wan
Wu Mei Wan
Zhi Zhu Wan

Treat Phlegm - rphlegm
Ban Xia Bai Zhu Tian Ma Tang
Bei Mu Gua Lou San
Chai Xian Tang
Dai Zhe Xuan Fu Tang
Dao Tan Tang
Er Chen Tang
Hai Zao Yu Hu Tang
Jin Fei Cao San
Ling Gan Wu Wei Jiang Xin Tang
Ling Gui Zhu Gan Tang
Qing Fei Yin
Qing Qi Hua Tan Wan
San Zi Yang Qing Tang
Wen Dan Tang
Xiao Luo Wan
Xiao Xian Xiong Tang
Zhi Sou San

Regulate Qi - rqi
Ban Xia Hou Po Tang
Bao An Shen
Ding Chuan Tang
Ding Xiang Shi Di Tang
Gua Lou Xie Bai Bai Jiu Tang
Huo Po Wen Zhong Tang
Jin Ling Zi San
Ju He Wan
Ju Pi Zhu Ru Tang
Liang Fu Wan
Nuan Gan Jian
Si Mo Tang
Su Zi Jiang Qi Tang
Tian Tai Wu Yao San
Xuan Fu Dai Zhe Tang
Yue Ju Wan

Stabilize and Bind - sab
Bao Can Wu Yu Fang
Fu Tu Dan

Stop Bleeding - stopxue
Huai Hua San
Huang Tu Tang
Jiao Ai Tang
Ke Xue Fang
Qing Re Zhi Beng Tang
Shi Hui San
Si Sheng Wang
Xiao Ji Yin Zi

Tonify Blood - tblood
Ai Fu Nuan Gong Wan
Dang Gui San
Di Dang Tang
Ren Shen Yang Ying Tang
Sheng Yu Tang
Shi Quan Da Bu Tang
Si Wu Tang
Tai Shan Pan Shi San
Tao Hong Si Wu Tang
Wen Qing Yin
Zhe Cong Yin

Tonify Qi - tqi
Bu Zhong Yi Qi Tang
Liu Jun Zi Tang
Ren Shen Yang Rong Tang
Shen Ling Bai Zhu San
Sheng Mai San
Shi Liu Wei Liu Qi Yin
Si Jun Zi Tang
Xiang Sha Liu Jun Zi Tang
Yi Qi Cong Ming Tang

Tonify Qi & Blood - tqiblood
Ba Zhen Tang
Dang Gui Bu Xue Tang
Gui Pi Tang
Zhi Gan Cao Tang

Xiao Feng San
Xiao Huo Luo Dan
Xiao Xu Ming Tang
Yu Zhen San
Zhen Gan Xi Feng Tang

Harmonize - harm
Ban Xia Xie Xin Tang
Chai Hu Shu Gan San
Da Chai Hu Tang
Da Yuan Yin
Dang Gui Shao Yao San
Gui Zhi Jia Long Gu Mu Li Tang
Hao Qin Qing Dan Tang
Si Ni San
Tong Xie Yao Fang
Xiang Sha Yang Wei Tang
Xiao Chai Hu Tang
Xiao Yao San

Invigorate the Blood - movexue
Bu Yang Huan Wu Tang
Da Huang Zhe Chong Wan
Dan Shen Yin
Fu Yuan Huo Xue Tang
Ge Xia Zhu Yu Tang
Gui Zhi Fu Ling Wan
Hong Hua Tao Ren Jian
Huo Luo Xiao Ling Dan
Nu Ke Bai Zi Ren Wan
Pai Nong San
Qi Li San
Shao Fu Zhu Yu Tang
Shen Tong Zhu Yu Tang
Sheng Hua Tang
Shi Xiao San
Shu Gan Tang
Shu Jing Huo Xue Tang
Tao He Cheng Qi Tang
Tong Qiao Huo Xue Tang
Wen Jing Tang
Xue Fu Zhu Yu Tang

Open the Orifices - open
An Gong Niu Huang Wan
Gun Tan Wan
Zhi Bao Dan
Zi Xue Dan

Purgative - purg
Da Cheng Qi Tang
Da Huang Fu Zi Tang
Da Xian Xiong Tang
Huang Long Tang
Ji Chuan Jian
Liang Ge San
Ma Zi Ren Wan
Run Chang Wan
San Wu Bei Ji Wan
Shi Zao Tang
Tiao Wei Cheng Qi Tang
Wen Pi Tang
Xiao Cheng Qi Tang
Xin Jia Huang Long Tang
Zeng Ye Cheng Qi Tang

Formulas
Formula Category

FORMULA

Calm the Spirit - ashen

Chai Hu Jia Long Gu Mu Li Tang
Ci Zhu Wan
Gan Mai Da Zao Tang
Huang Lian E Jiao Tang
Sheng Tie Luo Yin
Suan Zao Ren Tang
Tian Wang Bu Xin Dan
Zhu Sha An Shen Wan

Astringe - astringe

Gu Chong Tang
Gu Jing Wan
Jin Suo Gu Jing Wan
Jiu Xian San
Mu Li San
Sang Piao Xiao San
Si Shen Wan
Suo Quan Wan
Wan Dai Tang
Yi Huang Tang
Yu Ping Feng San

Clear the Heat - clht

Bai Hu Jia Gui Zhi Tang
Bai Hu Jia Ren Shen Tang
Bai Hu Tang
Bai Tou Weng Tang
Bao Yuan Chai Hu Qing Gan San
Dang Gui Liu Huang Tang
Dao Chi San
Dun Sou Tang
Huang Lian Jie Du Tang
Huang Lian Wen Dan Tang
Jian Er Wan
Jian Ying San
Jie Geng Tang
Jing Jei Lian Qiao Tang
Liu Yi San
Long Dan Xie Gan Tang
Ma Xing Shi Gan Tang
Pu Ji Xiao Du Yin
Qin Jiao Bie Jia San
Qing Gu San
Qing Hao Bie Jia Tang
Qing Luo Yin
Qing Shang Fang Feng Tang
Qing Shu Yi Qi Tang
Qing Wei San
Qing Xin Lian Zi Yin
Qing Yan Li Ge Tang
Qing Ying Tang
Ren Shen Xie Fei Tang
San Huang Xie Xin Tang
San Jia Fu Mai Tang
San Miao Wan
San Zhong Kui Jian Tang
Shao Yao Tang
Si Miao Yong An Tang
Sheng Long Tang
Wei Jing Tang
Wu Wei Xiao Du Yin
Yi Jiao Di Huang Tang
Xian Fang Huo Ming Yin
Xie Bai San
Xie Huang San

Xie Xin Tang
Yi Zi Tang
Yu Nu Jian
Zhi Zhuo Gu Ben Wan
Zhu Ye Shi Gao Tang
Zuo Jin Wan

Dry & Moisten - dry

Bai He Gu Jin Tang
Qing Zao Jiu Fei Tang
Sang Xing Tang
Sha Shen Mai Dong Tang
Xing Su San
Yang Yin Qing Fei Tang*
Yu Ye Tang

Expel Dampness - edamp

Ba Zheng San
Bei Xie Fen Qing Yin
Chai Ling Tang
Da Huang Mu Dan Pi Tang
Dang Gui Nian Tong Tang
Dao Shui Fu Ling Tang
Du Huo Ji Sheng Tang
Er Miao San
Er Zhu Tang
Fang Ji Huang Qi Tang
Fen Xiao Tang
Fu Ling Yin
Gan Lu Xiao Du Dan
Gui Zhi Shao Yao Zhi Mu Tang
Huo Xiang Zheng Qi Tang
Ji Ming San
Juan Bi Tang
Ping Wei San
Qi Pi Tang
Qiang Huo Sheng Shi Tang
San Bi Tang
San Ren Tang
Shen Zhuo Tang
Shi Pi Yin
Shu Jing Li An San
Shung Jie San
Si Miao Wan
Wei Ling Tang
Wei Su Ning
Wu Ling San
Wu Pi San
Xuan Bi Tang
Yi Yi Ren Tang
Yin Chen Hao Tang
Yin Chen Wu Ling San
Yue Bi Jia Zhu Tang
Zhen Wu Tang
Zhu Ling Tang

Expel Wind - ewind

Da Ding Feng Zhu
Da Qin Jiao Tang
Di Huang Yin Zi
E Jiao Ji Zi Huang Tang
Qian Zheng San
Shi Wei Bai Du San
Tian Ma Gou Teng Yin
Wu Tou Tang
Wu Yao Shun Qi San

Tonify Yang - tyang

Er Xian Tang
Gui Lu Er Xian Jiao
You Gui Wan

Tonify Yin - tyin

Ba Xian Chang Shou Wan
Bu Fei E Jiao Tang
Da Bu Yin Wan
Er Long Zuo Ci Wan
Er Zhi Wan
Gu Yin Jian
Hu Qian Wan
Jia Jian Fu Mai Tang
Jin Gui Shen Qi Wan
Liu Wei Di Huang Wan
Ming Mu Di Huang Wan
Qi Ju Di Huang Wan
Yi Guan Jian
Zhi Bai Di Huang Wan
Zuo Gui Yin

Warm Interior - wint

An Zhong San
Da Jian Zhong Tang
Dang Gui Si Ni Tang
Fu Zi Li Zhong Wan
Hei Xi Dan
Huang Qi Jian Zhong Tang
Li Zhong Wan
Shen Fu Tang
Si Ni Tang
Tao Hua Tang
Wu Zhu Yu Tang
Xiao Jian Zhong Tang
Yang He Tang

FORMULA

Formula	Herbs / Dosage	Indications / Functions
Ai Fu Nuan Gong Wan (mugwort & prepared aconite warming the womb pill) **C** - tblood	Xiang Fu 180g Ai Ye 90g Dang Gui 90g Huang Qi 60g Wu Zhu Yu 60g Chuan Xiong 60g Bai Shao 60g Shu Di Huang 30g Rou Gui 15g Xu Duan 45g	• **Warms and comforts the wombs.** • **Tonifies the blood, calms the fetus.** Cold, painful sensation in the lower abdominal, loose stools, abdominal distension, white coat during the second or third trimester of pregnancy. *Tongue:* pale, white coat.
An Gong Niu Huang Wan (calm palace with cattle gallstone pill) **C** - open	Niu Huang * 30g Xi Jiao * 30g She Xiang * 7.7g Huang Qin 30g Huang Lian 30g Zhi Zi 30g Xiong Huang 30g Bing Pian 7.5g Yu Jin 30g Zhen Zhu 15g Zhu Sha 30g	• **Clears heat and dispels toxins.** • **Opens orifices, calms the Spirit.** High fever, restlessness, difficulty speaking, coma from wind-stroke, cold limbs, stiff tongue. *Tongue:* red, deep red. *Pulse:* rapid.
An Zhong San (calm the middle powder) **C** - wint	Gui Zhi 4g Suo Sha 1g Gan Cao 4g Liang Jiang 1g Yan Hu Suo 3g Xiao Hui Xiang 1.5g Sha Ren 1.5g Mu Li 3.0g	• **Regulates and descends the Qi.** • **Warms and strengthens the Stomach.** Deficiency, emaciation, nausea, vomiting, pain beneath the heart, soft and weak abdomen. *Pulse:* weak, thready.
Ba Xian Chang Shou Wan AKA Mai Wei Di Huang Wan (longevity pill) **B** - tyin	*Liu Wei Di Huang Wan +* Mai Men Dong Wu Wei Zi	• **Tonifies Kidney and Lung Yin.** Coughing blood, tidal fever, asthma, night sweats. *Tongue:* red. *Pulse:* rapid, thready. • Contains *Liu Wei Di Huang Wan* + Mai Men Dong, Wu Wei Zi.
Ba Zhen Tang (eight corrections powder) **B** - tqiblood	Ren Shen * 6-9g Bai Zhu ** 9-12g Bai Shao 12-15g Dang Gui 12-15g Fu Ling ** 12-15g Chuan Xiong 6-9g Shu Di Huang * 15-18g Gan Cao 3-6g	• **Tonifies the Qi and Blood.** Pale complexion, dizziness, vertigo, palpitations, reduced appetite, shortness of breath, fatigue, scanty menstruation. *Tongue:* pale body, thin white coat. *Pulse:* weak, thready. • Contains *Si Wu Tang* + *Si Jun Zi Tang*. • **Formula for Qi and Blood deficiency disorders.**
Ba Zheng San (eight corrections powder) **A** - edamp	Mu Tong * 3-6g Qu Mai 6-12g Che Qian Zi 9-15g Bian Xu 6-12g Hua Shi 12-30g Shan Zhi Zi 3-9g Da Huang 6-9g Deng Xin Cao 3-6g Gan Cao 3-9g	• **Drains damp-heat from the lower burner.** • **Promotes urination and clears fire.** • **Clears fire and heat in Lin Syndrome diseases.** Burning, frequent, painful and obstructed urination, discomfort and bloating of the lower abdomen, chills and fever, bitter taste, thirst, dry mouth, nausea. *Tongue:* yellow, greasy coat. *Pulse:* rapid. • **Relieves frequent, painful and burning urination due to damp-heat in the lower burner or in the channels, resembles UTI.**
Bai Du San (ginseng powder to overcome pathogenic influences) AKA Ren Shen Bai Du San **C** - rext	Qiang Huo * 3.00 Fu Ling 3.00 Du Huo * 3.00 Jie Geng 3.00 Qian Hu 3.00 Gan Cao 1.50 Chai Hu 3.00 Sheng Jiang ** 3.00 Chuan Xiong ** 3.00 Bo He 0.50 Zhi Qiao 3.00	• **Clears heat from the Lungs and Stomach.** • **Releases the exterior.** Common cold, high fever without sweating, stiffness and pain of head, neck, and shoulder, stuffed nose, cough with phlegm. *Tongue:* white, greasy coat. *Pulse:* floating, soggy.

Formula	Herbs / Dosage	Indications / Functions
Bai He Gu Jin Tang (lily bulb to consolidate lung decoction) **C** - dry	Bai He 3g Shu Di Huang 9g Sheng Di Huang 6g Mai Men Dong 4.5g Bai Shao 3g Xuan Shen 2.4g Chuan Bei Mu 3g Dang Gui 3g Jie Geng 2.4g Gan Cao 3g	• **Clears heat, nourishes yin.** • **Moistens the Lungs, expels phlegm.** Dry and sore throat, five-center heat, blood streaked sputum, night sweats. *Tongue:* red, little or no coat. *Pulse:* rapid, thready. • **Formula for yin deficiency in the Lung and Kidneys. It nourishes Lungs as it strengthens weak fire.**
Bai Hu Jia Gui Zhi Tang (white tiger decoction plus cinnamon) **B** - clht	*Bai Hu Tang +* Gui Zhi	• **Clears excess internal heat, generates fluids.** • **Expels wind-damp, opens the channels.** Painful swollen burning joints, limited mobility in joints. Also with fever that is not relieved by sweating. *Tongue:* dry body, yellow, red coat. *Pulse:* slippery, rapid. • **Formula for excess heat in the Lungs and Stomach. It nourishes fluids as it sedates fire.** • Contains *Bai Hu Tang* + Gui Zhi.
Bai Hu Jia Ren Shen Tang (white tiger plus ginseng decoction) **C** - clht	Shi Gao 15-60g Zhi Mu 6-12g Gan Cao 2-10g Ren Shen 5-10g Jing Mi 15-30g	• **Clears Qi level heat, generates fluids.** • **Drains stomach fire, stops thirst.** High fever, severe sweating & thirst, overall weakness, dry mouth, profuse perspiration, increased urination. *Tongue:* red tip and sides. *Pulse:* empty, forceful, rapid. • Contains *Bai Hu Tang* + Ren Shen.
Bai Hu Tang (white tiger decoction) **A** - clht	Shi Gao * 30g Zhi Mu ** Geng Mi 9-15g Zhi Gan Cao 3g	• **Clears Qi level heat and Yangming excess.** • **Generates fluids.** Big four - big sweat, big fever, big thirst, big pulse, dry mouth, red face. *Tongue:* red body, dry coat. *Pulse:* big, strong, rapid.
Bai Tou Weng Tang (pulsatilla decoction) **B** - clht	Bai Tou Weng * 6g Huang Lian 9g Huang Bai 9g Qin Pi 9g	• **Clears heat and detoxifies.** • **Cools the blood, stops dysentery.** Abdominal pain, blood and pus in the stool, diarrhea, tenesmus, burning anus, irritability, thirst. *Tongue:* red body, yellow coat. *Pulse:* wiry, rapid. • **This formula clears damp-heat from the intestines to relieve intestinal disorders, perhaps due to infection.**
Ban Xia Bai Zhu Tian Ma Tang (pinellia, atractylodes & gastrodia decoction) **A** - rphlegm	Ban Xia * 4.5g Bai Zhu ** 9g Tian Ma * 3g Ju Hong 3g Fu Ling 3g Sheng Jiang 1slice Da Zao 2pc Gan Cao 1.5g	• **Expels wind and phlegm, dispels dampness.** • **Harmonizes the middle, strengthens the Spleen.** • **Formula for dizziness, headaches, and Meniere's due to wind-phlegm.** Dizziness, vertigo, headaches, sputum, heaviness of the head, fullness of the chest, nausea, vomiting. *Tongue:* greasy, white coat. *Pulse:* slippery, rapid.

FORMULA

FORMULA

Formula	Herbs / Dosage	Indications / Functions
Ban Xia Hou Po Tang (pinellia & magnolia decoction) A - rqi	Ban Xia * 9-12g Hou Po 9g Zi Su Ye 6g Fu Ling 12g Sheng Jiang 15g	• **Regulates and descends the Qi.** • **Expels phlegm.** Plum-pit throat, tightness of the throat, tightness of the chest and hypochondrium, nausea, vomiting, cough with phlegm. *Tongue:* white, moist, greasy coat. *Pulse:* slippery, wiry. • **Formula to resolve Qi and Phlegm and Liver qi stagnation attacking the Lung and Stomach. Special for plum-pit throat tightness from emotional stress or nervousness.**
Ban Xia Xie Xin Tang (pinellia drain epigastrium decoction) A - harm	Ban Xia * 9g Gan Jiang 9g Huang Qin 9g Huang Lian 3g Ren Shen 9g Da Zao 12pcs Gan Cao 9g	• **Harmonizes and tonifies the Stomach.** • **Descends Stomach Qi.** • **Expels masses.** Painless epigastric fullness or distention, dry vomiting, nausea, vomiting, borborygmus, diarrhea. *Tongue:* thin, greasy, yellow coat. *Pulse:* wiry, rapid, weak. • **Formula for Stomach deficiency that leads to stagnation heat and rebellious Qi.**
Bao An Shen (polyporus & pinellia combination) C - rqi	Fu Ling 3.00 Zhu Ling 2.00 Yu Mi Rui 5.00 Ban Xia 2.00 Hou Pu 3.00 Chen Pi 2.00 Gan Cao 1.00 Hua Shi 5.00 Cang Zhu 3.00 Ze Xie 2.00 Zhi Qiao 2.00	• **Regulates Qi, expels phlegm.** Dry mouth and throat, dry lungs, dry cough with difficult-to-expectorate phlegm, sore throat. *Tongue:* red. *Pulse:* thin, rapid. • Contains *Wu Ling San + Er Chen Tang.*
Bao Can Wu Yu Fang (dang gui & artemisia combination) C - sab	Dang Gui 3.00 Chuan Xiong 3.00 Jing Jie 1.60 Qiang Huo 1.00 Zhi Qiao 1.20 Bai Shao 4.00 Hou Pu 1.40 Tu Si Zi 2.00 Ai Ye 1.40 Huang Qi 1.60 Bei Mu 2.00 Gan Cao 1.00 Sheng Jiang 3.00	• **Stabilizes the fetus, nourishes the blood.** Fetal irritability, difficult labor, pain in the waist and abdomen during pregnancy, and habitual abortion. Mainly for cases that have abortive symptoms at first stage of pregnancy. *Tongue:* pale, weak. *Pulse:* smooth.
Bao He Wan (preserve harmony pill) A - rfood	Shan Zha * 9-15g Shen Qu ** 9-12g Lai Fu Zi ** 6-9g Ban Xia 9-12g Chen Pi 9-12g Fu Ling 9-12g Lian Qiao 3-6g (Mai Ya) dect.	• **Reduces food stagnation.** • **Harmonizes the Stomach.** Fullness of the stomach and chest, abdominal distention with occasional pain, pain that lessens after bowel movement, belching, sour regurgitation, nausea, vomiting, sour taste, no appetite. *Tongue:* greasy, yellow coat. *Pulse:* slippery. • **Main formula for overeating.**
Bao Yuan Chai Hu Qing Gan San (bupleurum & moutan formula) C - clht	Chai Hu 3.00 Huang Qin 3.00 Sheng Di Huang 3.00 Huang Lian 2.00 Dang Gui 3.00 Mu Dan Pi 3.00 Shan Zhi Zi 2.00 Chuan Xiong 1.50 Sheng Ma 2.50 Gan Cao 1.00	• **Clears heat and regulates blood.** • **Purges Liver fire.** For swelling and pain of the throat, toothache, and gingivitis. *Tongue:* red. *Pulse:* thin, rapid.

Formula	Herbs / Dosage	Indications / Functions
Bei Mu Gua Lou San (fritillary & trichosantes powder) **A** - rphlegm	Bei Mu * 4.5g Gua Lou ** 3g Tian Hua Fen 2.4g Fu Ling 2.4g Ju Hong 2.4g Jie Geng 2.4g	• **Moistens the Lung.** • **Clears damp-heat.** • **Regulates Qi, expels phlegm.** Dry mouth and throat, dry lungs, dry cough with difficult-to-expectorate phlegm, sore throat. *Tongue:* red body, thin dry coat. *Pulse:* thin, rapid. • **This formula expels phlegm that is sticky, stubborn, and difficult to spit or cough out.**
Bei Xie Fen Qing Yin (dioscorea hypoglauca to separate clear decoction) **B** - edamp	Bei Xie * 12g Yi Zhi Ren ** 9g Wu Yao 9g Shi Chang Pu 9g	• **Warms the Kidney Yang.** • **Promotes urination, drains damp.** • **Clears turbid water.** Frequent cloudy urination, painful urination, perhaps with heat, dribbling, and bleeding. *Tongue:* pale body, white coat. *Pulse:* sunken, slow, weak. • **Formula for cloudy urination (Gao Lin) syndrome, particularly for those due to Kidney Yang deficiency.**
Bu Fei E Jiao Tang (tonify lung with ass-hide gelatin decoction) **C** - tyin	E Jiao 4.5g Ma Dou Ling 1.5g Niu Bang Zi 7.5g Geng Mi 30g Xing Ren 6g Gan Cao 7.5g	• **Nourishes the Yin.** • **Tonifies the Lung, stops coughing.** Coughing and wheezing, dry throat, scanty or bloody sputum. *Tongue:* red body, little or no coat. *Pulse:* floating, thready, rapid.
Bu Yang Huan Wu Tang (tonify yang to restore five-tenths decoction) **B** - movexue	Huang Qi 120g Dang Gui 6g Chuan Xiong 3g Chi Shao 4.5g Tao Ren 3g Hong Hua 3g Di Long 3g	• **Promotes blood circulation, tonifies the Qi.** • **Regulates the channels.** Hemiplegia following a stroke, paraplegia, deviated mouth and face, speech difficulty, drooling, frequent urination or incontinence, weakness and paralysis of the lower limbs. *Tongue:* thin, white coat. *Pulse:* weak, perhaps wiry. • **Formula for paralysis due to deficient Qi that is unable to move blood sufficiently to nourish the limbs and head. For paralysis following strokes due to blockage but not due to hemorrhage.**
Bu Zhong Yi Qi Tang (tonify middle & increase qi decoction) **A** - tqi	Huang Qi * 1.5g Ren Shen ** 0.9g Zhi Gan Cao ** 1.5g Bai Zhu ** 0.9g Chen Pi 0.9g Dang Gui 6g Sheng Ma 0.9g Chai Hu 0.9g	• **Tonifies the Qi of the middle burner.** • **Raises sunken Yang.** Intermittent low-grade fever that is worse with exertion, headache, fatigue, spontaneous sweating, aversion to cold, impaired sense of taste, weak limbs, prolapsed organs, shortness of breath, slowed speech with weak activity, shiny pale complexion, reduced appetite, loose stools. *Tongue:* pale body, thin white coat. *Pulse:* weak, empty. • **Formula to raise sinking clear Qi, lifts prolapsed organs, relieves Qi-deficient fevers, and generally tonifies the Qi.**

FORMULA

Formula	Herbs / Dosage	Indications / Functions
Cang Er Zi San (xanthium powder) B - rext	Cang Er Zi 7.5g Xin Yi Hua 15g Bai Zhi 30g Bo He 1.5g	• **Expels wind, opens the nose.** • **Stops pain.** Copious purulent foul-smelling nasal discharge, nasal obstructions, dizziness, frontal headache. *Tongue:* normal, yellow coat. *Pulse:* floating, rapid.
Chai Ge Jie Ji Tang (bupleurum & kudzu release muscle layer decoction) A - rext	Chai Hu * 3-9g Gen Gen * 6-12g Qiang Huo 3-6g Bai Zhi 3-6g Huang Qin 6-9g Shi Gao 4.5-15g Jie Geng 3-6g Bai Shao 6-9g Gan Cao 3-6g Sheng Jiang 3-6g Da Zao 2-3pcs	• **Releases the surface, loosens the muscles.** • **Clears internal heat.** High fever, slight chills, body aches, aversion to cold, heaviness of the head, irritability, dry nose, red eyes, bitter taste, insomnia. *Tongue:* thin, yellow coat. *Pulse:* floating, slippery, rapid. • **Formula for wind-cold that becomes internal heat, with a combination of surface chills and fever from internal heat. Clears three-level-heat from the Taiyang, Shaoyang, and Yangming levels of febrile disease.**
Chai Hu Jia Long Gu Mu Li Tang (bupleurum, dragon bone & oyster shell decoction) C - ashen	Chai Hu * 12g Gui Zhi * 4.5g Huang Qin * 4.5g Ban Xia 6-9g Sheng Jiang 4.5g Ren Shen 4.5g Fu Ling 4.5g Long Gu 4.5g Mu Li 4.5g Da Huang * 6g Qian Dan 4.5g Da Zao 6pcs	• **Settles the Heart, calms the Spirit.** • **Unblocks three yang stages.** Fullness of the chest, irritability, palpitations, heaviness of the body, constipation, delirious speech, inability to rotate trunk. *Tongue:* red, little or no coat. *Pulse:* wiry, rapid.
Chai Hu Shu Gan San (bupleurum powder to spread liver) B - harm	Chai Hu 6g Chuan Xiong 4.5g Zhi Ke 4.5g Bai Shao 4.5g Zhi Gan Cao 1.5g Xiang Fu 4.5g	• **Harmonizes Liver Qi, regulates blood.** • **Formula for Liver Qi stagnation.** Alternating chills and fever, hypochondriac pain, flank pain, emotional imbalance, irregular menstruation. *Tongue:* thin, white coat. *Pulse:* wiry.
Chai Ling Tang (bupleurum & hoelen combination) C - edamp	Chai Hu 7.00 Fu Ling 3.00 Ban Xia 5.00 Huang Qin 3.00 Sheng Jiang 4.00 Da Zao 3.00 Gan Cao 2.00 Ren Shen 3.00 Bai Zhu 3.00 Ze Xie 5.00 Zhu Ling 3.00 Gui Zhi 2.00	• **Relieves chest distention, expels water retention.** • **Strengthens the Liver and Spleen.** Alternating chills and fever, chest distension, liver and gallbladder disorders, gastroenteritis, nephritis, edema, diarrhea, dysuria, scanty urine. *Tongue:* thin, white coat. *Pulse:* wiry. • Contains *Wu Ling San + Xiao Chai Hu Tang.*
Chai Xian Tang (bupleurum & scute combination) C - rphlegm	Chai Hu 4.00 Ban Xia 6.00 Huang Qin 2.00 Sheng Jiang 2.00 Gua Lou Ren 4.00 Gan Cao 1.00 Huang Lian 2.00 Ren Shen 1.50	• **Disperses heat and resolves phlegm.** • **Comforts the chest and relieves accumulation.** Alternating chills and fever, chest fullness, pressing chest pain and rapid respiration, pleurisy, bitter taste in the mouth, cholecystitis and infectious hepatitis. *Tongue:* yellow coat.

Formula	Herbs / Dosage	Indications / Functions
Chuan Xiong Cha Tiao San (ligusticum powder w/ green tea) **B -** rext	Chuan Xiong 120g Bo He 240g Qiang Huo 60g Bai Zhi 60g Xi Xin 30g Jing Jie 120g Fang Feng 45g Gan Cao 60g	• **Expels wind, relieves pain.** All types of headaches with fever and chills, sinus congestion, vertigo, dizziness, aversion to cold. *Tongue:* thin, white coat. *Pulse:* floating, tight. • **Formula for headaches from pathogenic wind: frontal, vertex, occipital.** Take this with tea to moderate the heat - black tea is cooling, but green tea is the most cooling.
Ci Zhu Wan (magnetite & cinnabar pill) **C -** ashen	Ci Shi * 60g Zhu Sha 30g Shen Qu 120g	• **Calms the Spirit, nourishes the Yang.** • **Brightens the eyes.** Palpitations, diminished vision and hearing, insomnia, tinnitus, dizziness.
Cong Chi Tang (scallion & prepared soybean decoction) **B -** rext	Cong Bai 3-5pcs Dan Dou Chi 12-30g	• **Releases the surface, induces sweating.** • **Unblocks Yang Qi.** Mild fever, mild chills, no sweating, headache, nasal congestion, sneezing, aversion to cold. *Tongue:* thin, white coat. *Pulse:* floating. • **Formula for mild colds, or colds in their early stages.**
Da Bu Yin Wan (great tonify yin pill) **B -** tyin	Shu Di Huang * 18g Gui Ban * 18g Huang Bai 12g Zhi Mu 12g	• **Tonifies the Yin.** • **Clears false heat.** • **Strengthens and nourishes weak and dry bones.** Afternoon tidal fever with *steaming bone syndrome,* night sweats, hot sensation of the ankles, knees and legs, hemoptysis, irritability, thirst, easily hungered. *Tongue:* red body, little or no coat. *Pulse:* thin, rapid, forceful.
Da Chai Hu Tang (major bupleurum decoction) **B -** harm	Chai Hu 24g Huang Qin 9g Da Huang 6g Zhi Shi 6-9g Bai Shao 9g Ban Xia 24g Sheng Jiang 15g Da Zao 12pcs	• **Harmonizes Shaoyang channels, sedates Yangming organ heat.** • **Clears interior heat.** Alternating chills and fever, irritability, bitter taste of the mouth, fullness of the chest and hypochondrium, nausea, vomiting, diarrhea, constipation. *Tongue:* yellow coat. *Pulse:* strong, wiry.
Da Cheng Qi Tang (major order qi decoction) **A -** purg	Da Huang * 12g Mang Xiao 9-12g Hou Po 24g Zhi Shi 12-15g	• **Purges stools.** • **Clears heat in the Stomach and Intestines.** Constipation, gas, afternoon tidal fever, abdominal distention and pain upon pressure, delirium, tight abdomen. *Tongue:* red body, dry, yellow and dark coat. *Pulse:* strong and deep pulse. • **A purgative formula for constipation due to internal heat, a Yangming organ disease.**
Da Ding Feng Zhu (big pearl for endogenous wind) **C -** ewind	E Jiao 6-9g Sheng Di Huang 10-15g Mai Men Dong 10-15g Bai Shao 9-12g Gui Ban 9-12g Bei Jia 9-12g Mu Li 9-12g Wu Wei Zi 6-9g Huo Ma Ren 6-9g Zhi Gan Cao 3-6g Ji Zi Huang 2pcs	• **Expels wind and nourishes the Yin.** Fatigue, convulsions, muscle spasms with alternating flexion and extension of the extremities. *Tongue:* greasy, yellow coat. *Pulse:* slow, thin, weak, deep.

Formula	Herbs / Dosage	Indications / Functions
Da Huang Fu Zi Tang (rhubarb & aconite decoction) **B -** purg	Da Huang 9g Fu Zi * 6-12g Xi Xin 6g	• **Warms the interior and expels cold.** • **Purges stools, stops pain.** Abdominal pain, constipation, cold limbs, aversion to cold. *Tongue:* white, greasy tongue. *Pulse:* wiry, tight. • **Purges "frozen stools" caused by internal cold stagnation.**
Da Huang Mu Dan Pi Tang (rhubarb & aconite decoction) **B -** edamp	Da Huang * 12g Mu Dan Pi 3g Mang Xiao ** 9-12g Tao Ren 9-15g Dong Gua Ren 15-30g	• **Clears damp-heat.** • **Promotes circulation, resolves blood stagnation.** Appendicitis - severe and intense pain in the lower right abdomen, rebound tenderness, inability to extend the right leg, fever, sweating. *Tongue:* white, greasy coat. *Pulse:* slippery, wiry, rapid. • **Formula for appendicitis.**
Da Huang Zhe Chong Wan (rhubarb & eupolypaga pill) **C -** movexue	Da Huang * 300g Zhe Chong * 30g Tao Ren 60g Gan Qi 30g Qi Cao 60g Shui Zhi 60g Meng Chong 60g Huang Qin 60g Xing Ren 60g Sheng Di Huang 300g Bai Shao 120g Gan Cao 90g	• **Dispels blood stagnation.** • **Generates new blood.** Dry blood clumping, emaciation, abdominal fullness, reduced appetite, dry rough scaly skin, dull dark eyes, tidal fever, amenorrhea. *Pulse:* weak.
Da Jian Zhong Tang (major strengthen middle decoction) **A -** wint	Chuan Jiao * 3-9g Yi Tang 18-30g Ren Shen 6g Gan Jiang ** 12g	• **Warms the middle and tonifies Qi.** • **Relieves pain.** • **Kills parasites.** Stomach pain, chest pain, stomach cold, vomiting, unable to hold food down, moving mass in the stomach, roundworms. *Tongue:* swollen. *Pulse:* wiry. • **Relieves excess stomach pain due to cold and deficiency of the middle burner.**
Da Qin Jiao Tang (major gentiana qinjiao combination) **C -** ewind	Qin Jiao 4.00 Shi Gao 4.00 Dang Gui 2.00 Bai Shao 2.00 Chuan Xiong 2.00 Sheng Di Huang 2.00 Shu Di Huang 2.00 Bai Zhu 2.00 Fu Ling 2.00 Gan Cao 2.00 Huang Qin 2.00 Fang Feng 2.00 Qiang Huo 2.00 Du Huo 2.00 Bai Zhi 2.00 Xi Xin 1.00	• **Expels wind and clears heat.** • **Nourishes and invigorates blood.** • **Strengthens and regulates Ying-Wei.** Deviation of eyes and mouth, joint pain, tingling of skin, dysphasia, hemiplegia, rheumatic arthritis, muscle spasms, chills and fever, cerebral accidents, facial paralysis. *Tongue:* yellow or white coat. *Pulse:* floating and tight, wiry, thin.
Da Qing Long Tang (major bluegrass dragon decoction) **B -** rext	Ma Huang 18g Gui Zhi 6g Xing Ren 60pcs Zhi Gan Cao 6g Shi Gao 1pc Sheng Jiang 9g Gui Zhi 6g Da Zao 12pcs	• **Releases the surface, induces sweating.** • **Clears interior heat.** Severe chills, high fever, body aches, no sweating, irritability. *Tongue:* thin, white or thin, yellow coat. *Pulse:* floating, tight, rapid. • **Formula for a combination of wind-cold on the surface (no sweating) and increasing internal heat (fever).** • Contains *Ma Huang Tang* + Shi Gao, Sheng Jiang, Da Zao.

Formula	Herbs / Dosage	Indications / Functions
Da Xian Xiong Tang (major sinking chest decoction) **B** - purg	Gan Sui 0.3- Da Huang 0.6g Mang Xiao 18g 9-12g	• **Purges interior heat, expels water.** • **Reduces masses.** • **Purges "frozen stools" caused by internal cold stagnation.** Hardness, fullness and pain in the chest and stomach, constipation, tidal fever, thirst. *Tongue:* dry, red. *Pulse:* deep, tight, forceful.
Da Yuan Yin (reach membrane source) **B** - harm	Cao Guo * 1.5g Bing Lang * 6g Hou Po * 3g Huang Qin 3g Bai Shao 3g Zhi Mu 3g Gan Cao 1.5g	• **Dispels dirty-damp stagnation.** Alternating chills and fever, fullness of the chest, nausea, vomiting, headache, irritability. *Tongue:* deep red sides, foul pasty yellow coat. *Pulse:* wiry, tight, rapid. • **Formula used exclusively to treat malaria.**
Dai Zhe Xuan Fu Tang (Inula & Hematite Combination) **C** - rphlegm	Xuan Fu Hua * 3.00 Dai She Zi * 5.00 Ban Xia 5.00 Da Zao 3.00 Ren Shen 2.00 Gan Cao 3.00 Dai Zhe Shi 1.00 Sheng Jiang 5.00	• **Descends flushing-up, disperses phlegm.** • **Nourishes Qi and harmonizes the Stomach.** Gastritis, gastroptosis, ulcer, sour stomach, initial stage of gastric cancer, gastric distention and vomiting. *Tongue:* white, furry coat. *Pulse:* wiry, weak.
Dan Shen Yin (salvia decoction) **B** - movexue	Dan Shen 30g Tan Xiang 4.5g Sha Ren 4.5g	• **Dispels blood stagnation, regulates blood.** • **Promotes qi circulation, stops pain.** Chest pain, flank pain, epigastric and abdominal pain that radiates upward, fullness of the chest, shortness of breath. *Tongue:* purple with purple spots. *Pulse:* choppy, hesitant, wiry.
Dang Gui Bu Xue Tang (tangkuei tonify blood decoction) **B** - tqiblood	Dang Gui 6g Huang Qi 30g	• **Tonifies Qi and Blood.** • **Promotes healing of wounds.** Anemia, hot sensation in muscles, fatigue, flushed face, headache, fever, yin boils, open sores, thirst without desire to drink, delayed or scanty menstruation. *Tongue:* pale. *Pulse:* full, but without a root. • **Formula for Liver blood and Spleen qi deficiency.**
Dang Gui Liu Huang Tang (angelica & six yellow decoction) **B** - clht	Dang Gui * 6-9g Sheng Di Huang 9-15g Shu Di Huang 9-15g Huang Lian 3-6g Huang Qin 6-12g Huang Bai 6-12g Huang Qi 30g	• **Nourishes the Yin, purges Liver fire.** • **Tonifies Qi and Blood, consolidates the exterior.** Fever, night sweats, dry mouth, red face, constipation, scanty urination. *Tongue:* dark red, dry coat. *Pulse:* rapid.
Dang Gui Nian Tong Tang (dang gui & anemarrhena combination) **C** - edamp	Dang Gui 1.25 Qiang Huo 1.25 Gan Cao 1.25 Huang Qin 1.25 Yin Chen 1.25 Ren Shen 0.75 Ku Shen Gen 0.75 Sheng Ma 0.75 Ge Gen 0.75 Cang Zhu 0.75 Bai Zhu 1.00 Ze Xie 1.00 Zhu Ling 1.00 Fang Feng 1.00 Zhi Mu 1.00	• **Dispels wind and clears heat.** • **Induces sweating, relieves inflammation, and stops pain.** Arthralgia with swelling, generalized swelling and painful joints, acute rheumatism, heaviness in the shoulders, eczema, gonorrhea, beriberi, and scabies. *Tongue:* yellow, greasy, furry coat. *Pulse:* soft, floating, slow.

FORMULA

Formula	Herbs / Dosage	Indications / Functions
Dang Gui San (dang gui powder) **C -** tblood	Dang Gui 4.00 Huang Qin 4.00 Bai Shao 4.00 Chuan Xiong 4.00 Bai Zhu 2.00	• **Stops the bleeding, calms restless fetus, and nourishes the blood.** Miscarriages, unstable gestation, and postpartum problems.
Dang Gui Shao Yao San (tangkuei & peony powder) **C -** harm	Dang Gui 10g Bai Shao 30g Fu Ling 15g Bai Zhu 12g Ze Xie 10g Chuan Xiong 10g	• **Nourishes Liver blood, tonifies the Spleen and Stomach.** • **Spreads Liver Qi, resolves dampness.** Continuous cramping in the abdomen, urinary difficulty, edema, anemia, low back pain, fatigue, irregular menstruation, chronic nephritis. *Tongue:* pale, thin coat. *Pulse:* deep, weak.
Dang Gui Si Ni Tang (tangkuei frigid extremity decoction) **B -** wint	Gui Zhi * 9g Dang Gui * 9g Bai Shao ** 9g Mu Tong 6g Xi Xin ** 6g Da Zao 25pcs Zhi Gan Cao 6g	• **Warms the channels and expels cold.** • **Nourishes the Blood, promotes circulation.** Cold and pale limbs, anemia, lower back pain. *Tongue:* pale body, thin, white coat. *Pulse:* deep, thin. • **Formula for Raynaud's disease.**
Dao Chi San (guide out red powder) **B -** clht	Sheng Di Huang* 15-30g Mu Tong 3-6g Dan Zhu Ye 3-6g Gan Cao 3-6g	• **Clears Heart fire.** • **Promotes urination.** Irritability, thirst, dark urination, red face, burning and painful urination, canker sores. *Tongue:* red body, dry coat. *Pulse:* rapid, slippery. • **Formula for canker sores and other heat signs in the Heart.** This formula drains heat from the Heart by way of the Small Intestine.
Dao Shui Fu Ling Tang (hoelen atractylodes & areca combination) **C -** edamp	Chi Fu Ling 4.80 Ze Xie 4.80 Bai Zhu 4.80 Mai Men Dong 4.80 Sang Bai Pi 1.60 Zi Su Ye 1.60 Da Fu Pi 1.20 Sha Ren 1.20 Mu Xiang 1.20 Deng Xin Cao 1.00 Bing Lang 1.60 Mu Gua 1.60 Chen Pi 1.20	• **Dispels water and edema.** • **Reduces swelling and distention.** Chronic nephritis, edema with asthma, ascites, and difficult urination. *Tongue:* white, thick, furry coat. *Pulse:* slow.
Dao Tan Tang (guide out phlegm decoction) **C -** rphlegm	Ju Hong 10g Ban Xia 15g Fu Ling 12g Gan Cao 3g Zhi Shi 3-10g Dan Nan Xing 12g Sheng Jiang 10g	• **Dries dampness, expels phlegm.** Obstructed phlegm, vertigo, headache, accumulation of congested fluids, stifling sensation and focal distention in the chest and diaphragm, reduced appetite, coughing and wheezing, copious sputum, difficult breathing, thick gummy nasal discharge. *Tongue:* white, greasy coat. *Pulse:* slippery, wiry.
Di Dang Tang (rhubarb & leech combination) **C -** tblood	Tao Ren 2.00 Da Huang 10.00 Shui Zhi 10.00 Meng Chong 1.00	• **Disperses stagnant blood.** • **Activates and regulates blood.** Abnormal menses, dark stools, stagnant blood in the face, lips and tongue, amenorrhea, menstrual irregularity, uterine myoma, and amnesia due to anemia.

Formula	Herbs / Dosage	Indications / Functions
Di Huang Yin Zi (rehmannia decoction) **B** - ewind	Sheng Di Huang 6-9g Shan Zhu Yu 9-12g Rou Cong Rong 9-12g Ba Ji Tian 6-9g Fu Zi 3-6g Rou Gui 1-3g Yuan Zhi 3-6g Fu Ling 6-9g Bo He 3-6g Shi Hu 6-9g Mai Men Dong 6-9g Wu Wei Zi 3-6g Sheng Jiang 3-6g Da Zao 3-5pcs Jiu Jie Chang Pu 3-6g	• **Tonifies Kidney Yang and Liver Yin.** • **Opens orifices, expels phlegm.** Difficulty talking, paralysis of the limbs due to stroke or MS, thirst without desire to drink, loss of mental clarity. *Tongue:* dark red body, greasy coat. *Pulse:* deep, weak, slow. • **Formula for paralysis due to Kidney Yin and Yang deficiency and phlegm misting the orifices.**
Ding Chuan Tang (stop wheezing decoction) **A** - rqi	Ma Huang 9g Bai Guo 9g Xing Ren 4.5g Su Zi 6g Ban Xia 9g Kuan Dong Hua 9g Huang Qin 4.5g Sang Bai Pi 9g Gan Cao 3g	• **Opens the Lungs and descends Lung Qi.** • **Stops cough and asthma.** • **Clears hot phlegm from the Lungs.** Asthma, shortness of breath, cough, sticky yellow mucus, perhaps some slight chills and fever. *Tongue:* greasy, yellow coat. *Pulse:* slippery, rapid.
Ding Xiang Shi Di Tang (clove & persimmon calyx decoction) **B** - rqi	Ding Xiang 6g Shi Di 6-9g Ren Shen 3-6g Sheng Jiang 6-9g	• **Tonifies Stomach Qi.** • **Warms the Stomach.** • **Suppresses rebellious Stomach Qi.** Hiccups, nausea, vomiting, belching, fullness of the stomach and chest, reduced appetite. *Tongue:* white coat. *Pulse:* deep, slow, weak. • **Formula for excess cold in the middle burner due to Stomach Qi and Yang deficiency.**
Du Huo Ji Sheng Tang (angelica & sangjisheng decoction) **A** - edamp	Du Huo * 9g Qin Jiao ** 6g Fang Feng ** 6g Xi Xin ** 6g Du Zhong 6g Niu Xi 6g Sang Ji Sheng 6g Dang Gui 6g Chuan Xiong 6g Sheng Di Huang 6g Bai Shao 6g Fu Ling 6g Gan Cao 6g Rou Gui 6g	• **Dispels wind-damp, stops pain.** • **Tonifies the Liver and Kidney.** • **Tonifies Qi and Blood.** Weak cold painful back, stiffness and numbness of the joints, weak muscles, palpitations, gets cold easily but loves warmth, chronic joint pain, shortness of breath. *Tongue:* swollen body, thin white coat. *Pulse:* weak. • **Formula for bi pain with underlying deficiency.**
Dun Sou Tang (morus & platycodon combination) **C** - clht	Chai Hu 5.00 Jie Geng 2.50 Huang Qin 2.50 Shan Zhi Zi 1.00 Gan Cao 1.00 Sang Bai Pi 2.50 Shi Gao 5.00	• **Disperses Lung heat.** Cough with heat, hacking cough, whooping cough, and bronchial cough with less sputum.
E Jiao Ji Zi Huang Tang (ass-hide gelatin & egg yolk decoction) **B** - ewind	E Jiao 6g Ji Zi Huang 7yks Sheng Di Huang 12g Bai Shao 9g Gou Teng 6g Shi Jue Ming 15g Mu Li 12g Fu Shen 12g Luo Shi Teng 9g Gan Cao 1.8g	• **Nourishes the Yin and Blood.** • **Dispels wind, calms the Liver.** Rigid extremities, muscle spasms, dizziness, vertigo, alternating flexion and extension. *Tongue:* dark red body, little or no coat. *Pulse:* thin, rapid.

Formula	Herbs / Dosage	Indications / Functions
Er Chen Tang (two aged decoction) A - rphlegm	Ban Xia * 15g Ju Hong * 15g Fu Ling ** 9g Gan Cao 4.5g Sheng Jiang 7pcs Wu Mei 1pc	• **Dries dampness, expels phlegm.** • **Harmonizes the middle burner.** • **Descends Stomach Qi.** Fullness of the chest and stomach, coughing with copious white phlegm, nausea, vomiting, dizziness, palpitations. *Tongue:* swollen body, greasy white coat. *Pulse:* slippery. • **Basic formula for treating damp and phlegm conditions.**
Er Long Zuo Ci Wan (pills for the deaf) B - tyin	Pill	• **Replenishes Kidney Yin, opens the ears and improves hearing.** Difficult hearing, tinnitus, vertigo, deafness. *Tongue:* red. *Pulse:* thready, rapid.
Er Miao San (two-marvel powder) B - edamp	Huang Bai 9-12g Cang Zhu 6-9g	• **Clears damp-heat from the lower burner.** Pain or lack of strength in the legs and lower back (esp. sinews, bones), yellow scanty urine, paralysis, swollen ankles, odorous vaginal discharge, boils on the lower body, itchy skin on the genitals. *Tongue:* greasy, yellow coat. *Pulse:* slippery, deep. • **Formula for damp-heat in the lower burner, with signs of leg Qi disorders like swollen ankles or open sores that don't heal.**
Er Xian Tang (two immortal decoction) C - tyang	Xian Mao 4.50 Ba Ji Tian 4.50 Yin Yang Huo 4.50 Zhi Mu 3.00 Huang Bai 3.00 Dang Gui 4.50	• **Warms Kidney Yang, Tonifies Yin and Essence.** • **Regulates penetrating and conception vessels, drains Kidney fire.** Headache, amenorrhea, sweating, irritability, insomnia, dizziness and heart palpitations cause by hypertension, menopause, PMS, hot flashes, UTI. *Tongue:* pale. *Pulse:* thready, rapid.
Er Zhi Wan (two-ultimate pill) B - tyin	Nu Zhen Zi Pill Han Lian Cao	• **Tonifies Kidney and Liver.** Weakness and soreness of the lower back and knees, weakness and atrophy of lower limbs, dry mouth and throat, insomnia, dizziness, premature graying, hair loss. *Tongue:* red, dry coat.
Er Zhu Tang (atractylodes & arisaema combination) C - edamp	Bai Zhu 2.50 Fu Ling 2.50 Chen Pi 2.50 Xiang Fu 2.50 Tian Nan Xing 2.50 Huang Qin 2.50 Wei Ling Xian 2.50 Qiang Huo 2.50 Ban Xia 4.00 Cang Zhu 3.00 Gan Cao 1.00 Sheng Jiang 3.00	• **Dispels wind and dampness.** • **Resolves phlegm and stops pain.** Aching arms due to phlegm and water, poor muscle tone, shoulder bursitis and forearm neuralgia. *Tongue:* white, greasy, sticky coat. *Pulse:* slippery, wiry.

Formula	Herbs / Dosage	Indications / Functions
Fang Feng Tong Sheng San (ledebouriella powder sagely unblocks) **B -** rext	Fang Feng 15g Ma Huang 15g Huang Qin 30g Gan Cao 15g Sheng Jiang 3pcs Da Huang 15g Mang Xiao 15g Jing Jie 15g Bo He 15g Zhi Zi 15g Hua Shi 90g Shi Gao 30g Lian Qiao 15g Jie Geng 30g Chuan Xiong 15g Bai Shao 15g Bai Zhu 15g Dang Gui 15g	• **Expels wind, clears heat.** • **Opens the bowels, drains damp.** Chills, fever, headache, soreness of the joints, migrating pain, red and sore eyes, bitter taste, fullness of the chest and diaphragm, dry throat, constipation. *Tongue:* yellow, greasy coat. *Pulse:* rapid, slippery, wiry. • **Expels wind-damp or wind-water.**
Fang Ji Huang Qi Tang (stephania & astragalus decoction) **B -** edamp	Huang Qi * 3.8g Han Fang Ji * 3g Bai Zhu 2.3g Sheng Jiang 4pcs Da Zao 1pc Gan Cao 1.5g	• **Strengthens the Qi and the Spleen.** • **Expels wind-damp or wind water.** • **Promotes urination.** Chills, aversion to wind, sweating, heaviness of the body, difficult urination, edema. *Tongue:* pale, thin white coat. *Pulse:* floating, slippery. • **Formula for expelling wind-damp or wind-water.**
Fen Xiao Tang (hoelen & alisma combination) **C -** edamp	Cang Zhu 3.00 Fu Ling 3.00 Bai Zhu 3.00 Chen Pi 2.00 Hou Pu 2.00 Xiang Fu 2.00 Zhu Ling 2.00 Ze Xie 2.00 Zhi Shi 1.00 Mu Xiang 1.00 Da Fu Pi 1.00 Sha Ren 1.00 Sheng Jiang 2.00 Deng Xin Cao 1.00	• **Dispels Qi and food stagnation.** • **Dispels water and edema and tonifies the Spleen.** Peritonitis, nephritis, scanty or yellow urination, constipation, distention and abdomen discomfort, pitting edema, initial stage of ascites, and cirrhosis. *Tongue:* white, slippery, greasy, dirty coat. *Pulse:* soft.
Fu Ling Yin (hoelen combination) **C -** edamp	Fu Ling 5.00 Zhi Shi 1.50 Cang Zhu 4.00 Ren Shen 3.00 Chen Pi 3.00 Sheng Jiang 3.00	• **Harmonizes the Stomach and disperses phlegm.** • **Dispels dampness.** Retention of phlegm in the stomach, belching, gastroptosis, gastritis, gas, stomach water stagnancy.
Fu Tu Dan (hoelen & cuscuta formula) **C -** sab	Tu Si Zi 10.00 Wu Wei Zi 8.00 Fu Ling 3.00 Shan Yao 6.00 Shi Lian Zi 3.00	• **Strengthens the Spleen and astringes the Kidney.** • **Dispels damp, supports the Heart and Spleen.** Nocturnal emission, enuresis, leukorrhagia with thin discharge, or prolonged diarrhea, accompanied with lumbago, fatigue which is attributive to weakness of kidney-energy and failure of preserving essence by the spleen. *Tongue:* pale, whitish furry coat. *Pulse:* slow, weak, deep.
Fu Yuan Huo Xue Tang (revive health by invigorating blood decoction) **B -** movexue	Dang Gui 9g Tao Ren 9g Hong Hua 6g Chuan Shan Jia 6g Da Huang 30g Tian Hua Fen 9g Chai Hu 15g Gan Cao 6g	• **Promotes blood circulation.** • **Unblocks the channels, soothes Liver Qi.** Acute severe pain in the hypochondria, chest or flank area due to trauma. *Tongue:* purple spots on the sides. *Pulse:* wiry. • **Formula for acute chest pain due to trauma.**

FORMULA

Formula	Herbs / Dosage	Indications / Functions
Fu Zi Li Zhong Wan (prepared aconite pill to regulate the middle) **C** - wint	Fu Zi 3-15g Gan Jiang Ren 3-10g Shen 5-10g Bai Zhu 5-15g Zhi Gan Cao 2-10g	• **Warms the middle, dispels cold.** • **Regulates Spleen and Stomach.** Abdominal and epigastric pain better with pressure, vomiting, diarrhea, inability to keep food down, cold body, hands, and feet, mild sweating, rigidity, spasms, lockjaw. *Tongue:* light red, white coat. *Pulse:* deep, slow, faint.
Gan Lu Xiao Du Dan (sweet dew eliminate toxin pill) **B** - edamp	Hua Shi 15-20g Yin Chen Hao 10-15g Mu Tong 5-10g Huang Qin 10-15g Lian Qiao 5-10g Chuan Bei Mu 5-10g She Gan 5-10g Shi Chang Pu 6-10g Bai Dou Kou 5-10g Bo He 3-6g Huo Xiang 5-10g	• **Clears damp-heat and detoxifies.** • **Clears up turbid water.** Fever, swollen, sore, and puffy body, fullness of the chest, lethargy, yellow complexion, swollen throat, thirst, dark scanty urination, diarrhea, or vomiting, jaundice. *Tongue:* thick, greasy, yellow coat. *Pulse:* slippery, rapid. • **Formula for damp-heat stuck in the Qi level, or for Pig Head syndrome, in which damp-heat rises to the head.**
Gan Mai Da Zao Tang (licorice, wheat & jujube decoction) **A** - ashen	Fu Xiao Mai * 9-15g Gan Cao 9g Da Zao 10pcs	• **Nourishes the Heart, calms the Spirit.** • **Harmonizes the middle burner.** • **Relieves depression.** Disorientation, depression, abnormal behavior, irritability, insomnia, absent-mindedness, excessive worry, restlessness, short attention span, crying spells, low energy, fatigue, excessive yawning. *Tongue:* red, little or no coat. *Pulse:* thready, rapid. • **Formula for restless organ disorder "zang zao", Heart Yin and Heart Qi deficiency with Liver Qi stagnation, resulting in emotional and mental imbalance.**
Ge Gen Huang Lian Huang Qin Tang (kudzu, scutellaria, & coptis decoction) **B** - rext	Ge Gen * 15-24g Huang Lian ** 6g Huang Qin ** 9g Zhi Gan Cao 6g	• **Clears damp-heat.** • **Releases the surface.** Fever, slight chills, sweating, diarrhea with burning sensation in the anus, thirst, dry mouth, foul smelling stools, irritability, heat in the chest. *Tongue:* red body, yellow coat. *Pulse:* floating, rapid. • **Formula for common cold syndromes accompanied by diarrhea, perhaps due to Stomach heat, or heat in the intestines.**
Ge Gen Tang (kudzu decoction) **A** - rext	Gen Gen * 12g Ma Huang ** 9g Gui Zhi ** 6g Bai Shao 6g Sheng Jiang 9g Da Zao 12pcs Gan Cao 6g	• **Releases the surface and loosens the muscles.** • **Generates fluids.** Stiff neck, slight fever, slight chills, no sweating, pain in the upper back, body aches, headache. *Tongue:* thin, white coat. *Pulse:* floating, tight. • **Formula for wind-cold with joint pain and body aches.**

FORMULA

Formula	Herbs / Dosage	Indications / Functions
Ge Xia Zhu Yu Tang (drive out blood stasis below diaphragm decoction) **B** - movexue	Dang Gui 9g Chuan Xiong 6g Chi Shao 6g Hong Hua 9g Tao Ren 9g Wu Ling Zhi 9g Yan Hu Suo 3g Xiang Fu 4.5g Zhi Ke 4.5g Wu Yao 6-12g Mu Dan Pi 6g Gan Cao 9g	• **Regulates Liver, dispels blood stagnation.** • **Regulates Qi, relieves pain.** Pain and cramping in the lower abdomen, delayed and scanty menstruation, breast distention, abdominal distention. *Tongue:* purple body. *Pulse:* wiry, tight. • **Formula for menstrual difficulties, including painful cramping, due to blood stagnation.**
Gu Chong Tang (stabilize flooding decoction) **B** - astringe	Bai Zhu 30g Huang Qi 18g Shan Zhu Yu 24g Bai Shao 12g Duan Long Gu 24g Mu Li 24g Hai Piao Xiao 12g Zong Lu Tan 6g Wu Bei Zi 1.5g Xi Cao 9g	• **Nourishes the Liver, regulates Spleen Qi.** • **Strengthens the Chong, stops the bleeding.** Excessive menstrual bleeding, spotting, palpitations, shortness of breath. *Tongue:* pale. *Pulse:* weak.
Gu Jing Wan (stabilize menses pill) **A** - astringe	Gui Ban * 30g Bai Shao * 30g Huang Bai 9g Huang Qin 30g Chun Pi 21g Xiang Fu 7.5g	• **Regulates the Chong and Ren channels.** • **Nourishes the Yin.** • **Clears heat, stops bleeding.** Excess menstrual bleeding, abnormal menstrual cycle, spotting between period, irritability, leukorrhea with yellow discharge, abdominal pains and cramps, chest discomfort due to heat, dark urine. *Tongue:* purple or red body, greasy coat. *Pulse:* wiry, slippery.
Gu Yin Jian (stabilize yin decoction) **B** - tyin	Ren Shen 3-6g Shu Di Huang 9-15g Shan Yao 6g Shan Zhu Yu 4.5g Yuan Zhi 2.1g Zhi Gan Cao 3-6g Wu Wei Zi 3-6g Tu Si Zi 6-9g	• **Tonifies the Kidney.** • **Regulates the Chong and Ren.** Irregular menstruation, scanty and pale menstrual flow, dizziness, tinnitus, lower back pain, frequent urination. *Tongue:* pale body. *Pulse:* deep, weak.
Gua Lou Xie Bai Bai Jiu Tang (trichosantes, chive & wine decoction) **B** - rqi	Gua Lou 12g Xie Bai 9g Bai Jui 60ml	• **Penetrates the Yang.** • **Regulates Qi.** • **Expels phlegm, resolves stagnation.** Chest pain that radiates to the upper back, palpitations, shortness of breath, cough with mucus, asthma. *Tongue:* thick, greasy coat. *Pulse:* wiry, slippery, deep. • **Relieves chest pain by expelling phlegm from the chest. Also for chronic bronchitis and other phlegm disorders of the chest.**
Gui Lu Er Xian Jiao (turtle shell & deer antler syrup) **C** - tyang	Gui Ban 5-10g Lu Jiao 10-20g Ren Shen 3-6g Gou Qi Zi 3-6g	• **Nourishes the Kidney Yin, strengthens the Kidney Yang.** Lower back soreness and pain, cock's crow diarrhea, diminished vision, impotence, emaciation. *Tongue:* pale, white coat. *Pulse:* deep, slow, weak.

FORMULA

Formula	Herbs / Dosage	Indications / Functions
Gui Pi Tang (restore spleen decoction) A - tqiblood	Huang Qi 9-12g Ren Shen 3-6g Bai Zhu * 9-12g Fu Ling 9-12g Dang Gui 6-9g Mu Xiang 3-6g Long Yan Rou 6-9g Suan Zao Ren 9-12g Yuan Zhi 3-6g Sheng Jiang 5pcs Da Zao 1pc Gan Cao 3-6g	• **Tonifies Spleen Qi and Heart Blood.** Fatigue, irritability, palpitations, anxiety, insomnia, forgetfulness, frequent and heavy excessive dreaming, fear and anxiety, low-grade fever, reduced appetite, diarrhea, pale face, scanty menses, yellow complexion. *Tongue:* pale swollen body, thin white coat. *Pulse:* floating, tight. • **Formula for deficiencies due to over-thinking, with fatigue, reduced appetite, soft stools and the inability of Spleen to control the blood.**
Gui Zhi Fu Ling Wan (cinnamon & poria pill) A - movexue	Gui Zhi * 9-12g Fu Ling * 9-12g Bai Shao ** 9-15g Tao Ren 9-12g Mu Dan Pi 9-12g	• **Reduces blood stagnation in the Uterus.** • **Promotes blood circulation, softens masses.** Uterine bleeding during pregnancy, abdomen pain upon pressure, ovarian cysts, groin pain, difficult labor, lumps or masses in the lower abdomen, swelling, spasms, amenorrhea, dysmenorrhea, lochia retention. *Tongue:* purple body, greasy coat. *Pulse:* slippery, choppy, wiry. • **Formula for ovarian cysts and masses in the lower abdomen.**
Gui Zhi Jia Long Gu Mu Li Tang (cinnamon twig decoction plus dragon bone & oyster shell) C - harm	Gui Zhi 3-10g Bai Shao 5-10g Long Gu 15-30g Mu Li 15-30g Sheng Jiang 2-3pc Da Zao 3-12g Gan Cao 2-10g	• **Restrains Jing, anchors rebellion.** • **Regulates and harmonizes Ying and Wei Qi.** Nocturnal emission, excessive dreaming, cold sensation in the lower body, dizziness, hair loss, lower abdominal contraction and pain. *Tongue:* red tip, thin, white coat. *Pulse:* thin, deep, rapid.
Gui Zhi Shao Yao Zhi Mu Tang (cinnamon twig, peony & anemarrhena decoction) C - edamp	Gui Zhi 12g Ma Huang 6g Fu Zi 6g Zhi Mu 12g Bai Zhu 15g Bai Shao 9g Sheng Jiang 15g Fang Feng 12g Gan Cao 6g	• **Dispels wind and damp.** • **Promotes flow of Yang Qi.** Swollen painful joints, reduced range of motion in joints, no sweating, weight loss, headache, dizziness. *Tongue:* white, greasy coat. *Pulse:* wiry, slippery. • **Formula for recurrent painful obstruction with heat.**
Gui Zhi Tang (cinnamon decoction) A - rext	Gui Zhi * 9g Bai Shao ** 9g Sheng Jiang 9g Da Zao 12pcs Zhi Gan Cao 6g	• **Releases the surface and loosens muscles.** • **Regulates the Ying and Wei Qi.** • **Promotes or stops sweating.** Chills and fever with or without sweating, stiff neck, aversion to wind, headache, nasal congestion, no thirst. *Tongue:* thin, white coat. *Pulse:* soft, floating. • **Formula for wind-cold with deficiency.** Milder than Ma Huang Tang.

Formula	Herbs / Dosage	Indications / Functions
Gun Tan Wan (vaporize phlegm pill) **B** - open	Meng Shi * 30g Da Huang ** 240g Huang Qin 240g Chen Xiang 15g	• **Clears and descends fire.** • **Expels phlegm and opens orifices.** Mental imbalance with palpitations, anxiety, palpitations leading to coma, coughing with phlegm that's difficult-to-expectorate, tinnitus, fullness of the chest, dizziness, vertigo, constipation. *Tongue:* thick and greasy, yellow coat. *Pulse:* slippery, strong, rapid. • **Formula to clear phlegm-fire and open Heart orifices.**
Hai Zao Yu Hu Tang (seaweed decoction) **C** - rphlegm	Hai Zao * 9g Kun Bu * 9g Hai Dai * 9g Bei Mu 9g Ban Xia 9g Du Huo 9g Chuan Xiong 6g Dang Gui 9g Qing Pi 6g Chen Pi 6g Lian Qiao 9g Gan Cao 3g	• **Reduces goiters.** • **Resolves phlegm, softens hardness.** Goiter, hard masses and nodules, fullness in the chest, deep breathing, sighing. *Tongue:* thin, greasy coat. *Pulse:* wiry, slippery.
Hao Qin Qing Dan Tang (artemisia annua & scutellaria decoction) **B** - harm	Qing Hao * 4.5-6g Huang Qin * 4.5-9g Zhu Ru 9g Chen Pi 4.5g Zhi Ke 4.5g Ban Xia 4.5g Chi Fu Ling 9g Bi Yu San 9g	• **Clears Gallbladder heat and Shaoyang damp-heat.** • **Harmonizes the Stomach, expels phlegm.** High fever, slight chills, bitter taste, vomiting sticky yellow fluids, fullness of the chest and hypochondriac regions. *Tongue:* red body, greasy yellow coat. *Pulse:* slippery, soggy, wiry, rapid. • **Formula for Shaoyang chills and fever, with vomiting.**
Hei Xi Dan (lead special pill) **C** - wint	Jin Ling Zi 30g Hu Lu Ba 30g Mu Xiang 30g Rou Dou Kou 30g Bu Gu Zi 30g Chen Xiang 30g Hui Xiang 30g Yang Qi Shi 30g Rou Gui 15g Hei Xi 60g Liu Huang 60g	• **Warms and tonifies lower burner Yang Qi.** • **Forces floating Yang downward.** Profuse wheezing, gasping for breath, incessant coldness, oily sweat. *Tongue:* pale, white coat. *Pulse:* deep, weak, slow. • **Formula for excess above and deficiency below and syndromes near Yang collapse.**
Hong Hua Tao Ren Jian (safflower & peach kernel decoction) **C** - movexue	Hong Hua 6-9g Tao Ren 6-9g Sheng Di Huang 9-12g Bai Shao Yao 6-9g Dang Gui 6-9g Chuan Xiong 3-6g Dan Shen 6-9g Yan Hu Suo 6-9g Xiang Fu 3-6g Qing Pi 3-6g	• **Moves and nourishes blood.** • **Removes blood stagnation.** Abdominal pain and distension worse with pressure, hypochondriac distention, irregular menstruation, amenorrhea, dysmenorrhea, mental depression. *Tongue:* purple spots, thin coat. *Pulse:* deep, hesitant, wiry.
Hu Qian Wan (hidden tiger pill) **B** - tyin	Huang Bai * 150g Shu Di Huang ** 60g Gui Ban ** 120g Zhi Mu * 30g Bai Shao 60g Hu Gu 60g Suo Yang 45g Gan Jiang 15g Chen Pi 60g	• **Nourishes the Yin, sedates false heat.** • **Strengthens the sinews, tendons, and bones.** • **Descends fire.** Weakness of the sinews, muscles and lower back, muscle wasting, difficulty walking, dizziness, tinnitus, paralysis. *Tongue:* red body, little or no coat. *Pulse:* thready, weak. • **Formula for atrophy disorders, especially for elderly patients with difficulty walking due to undernourished muscles and tendons.**

FORMULA

Formula	Herbs / Dosage	Indications / Functions
Huai Hua San (sophora powder) B - stopxue	Huai Hua * 9-30g Ce Bai Ye ** 9-15g Zhi Ke 6-9g Jing Jie 6-9g	• **Stops bleeding in the Intestines.** • **Expels intestinal wind.** • **Cools heat.** Bright red or dark red anal bleeding, bleeding hemorrhoids. *Tongue:* red body, little or no coat. *Pulse:* thin, weak.
Huang Lian E Jiao Tang (coptis & ass-hide gelatin decoction B - ashen	Huang Lian * 12g Huang Qin * 6g E Jiao * 9g Bai Shao 6g Ji Zi Huang 2pcs	• **Nourishes the Yin and Blood.** • **Clears damp-heat, calms the Spirit.** Irritability with heat in the chest, insomnia, palpitations, dry mouth and throat, anxiety. *Tongue:* red body, dry yellow coat. *Pulse:* thin, rapid. • **Formula for damage to the Yin fluids due to febrile disease at the blood level.**
Huang Lian Jie Du Tang (coptis decoction relieve toxicity) A - clht	Huang Lian * 9g Huang Qin ** 6g Huang Bai 6g Zhi Zi 6-12g	• **Clears heat and fire toxins in all three burners.** • **Dispels damp-heat in the San Jiao.** Big fever, irritability, thirst, dry throat, delirium, disturbed spirit, nosebleeds, pimples, boils, sores. *Tongue:* red body, yellow coat. *Pulse:* strong, rapid.
Huang Lian Wen Dan Tang (coptis warm the gallbladder decoction) C - clht	Huang Lian 3g Ban Xia 6g Chen Pi 6g Fu Ling 9g Gan Cao 3g Zhu Ru 9g Zhi Shi 6g	• **Clears heat, promotes qi movement, and transforms phlegm and damp.** Bitter taste in the mouth, profuse sputum, nausea and vomiting, dizziness, palpitations, insomnia, restlessness, lower abdominal contraction and pain, cold sensation at the tip of penis, watery diarrhea, dream disturbed sleep, hair loss. *Tongue:* greasy, yellow, sticky coat. *Pulse:* hollow, slow. • Contains **Wen Dan Tang** + Huang Lian.
Huang Long Tang (yellow dragon decoction) B - purg	Da Huang * 9g Mang Xiao * 12g Hou Po 3g Zhi Shi 6g Ren Shen 6g Dang Gui 9g Jie Geng 3g Sheng Jiang 9g Da Zao 2pcs Gan Cao 3g	• **Purges heat, promotes bowel movement.** • **Tonifies Qi and Blood.** • **Formula for Yang Ming Fu excess.** Green watery diarrhea, constipation, fullness of stomach, fever, thirst, shortness of breath. *Tongue:* yellow or black coat. *Pulse:* weak. • Contains **Da Cheng Qi Tang** + Ren Shen, Dang Gui, Jie Geng, Sheng Jiang, Da Zao, Gan Cao.
Huang Qi Jian Zhong Tang (astragalus decoction to construct the middle) C - wint	Huang Qi 10-15g Yi Tang 18-30g Gui Zhi 9g Shao Yao 18g Zhi Gan Cao 6g Sheng Jiang 9g Da Zao 12pc	• **Warms and tonifies middle burner.** • **Moderate spasmodic abdominal pain.** Impaired defensive Wei Qi, alternating chills and fever, stifling sensation in the chest, abdominal pain due to cold, fatigue, spontaneous sweating, pale face. *Tongue:* pale, white coat. *Pulse:* deep, slow.

Formula	Herbs / Dosage	Indications / Functions
Huang Tu Tang (yellow earth decoction) **B - stopxue**	Zao Xin Tu * 18g Bai Zhu 9g Fu Zi 9g Sheng Di Huang 9g E Jiao 9g Huang Qin 9g Zhi Gan Cao 9g	• **Stops bleeding, nourishes the blood.** • **Tonifies Yang, strengthens the Spleen.** Bloody stools, hemorrhoids, vomiting blood, nosebleeds, dark blood, cold limbs. *Tongue:* swollen, pale, white coat. *Pulse:* weak, deep. • **Formula for LI bleeding due to inability of the Spleen to secure blood.**
Huo Luo Xiao Ling Dan (invigorate collaterals wonder pill) **C - movexue**	Dang Gui 15g Dan Shen 15g Ru Xiang 15g Mo Yao 15g	• **Moves the blood, dispels blood stagnation.** • **Unblocks the channels, stops pain.** Pain at various locations, bruising and swelling due to trauma, rheumatic pain, masses, nodules, accumulations, ulcerations. *Tongue:* dark. *Pulse:* wiry.
Huo Po Wen Zhong Tang (magnolia warm middle decoction) **C - rqi**	Hou Po * 9-15g Cao Dou Kou ** 6-9g Chen Pi 9-15g Mu Xiang 6-9g Gang Jiang 1.5-6g Sheng Jiang 3pcs Fu Ling 9-12g Gan Cao 3-9g	• **Regulates Qi and warms the middle.** Epigastric and abdominal distention and pain, reduced appetite, fatigue in the limbs. *Tongue:* white, greasy coat. *Pulse:* deep, wiry. • **Formula for damp-cold invading Spleen and Stomach.**
Huo Xiang Zheng Qi Tang (agastache correct qi powder) **A - edamp**	Huo Xiang * 90g Hou Po 60g Zi Su Ye 30g Bai Zhi 30g Chen Pi 60g Fu Ling 30g Bai Zhu 60g Da Fu Pi 30g Jie Geng 60g Ban Xia 60g Gan Cao 75g Sheng Jiang 3-6g Da Zao 1pc	• **Releases the surface and expels damp.** • **Regulates Qi, harmonizes the middle burner.** • **Classic formula for stomach flu.** Nausea, vomiting, chills and fever, diarrhea, fullness of the stomach, borborygmus, headache. *Tongue:* greasy, white coat. *Pulse:* floating, slippery.
Ji Chuan Jian (benefit river flow decoction) **B - purg**	Rou Cong Rong 6-9g Dang Gui 9-15g Niu Xi 6g Ze Xie 4.5g Zhi Ke 3g Sheng Ma 1.5-3g	• **Moistens the intestines, warms the Kidney.** • **Promotes bowel movement.** Constipation, clear urination, coldness and pain of the lower back. *Tongue:* swollen, pale, thin, white coat. *Pulse:* weak. • **Formula for constipation due to Kidney Qi and Yang deficiency, perhaps after a long-term illness.**
Ji Ming San (cock's crow powder) **C - edamp**	Bing Lang 8.00 Chen Pi 5.00 Mu Gua 5.00 Wu Zhu Yu 1.50 Zi Su Ye 1.50 Jie Geng 2.50 Sheng Jiang 2.50	• **Dispels cold-dampness.** • **Promotes vital qi flow, clears channels and collaterals.** Dampness and excess conditions, fever, intolerance to cold, difficult movement, beriberi, chest fullness, palpitations, irritability, shortness of breath, edema, oppression of chest, nausea and vomiting. *Tongue:* white, greasy, furry coat. *Pulse:* soft, slow, floating.
Jia Jian Fu Mai Tang (modified baked licorice decoction) **C - tyin**	Zhi Can Cao 9-12g Sheng Di Huang 15-20g Bai Shao Yao 6-9g Mai Men Dong 6-9g Huo Ma Ren 9-12g E Jiao 6-9g	• **Nourishes the blood, preserves Yin.** • **Generates fluids, moistens dryness.** Chronic late-stage fever, red face, restlessness, palpitations, dry mouth, cracked lips, black teeth. *Tongue:* red, dry, little or no coat. *Pulse:* weak, forceful.

Formula	Herbs / Dosage	Indications / Functions
Jia Jian Wei Rui Tang (modified polygonatum decoction) **B** - rext	Yu Zhu 6-9g Cong Bai 6g Jie Geng 3-4.5g Dan Dou Chi 9-12g Bo He 3-4.5g Bai Wei 1.5-3g Zhi Gan Cao 1.5g Da Zao 2pcs	• **Releases the surface, clears heat.** • **Tonifies the Yin.** Slight chills, fever, no sweating, headache, sore throat, coughing, sticky phlegm that is difficult-to-expectorate, thirst, irritability. *Tongue:* dark red. *Pulse:* thin, rapid, floating. • **Formula for wind-cold invasion with underlying Yin deficiency.**
Jian Er Wan (atractylodes & pogostemonis combination) **C** - clht	Rou Dou Kou 2.00 Shi Jun Zi 2.00 Mai Ya 2.00 Huang Lian 2.00 Shen Qu 4.00 Bing Lang 2.00 Mu Xiang 1.00 Hu Huang Lian 2.00 Bai Zhu 2.00 Shan Zha 2.00 Zhi Shi 2.00	• **Clears heat, expels intestinal parasites and promotes digestion.** • **Relieves infantile malnutrition, strengthens the Spleen.** Infantile malnutrition, abdominal pain, sallow complexion, emaciation, abdominal fullness, fever, foul breath.
Jian Pi Wan (strengthen spleen pill) **B** - rfood	Bai Zhu * 75g Fu Ling* 60g Ren Shen * 45g Shan Yao ** 30g Rou Dou Kou ** 30g Shan Zha 30g Shen Qu 30g Mai Ya 30g Mu Xiang 22.5g Chen Pi 30g Sha Ren 30g Gan Cao 22.5g Huang Lian 22.5g	• **Harmonizes Spleen and Stomach.** • **Resolves food stagnation, stops diarrhea.** • **Classic formula for stomachaches.** Bloating and distension in the stomach, reduced appetite, loose stools, indigestion. *Tongue:* greasy, yellow coat. *Pulse:* weak.
Jian Ying San (inphantrans formula) **C** - clht	Jiang Chan 1.00 Gou Teng 1.00 Shi Chang Pu 2.50 Shan Zhi Zi 2.50 Tian Ma 2.50 Huang Lian 2.50 Bei Mu 2.50 Niu Huang 0.10 Bo He 1.00 Ju Hong 2.50 Gan Cao 1.00 Zhu Sha 0.10 Bing Pian 0.10	• **Clears Lungs and expels heat and sputum.** • **Calm the shen.** Fever, shortness of breath, eczema, bronchitis, cough, sore throat, influenza.
Jiao Ai Tang (ass-hide gelatin & mugwort decoction) **B** - stopxue	Ai Ye * 9g E Jiao * 6g Sheng Di Huang 18g Dang Gui 9g Bai Shao 12g Chuan Xiong 6g Gan Cao 6g	• **Tonifies the Blood, stops bleeding.** • **Regulates the channels, calms the fetus.** Excessive menstruation, restless fetus, spotting, bleeding during pregnancy, continuous bleeding after delivery, abdominal pain. *Tongue:* pale, thin, white coat. *Pulse:* empty, wiry. • **Formula for uncontrolled bleeding disorders due to deficiency of Blood and Yang.**
Jie Geng Tang (platycodon combination) **C** - clht	Jie Geng 2.00 Gan Cao 3.00	• **Dispels stagnation, detoxifies, and expels phlegm and pus.** Sore throat, cough with mucus or thick pus with blood, oppression of chest, dry throat but not thirst, tonsillitis, bronchitis, pneumonia.
Jin Fei Cao San (schizonepeta & pinellia formula) **C** - rphlegm	Xuan Fu Hua 4.50 Qian Hu 4.50 Jing Jie 6.00 Ban Xia 1.50 Gan Cao 1.50 Ma Huang 4.50 Chi Shao 1.50 Sheng Jiang 3.00 Da Zao 1.00	• **Dispels wind and cold.** • **Resolves phlegm and stops cough.** Common cold manifesting cough with headache and profuse yellowish thick sputum, stuffy nose, deep voice, chest discomfort; bronchitis, tracheitis, and bronchial asthma. *Tongue:* white, smooth, furry coat. *Pulse:* floating, tight.

FORMULA

Formula	Herbs / Dosage	Indications / Functions
Jin Gui Shen Qi Wan AKA Ba Wei Di Huang Wan golden-cabinet kidney qi pill) A - tyin	Sheng Di Huang * 24g Fu Zi 3g Gui Zhi 3g Shan Zhu Yu ** 12g Shan Yao ** 12g Mu Dan Pi 9g Ze Xie 9g Fu Ling 9g (3g for Sheng Di, 3g Fu Zi)	• **Tonifies Kidney Yang.** • **Drains water-damp, promotes urination.** Lower back pain, weak knees, cold legs, frequent or difficult urination, thirst, leg qi syndrome with swollen, numb, and weak lower limbs. *Tongue:* pale, swollen, thin, white, moist coat. *Pulse:* weak, slow. • Contains *Liu Wei Di Huang Wan* – replace Shu Di Huang with Sheng Di Huang + Fu Zi + Gui Zhi.
Jin Ling Zi San (melia powder) B - rqi	Chuan Lian Zi 30g Yan Hu Suo 30g	• **Regulates Liver Qi, promotes circulation.** • **Clears heat, stops pain.** Chest pain, epigastric pain, hypochondriac pain, pain aggravated by spicy foods, groin pain, hernia pain, dysmenorrhea. *Tongue:* red body, yellow coat. *Pulse:* wiry, rapid. • **Formula for Liver Qi stagnation with fire, presenting with painful menstruation and hernias due to long-term stagnation.**
Jin Suo Gu Jing Wan (metal lock stabilize essence pill) B - astringe	Sha Yuan Ji Li * 60g Qian Shi ** 60g Lian Zi ** 120g Long Gu 30g Mu Li 30g Lian Xu 60g	• **Stabilizes the Kidneys, binds the essence.** Seminal emissions, lower back pain, frequent urination, fatigue, tinnitus. *Tongue:* pale body, white coat. *Pulse:* weak. • **Formula for Kidney Jing and Yang deficient symptoms due to the Kidney gate not closing. It binds the essence and stops seminal emissions, frequent urination.**
Jing Fang Bai Du San (schizonepeta & ledebouriella powder to overcome pathogenic influences) C - rext	Jing Jie 3-10g Fang Feng 3-9g Chuan Xiong 3-10g Qiang Huo 3-10g Du Huo 3-10g Chai Hu 3-10g Fu Ling 10-15g Qian Hu 3-9g Zhi Ke 3-10g Jie Geng 3-9g Sheng Jiang 2-3pc Gan Cao 2-10g Bo He 1.5-6g	• **Promotes sweating, releases the exterior.** • **Dispels wind, stops pain.** Fever, muscle ache, intolerance to cold, stuffy nose, bloodshot eyes, common colds affected by wind, damp and cold. *Tongue:* thin, white coat. *Pulse:* floating, rapid.
Jing Jei Lian Qiao Tang (schizonepeta & forsythia combination) C - clht	Dang Gui 2.00 Bai Shao 2.00 Chuan Xiong 2.00 Huang Qin 2.00 Shan Zhi Zi 2.00 Lian Qiao 2.00 Jing Jie 2.00 Fang Feng 2.00 Zhi Qiao 2.00 Gan Cao 1.50 Bai Zhi 2.00 Jie Geng 2.00 Chai Hu 2.00	• **Clears heat and fire.** • **Nourishes blood and soothes the Liver.** Suppurative diseases in the upper body including ears or nose, otitis, rhinitis, sinusitis, nosebleeds, TB, tonsillitis, epistaxis, and acne.
Jiu Wei Qiang Huo Tang (nine-herb notopterygium decoction) B - rext	Qiang Huo 4.5g Fang Feng 4.5g Cang Zhu 4.5 Xi Xin 1.5g Chuang Xiong 3g Bai Zhi 3g Huang Qin 3g Sheng Di Huang 3g Gan Cao 3g	• **Dispels exterior wind-cold-damp.** • **Eliminates interior heat.** Predominant chills, slight fever without sweating, headache, stiff neck, aches and pains, bitter taste, slight thirst. *Tongue:* white, slight yellow coat. *Pulse:* floating.

Formula	Herbs / Dosage	Indications / Functions
Jiu Xian San (nine-immortal pill) C - astringe	Ren Shen * 1.5g Zi Ying Sue Ke * 6g Wu Mei ** 6g Wu Wei Zi ** 1.5g E Jiao 1.5g Kuan Dong Hua 1.5g Bei Mu 1.5g Jie Geng 1.5g Sang Bai Pe 1.5g Sheng Jiang 2pcs Da Zao 1pc	• **Tonifies Lung Qi, nourishes Lung Yin.** Chronic cough, spontaneous sweating, wheezing, pale complexion, shortness of breath. *Tongue:* pale. *Pulse:* rapid.
Ju He Wan (tangerine seed pill) B - rqi	Ju He 9-12g Lian Zi 3-6g Yan Hu Suo 6-9g Hou Po 6-9g Zhi Shi 6-9g Rou Gui 1-3g Kun Bu 6-9g Hai Zao 6-9g Hai Dai 6-9g Tao Ren 3-6g Mu Tong 6-9g Mu Xiang 3-6g	• **Regulates Qi, stops pain.** • **Softens hardness.** Swollen testis, distension and pain in lower abdomen, hernia, radiating pain to lower spine. *Tongue:* white coat. *Pulse:* deep, wiry.
Ju Pi Zhu Ru Tang (tangerine peel & bamboo shavings decoction) A - rqi	Chen Pi * 9-12g Zhu Ru * 9-12g Ren Shen 3g Sheng Jiang 18g Da Zao 30pcs Gan Cao 15g	• **Descends Stomach Qi.** • **Harmonizes the middle burner.** • **Clears Stomach heat, tonifies Qi.** Belching, nausea, hiccups, vomiting, dry mouth, thirst. *Tongue:* red body, thin yellow coat. *Pulse:* thin, rapid. • **Suppresses rebellious Stomach Qi.**
Juan Bi Tang (remove painful obstruction decoction) B - edamp	Qiang Huo * 3g Du Huo * 3g Hai Feng Tang ** 9g Qin Jiao ** 3g Chuan Xiong 2.1g Mu Xiang 2.4g Ru Xiang 2.4g Rou Gui 1.5g Gan Cao 1.5g Sang Zhi ** 9g Dang Gui 9g	• **Dispels wind-damp, relieves pain.** Joint pain worse with cold, better with warmth, heaviness and numbness in the limbs. *Tongue:* thick, white coat. *Pulse:* slow, slippery. • **Formula for early stage painful obstruction.**
Ke Xue Fang (coughing blood formula) B - stopxue	Qing Dai * 6-9g Zhi Zi * 9g Gua Lou Ren 9g Fu Hai Shi 9g He Zi 6-9g	• **Cools the blood, stops bleeding.** • **Clears heat, resolves phlegm.** Coughing blood, pain in the chest and hypochondrium, irritability, constipation, red cheeks. *Tongue:* red, yellow coat. *Pulse:* wiry, rapid.
Li Zhong Wan (regulate middle pill) A - wint	Dang Shen ** 9g Gan Jiang * 9g Bai Zhu 9g Zhi Gan Cao 9g	• **Tonifies Spleen and Stomach.** • **Warms the middle burner, dispels cold.** 1. <u>Cold in the abdomen:</u> nausea, vomiting, bloating, no thirst, pale tongue, weak pulse. 2. <u>Yang deficient bleeding</u>: vomiting blood, bloody stools, abnormal uterine bleeding, nose bleeding, swollen tongue and slow weak pulse. 3. <u>Infantile convulsions due to Spleen Qi and Yang deficiency:</u> excessive saliva, drooling, no appetite, swollen tongue, wiry and weak pulse. • **Formula for nausea and vomiting due to bleeding and convulsions-disorders of Spleen and Stomach Yang deficiency.**

Formula	Herbs / Dosage	Indications / Functions
Liang Fu Wan (galangal & cypress pill) B - rqi	Gao Liang Jiang 6g Xiang Fu 6g	• **Warms the middle burner.** • **Regulates Liver Qi and stops pain.** Stomach pain, coldness of the stomach relieved by warmth and pressure, stiffness in the chest, hypochondriac pain, groin pain, no thirst, dysmenorrhea. *Tongue:* pale, swollen, white coat. *Pulse:* wiry, slow. • **This formula warms the Stomach and regulates Qi. It relieves pain in the epigastrium and hypochondria caused by Stomach cold and Liver Qi stagnation respectively.**
Liang Ge San (cools diaphragm powder) B - purg	Lian Qiao 1200g Huang Qin 300g Zhi Zhi 300g Da Huang 600g Mang Xiao 600g Bo He 300g Gan Cao 600g	• **Clears heat and fire in the upper burner.** • **Purges heat in the middle burner.** Heat sensations in the chest, thirst, dry mouth, red face, sore throat, nose bleeding, constipation, dark scanty urine. *Tongue:* red, yellow, greasy coat. *Pulse:* slippery, rapid.
Ling Gan Wu Wei Jiang Xin Tang (poria, licorice, schisandra, ginger & asarum decoction) B - rphlegm	Gan Jiang 9g Xi Xin 9g Fu Ling 12g Wu Wei Zi 6-12g Gan Cao 9g	• **Warms the Lung, expels phlegm, stops cough.** Coughing, thin and clear mucus, fullness or discomfort in the chest, excess saliva, hiccups, nausea. *Tongue:* greasy, white coat. *Pulse:* slow, slippery. • **Formula for coughing due to cold phlegm in the Lungs, resulting from deficiency of Yang.**
Ling Gui Zhu Gan Tang (poria, cinnamon, atractylodes & licorice decoction) B - rphlegm	Fu Ling 12g Bai Zhu 6g Zhi Gan Cao 6g Gui Zhi 9g	• **Strengthens the Spleen.** • **Expels damp and phlegm.** Fullness of the chest and stomach, palpitations, dizziness, shortness of breath, coughing excess mucus. *Tongue:* greasy, white coat. *Pulse:* wiry, slippery. • **Formula for phlegm stagnation in the Lungs, Heart, and in the head, with symptoms of dizziness and fullness of the chest.**
Liu Jun Zi Tang (six-ingredient rehmannia pill) B - tqi	Ren Shen 3g Bai Zhu 4.5g Fu Ling 3g Gan Cao 3g Ban Xia 4.5g Chen Pi 3g	• **Tonifies Qi and expels phlegm.** • **Strengthens the Spleen, stops vomiting.** Reduced appetite, nausea, vomiting, fullness of the chest, palpitations, dizziness, shortness of breath. *Tongue:* greasy, white coat. *Pulse:* wiry, slippery. • Contains *Si Jun Zi Tang* + Chen Pi, Ban Xia.
Liu Shen Wan (six miracle pill) C - rext	Pill	• **Relieves fire toxicity, reduces swelling, stops pain.** Sore throat, boils, carbuncles and furuncles, acute tonsillitis, all kinds of abscesses, difficult swallowing.

FORMULA

Formula	Herbs / Dosage	Indications / Functions
Liu Wei Di Huang Wan (six-ingredient rehmannia pill) A - tyin	Shu Di Huang * 24g Shan Zhu Yu ** 12g Shan Yao ** 12g Mu Dan Pi 9g Fu Ling 9g Ze Xie 9g	• **Nourishes the Yin, strengthens the Kidneys.** • **Sedates deficient heat.** • **Formula to tonify Kidney Yin.** Soreness and weakness of lower back and knees, dizziness, deafness, dry mouth and throat, tinnitus, night sweats, seminal emissions, *steaming bone syndrome*, five-center heat, loose teeth, frequent urination, incontinence, *wasting & thirsting syndrome* (diabetes). *Tongue:* red body, little or no coat. *Pulse:* deep, thin, rapid.
Liu Yi San (six-to-one powder) B - clht	Hua Shi * 6:1 ratio Gan Cao (9-18g dosage)	• **Clears summer-heat, drains dampness.** Fever, thirst, irritability, nausea, vomiting, diarrhea, difficult urination. *Tongue:* thin, yellow, greasy coat. *Pulse:* rapid, slippery.
Long Dan Xie Gan Tang (drain liver decoction) A - clht	Long Dan Cao * 3-9g Huang Qin ** 6-12g Zhi Zi ** 6-12g Ze Xie 6-12g Mu Tong 3-6g Che Qian Zi 9-15g Dang Gui Wei 6-12g Sheng Di Huang 9-15g Chai Hu 3-9g Gan Cao 3-6g	• **Clears Liver and Gallbladder fire.** • **Clears damp-heat in the Lower Burner.** Headache, hypochondriac pain, dizziness, deafness, red eyes, bitter taste, ear infection, dark menstrual flow, breast lumps, shingles, herpes, leukorrhea, UTI. *Tongue:* red body, yellow coat. *Pulse:* wiry, rapid.
Ma Huang Tang (ephedra decoction) A - rext	Ma Huang * 9g Gui Zhi ** 6g Xing Ren 9-12g Zhi Gan Cao 3g	• **Releases the surface, promotes sweating to expel cold.** • **Opens the Lungs, calms the wheezing.** • **Formula for wind-cold common cold, with more chills than fever.** Chills more than fever, no sweating, headache, runny nose, body aches, wheezing, shortness of breath. *Tongue:* thin, white coat. *Pulse:* floating, tight.
Ma Huang Xi Xin Fu Zi Tang (ephedra, asarum & aconite decoction) B - rext	Ma Huang 6g Fu Zi 9g Xi Xin 6g	• **Tonifies the Yang.** • **Releases the surface, dispels wind-cold.** Chills and fever without sweating, internal cold feeling with chills and fever on top, fatigue, weakness, cold limbs, heart rate. *Tongue:* thin, swollen, white coat. *Pulse:* deep, slow. • **Formula for patients who contract wind-cold on the surface, with an underlying Yang deficient cold in the interior.**
Ma Xin Yi Gan Tang (ma huang & coix combination) C - rext	Ma Huang 5.00 Xing Ren 4.00 Yi Yi Ren 5.00 Zhi Gan Cao 10.00	• **Releases the exterior.** • **Dispels wind-dampness.** Muscular rheumatism with body aches, muscle pain, fever, arthritis, edema during pregnancy, asthmatic cough with fever, corns and calluses of the palms and fingers. *Tongue:* thin, white, furry coat. *Pulse:* floating, rapid.

FORMULA

Formula	Herbs / Dosage	Indications / Functions
Ma Xing Shi Gan Tang (ephedra, apricot, gypsum & licorice decoction) **A** - clht	Shi Gao * 48g Ma Huang * 12g Xing Ren 18g Gan Cao 6g	• **Releases the surface.** • **Clears the Lungs.** • **Clears heat.** Shortness of breath, coughing, wheezing, asthma, thirst, fever with or without sweating, nasal flaring. *Tongue:* red body, red tip, yellow coat. *Pulse:* floating, rapid. • **Formula for wind-cold surface conditions that begin to penetrate into the interior.**
Ma Zi Ren Wan (hemp seed pill) **B** - purg	Huo Ma Ren * 20-30g Xing Ren ** 6-9g Bai Shao 10-15g Zhi Shi 6-9g Hou Po 6-9g Da Huang 6-9g	• **Moistens the intestines, promotes bowel movement.** Constipation with hard and dry stools, frequent urination. *Tongue:* yellow, dry coat. *Pulse:* floating, rapid, choppy. • **Formula for chronic constipation due to deficiency of Yin, which frequently occurs in the elderly.**
Mai Men Dong Tang (Ophiopogonis Decoction) **C** - rext	Mai Men Dong 10-15g Ren Shen 5-10g Da Zao 3-12g Gan Cao 2-10g Ban Xia 5-10g Geng Mi 15-20g	• **Benefits the Stomach, generates fluids.** • **Directs Rebellious Qi downward.** Cough with thin sputum, hiccups, dry throat, thirst, shortness of breath. *Tongue:* red tip, dry, little or no coat. *Pulse:* rapid, deficient.
Ming Mu Di Huang Wan (improve vision pill with rehmannia) **C** - tyin	Pill	• **Nourishes the Liver, enriches the Kidney.** • **Improves vision, disperses wind and heat.** Blurry vision, dry eyes, night blindness, pain in the eyes. *Tongue:* red, thin coat. *Pulse:* thready, rapid.
Mu Li San (oyster shell powder) **B** - astringe	Mu Li * 15-30g Huang Qi ** 9-15g Ma Huang Gen 3-9g Fu Xiao Mai 15-30g	• **Stabilizes the surface, stops sweating.** • **Formula for excess sweating due to Qi and Yin deficiency.** Spontaneous sweating, palpitations, insomnia, shortness of breath, fatigue. *Tongue:* red, pale. *Pulse:* thin, weak.
Mu Xiang Bing Lang Wan (aucklandia & betel nut pill) **B** - rfood	Mu Xiang 30g Bing Lang 30g Xiang Fu 12g Chen Pi 30g E Zhu 30g Qing Pi 30g Qian Niu Zi 120g Da Huang 90g Huang Lian 30g Huang Bai 90g	• **Regulates Qi, resolves food stagnation.** • **Resolves damp-heat stagnation, purges interior-heat.** Fullness and pain in stomach, diarrhea, constipation, amoebic dysentery, red and white diarrhea, tenesmus. *Tongue:* greasy coat. *Pulse:* strong. • **Formula for stomach pains and digestive discomforts due to food stagnation and food poisoning.**
Nu Ke Bai Zi Ren Wan (biota & achyranthes formula) **C** - movexue	Bai Zi Ren 4.00 Fai Niu Xi 4.00 Wan Nian Song 4.00 Ze Xie 4.00 Xu Duan 4.00 Shu Di Huang 6.00	• **Eliminates blood stagnation.** • **Regulates menstruation, nourishes Qi and Blood.** Menstrual irregularity and amenorrhea.

Formula	Herbs / Dosage	Indications / Functions
Nuan Gan Jian (warm liver decoction) **B** - rqi	Dang Gui * 6-9g Gou Qi Zi 6g Rou Gui 3-6g Chen Xiang ** 3g Fu Ling 6g Wu Yao ** 6g Sheng Jiang 3-5pcs Xiao Hui Xiang 6g	• **Warms the Kidney and Liver.** • **Regulates Qi, stops pain.** Sharp lower abdomen pain aggravated by cold, swelling, distension, painful scrotum. *Tongue:* pale. *Pulse:* tight. • **Formula for Kidney and Liver cold deficiencies.**
Pai Nong San (platycodon & aurantium formula) **C** - movexue	Bei Mu * 4.5g Gua Lou ** 3g Tian Hua Fen 2.4g Fu Ling 2.4g Ju Hong 2.4g Jie Geng 2.4g	• **Activates blood, disperses hardness and accumulations.** • **Dispels pus.** Suppurative and inflammatory diseases, hardness in the upper abdomen, mastitis, carbuncles, hemorrhoids, boils, gangrene, and lymphadenitis.
Ping Wei San (calm stomach powder) **A** - edamp	Cang Zhu * 12-15g Hou Po ** 9-12g Chen Pi 9-12g Sheng Jiang 3-9g Da Zao 3-12pcs Gan Cao 3-6g	• **Dispels dampness, strengthens the Spleen.** • **Regulates Qi, harmonizes the Stomach.** Fullness of the stomach and abdomen, indigestion, reduced appetite, no taste, heaviness of the body, vomiting, nausea, fatigue, frequent urination. *Tongue:* swollen body, thick, white, greasy coat. *Pulse:* slippery. • **Formula for Stomach disorders due to dampness.**
Pu Ji Xiao Du Yin (universal benefit to eliminate toxin decoction) **B** - clht	Huang Lian * 15g Huang Qin* 15g Niu Bang Zi 3g Lian Qiao 3g Bo He 3g Jiang Can 1.5g Xuan Shen 6g Ma Bo 3g Ban Lang Gen 3g Jie Geng 6g Chen Pi 6g Gan Cao 6g Sheng Ma 1.5g Chai Hu 6g	• **Clears heat and detoxifies.** • **Dispels wind-heat.** Chills and fever, hot painful swelling of the face, allergic reactions, sore throat, sinus infection. *Tongue:* red body, white or yellow coat. *Pulse:* floating, strong, rapid. • **Formula for swelling and pain of the face due to rising heat (Big Head Syndrome).**
Qi Ju Di Huang Wan (lycium, chrysanthemum & rehmannia pill) **B** - tyin	*Liu Wei Di Huang Wan +* Gou Qi Zi Ju Hua	• **Tonifies Kidney Yin, tonifies blood, clears the eyes.** Liver Yin deficiency with blurry vision, dry eyes, dizziness, and tearing up easily in windy conditions. *Tongue:* red, thin coat. *Pulse:* thready, rapid. • Contains ***Liu Wei Di Huang Wan*** + Gou Qi Zi, Ju Hua.
Qi Li San (seven-thousandths teal powder) **C** - movexue	Xue Jie * 30g Hong Hua ** 4.5g Ru Xiang 4.5g Mo Yao 4.5g She Xiang .36g Bing Pian .36g Er Cha 7.5g Zhu Sha 3-6g	• **Dispels blood stagnation, stops pain and bleeding.** • **Promotes Qi movement, reduces swelling.** Bruising, pain with trauma of broken bones and torn sinews, laceration, burns, scalds, unknown swelling. • **Formula for trauma, especially for internal or external injuries.**

Formula	Herbs / Dosage	Indications / Functions
Qi Pi Tang (lotus & citrus combination) C - edamp	Ren Shen 3.00 Bai Zhu 4.00 Fu Ling 4.00 Lian Zi 4.00 Shan Yao 4.00 Shan Zha 2.00 Chen Pi 2.00 Ze Xie 2.00 Gan Cao 2.00	• **Eliminates food stagnation, strengthens the Spleen and Stomach.** Indigestion, reduced appetite, chronic diarrhea, gastritis, malnutrition in children, intestinal TB. *Tongue:* greasy, yellow, furry coat. *Pulse:* weak.
Qian Zheng San (restore symmetry powder) B - ewind	Bai Fu Zi * 6g Jiang Can 6g Quan Xie 6g	• **Expels wind-phlegm.** Facial twitching or paralysis, deviation of the eyes and mouth, difficulty speaking, salivation, lacrimation, joint pain, spasms of the limbs, hemiplegia, aversion to wind. • **Primarily used for Bell's Palsy-facial paralysis due to wind-phlegm in the channels.**
Qiang Huo Sheng Shi Tang (notopterygium to overcome dampness decoction) B - edamp	Qiang Huo * 3g Du Huo * 3g Fang Feng ** 1.5g Gao Ben ** 1.5g Chuan Xiong 1.5g Man Jing Zi 0.9g Zhi Gan Cao 1.5g	• **Dispels wind-damp, releases the surface.** Headache, body ache, heaviness of the body, chills and fever without sweating. *Tongue:* white coat. *Pulse:* floating. • **Formula for wind-damp attack in the exterior with body aches and heavy damp retention.**
Qin Jiao Bie Jia San (gentiana macrophlla & turtle shell formula) C - clht	Qin Jiao 2.50 Bie Jia 5.00 Chai Hu 5.00 Zhi Mu 2.50 Di Gu Pi 5.00 Dang Gui 2.50 Wu Mei 2.00 Qing Hao 1.50	• **Nourish the Yin, cools blood.** • **Resolves chronic consumptive heat.** Fatigue, flushed complexion, night sweating, five-center heat, TB, pneumonia, generalized debility due to prolonged illness, emaciation, high fever accompanied by cough, lassitude of the limbs. *Tongue:* red. *Pulse:* rapid, weak.
Qing Fei Yin (platycodon & citrus formula) C - rphlegm	Xing Ren 3.00 Bei Mu 3.00 Fu Ling 3.00 Ju Hong 1.50 Ma Huang 2.00 Jie Geng 1.50 Gan Cao 1.50 Fang Feng 2.00 Sheng Jiang 3.00 Wu Wei Zi 1.50 Bo He 2.00	• **Clears and moistens the Lungs.** • **Dissolves phlegm, stops cough.** Chronic respiratory disease, dry throat, extreme thirst, cough, hoarseness, abundant phlegm which is sticky yellow or white, shortness of breath, chronic inflammation which are attributive to accumulation of heat in the lungs. *Tongue:* yellow, thin, furry coat.
Qing Gu San (cool bones powder) - clht	Yin Chai Hu 4.5g Zhi Mu 3g Hu Huang Lian 3g Di Gu Pi 3g Qing Hao 3g Bie Jia 3g Gan Cao 1.5g Qin Jiao 3g	• **Clears false heat.** • **Formula for *Steaming Bone Syndrome*.** Long-standing low-grade fever, *steaming bone* pain, night sweating, malar flush, red lips, emaciation, dry mouth, thirst. *Tongue:* red body, little or no coat. *Pulse:* thin, rapid.
Qing Hao Bie Jia Tang (artemisia annua & soft shelled turtle decoction) - clht	Qing Hao * 6g Bie Jia * 15g Sheng Di Huang 12g Zhi Mu 6g Mu Dan Pi 9g	• **Nourishes the Yin, clears deficient heat.** Low-grade fever that is cooler in the a.m. and hotter in the p.m., malar flush, red lips, emaciation, no sweating. *Tongue:* red body, little or no coat. *Pulse:* thin, rapid. • **Formula for deep internal heat that lingers following a bout with long-term febrile disease.**

FORMULA

Formula	Herbs / Dosage	Indications / Functions
Qing Luo Yin (clear collaterals decoction) B - clht	Jin Yin Hua * 6g Bian Dou Hua * 6g Xi Gua Shuang 6g He Ye 6g Dan Zhu Ye 6g	• **Clears summer-heat.** • **Clears Lung heat.** Mild fever, thirst, fuzzy head and vision, dizziness. *Tongue:* pink, thin, white coat.
Qing Qi Hua Tan Wan (clear qi & resolve phlegm) B - rphlegm	Dan Nan Xing 45g Huang Qin 30g Gua Lou Ren 30g Zhi Shi 30g Chen Pi 30g Fu Ling 30g Xing Ren 30g Ban Xia 45g	• **Clears heat, expels phlegm.** • **Descends Qi and stops cough.** • **Formula for bronchitis and pneumonia.** Cough with yellow, sticky phlegm, fullness of the chest, shortness of breath, nausea, vomiting. *Tongue:* red body, greasy, yellow coat. *Pulse:* slippery, rapid.
Qing Re Zhi Beng Tang (clears heat & stop excess bleeding decoction) B - stopxue	Zhi Zi * 9g Huang Qin * 15g Huang Bai * 9g Sheng Di Huang 24g Mu Dan Pi 9g Di You 24g Bai Shao 30g Ce Bai Ye Tan 30g Chun Gen Bai Pi 30g Duan Gui Ban 15g	• **Clears heat, stops bleeding.** Profuse uterine bleeding, dry mouth, parched lips. *Tongue:* yellow coat. *Pulse:* rapid. • **Formula for reckless movement of hot blood.**
Qing Shang Fang Feng Tang (ledebouriella combination) C - clht	Chuan Xiong 2.00 Huang Qin 2.00 Lian Qiao 2.50 Bai Zhi 2.50 Fang Feng 3.00 Jie Geng 2.50 Shan Zhi Zi 1.50 Jing Jie 1.50 Huang Lian 1.50 Zhi Qiao 1.50 Gan Cao 1.00 Bo He 1.50 Zhu Ru 3.00	• **Dispels wind and clears fire in the upper burner.** • **Expels toxins.** Heat and toxins in the upper body, pimples, head and facial boils, red nose, red eyes, flushed face, any types of suppurative inflammation or toxin swelling in the head and face. *Tongue:* red. *Pulse:* rapid, excess.
Qing Shu Yi Qi Tang (clear summer-heat & augment qi decoction) B - clht	Xi Yang Shen * 4.5-6g Xi Gua Pi 24-30g Lian Geng 12-15g Shi Hu 12-15g Mai Men Dong 6-9g Huang Lian 2-3g Zhi Mu 4.5-6g Dan Zhu Ye 4.5-6g Geng Mi 12-15g Gan Cao 2-3g	• **Clears summer-heat, strengthens the Qi.** • **Nourishes the Yin, generates fluids.** Fever, excessive sweating, thirst, fatigue, scanty dark urine, irritability, shortness of breath. *Tongue:* red. *Pulse:* empty, rapid. • **Formula for summer-heat with depleted Qi and Yin.**
Qing Wei San (clear stomach powder) B - clht	Huang Lian * 3-6g Sheng Ma ** 3-6g Sheng Di Huang 6-12g Mu Dan Pi 6-9g Dang Gui 6-12g	• **Clears Stomach heat.** • **Cools the Blood and nourishes the Yin.** Toothache, bleeding gums, dry mouth, bad breath, puffy face, red eyes. *Tongue:* red. *Pulse:* rapid, big.
Qing Xin Lian Zi Yin (lotus seed combination) C - clht	Mai Men Dong 3.00 Che Qian Zi 3.00 Di Gu Pi 3.00 Ren Shen 4.50 Shi Lian Rou 4.50 Huang Qin 3.00 Huang Qi 4.50 Fu Ling 4.50 Zhi Gan Cao 3.00	• **Dispels dampness, clears Heart heat.** • **Nourishes the Yin and tonifies Qi.** Mental stress, fever, turbid urine, urine frequency, chronic cystitis, chronic nephritis, diabetes, leukorrhea, UTI, impotence. *Tongue:* red. *Pulse:* rapid, submerged.

Formula	Herbs / Dosage	Indications / Functions
Qing Yan Li Ge Tang (arctium combination) C - clht	Jin Yin Hua 2.00 Jing Jie 3.00 Bo He 3.00 Jie Geng 3.00 Fang Feng 3.00 Huang Qin 3.00 Huang Lian 3.00 Shan Zhi Zi 1.50 Lian Qiao 1.50 Xuan Shen 1.50 Da Huang 1.50 Mang Xiao 1.50 Niu Bang Zi 1.50 Gan Cao 1.50	• **Purges Lung and Stomach heat, dispels toxins.** Tonsillitis, laryngitis, excessive phlegm and saliva, fever, sore throat.
Qing Ying Tang (clear nutritive level decoction) B - clht	Xi Jiao * 9g Xuan Shen 9g Sheng Di Huang 15g Mai Men Dong 9g Huang Lian 2-3g Dan Zhu Ye 4.5-6g Lian Qiao 6g Jin Yin Hua 9g Dan Shen 6g	• **Clears heat toxins from the Ying & Xue levels of the Wen Bing.** Nighttime fever, irritability, bruises, delirium, skin macula, insomnia, chills. *Tongue:* dark red, dry. *Pulse:* thin, rapid.
Qing Zao Jiu Fei Tang (eliminate dryness & rescue lung decoction) C - dry	Sang Ye 9g Shi Gao 7.5g E Jiao 2.4g Mai Men Dong 3.6g Ren Shen 2.1g Xing Ren 2.1g Pi Pa Ye 3g Gan Cao 3g Hei Zhi Ma 3g	• **Moistens the Lungs, clears dryness.** Headache, fever, hacking cough, wheezing, dry and parched throat, fullness of the chest, irritability, thirst, hypochondriac pain. *Tongue:* dry, little or no coat. *Pulse:* big, rapid, weak.
Ren Shen Bai Du San (ginseng powder to overcome pathogenic influences powder) A - rext	Ren Shen 30g Qiang Huo * 30g Du Huo * 30g Chuan Xiong 30g Chai Hu 30g Qian Hu 30g Zhi Ke 30g Jie Geng 30g Fu Ling 30g Sheng Jiang 6g Bo He 6g Gan Cao 15g	• **Dispels wind and cold.** • **Releases the surfaces, tonifies Qi.** Chills and fever, no sweating, shoulder pain, headache, body ache, fullness of the chest, heaviness of the head, obstructed nasal passages, cough with phlegm. *Tongue:* greasy, white coat. *Pulse:* floating, slippery, soggy. • **Formula for wind-cold with muscle stiffness and joint pain.**
Ren Shen Xie Fei Tang (ginseng & platycodon combination) C - clht	Ren Shen 2.00 Jie Geng 2.00 Lian Qiao 2.00 Zhi Qiao 2.00 Huang Qin 2.00 Bo He 2.00 Xing Ren 2.00 Da Huang 2.00 Shan Zhi Zi 2.00 Gan Cao 2.00 Sang Bai Pi 2.00	• **Dispels heat, moistens the Lungs.** • **Resolves phlegm, regulate Qi circulation.** Cough, wheezing, profuse yellow or thick phlegm, dry stool or constipation, pneumonia, pharyngitis, laryngitis, tonsillitis, bronchitis, pulmonary tuberculosis, sore throat, asthma, loss of voice. *Tongue:* yellow coat. *Pulse:* slippery, rapid.
Ren Shen Yang Rong Tang (ginseng nourish nutritive qi decoction) B - tqi	Bai Shao 90g Dang Gui 30g Chen Pi 30g Huang Qi 30g Rou Gui 30g Ren Shen 30g Bai Zhu 30g Zhi Gan Cao 30g Shu Di Huang 22.5g Wu Wei Zi 22.5g Fu Ling 22.5g Yuan Zhi 15g Sheng Jiang 3pcs Da Zao 2pcs	• **Tonifies the Qi and Blood.** • **Nourishes the Heart, calms the Spirit.** Palpitations, poor memory, fever, reduced appetite, fatigue, shortness of breath, weight loss, dry skin, dry mouth. *Tongue:* pale body. *Pulse:* deficient. • **Formula for dry constipation due to blood deficiency.**
Ren Shen Yang Ying Tang (ginseng decoction to nourish nutritive qi) C - tblood	Bai Shao 5-10g Dang Gui 5-15g Chen Pi 3-10g Huang Qi 9-30g Rou Gui 1-6g Ren Shen 5-10g Bai Zhu 5-15g Zhi Gan Cao 2-10g Shu Di Huang 10-20g Wu Wei Zi 2-6g Fu Ling 10-15g Yuan Zhi 3-10g	• **Augment the Qi, tonifies blood.** • **Nourishes Heart, calms the Spirit.** Emaciation, pale face, loss of appetite, insomnia, palpitations, forgetfulness, irregular menstruation. *Tongue:* pale. *Pulse:* thready, weak.

Formula	Herbs / Dosage	Indications / Functions
Run Chang Wan (moisten intestine pill from master shen's book) **B -** purg	Huo Ma Ren* 15g Tao Ren * 9g Dang Gui 9g Sheng Di Huang 30g Zhi Ke 9g	• **Moistens the intestines, promotes bowel movement.** Constipation, pale skin & nails, dry mouth with big thirst. *Tongue:* dry. *Pulse:* thin.
San Ao Tang (three-unbinding decoction) **B -** rext	Ma Huang 6-9g Xing Ren 6-9g Gan Cao 3-6g	• **Releases the surface, opens Lung Qi.** • **Relieves coughing and wheezing.** Coughing, wheezing, head and body ache, surface cold signs, fullness of the chest. *Tongue:* thin, white coat. *Pulse:* floating. • **Effective auxiliary formula for many cases of cough.**
San Bi Tang (three painful obstruction decoction) **C -** edamp	Xu Duan 1.50 Du Zhong 1.50 Fang Feng 1.50 Rou Gui 1.50 Xi Xin 1.50 Ren Shen 1.50 Fu Ling 1.50 Dang Gui 1.50 Bai Shao 1.50 Huang Qi 1.50 Fai Niu Xi 1.50 Gan Cao 1.50 Qin Jiao 1.50 Sheng Di Huang 1.50 Chuan Xiong 1.50 Du Huo 1.50 Sheng Jiang 1.50 Da Zao 1.50	• **Tonifies the Liver and Kidney.** • **Nourishes the Blood, dispels wind and dampness.** Tremors of the hands and feet, muscle pain, muscle spasm, arthritis, sciatica, paralysis, fibromyalgia. *Tongue:* pale, trembling, white, fur coat. *Pulse:* thin, weak, slow.
San Huang Shi Gao Tang (coptis & scute combination) **C -** rext	Huang Qin 2.50 Huang Lian 2.50 Huang Bai 2.50 Shan Zhi Zi 2.50 Ma Huang 2.50 Shi Gao 5.00 Dan Dou Chi 2.50 Da Zao 2.00 Sheng Jiang 3.00 Xi Cha 2.00	• **Clears toxic heat, relieves inflammation.** Acute febrile disease manifesting flushed complexion, dry nose and tongue, irritability, thirst, listlessness, insomnia, delirium, and skin eruption, black measles, epistaxis, and hemorrhages due to inflammation. *Tongue:* red, yellow, furry coat. *Pulse:* floating, bounding, rapid.
San Huang Xie Xin Tang (coptis & rhubarb combination) **C -** clht	Da Huang 1.00 Huang Qin 1.00 Huang Lian 1.00	• **Clears heat, stops bleeding.** • **Calms the shen, purges excess.** Anxiety, congestion, stiff and achy shoulders, habitual constipation, dysentery, epistaxis, nosebleeds, hemoptysis, hypertension, liver disorders, gastritis, and hemorrhoidal bleeding. *Tongue:* red. *Pulse:* strong. • **Formula for treating bleeding in the upper torso.**
San Jia Fu Mai Tang (three shells to restore the pulse decoction) **C -** clht	Mu Li 15g Bie Jia 24g Gui Ban 30g Zhi Gan Cao 18g Sheng Di Huang 18g Bai Shao Yao 18g Mai Men Dong 15g E Jiao 9g Huo Ma Ren 9g	• **Nourishes Yin and Blood, anchors the Yang.** • **Extinguishes Wind.** Fever, hand and feet spasms, convulsions, severe palpitations, fatigue, heat sensations in the hand sand feet, bleeding, dizziness, vertigo, tinnitus, dry throat, black teeth due to severe dryness. *Tongue:* dark red, dry, furry. *Pulse:* thready, rapid, weak, wiry.
San Miao Wan (three marvel pill) **C -** clht	Huang Bai 2-10g Cang Zhu 5-10g Niu Xi 6-15g	• **Clears heat, dries dampness.** Numbness or burning of the feet, low back pain, extremity weakness.

Formula	Herbs / Dosage	Indications / Functions
San Ren Tang (three-nut decoction) **B** - edamp	Xing Ren * 15g Bai Dou Kou * 6g Yi Yi Ren 18g Ban Xia ** 9g Hou Po ** 6g Hua Shi 18g Tong Cao 6g Dan Zhu Ye 6g	• **Clears damp-heat.** • **Opens Lung Qi, relieves coughing and wheezing.** Headache, chills, tidal fever higher in the afternoon (3-5p.m.), heavy feeling of the body, body aches, reduced appetite, fullness of the chest, yellow complexion, thirst but no desire to drink. *Tongue:* white or yellow coat. *Pulse:* floating, slippery, wiry, soggy. • **Formula for damp-heat attack with more dampness than heat.**
San Wu Bei Ji Wan (three substance emergency pill) **B** - purg	Ba Dou * 30g Gan Jiang 30g Da Huang 30g	• **Purges cold stagnation.** Sharp stomach pain, constipation, fullness in the stomach, lockjaw, pale complexion, coma. *Tongue:* bluish purple, white coat. *Pulse:* tight, weak.
San Zhong Kui Jian Tang (forsythia & laminaria combination) **C** - clht	Huang Bai 4.00 Zhi Mu 2.50 Jie Geng 2.50 Jing San Ling 1.50 E Zhu 1.50 Lian Qiao 1.50 Huang Lian 1.00 Zhi Gan Cao 1.50 Huang Qin 4.00 Bai Shao 1.00 Ge Gen 1.50 Chai Hu 2.50 Dang Gui Wei 1.00 Long Dan 2.50 Sheng Ma 0.50 Gua Lou Gen 2.50	• **Clears heat and detoxifies.** • **Dispels damp-heat, reduces swelling.** Lymphadenitis in the neck, scrofula, carbuncles, swollen thyroid glands, goiter, unknown tumors. *Tongue:* red, yellow, white coat. *Pulse:* rapid, wiry.
San Zi Yang Qing Tang (three-seed nourish parents decoction) **B** - rphlegm	Zi Su Zi 6-9g Bai Jie Zi 6-9g Lai Fu Zi 6-9g	• **Descends rebellious Qi.** • **Warms the interior, expels cold phlegm.** • **Reduces food stagnation.** Coughing and wheezing with white phlegm, shortness of breath, fullness of the stomach, digestive difficulties, reduced appetite, nausea. *Tongue:* greasy, white coat. *Pulse:* slippery. • **For cold-damp in the Lungs, with coughing and mucus. Also resolves food stagnation.**
Sang Ju Yin (mulberry leaf & chrysanthemum decoction) **A** - rext	Sang Ye * 7.5g Ju Hua * 3g Bo He 2.4g Xing Ren 6g Jie Geng 6g Lian Qiao 4.5g Lu Gen 6g Gan Cao 2.4g	• **Dispels wind-heat.** • **Opens the Lung, stops cough.** Cough, fever, chills, headache, sore throat, thirst. *Tongue:* thin, white or yellow coat. *Pulse:* floating, rapid. • **Special for wind-heat common cold with coughing.**
Sang Piao Xiao San (mantis egg-case powder) **C** - astringe	Sang Piao Xiao * 9-12g Long Gu ** 12-30g Ren Shen** 9-12g Fu Shen 9-12g Yuan Zhi 3-6g Chang Pu 6-9g Gui Ban 9-15g Dang Gui 6-9g	• **Regulates the Heart and Kidney.** • **Consolidates Essence, stops leakages.** Frequent urination, cloudy urination, incontinence, absent-mindedness, seminal discharge. *Tongue:* pale, white coat. *Pulse:* deep, weak, slow.

Formula	Herbs / Dosage	Indications / Functions
Sang Xing Tang (mulberry leaf & apricot kernel decoction) **B -** dry	Sang Ye * 3g Zhi Zi ** 3g Dan Dou Chi ** 3g Xing Ren 4.5g Zhe Bei Mu 3g Sha Shen 3g Li Pi 3g	• **Dispels wind and dryness.** • **Relieves coughing.** Fever, headache, thirst, dry nose and throat, dry hacking cough, perhaps with thin and sticky phlegm. *Tongue:* red body, thin, dry, white coat. *Pulse:* floating, rapid. • **Formula for dry lungs and coughing.**
Sha Shen Mai Dong Tang (glehnia & ophiopogonis decoction) **B -** dry	Sha Shen 9g Mai Men Dong 9g Yu Zhu 6g Sang Ye 4.5g Tian Hua Fen 4.5g Bai Bian Dou 4.5g Gan Cao 3g	• **Nourishes the Lungs and Stomach.** • **Generates fluids.** Dry cough, dry throat, thirst, headache, fever. *Tongue:* dry body, no coat. *Pulse:* big, rapid. • **Formula for dry Lungs and Stomach.**
Shao Fu Zhu Yu Tang (drive out blood stasis in lower abdomen decoction) **B -** movexue	Yan Hu Suo 3g Mo Yao 3g Chuan Xiong 3g Dang Gui 9g Chi Shao 6g Pu Huang 9g Wu Ling Zhi 6g Xiao Hui Xiang 1.5g Gan Jiang 0.6g Rou Gui 3g	• **Promotes blood circulation, stops pain.** • **Warms the channels, stops pain.** • **Resolves blood stagnation in the lower burner.** Dysmenorrhea, clotting, fullness or pain of the lower abdomen, irregular menstruation, dark complexion. *Tongue:* purple. *Pulse:* wiry, choppy, slow. • **Formula for many menstrual disorders with pain. Also for Liver channel disorders with testicular and hernia pains.**
Shao Yao Tang (peony decoction) **B -** clht	Shao Yao * 15-20g Dang Gui ** 6-9g Mu Xiang 4.5g Bing Lang 4.5g Huang Lian 6-9g Huang Qin 9-12g Da Huang 6-9g Rou Gui 1.5-3g Gan Cao 4.5g (15g dosages)	• **Clears damp-heat and toxins.** • **Regulates Qi and Blood, stops pain.** Abdominal pain, diarrhea with pus and blood, tenesmus, burning sensation in the anus, dark scanty urine. *Tongue:* thick, yellow, greasy coat. *Pulse:* floating, wiry, rapid.
She Gan Ma Huang Tang (belamcanda & ephedra decoction) **B -** rext	She Gan 9g Ma Huang 12g Zi Wan 9g Kuan Dong Hua 9g Ban Xia 9g Xi Xin 9g Sheng Jiang 12g Wu Wei Zi 3g Da Zao 3pcs	• **Warms the Lungs.** • **Promotes fluid movement in the chest.** • **Descends rebellious Qi, relieves cough.** Coughing, wheezing with a rattling or gurgling sound. *Tongue:* greasy, white coat. *Pulse:* tight, slippery. • **Formula for cold-phlegm asthma.**
Shen Fu Tang (ginseng & prepared aconite decoction) **B -** wint	Ren Shen * 12g Fu Zi 9g	• **Rescues collapsed Yang.** Shock, cold hands and feet, spontaneous sweating, aversion to cold, loose stools, shortness of breath, dizziness, pale complexion. *Tongue:* pale. *Pulse:* faint.
Shen Ling Bai Zhu San (ginseng, poria & atractylodes powder) **B -** tqi	Ren Shen 9-12g Shan Yao 10-15g Lian Zi 15-20g Bai Zhu 9-12g Fu Ling 10-15g Yi Yi Ren 20-30g Bai Bian Dou 15-20g Zhi Gan Cao 3-6g Sha Ren 3-6g Jie Geng 6-9g	• **Tonifies the Spleen, reduces dampness.** • **Harmonizes the Stomach, stops diarrhea.** Weakness of the limbs, emaciation, reduced appetite, vomiting, diarrhea, fullness of the epigastrium, pale or yellow complexion. *Tongue:* greasy, white coat. *Pulse:* weak, slippery. • **Formula for chronic diarrhea due to Spleen Qi deficiency with dampness. Also for leukorrhea, edema, coughing.**

Formula	Herbs / Dosage	Indications / Functions
Shen Su Yin (ginseng & perilla combination) **C** - rext	Ren Shen 3.00 Zi Su Ye 3.00 Ban Xia 3.00 Fu Ling 3.00 Chen Pi 2.00 Ge Gen 3.00 Jie Geng 2.00 Qian Hu 3.00 Zhi Qiao 2.00 Da Zao 1.00 Mu Xiang 2.00 Gan Cao 2.00 Sheng Jiang 2.00	• **Releases the exterior, stops cough.** • **Regulates Qi, transforms phlegm.** Common cold in elderly or weak persons manifesting headache, chills, cough with thick sputum, chest distress, pneumonia, toxemia during pregnancy, and bronchitis. *Tongue:* pale, white, furry coat. *Pulse:* weak.
Shen Tong Zhu Yu Tang (drive out blood stasis from painful body decoction) **B** - movexue	Tao Ren 9g Hong Hua 9g Mo Yao 6g Ling Zhi 6g Dang Gui 9g Di Long 6g Qiang Huo 3g Qin Jiao 3g Niu Xi 9g Xiang Fu 3g Gan Cao 6g Chuan Xiong 6g	• **Promotes blood circulation.** • **Expels bi pain.** Joint pain, shoulder pain, hip pain, back pain, elbow pain. *Tongue:* purple, thin, white coat. *Pulse:* wiry. • **Formula for bi pain in the joints due to stagnation of Qi and Blood.**
Shen Zhuo Tang (hoelen, atractylodes, combination) **C** - edamp	Fu Ling 6.00 Gan Jiang 6.00 Bai Zhu 3.00 Gan Cao 3.00	• **Warms the Spleen, expels damp-heat of the Kidney and Spleen.** Releases pain of lower waist, bed-wetting, and edema below the waist. • **Formula for treating lower jiao problems.**
Sheng Hua Tang (generation & transformation decoction) **B** - movexue	Dang Gui 24g Chuan Xiong 9g Tao Ren 14pcs Pao Jiang 1.5g Gan Cao 1.5g	• **Regulates the Blood, stops pain.** Dark purplish blood, coldness and pain in lower abdomen after childbirth, retention of lochia, postpartum. *Tongue:* thin, purple spots, pale-purple. *Pulse:* deep, choppy.
Sheng Ma Ge Gen Tang (cimicifuga & kudzu decoction) **B** - rext	Sheng Ma 3-6g Ge Gen 3-9g Chi Shao 6-9g Zhi Gan Cao 3g	• **Releases the surface, dispels rashes.** Measles, skin rashes, fever, chills, body aches, sneezing, coughing, red eyes, thirst. *Tongue:* red body, dry coat. *Pulse:* floating, rapid. • **Encourages rashes and measles to the surface.**
Sheng Mai San (generate pulse powder) **A** - tqi	Ren Shen * 9-15g Mai Men Dong ** 9-12g Wu Wei Zi 3-6g	• **Tonifies Qi and Yin.** • **Generates fluids and stops excessive sweating.** Profuse sweating, fatigue, chronic or dry cough, low voice, shortness of breath, big thirst, insomnia, sore throat, palpitations. *Tongue:* red body, dry, thin coat. *Pulse:* floating, rapid, weak. • **Formula for Lung Qi and Lung Yin deficiency.**
Sheng Tie Luo Yin (iron fillings decoction) **C** - ashen	Sheng Tie Luo * 30-60g Dan Nan Xing 3g Bei Mu 3g Xuan Shen 4.5g Mai Men Dong 9g Lian Qiao 3g Tian Men Dong 9g Gou Teng 4.5g Dan Shen 4.5g Fu Ling 4g Fu Shen 3g Chen Pi 3g Shi Chang Pu 3g Yuan Zhi 3g Zhu Sha * 0.9g	• **Settles the Heart, calms the Spirit.** • **Clears Heart phlegm and Heart fire.** Manic behavior, restlessness, agitation, bad temper, severe throbbing headache, severe emotional instability, yelling at people for no reason. *Tongue:* scarlet, yellow, greasy coat. *Pulse:* wiry, rapid.

Formula	Herbs / Dosage	Indications / Functions
Sheng Yu Tang (dang gui four plus combination) **C** - tblood	Shu Di Huang 4.00 Bai Shao 4.00 Huang Qi 4.00 Ren Shen 4.00 Dang Gui 2.00 Chuan Xiong 2.00	• **Nourishes the Qi and Blood, tonifies Yin.** Anemia, oligomenorrhea, loss of blood manifesting thirst, listlessness, sensation of heat, and insomnia. *Tongue:* pale, thin, white coat. *Pulse:* thin, weak.
Shi Hui San (ten-ingredient partially charred powder) **B** - stopxue	Da Ji * 9g Xiao Ji ** 15g He Ye 9g Qian Cao 9g Ce Bai Ye 9g Bai Mao Gen 30g Zhong Lu Pi 6g Zhi Zi 12g Da Huang 9g Mu Dan Pi 9g	• **Cools the Blood.** • **Stops bleeding in the upper burner.** Acute bleeding in upper and middle orifices, coughing blood, vomiting blood, bright red blood, nose bleeding. *Tongue:* red. *Pulse:* floating, strong, rapid. • **Formula for Liver fire attacking the Stomach.**
Shi Liu Wei Liu Qi Yin (dang gui sixteen herb combination) **C** - tqi	Hou Po 1.50 Huang Qi 1.50 Mu Xiang 1.50 Wu Yao 1.50 Ren Shen 2.50 Bai Shao 2.50 Dang Gui 2.50 Rou Gui 2.50 Jie Geng 2.50 Chuan Xiong 2.50 Bai Zhi 1.50 Zhi Qiao 1.50 Fang Feng 1.50 Bing Lang 1.50 Zi Su 1.50 Gan Cao 1.50	• **Tonifies and regulates Qi and Blood.** • **Reduces swelling and drains pus.** Tumors of unknown cause, sores, carbuncles, fibroid disease, breast cancer, swollen lymph nodes, goiter, cervical lymph adenoma.
Shi Pi Yin (bolster spleen decoction) **B** - edamp	Fu Zi * 30g Gan Jiang * 30g Hou Po 30g Mu Xiang 30g Da Fu Pi 30g Cao Guo 30g Fu Ling ** 30g Bai Zhu** 30g Mu Gua 30g Gan Cao 15g Sheng Jiang 5pcs Da Zao 1pc	• **Warms the Yang, strengthens the Spleen.** • **Regulates Qi, promotes urination.** Edema – more prominent in lower body, fullness in the abdomen, reduced appetite, heavy feeling of the body, cold limbs, no thirst, scanty urination, unformed stools, diarrhea. *Tongue:* pale body, thick, greasy coat. *Pulse:* thin, slow, deep. • **Formula for edema due to Spleen and Kidney Yang deficiency, especially in the lower burner, perhaps with diarrhea.**
Shi Quan Da Bu Tang (ten complete great tonic decoction) **A** - tblood	Ren Shen * 6-9g Bai Zhu 9-12g Fu Ling 12-15g Shi Di Huang 15-18g Bai Shao 12-15g Dang Gui 12-15g Chuan Xiong 6-9g Rou Gui 6-9g Huang Qi 15-18g Gan Cao 3-6g	• **Tonifies the Qi, Blood, and Yang.** • **More warming than Ba Zhen Tang.** Reduced appetite, weakness of the lower limbs, fatigue, pale complexion, shortness of breath, hair loss. *Tongue:* pale, swollen, white coat. *Pulse:* thin.
Shi Shen Tang (ma huang & cimicifuga combination) **C** - rext	Ma Huang 2.50 Ge Gen 2.50 Sheng Ma 2.50 Chuan Xiong 2.50 Bai Zhi 2.50 Zi Su Ye 2.50 Gan Cao 2.50 Chen Pi 2.50 Xiang Fu 2.50 Sheng Jiang 3.00 Chi Shao 2.50	• **Dispels wind and cold, releases exterior.** • **Soothes channels and meridians.** Influenza, chills, fever, headache, stuffy nose, cough, oppression of chest. *Tongue:* white, furry coat. *Pulse:* floating, tense.
Shi Wei Bai Du San (bupleurum & schizonepeta formula) **C** - ewind	Chai Hu 3.00 Du Huo 1.50 Jie Geng 3.00 Chuan Xiong 3.00 Ying Pi 3.00 Fang Feng 1.50 Fu Ling 3.00 Jing Jie 1.00 Gan Cao 1.00 Sheng Jiang 3.00	• **Dispels wind, removes toxins.** Various skin ailments, carbuncles, furuncles, boils, urticaria, eczema, acne, dermatitis, mastitis, lymphadenitis, athlete's foot, allergic ophthalmia, external otitis, and suppurative diseases.

Formula	Herbs / Dosage	Indications / Functions
Shi Wei Xiang Ru Yin (elsholtzia ten combination) **C** - rext	Ren Shen 2.00 Huang Qi 2.00 Chen Pi 2.00 Mu Gua 2.00 Hou Pu 2.00 Bai Bian Dou 2.00 Fu Ling 2.00 Xiang Ru 4.00 Bai Zhu 2.00 Gan Cao 2.00	• **Dispels dampness, releases the exterior.** • **Harmonizes the Stomach and Spleen.** Common cold in the summer exhibiting lack of appetite, indigestion, heaviness of the head, lassitude, profuse sweating, vomiting or diarrhea. *Pulse:* weak
Shi Xiao San (sudden smile powder) **B** - movexue	Wu Ling Zhi 3g Pu Huang 3g	• **Dispels blood stagnation, regulates the Blood.** • **Promotes circulation, stops pain.** Chest pain, epigastrium and abdominal pain, postpartum pain, irregular menstruation, clotting, lochia retention. *Tongue:* purple. *Pulse:* wiry. • Note: administer with rice wine or vinegar.
Shi Zao Tang (ten jujube decoction) **B** - purg	Gan Sui 20g Da Ji 20g Yuan Hua 20g Da Zao 20g	• **Dispels water, promotes bowel movements.** Fluid in hypochondrium, pain in the chest during coughing, dry vomiting, shortness of breath, headache, dizziness. *Tongue:* white coat. *Pulse:* wiry, deep.
Shu Gan Tang (bupleurum & evodia combination) **C** - movexue	Chai Hu 3.00 Dang Gui 3.00 Tao Ren 2.00 Bai Shao 1.50 Qing Pi 2.00 Chuan Xiong 1.50 Zhi Qiao 2.00 Huang Lian 3.00 Hong Hua 1.00 Wu Zhu Yu 1.00	• **Soothes the Liver, regulates the Qi and Blood.** • **Eliminates stagnant blood in the chest, stops pain.** Chest pain due to blood stasis, pain of the lower left ribs, hypochondriac pain, acid regurgitation, intercostal neuralgia, rib pain, costal pain due to contusion, and pancreatitis. *Tongue:* white, yellow or greasy coat. *Pulse:* rapid, wiry.
Shu Jing Huo Xue Tang (relax channels & invigorate blood decoction) **C** - movexue	Dang Gui 2.00 Sheng Di Huang 2.00 Cang Zhu 2.00 Chuan Xiong 1.00 Tao Ren 2.00 Fu Ling 1.00 Bai Shao 2.50 Fai Niu Xi 2.00 Wei Ling Xian 2.00 Fang Ji 1.00 Qiang Huo 1.00 Fang Feng 1.00 Long Dan 1.00 Sheng Jiang 3.00 Chen Pi 2.00 Bai Zhi 1.00 Gan Cao 1.00	• **Unblocks and relaxes channels.** • **Eliminates stagnant blood.** • **Dispels wind-dampness.** Severe pain in the muscles, neuralgia, sciatica, low back pain, numbness and pain of the lower limbs, hypertension, paraplegia, gout, mucoid arthritis, and edema. *Tongue:* pale, pink, purple spots. *Pulse:* hesitant, tight.
Shu Jing Li An San (clematis & carthamus formula) **C** - edamp	N/A	• **Relieves pain induced by wind-dampness.** Severe joint pain, pain of the limbs, swelling and pain of the knee joints, palsy, chronic rheumatoid arthritis, hemiplegia, chronic beriberi.
Shung Jie San (modified ledebouriella & platycodon formula) **C** - edamp	Fang Feng 1.00 Jing Jie 1.00 Dang Gui 1.00 Bai Shao 1.00 Lian Qiao 1.00 Chuan Xiong 1.00 Bo He 1.00 Ma Huang 1.00 Shan Zhi Zi 1.00 Bai Zhu 1.00 Huang Qin 2.00 Jie Geng 2.00 Gan Cao 4.00 Shi Gao 2.00 Hua Shi 6.00	• **Expels superficial evils.** • **Promotes bowel movement.** Obesity, hypertension, arteriosclerosis, cardiac asthma, hemorrhoids, alcoholism, chronic nephritis, and scabies. *Tongue:* red, white or yellow coat. *Pulse:* rapid, floating, slippery.

Formula	Herbs / Dosage	Indications / Functions
Si Jun Zi Tang (four gentlemen decoction) **A -** tqi	Ren Shen * 3-9g Bai Zhu ** 6-9g Fu Ling 6-9g Gan Cao 3-6g	• **Tonifies Spleen Qi, dries the Spleen.** • **Formula for tonifying Spleen Qi.** Withered and pale face, reduced appetite, loose stools, soft voice, weakness of the limbs. *Tongue:* pale. *Pulse:* thin, weak.
Si Miao Wan (four-marvel pill) **B -** edamp	Huang Bai 200g Cang Zhu 120g Yi Yi Ren 200g Niu Xi 120g	• **Clears damp-heat.** • **Promotes circulation, relieves pain.** Numbness and weakness in the lower body, swollen feet, ulcerated sores on hot swollen areas painful to the touch, fever, thirst. *Tongue:* red body, greasy, yellow coat. *Pulse:* slippery, wiry.
Si Miao Yong An Tang (four valiant for well-being decoction) **B -** clht	Jin Yin Hua * 90g Dang Gui 60g Xuan Shen ** 90g Gan Cao 30g	• **Clears heat and detoxifies.** • **Promotes blood circulation, relieves pain.** Ulcerated sores on hot swollen regions that are painful to the touch, fever, thirst. *Tongue:* red. *Pulse:* rapid. • **Formula for poor circulation with heat-toxins, for bone marrow infections, and especially for diabetes.**
Si Mo Tang (four milled-herb decoction) **B -** rqi	Ren Shen 3g Bing Lang 9g Che Xiang 3g Wu Yao 9g	• **Regulates Qi, descends rebellious Qi.** • **Opens the chest.** Fullness in the chest and diaphragm, labored breathing, fullness and distension in the stomach, reduced appetite.
Si Ni San (frigid extremities powder) **A -** harm	Chai Hu * 9-12g Bai Shao 12-24g Zhi Shi ** 9-12g Gan Cao 6-9g	• **Regulates Liver Qi, harmonizes the Spleen.** • **Resolves stagnation, clears heat.** Cold limbs with warm body, abdominal pain, fullness of the chest and stomach, diarrhea with tenesmus, bitter taste. *Tongue:* red. *Pulse:* wiry. • **Formula for Qi and heat stagnation that results in coldness of the limbs. Also for Liver and Spleen disharmony and Liver invading Stomach.**
Si Ni Tang (frigid extremities decoction) **A -** wint	Sheng Fu Zi 1pc Gan Jiang 4.5g Zhi Gan Cao 6g	• **Restores the Yang, warms the interior.** Coldness of the body and limbs, aversion to cold, fatigue, irritability, nausea, vomiting, diarrhea with undigested food, no thirst. *Tongue:* pale. *Pulse:* deep, weak. • **Restores the Yang-for Yang deficiency with cold, or emergency cases of Yang collapse.**
Si Shen Wan (four miracle pill) **A -** astringe	Bu Gu Zhi * 120g Wu Zhu Yu 30g Rou Dou Kou ** 60g Wu Wei Zi 60g Sheng Jiang 240g Da Zao 100pcs	• **Tonifies the Kidney Yang and Spleen Yang.** *Cock's Crow diarrhea* syndrome, nausea, vomiting, coldness of the body and limbs, fatigue, irritability, diarrhea with undigested food, no thirst. *Tongue:* pale, thin or white coat. *Pulse:* deep, weak, slow.

Formula	Herbs / Dosage	Indications / Functions
Si Sheng Wan (four fresh pill) **C -** stopxue	Ce Bai Ye * 12g Sheng Di Huang 15-24g Sheng He Ye 9-12g Sheng Ai Ye 6-9g	• **Cools the Blood, stops the bleeding.** Coughing blood, spitting blood, vomiting blood, nosebleeds, dry mouth and throat. *Tongue:* red, deep-red. *Pulse:* rapid, wiry, forceful. • **Formula for blood heat in the upper burner.**
Si Wu Tang (four-substances decoction) **A -** tblood	Shu Di Huang * 9-21g Dang Gui 9-12g Bai Shao 9-15g Chuan Xiong 3-6g	• **Tonifies and regulates the Blood.** • **Regulates the Liver.** Dizziness, blurry vision, irregular menstruation, PMS, palpitations, insomnia, pale face and nails, scanty menstruation, easily frightened, tinnitus, dysmenorrhea, amenorrhea, lochia retention. *Tongue:* pale. *Pulse:* thready, weak, choppy. • **Notes:** double the following according to season: summer – Bai Shao, fall – Shu Di Huang, winter – Dang Gui, spring – Chuan Xiong. • **Formula for blood deficiency with blood stagnation.**
Su Zi Jiang Qi Tang (perilla descend qi decoction) **A -** rqi	Su Zi * 9-12g Ban Xia 6-9g Hou Po 3-6g Qian Hu 6-9g Rou Gui 1.5-3g Dang Gui 6-9g Gan Cao 3-4.5g Chen Pi 6-9g Zi Su Ye 6-9g Sheng Jiang 1-3g Da Zao 3pcs	• **Expels phlegm, descends rebellious Qi.** • **Warms the Kidney.** Wheezing, asthma, excess mucus in the lungs, shortness of breath, cough, fullness of the diaphragm region, edema, excess yellow phlegm. *Tongue:* white, greasy coat. *Pulse:* slippery, weak. • **Stops wheezing and asthma due to Kidney not grasping the Lung Qi-excess above and deficiency below.**
Suan Zao Ren Tang (sour jujube decoction) **A -** ashen	Suan Zao Ren * 15-18g Chuan Xiong ** 6g Fu Ling 6g Zhi Mu 6g Gan Cao 3g	• **Nourishes Heart blood and Liver blood.** • **Calms the Spirit, clears heat.** • **Nourishes the Yin.** Insomnia, irritability, anxiety, nervousness, forgetfulness, excessive dreaming, palpitations, night sweats, thirst, dizziness, dry mouth and throat. *Tongue:* dry, red tip. *Pulse:* thready, wiry rapid. • **Formula for insomnia due to Yin and Blood deficiencies of the Heart and Liver.**
Suo Quan Wan (enuresis pills) **B -** astringe	Yi Zhi Ren * 9-12g Wu Yao 6-12g Shan Yao 9-15g	• **Warms the Spleen and Kidney.** • **Stops leakages and urination.** Urination difficulties, lower back pain, incontinence, profuse urination, bedwetting, spermatorrhea, leukorrhea. *Tongue:* pale, white coat. *Pulse:* deep, weak.
Tai Shan Pan Shi San (powder that gives stability to mount tai) **B -** tblood	Ren Shen * 3g Huang Qi 3g Xu Duan 3g Huang Qin 3g Chuan Xiong 2.4g Shu Di Huang 2.4g Bai Shao 2.4g Bai Zhu 6g Sha Ren 1.5g Nuo Mi pinch Gan Cao 1.5g	• **Regulates the Qi and Blood.** • **Strengthens Spleen, calms the fetus.** • **Prevents miscarriages.** Restless fetus, history of abortion, malaise, pale complexion, fatigue, no appetite. *Tongue:* pale, thin, white coat. *Pulse:* weak, slippery, forceless.

FORMULA

Formula	Herbs / Dosage	Indications / Functions
Tao He Cheng Qi Tang (peach pit order qi decoction) **A -** movexue	Tao Ren * 12-15g Da Huang * 12g Gui Zhi 6g Mang Xiao 6g Zhi Gan Cao 6g	• **Resolves blood stagnation in lower burner.** • **Clears heat.** Lower abdominal pain, incontinence, constipation, delirium, night fever, restlessness, thirst, painful or absent menstruation. *Tongue:* red-purple body, dry, yellow coat. *Pulse:* strong, deep, choppy. • **Formula for painful blood stagnation in the lower abdomen, and for constipation that can result from lower burner stagnation.**
Tao Hong Si Wu Tang (four substance w/ safflower & peach pit decoction) **B -** tblood	*Si Wu Tang +* Tao Ren Hong Hua	• **Regulates blood, promotes circulation.** Cramps, lower abdominal pain, irregular menstruation, dark purple bleeding, clotting. *Tongue:* red-purple body. *Pulse:* wiry, choppy. • **Widely used to resolve blood stagnation, but particularly for menstrual disorders and for traumatic injuries.** • Contains *Si Wu Tang* + Tao Ren, Hong Hua.
Tao Hua Tang (peach blossom decoction) **C -** wint	Chi Shi Zhi 9-30g Gan Jiang 3-10g Geng Mi 20-30g	• **Warms the middle burner, astringes the intestines.** Chronic diarrhea, dark bloody stools, pus in the stools, abdominal pain better with heat and pressure. *Tongue:* pale, white coat. *Pulse:* slow, weak.
Teng Long Tang (moutan & persica combination) **C -** clht	Yi Yi Ren 8.00 Dong Gua Zi 5.00 Mang Xiao 5.00 Mu Dan Pi 4.00 Tao Ren 4.00 Cang Zhu 4.00 Da Huang 1.50 Gan Cao 1.00	• **Clears heat, reduces inflammation.** • **Dispels blood stagnation and promotes blood circulation.** Various inflammations in the lower abdomen, periproctitis, testitis, prostatitis, endometriosis, peritonitis, uterine tumor, and intestinal abscess. *Tongue:* red, yellow, dry coat. *Pulse:* rapid, overflowing.
Tian Ma Gou Teng Yin (gastrodia & uncaria decoction) **A -** ewind	Tian Ma * 9g Gou Teng * 12-15g Shi Jue Ming * 18-24g Niu Xi 12g Sang Ji Shang 9-24g Ye Jiao Teng 9-30g Fu Shen 9-15g Du Zhong 9-12g Zhi Zi 9g Huang Qin 9g Yi Mu Cao 9-12g	• **Dispels internal wind.** • **Soothes the Liver, calms the Spirit.** • **Clears heat, promotes blood circulation.** Headache, dizziness, vertigo, insomnia, tremors, blurry vision, hemiplegia, tinnitus. *Tongue:* red. *Pulse:* wiry, rapid. • **Formula for headaches, dizziness, blurry vision due to internal Liver wind.** • **Formula for Parkinson's disease.**
Tian Tai Wu Yao San (top quality lindera powder) **B -** rqi	Mu Xiang 15g Wu Yao * 15g Hui Xiong ** 15g Qing Pi 15g Gao Liang Jiang 15g Bing Lang 12-15g Jin Ling Zi 12-15g Ba Dou 15g Chuan Lian Zi 15g	• **Tonifies Liver Qi.** • **Dispels cold, stops pain.** Lower abdominal pain radiating to testicles. *Tongue:* pale, white. *Pulse:* slow, wiry. • **Formula for cold invading the Liver channels.**

Formula	Herbs / Dosage	Indications / Functions
Tian Wang Bu Xin Dan (heavenly emperor's heart tonic pill) **A** - ashen	Sheng Di 120g Huang * 15g Dan Shen ** 30g Dang Gui ** 15g Xuan Shen 30g Tian Men Dong 30g Mai Men Dong 15g Dang Shen 15g Fu Ling 30g Bai Zi Ren 30g Suan Zao Ren 15g Yuan Zhi 30g Wu Wei Zi 15g Jie Geng 15g Zhu Sha	• **Nourishes the Heart and Kidney.** • **Tonifies the Yin and Blood.** • **Calms the Spirit, clears empty-heat.** Poor memory, palpitations, insomnia, five-center heat, irritability, forgetfulness, excessive dreaming, nocturnal emissions, fatigue, constipation, mouth ulcers, dry stools. *Tongue:* red, little coat. *Pulse:* thin, rapid. • **Formula for Heart & Kidney not communicating.**
Tiao Wei Cheng Qi Tang (regulate stomach & order qi decoction) **A** - purg	Da Huang * 12g Mang Xiao 9-12g Gan Cao 6g	• **Purges heat stagnation.** Mild constipation, aversion to heat, thirst, fullness of the stomach, canker sores, nosebleed, toothache, foul breath. *Tongue:* yellow coat. *Pulse:* slippery, rapid. • **A moderate purgative for constipation due to Yangming organ heat disorder, Stomach heat.**
Tong Qiao Huo Xue Tang (invigorate blood circulation & open orifices decoction) **B** - movexue	Chi Shao 3g Chuan Xiong 3g Tao Ren 9g Hong Hua 9g Cong Bai 3g Da Zao 7pcs Sheng Jiang 9g She Xiang 0.15g	• **Promotes blood circulation, dispels stagnation.** • **Opens the orifices.** • **Formula for blood stagnation in the upper jiao and in the head.** Headache, vertigo, tinnitus, hair loss, dark complexion, dark around the eyes, brandy colored nose. *Tongue:* dark red-purple body. *Pulse:* wiry, choppy.
Tong Xie Yao Fang (painful diarrhea formula) **B** - harm	Bai Zhu 90g Bai Shao 60g Chen Pi 45g Fang Feng 30-60g	• **Regulates Liver Qi.** • **Tonifies the Spleen.** Abdominal pain following diarrhea, borborygmus, gas, diarrhea. *Tongue:* thin white coat. *Pulse:* wiry, weak.
Wan Dai Tang (end discharge decoction) **B** - astringe	Bai Zhu * 30g Shan Yao * 30g Dang Shen * 6g Cang Zhu 9g Chen Pi 1.5g Che Qian Zi 9g Chai Hu 1.8g Bai Shao 15g Jie Sui Tan 1.5g Gan Cao 3g	• **Regulates the Dai channels.** • **Tonifies the middle.** • **Strengthens the Spleen, dispels damp.** Vaginal discharge that is clear, profuse, and sticky without smell, pale complexion, fatigue, poor appetite, diarrhea. *Tongue:* pale, swollen body, thin, white, greasy coat. *Pulse:* weak, slippery, soft. • **Formula for leukorrhea due to Spleen Qi deficiency. Expels dampness in the lower burner and clears up clear white discharge by strengthening the Spleen.**
Wei Jing Tang (reed decoction) **B** - clht	Lu Gen * 30g Yi Yi Ren 30g Dong Gua Ren 24g Tao Ren 9g	• **Clears Lung-heat and Lung-phlegm.** • **Promotes Qi circulation, reduces pus.** Coughing, foul smelling yellow mucus, bloody mucus, dry skin, chest pain. *Tongue:* red, greasy, yellow coat. *Pulse:* slippery, rapid. • **Formula for bronchitis, lung abscess, and lung infections with yellow mucus due to heat.**

Formula	Herbs / Dosage	Indications / Functions
Wei Ling Tang (calm the stomach & poria decoction) C - edamp	Ze Xie 9-12g Fu Ling 6-9g Zhu Ling 6-9g Gui Zhi 3-6g Bai Zhu 6-9g Cang Zhu 6-9g Hou Po 6-9g Chen Pi 3-6g Gan Cao 1-3g Sheng Jiang 1-3g Da Zao 3-5pcs	• **Dispels dampness, promotes urination.** • **Regulates Spleen and Stomach.** Abdominal fullness, loss of appetite, heaviness in the head and body, edema in the face and body, urinary difficulty, watery diarrhea. *Tongue:* white, greasy coat. *Pulse:* soft, thready. • Contains ***Wu Ling San*** + ***Ping Wei San.***
Wei Su Ning (galanga & pinellia formula) C - edamp	Ren Shen 2.40 Bai Zhu 2.40 Fu Ling 2.40 Ban Xia 2.40 Sheng Jiang 1.20 Da Zao 1.20 Gan Cao 2.40 Rou Gui 1.20 Mu Li 1.20 Yan Hu Suo 1.20 Xiao Hui Xiang 1.20 Sha Ren 1.20 Gao Liang Jiang 1.20	• **Dispels cold, strengthens the Stomach.** Stomachache, gastralgia, gastric ulcer, duodenal ulcer, chronic gastritis, gastroptosis, loss of appetite, indigestion, and vomiting.
Wen Dan Tang (warm gallbladder decoction) A - rphlegm	Zhu Ru * 6g Zhi Shi ** 6g Ban Xia 6g Chen Pi 9g Fu Ling 4.5g Gan Cao 3g Da Zao 3-4pcs	• **Dries dampness and expels phlegm.** • **Clears heat, opens the Heart and Gallbladder.** Dizziness, irritability, insomnia, nausea, vomiting, depression, bitter taste, thirst, mental imbalances. *Tongue:* greasy, yellow coat. *Pulse:* slippery, wiry. • **Formula for mental imbalance due to phlegm obstruction of the Heart and Gallbladder.**
Wen Jing Tang (warm menses decoction) A - movexue	Wu Zhu Yu * 9g Gui Zhi * 6g Dang Gui 9g Bai Shao 6g Chuan Xiong 6g E Jiao 6g Mai Men Dong 9g Mu Dan Pi 6g Ban Xia 6g Sheng Jiang 6g Gan Cao 6g Ren Shen 6g	• **Warms the channels, dispels cold.** • **Tonifies Qi and Blood.** • **Resolves blood stagnation.** Irregular menstruation, low-grade fever, infertility, spotting, cold abdomen, thirst, dry lips and mouth, warm palms and soles, low-grade evening fever or sense of body heat. *Tongue:* red body with pale, swollen sides. *Pulse:* thin, rapid. • **Formula for symptoms caused by deficient cold and blood stagnation affecting the Chong and Ren, two channels that figure prominently in women's disorders.**
Wen Pi Tang (warm spleen decoction) B - purg	Da Huang * 12g Ren Shen 6g Gan Jiang 6g Fu Zi 9g Gan Cao 6g	• **Tonifies and warms Spleen yang.** Chronic constipation or diarrhea, abdominal pain, cold hands and feet. *Tongue:* pale, white coat. *Pulse:* wiry, deep.
Wen Qing Yin (warming & clearing decoction) C - tblood	Dang Gui 3.00 Chuan Xiong 3.00 Shu Di Huang 3.00 Bai Shao 3.00 Huang Qin 3.00 Huang Bai 3.00 Shan Zhi Zi 3.00 Huang Lian 3.00	• **Nourishes the blood, removes toxins.** Irregular menstruation, uterine bleeding, dry mouth and lips, dermal disease due to anemia, eczema, metrorrhagia, menorrhagia, urticaria, and leukorrhea.

Formula	Herbs / Dosage	Indications / Functions
Wu Ji San (five accumulation powder) **C** - rext	Cang Zhu 8.00 Ma Huang * 2.00 Fu Ling 1.00 Ban Xia 1.00 Dang Gui 1.00 Hou Pu 1.50 Bai Shao 1.00 Chuan Xiong 1.00 Sheng Jiang 2.00 Chen Pi 2.00 Bai Zhi * 1.00 Jie Geng 4.00 Gan Jiang ** 1.50 Rou Gui ** 1.00 Zhi Gan Cao 1.00 Zhi Qiao 2.00	• **Dispels Qi, Blood, phlegm, cold, and food.** Heat in the upper body with chills in the lower body, stiff neck and back, abdominal pain and cold, gastroenteritis, lumbago, sciatica, gastritis, hernia pain, chill disease, menstrual pain, neuralgia, and rheumatism. *Pulse:* floating.
Wu Ling San (five fungus powder) **A** - edamp	Ze Xie * 4g Fu Ling ** 2.3g Zhu Ling ** 2.3g Bai Zhu 2.3g Gui Zhi 1.5g	• **Promotes urination, reduces dampness.** • **Warms the Yang.** 1. <u>Wind-Damp:</u> edema, headache, fever, thirst with inability to hold down water, difficult urination, white tongue coat, floating pulse. 2. <u>Internal Damp:</u> edema, diarrhea, difficult urination, vomiting. 3. <u>Dampness rising:</u> nausea, vomiting with shortness of breath, belching, coughing, dizziness (*running piglet syndrome*). • **Formula for three patterns of damp disorders.**
Wu Mei Wan (mume formula) **C** - rfood	Wu Mei 10.00 Xi Xin 3.00 Gan Jiang 6.00 Shu Jiao 3.00 Gui Zhi 6.00 Fu Zi 6.00 Huang Lian 3.00 Huang Bai 6.00 Ren Shen 6.00 Dang Gui 6.00	• **Warms the internal organs.** • **Dispels parasites.** Recurring abdomen pain, vomiting, cold hands and feet, chronic diarrhea, chronic dysentery, gastritis, biliary ascariasis. *Tongue:* geographic. *Pulse:* hidden, wiry, tight.
Wu Pi San AKA (Wu Pi Yin) (five peel powder) **A** - edamp	Fu Ling Pi 15g Sheng Jiang Pi 6g Da Fu Pi 15g Chen Pi 9g Sang Bai Pi 15g	• **Promotes urination, strengthens the Spleen.** • **Regulates Qi, dispels dampness.** Whole body edema (swollen and puffy), heaviness of the limbs, difficult urination, shortness of breath, fullness of the abdomen and stomach. *Tongue:* pale, swollen body, white greasy coat. *Pulse:* floating, slippery. • **Formula for pitting skin edema due to wind-damp or Spleen deficiency.**
Wu Tou Tang (aconite decoction) **B** - ewind	Chuan Wu * 9-12g Ma Huang 9g Bai Shao 9g Huang Qi 9g Gan Cao 9g	• **Warms the channels, relieves pain.** • **Expels wind.** Pain and limited mobility of the joints, particularly of the hands and feet. • **Formula for chronic wind-damp bi pain in the smaller joints.**
Wu Wei Xiao Du Yin (five ingredient eliminate toxin decoction) **B** - clht	Jin Yin Hua * 9g Pu Gong Ying 3.6g Zi Hua Di Ding 3.6g Ye Ju Hua 3.6g Tian Kui Zi 3.6g	• **Clears heat and toxins.** Boils, carbuncles, local inflammation with pus, skin lesions, fever, chills. -- *Tongue:* yellow, greasy coat. *Pulse:* rapid.
Wu Yao Shun Qi San (lindera formula) **C** - ewind	Wu Yao 4.00 Ma Huang 4.00 Chen Pi 4.00 Bai Jiang Chan 2.00 Gan Jiang 1.00 Chuan Xiong 2.00 Zhi Qiao 2.00 Jie Geng 2.00 Bai Zhi 2.00 Gan Cao 2.00 Sheng Jiang 3.00 Da Zao 1.00	• **Dispels wind-dampness,** • **Regulates Qi and stops pain.** Arthralgia, CVA, apoplexy, numbness, headache, dizziness, hemiplegia, tennis elbow, frozen shoulder, facial palsy, and trigeminal neuralgia.

FORMULA

Formula	Herbs / Dosage	Indications / Functions

Wu Zhu Yu Tang
 	
(evodia decoction)
 	
A - wint
	Wu Zhu Yu * 9-12g
	Sheng Jiang ** 18g
	Ren Shen 9g
	Da Zao 12pcs
		• **Warms the middle, tonifies Spleen.**
		• **Descends rebellious Stomach Qi.**
		  1. <u>Stomach Cold:</u> nausea, vomiting, stomach pain, sour taste, pale, white, swollen tongue, slow pulse.
		  2. <u>Liver & Stomach Disharmony:</u> vertex headache, vomiting, excess saliva, pale, white coat, wiry pulse.
		  3. <u>Kidney Yang Deficiency:</u> watery diarrhea, vomiting, cold limbs, irritability, swollen tongue, deep, slow and weak pulse.
		• **Formula for vomiting associated with three syndrome patterns.**

Xi Jiao Di Huang Tang (rhinoceros horn & rehmannia decoction) **B - clht**	Xi Jiao 3g Sheng Di Huang 24g Ci Shao 9g Mu Dan Pi 6g	• **Cools the Blood and clears heat toxins.** • **Resolves blood stagnation, stops bleeding.** Nosebleed, bloody vomit, bloody urination, bloody stools, black stools, bruising, thirst without desire to drink, fever, delirium. *Tongue:* dark red with red bumps. *Pulse:* strong, rapid. • **Formula for heat in the blood that causes bleeding and mental disorders.**
Xian Fang Huo Ming Yin (sublime formula for sustaining life) **C - clht**	Jin Yu Hua * 9g Chen Pi ** 9g Zhe Bei Mu 3g Tian Hua Fen 3g Dang Gui ** 6-12g Chi Shao** 3g Ru Xiang 3g Mo Yao 3g Fang Feng 3g Bai Zhi 3g Chuang Shan Jia 3g Zao Jia Ci 3g Gan Cao 3g	• **Relieves Toxicity, clears heat.** • **Promotes blood circulation, stops pain.** Painful red swollen sores and carbuncles, skin lesions, fever, chills, headache. *Tongue:* white, yellow, thin coat. *Pulse:* surging.
Xiang Ru San (elsholtzia powder) **B - rext**	Xiang Ru 480g Hou Po 240g Bai Bian Dou 240g	• **Releases the surface, expels cold-damp.** • **Harmonizes the middle burner.** Chills and fever, aversion to cold, headache, heaviness of the head, no sweating, fullness of the chest and stomach, weak limbs, diarrhea, vomiting. *Tongue:* thick, greasy, white coat. *Pulse:* floating, slippery. • **Formula for summer-time wind-damp attack.**
Xiang Sha Liu Jun Zi Tang (six gentlemen w/ aucklandia & amomum decoction) **B - tqi**	*Liu Jun Zi Tang +* Mu Xiang Sha Ren	• **Tonifies Qi.** • **Regulates Qi and harmonizes the Stomach.** Bloating and distention of the chest and stomach, stomach pain, diarrhea. *Tongue:* thick greasy white coat. *Pulse:* slippery. • **Regulates Qi of the chest and stomach areas to relieve pain.** • Contains *Liu Jun Zi Tang* + Mu Xiang, Sha Ren.
Xiang Sha Yang Wei Tang (cyperus & cluster combination) **C - harm**	Bai Zhu 3.00 Fu Ling 3.00 Cang Zhu 2.00 Hou Pu 2.00 Chen Pi 2.00 Xiang Fu 2.00 Ren Shen 2.00 Mu Xiang 1.50 Sha Ren 1.50 Gan Cao 1.50 Da Zao 1.50 Sheng Jiang 2.00 Bai Dou Kou 2.00	• **Harmonizes the Spleen and Stomach.** • **Dispels stagnant food and water, resolves dampness.** Anorexia, loss of appetite after illness, chronic gastritis, gastrectasis, gastrointestinal weakness, lack of nutrition, developmental failure in children. *Tongue:* pale, greasy, white coat. *Pulse:* soft, slippery.

Formula	Herbs / Dosage	Indications / Functions
Xiang Su San (cyperus & perilla leaf powder) **B -** rext	Zi Su Ye 120g Xiang Fu 120g Chen Pi 60g Zhi Gan Cao 30g	• **Releases the surface, dispels wind-cold.** • **Regulates Qi and harmonizes the middle.** Chills and fever without sweating, headache, fullness of the chest and stomach, reduced appetite. *Tongue:* thin, white coat. *Pulse:* floating, slippery, wiry. • **Formula for stomach flues due to wind-damp attack, with surface signs and dampness causing nausea, vomiting, and diarrhea.**
Xiao Chai Hu Tang (minor bupleurum decoction) **A -** harm	Chai Hu * 24g Huang Qin ** 9g Ren Shen 9g Ban Xia 24g Sheng Jiang 9g Da Zao 12pcs Zhi Gan Cao 9g	• **Harmonizes the Shaoyang channel.** Alternating chills and fever, bitter taste, irritability, fullness of the chest and hypochondrium, dry throat, dizziness, nausea, vomiting, low energy. *Tongue:* thin, white or yellow coat. *Pulse:* wiry. • **Formula for Shaoyang syndromes, with alternating chills and fever (malaria), or for damp-heat syndromes resulting from alcohol abuse.**
Xiao Cheng Qi Tang (minor order qi decoction) **A -** purg	Da Huang * 12g Hou Po 6g Zhi Shi 6-9g	• **Purges heat stagnation.** Afternoon tidal fever, abdominal pain increases upon pressure, constipation, distension, tenesmus, sweating, delirium. *Tongue:* yellow coat. *Pulse:* strong, slippery. • **Purgative for excess Yangming organ syndrome.**
Xiao Feng San (eliminate wind powder) **A -** ewind	Jing Jie * 3g Fang Feng * 3g Niu Bang Zi * 3g Chan Tui * 3g Cang Zhu 3g Ku Shen 3g Mu Tong 1.5g Shi Gao 3g Zhi Mu 3g Dang Gui 3g Sheng Di Huang 3g Hei Zhi Ma 3g Gan Cao 1.5g	• **Expels wind and clears heat.** • **Dispels dampness, stops itching.** • **Nourishes the blood.** Itching, rash, red skin, lesions, skin discharge from scratching, eczema, urticaria. *Tongue:* thin, white or yellow coat. *Pulse:* floating, strong. • **For itchy skin caused by wind, heat, dampness. Good for beginning stages of poison oak.**
Xiao Huo Luo Dan (minor invigorate collaterals pill) **A -** ewind	Chuan Wu * 180g Cao Wu * 180g Tian Nan Xing 180g Di Long 180g Ru Xiang 66g Mo Yao 66g	• **Warms the channels.** • **Expels wind, damp, and phlegm.** • **Promotes blood circulation, relieves pain.** Red skin, itching, rash, numbness, spasm, joint pain, heaviness in lower back and legs, skin discharge. *Tongue:* thin, white or moist coat. *Pulse:* floating, strong. • **Formula for Bi syndrome due to wind-damp, or qi and blood stagnation, or phlegm stagnation.**
Xiao Ji Yin Zi (cephalanoplos decoction) **B -** stopxue	Xiao Ji * 15g Ou Jie ** 15g Pu Huang ** 15g Sheng Di Huang 120g Hua Shi 15g Dan Zhu Ye 15g Mu Tong 15g Zhi Zi 15g Dang Gui 15g Gan Cao 15g	• **Cools the blood, promotes circulation.** • **Stops bleeding and urination.** Bloody urine, painful and frequent urination, feeling of heat in the body. *Tongue:* red body, thin, white coat. *Pulse:* rapid, full. • **Stops bloody urination. For bleeding UTI.**

FORMULA

Formula	Herbs / Dosage	Indications / Functions
Xiao Jian Zhong Tang (minor strengthen middle decoction) **B** - wint	*Gui Zhi Tang* + Yi Tang	• **Tonifies the Spleen and Stomach.** • **Warms and harmonizes the middle, stops pain.** Abdominal pain that responds well to heat and pressure, pale face, low-grade fever. *Tongue:* swollen. *Pulse:* weak. • **Formula for pain in the abdomen that comes and goes, and feels better with warmth.** • Contains *Gui Zi Tang* + Yi Tang.
Xiao Luo Wan (reduce scrofula pill) **B** - rphlegm	Xuan Shen 120g Mu Li 120g Zhe Bei Mu 120g	• **Clears heat and expels phlegm.** • **Reduces stagnation and nodules.** Neck nodules, plum-pit throat, cysts, sore and dry throat. *Tongue:* red. *Pulse:* wiry, slippery. • **Formula for hot-phlegm stagnation with nodules, plum-pit throat, cysts, dry throat.**
Xiao Qing Long Tang (minor bluegrass dragon decoction) **B** - rext	Ma Huang * 9g Gui Zhi * 9g Bai Shao 9g Wu Wei Zi 9g Gan Jiang ** 9g Xi Xin ** 9g Ban Xia 9g Zhi Gan Cao 9g	• **Releases the surface, expels wind and damp.** • **Warms the Lungs, dispels cold.** Predominant chills, fever, no sweating, wheezing, coughing, no thirst, heavy feeling of the body, edema, fullness of the epigastrium, mucus in the Lungs, asthma. *Tongue:* white, moist coat. *Pulse:* floating, tight, slippery. • **Treats wheezing and coughing due to wind invasion and damp stagnation. For asthma and bronchitis.**
Xiao Xian Xiong Tang (minor sinking chest decoction) **C** - rphlegm	Gua Lou Ren 9-12g Huang Lian 1-3g Ban Xia 3-6g	• **Clears heat and phlegm in the chest.** Painful distension in the chest and epigastrium when pressed, coughing yellow sputum, bitter taste, constipation. *Tongue:* yellow, greasy coat. *Pulse:* rapid, slippery, floating.
Xiao Xu Ming Tang (minor prolong life decoction) **C** - ewind	Ma Huang 3-6g Chuan Xiong 3-6g Fang Ji 6-12g Xing Ren 9-12g Fang Feng 9-12g Sheng Jiang 9-12g Ren Shen 3-6g Fu Zi 3-9g Rou Gui 3-6g Bai Shao 6-12g Huang Qin 4.5-9g Gan Cao 3-6g	• **Warms the channels, unblocks Yang Qi.** • **Dispels wind.** Hemiplegia, asymmetry of the face, slow and slurred speech, chills and fever, deviated mouth, loss of consciousness. *Tongue:* pale, thin, white coat. *Pulse:* weak, floating. • **Formula for wind-damp bi syndrome with hemiplegia.**
Xiao Yao San (rambling powder) **A** - harm	Chai Hu * 9g Dang Gui ** 9g Bai Shao ** 9g Fu Ling 9g Bai Zhu 9g Bo He 3g Zhi Gan Cao 6g Wei Jiang 6g	• **Regulates Liver Qi.** • **Strengthens the Spleen and tonifies blood.** Irritability, hypochondriac pain, headache, dizziness, vertigo, thirst, dry mouth, fatigue, no appetite, occasional chills and fever, PMS, irregular menstruation, breast distention. *Tongue:* red. *Pulse:* wiry, empty.

FORMULA

Formula	Herbs / Dosage	Indications / Functions
Xie Bai San AKA (Xie Fei San) (drain white powder) **B -** clht	Sang Bai Pi * 30g Di Gu Pi 30g Zhi Gan Cao 3g Geng Mi 15-30g	• **Clears Lung-heat.** Coughing, wheezing, fever with hot skin symptoms aggravated during late afternoon, dry mouth, scanty expectoration. *Tongue:* red body, yellow coat. *Pulse:* thin, rapid. • **Formula for coughing due to Lung-heat.**
Xie Huang San (drain yellow powder) **C -** clht	Fang Feng 6.00 Shi Gao * 7.00 Zhi Zi * 7.00 Huo Xiang 2.50 Gan Cao 3.00	• **Purges Spleen and Stomach fire.** Bad breath, thirst, acute gastritis with halitosis, ulcerative stomatitis, rosacea, dry mouth and lips. *Tongue:* red, protruded tongue. *Pulse:* rapid
Xie Xin Tang (drain epigastrium decoction) **C -** clht	Da Huang 6g Huang Lian 3g Huang Qin 3g	• **Clears heat and toxins from the Heart and Stomach.** 1. <u>Heart fire:</u> nosebleeds, vomiting blood, dark urination, constipation, red tongue, rapid pulse. 2. <u>Damp-heat:</u> jaundice, irritability, chest discomfort due to heat, red, greasy coat, rapid, slippery pulse. 3. <u>Full-heat:</u> fever, irritability, red eyes and face, chest heat, constipation, red, yellow coat, rapid pulse.
Xin Jia Huang Long Tang (newly augmented yellow dragon decoction) **B -** purg	Sheng Di Huang 15g Ren Shen 4.5g Da Huang 9g Mang Xiao 3g Xuan Shen 15g Mai Men Dong 15g Dang Gui 4.5g Hai Shen 2g Gan Cao 6g	• **Nourishes the Yin, Qi, and fluids.** • **Clears heat.** Constipation, fullness of stomach, fatigue, shortness of breath, dry mouth and throat, cracked lips, burned tongue. *Tongue:* dry, yellow, cracks, black coat. *Pulse:* deep, excess.
Xin Jia Xiang Ru Yin (newly-augmented elsholtzia decoction) **C -** rext	Xiang Ru 6g Jin Yu Hua 9g Bai Bian Dou 9g Hou Po 6g Lian Qiao 6g	• **Releases the exterior, expels wind, transforms dampness.** • **Clears summerheat.** Chills and fever, cough, headache, body ache, stifling sensation and oppression in the chest, irritability. *Tongue:* thin, greasy coat. *Pulse:* soggy, rapid.
Xing Su San (apricot kernel & perilla Leaf) **B -** dry	Zi Su Ye 6g Qian Hu 6g Xing Ren 6g Jie Geng 6g Zhi Ke 6g Chen Pi 6g Fu Ling 6g Ban Xia 6g Sheng Jiang 6g Gan Cao 3g Da Zao 2pcs	• **Warms the Lungs, opens Lung Qi.** • **Relieves coughing, transforms phlegm.** Cough with watery sputum, chills without sweating, headache, nasal congestion, dry throat. *Tongue:* dry body, white coat. *Pulse:* wiry. • **Formula for cough due to wind-cold-dry in the Lungs.**
Xuan Bi Tang (disband painful obstruction decoction) **C -** edamp	Fang Ji * 15g Xing Ren 15g Yi Yi Ren 15g Cha Sha 9g Ban Xia 9g Lian Qiao 9g Hua Shi 15g Chi Xiao Dou 9g Zhi Zi 9g	• **Clears and resolves damp-heat.** • **Unblocks the channels, stops pain.** Painful joints with heat, immobility, fever, chills, yellow, complexion, scanty dark urine. *Tongue:* gray, thick, yellow greasy coat. *Pulse:* rapid, wiry • **Formula for painful damp-heat obstruction.**

Formula	Herbs / Dosage	Indications / Functions
Xuan Fu Dai Zhe Tang (inula & hematite decoction) **B -** rqi	Xuan Fu Hua 9g Dai Zhe Shi 3g Ren Shen 6g Ban Xia 9g Da Zao 12g Sheng Jiang 15g Gan Cao 9g	• **Descends Stomach Qi.** • **Expels cold phlegm from the Stomach.** Hiccups, fullness in the stomach and chest area, belching, nausea, vomiting. *Tongue:* greasy white coat. *Pulse:* weak, slightly wiry. • **Relieves hiccups, belching, and nausea.**
Xue Fu Zhu Yu Tang (blood mansion eliminate stasis decoction) **A -** movexue	Tao Ren * 12g Hong Hua * 9g Chuan Xiong * 4.5g Sheng Di Huang 9g Dang Gui 9g Chi Shao 6g Niu Xi 9g Chai Hu 3g Jie Geng 4.5g Zhi Ke 6g Gan Cao 3g	• **Promotes blood circulation, regulates Qi.** • **Resolves blood stagnation, stops pain.** Palpitations, chest pain, sharp fixed headaches, pain in fixed locations on the chest or head, evening tidal fever, insomnia, irritability, dark and baggy eyes, dark purple lips, hiccups, inability to hold down water, dry vomiting. *Tongue:* purple body, purple dots, no coat. *Pulse:* wiry, choppy. • **Resolves blood stagnation that causes headaches and chest pain.**
Yang He Tang (yang heartening decoction) **B -** wint	Shu Di Huang * 30g Lu Jiao Jiao * 9g Rou Gui 3g Pao Jiang 1.5g Ma Huang 1.5g Bai Jie Zi 6g Gan Cao 3g	• **Tonifies the Yang and Blood.** • **Dispels cold.** Open sores, painful swellings without discoloration and are not hot to the touch. *Tongue:* pale body, white coat. *Pulse:* thin, deep. • **Formula for Yin boils due to Qi and Blood, and cold stagnation or for bone infections that are difficult to heal, and open sores that won't close up.** • **Tonifies Yang and Blood to help the body close up its open sores, especially following surgery.**
Yang Yin Qing Fei Tang (nourish the yin & clear lungs decoction) **C -** dry	Sheng Di Huang* 30g Xuan Shen * 24g Mai Men Dong ** 20g Bei Mu 10g Bai Shao ** 12g Mu Dan Pi ** 12g Bo He 6g Gan Cao 6g	• **Nourishes Kidney and Lung Yin, clears heat.** • **Cools the blood, relieves toxins.** Painful throat, throat with curd deposits which are difficult to scrape off, fever, dry nose, dry lips, heavy breathing with sounds of wheezing. *Tongue:* red, little or no coat. *Pulse:* floating, rapid.
Yi Guan Jian (one link decoction) **B -** tyin	Sheng Di Huang* 18-45g Sha Shen 9g Dang Gui 9g Gou Qi Zi * 9-18g Chuan Lian Zi 4.5g Mai Men Dong 9g	• **Tonifies Liver and Kidney Yin.** • **Regulates Liver Qi.** Chest and hypochondriac pain, heartburn, acid regurgitation, abdominal and epigastric distention, dry mouth and throat, thirst. *Tongue:* red and dry with little or no coat. *Pulse:* thin, wiry, perhaps rapid. • **Formula for a combination of Yin deficiency signs and Liver Qi stagnation.**
Yi Huang Tang (change yellow discharge decoction) **B -** astringe	Chan Shan Yao * 30g Qian Shi 30g Huang Bai ** 6g Che Qian Zi ** 3g Yin Xing 10pcs	• **Tonifies the Spleen and Kidney.** • **Clears damp-heat in the Lower Burner.** Vaginal discharge that is yellow or white, sticky with fishy smell, pale complexion, heaviness of the body, loose stools, reduced appetite, profuse yellow urine, lower back pain. *Tongue:* pale, thin, white coat. *Pulse:* slippery.

Formula	Herbs / Dosage	Indications / Functions
Yi Qi Cong Ming Tang (augment qi & increase acuity decoction) **C** - tqi	Huang Qi 6.00 Ren Shen 6.00 Ge Gen 3.50 Huang Bai 2.50 Man Jing Zi 3.50 Bai Shao 2.50 Sheng Ma 2.00 Gan Cao 2.00	• **Improves eyes and ears.** • **Tonifies Qi and raises Yang Qi.** Chronic fatigue, loss of appetite, prolapse of internal organs, chronic diarrhea, tinnitus, dizziness, blurring vision due to anemia, deafness, and primary stage of cataract.
Yi Yi Ren Tang (enlightened physician coicis decoction) **B** - edamp	Yi Yi Ren 24g Bai Shao 9g Ma Huang 6g Dang Gui 9g Cang Zhu 9g Gui Zhi 6g Gan Cao 6g	• **Drains damp while moistening the intestine.** • **Promotes circulation, relieves pain.** Swelling and painful joints, abdominal pain and fullness, reduced appetite, difficult urination, irregular menstruation, painful menstruation. *Tongue:* red and dry with little or no coat. *Pulse:* thin, wiry, perhaps rapid. • **Formula for damp-stagnation and blood stagnation in the lower abdomen.**
Yi Zi Tang (cimicifuga combination) **C** - clht	Da Huang 1.00 Sheng Ma 1.50 Chai Hu 4.00 Huang Qin 3.00 Dang Gui 4.00 Gan Cao 2.00	• **Dispels damp-heat in the lower burner.** • **Promotes bowel movements and relieves hemorrhoids.** Hemorrhoids, hemorrhoidal pain and bleeding, anal ache, rectal prolapse, and vaginal itching.
Yin Chen Hao Tang (artemisia decoction) **B** - edamp	Yin Chen Hao * 18g Zhi Zi 9g Da Huang 6g	• **Clears damp-heat.** • **Relieves jaundice.** Jaundice with "fresh yellow" eyes, yellow-tangerine skin, thirst, abdominal distention, difficult urination, dark scanty urination. *Tongue:* greasy, yellow coat. *Pulse:* slippery, rapid. • **Formula for damp-heat Yang-type jaundice.**
Yin Chen Wu Ling San (capillaris & hoelen formula) **C** - edamp	Yin Chen Hao 16.00 Ze Xie 2.50 Fu Ling 1.50 Zhu Ling 1.50 Bai Zhu 1.50 Gui Zhi 1.00	• **Dispels damp-heat, relieves jaundice.** Jaundice, sallow complexion, dark and deep reddish urine, hepatitis, nephritis, lingering thirst and fever, peritonitis, and water stagnation in the stomach. • Contains ***Wu Ling San*** + Yin Chen Hao.
Yin Qiao San (honeysuckle & forsythia powder) **A** - rext	Jin Yin Hua * 30g Lian Qiao * 30g Jie Geng 18g Niu Bang Zi 18g Bo He 18g Dan Dou Chi 15g Jing Jie 12g Dan Zhu Ye 12g Lu Gen 15-30g Gan Cao 15g	• **Dispels wind-heat.** • **Clears heat and detoxifies.** Fever, slight chills, sore throat, headache, nasal congestion, yellow mucus, cough. *Tongue:* red tip, thin-white or thin-yellow coat. *Pulse:* floating, rapid. • **Formula for common colds with sore throat and fever more than chills.**
You Gui Wan (restore right kidney pill) **B** - tyang	Shu Di Huang 20-30g Shan Yao 10-15g Shan Zhu Yu 10-15g Gou Qi Zi 10-15g Gan Cao 3-6g Du Zhong 6-9g Rou Gui 3-6g Fu Zi 6-9g	• **Tonifies Kidney yang and nourishes Essence.** Fatigue, aversion to cold, cold limbs, lower back pain, impotence, premature ejaculation, reduced appetite, loose stools, edema in lower extremities. *Tongue:* pale. *Pulse:* deep, weak. • **Formula for Kidney yang deficiency with waning fire at Ming-men.**

Formula	Herbs / Dosage	Indications / Functions
Yu Nu Jian (jade woman decoction) **B -** clht	Shi Gao 15-30g Shu Di Huang 9-30g Zhi Mu 3-6g Mai Men Dong 6-9g Niu Xi 3-6g	• **Clears Stomach heat.** • **Nourishes the Yin, moistens dryness.** Toothache, bleeding gums, headache, loose teeth, irritability, dry mouth, thirst, desire for cold drinks, fever. *Tongue:* red, dry, yellow coat. *Pulse:* floating, slippery.
Yu Ping Feng San (jade windscreen powder) **A -** astringe	Huang Qi * 30g Bai Zhu ** 60g Fang Feng 60g	• **Tonifies Qi, stops sweating.** Spontaneous sweating with aversion to cold, fatigue, pale complexion. *Tongue:* pale, thin or white coat. *Pulse:* floating, weak. • Formula for spontaneous sweating due to exterior deficiencies.
Yu Ye Tang (jade fluid decoction) **C -** dry	Shan Yao 30g Huang qi 15g Zhi Mu 18g Tian Hua Fen 9g Ji Nei Jin 6g Ge Gen 4.5g Wu Wei Zi 9g	• **Tonifies Qi, generates fluids.** • **Moistens dryness, alleviates thirst.** Excessive thirst not quenched by fluid intake, frequent copious turbid urination, shortness of breath, lassitude. *Pulse:* weak, thin.
Yu Zhen San (true jade powder) **C -** ewind	Bai Fu Zi * Equal Fang Feng amount Tian Nan Xing * Qiang Huo Tian Ma Bai Zhi	• **Dispels exterior wind.** • **Relieves spasms.** Lock jaw, stiff body, muscle spasms, lip spasms. *Pulse:* wiry, tight.
Yue Bi Jia Zhu Tang (atractylodes combination) **C -** edamp	Ma Huang 6.00 Bai Zhu 4.00 Sheng Jiang 3.00 Da Zao 3.00 Shi Gao 8.00 Gan Cao 2.00	• **Dispels wind-damp, moves body fluids.** • **Reduces swelling.** Edema, spontaneous sweating, dysuria, weakness in the lower back and legs, acute nephritis, beriberi, eczema, acute arthritis, acute conjunctivitis, polyps, keratitis, and jaundice. • Contains *Yue Bi Tang* + Bai Zhu.
Yue Ju Wan (escape restraint pill) **A -** rqi	Xiang Fu * 6-12g Chuan Xiong 6-12g Zhi Zi 6-12g Cang Zhu 6-12g Shen Qu 6-12g	• **Regulates Qi, releases constraint.** • **Reduces stagnation.** Fullness in the chest and diaphragm, epigastric and abdominal distension and pain, reduced appetite, indigestion, belching, nausea, vomiting. *Tongue:* dusky, purple, yellow, greasy coat. *Pulse:* wiry, slippery, rapid. • **Formula for mild constrained Qi.**
Zai Zao San (renewal powder) **C -** rext	Huang Qi * 6g Ren Shen * 3g Fu Zi 3g Gui Zhi 3g Xi Xin 3g Qiang Huo 3g Chuan Xiong 3g Fang Feng 3g Chuan Shi Shao 3g Gan Cao 1.5g Sheng Jiang 3g Da Zao 2pcs	• **Releases the surface.** • **Tonifies the Yang and Qi.** Fever, chills, no sweating, headache, cold limbs, fatigue, desire to lie down, pale complexion, weak voice. *Tongue:* pale, white coat. *Pulse:* floating, weak.

Formula	Herbs / Dosage	Indications / Functions
Zeng Ye Cheng Qi Tang (increase fluids & order qi decoction) **B -** purg	Xuan Shen 30g Sheng Di Huang 24g Mai Men Dong 24g Mang Xiao 4.5g Da Huang 9g	• **Nourishes the Yin, generates fluids.** • **Clears heat, moves dry stools.** Dry constipation, thirst. *Tongue:* red body. *Pulse:* thin, rapid. • **Formula for constipation caused by extreme dryness in the system, perhaps after loss of blood, or after long-term diarrhea that severely depletes the fluids, or due to excess Yangming fevers. It moistens the body, tonifies blood and purges dry stools.**
Zhe Cong Yin (cinnamon & persica combination) **C -** tblood	Mu Dan Pi 3.00 Bai Shao 3.00 Chuan Xiong 3.00 Gui Zhi 3.00 Dang Gui 5.00 Tao Ren 5.00 Yan Hu Suo 3.00 Niu Xi 3.00 Hong Hua 2.00	• **Tonifies and nourishes the blood.** • **Eliminates blood stagnation in the lower burner, stops pain.** Irregular menstruation, peritonitis, and abdominal pain due to uterine inflammation, pelvic inflammation.
Zhen Gan Xi Feng Tang (sedate liver & extinguish wind decoction) **B -** ewind	Huai Niu Xi * 30g Zhe Shi ** 30g Long Gu 15g Mu Li 15g Gui Ban 15g Xuan Shen 15g Tian Men Dong 15g Bai Shao 15g Chuan Lian Zi 15g Mai Ya 6g Gan Cao 4-5g	• **Settles Liver Yang Rising.** • **Dispels internal wind.** • **Nourishes Liver Yin.** Dizziness, vertigo, headache, tinnitus, heaviness of the head, mental confusion, irritability, flushed red face, facial paralysis. *Tongue:* slight-dark red body. *Pulse:* wiry, strong. • **Settles the Liver Yang to dispel internal wind. For syndromes of Liver Yang rising due to Yin deficiency, which do not always present with heat signs.**
Zhen Wu Tang (true warrior decoction) **A -** edamp	Fu Zi * 9g Fu Ling ** 9g Bai Zhu ** 6g Bai Shao 9g Sheng Jiang 9g	• **Warms the Kidney Yang.** • **Dispels dampness, promotes urination.** Difficult urination, heaviness of the body and limbs, edema, abdominal pain, no thirst, head heaviness, stomach pain, intolerance to cold, diarrhea. *Tongue:* greasy, white coat. *Pulse:* deep, thin, weak. • **Formula for water retention due to Spleen and Kidney Yang.**
Zhi Bai Di Huang Wan (anemarrhena, phellodendron & rehmannia pill) **B -** tyin	*Liu Wei Di Huang Wan +* Huang Bai Zhi Mu	• **Tonifies the Kidney Yin.** • **Clears deficient heat.** Night sweats, flushed face, low-grade fever, hematuria, hot flashes, dry mouth. *Tongue:* dry, red body. *Pulse:* big pulse. • **Formula for *Steaming Bone Syndrome*, menopausal symptoms. Popularly used for patients of AIDS, Lung TB, cancer.** • Contains *Liu Wei Di Huang Wan* + Huang Bai, Zhi Mu.

Formula	Herbs / Dosage	Indications / Functions
Zhi Bao Dan (greatest treasure special pill) **C -** open	She Xiang .1-.3g Bing Pian .3-.5g An Xi Xiang 1-3g Xi Jiao .5-1g Niu Huang 1-3g Dai Mao 3-6g Xiong Huang .2-.5g Zhu Sha .2-.5g Hu Po 3-6g	• **Clears heat and toxicity.** • **Opens orifices, resuscitates, anti-convulsive.** Stroke, coma, fever, irritability, restlessness, impaired speech, labored breathing, spasms, convulsions. *Tongue:* red, deep-red, greasy, yellow coat. *Pulse:* slippery, rapid.
Zhi Gan Cao Tang AKA: Fu Mai Tang (honey fried licorice decoction) **B -** tqiblood	Zhi Gan Cao 12g Ren Shen 6g E Jiao 6g Sheng Di Huang 48g Mai Men Dong 9g Huo Ma Ren 9g Gui Zhi 9g Sheng Jiang 9g Da Zao 30pcs Wine/brandy	• **Tonifies Qi, Blood, and Yin.** • **Restores irregular pulse.** • **Stops palpitations.** Exhaustion, palpitations, irregular pulse, insomnia, night sweats, constipation, shortness of breath, anxiety, dry mouth and throat. *Tongue:* red body, shiny coat. *Pulse:* weak, irregular, knotted. • **Formula to tonify Heart – Qi, Yang, and Yin.**
Zhi Sou San (stop cough powder) **A -** rphlegm	Zi Wan * 960g Bai Qian * 960g Bai Bu * 960g Chen Pi 480g Jie Geng 960g Jing Jie 960g Gan Cao 360g	• **Opens Lung Qi and stops coughing.** • **Releases the surface, expels wind and phlegm.** Itchy throat, coughing, chills, fever, aversion to wind, sputum. *Tongue:* thin, white coat. *Pulse:* floating. • **Formula for stopping coughs caused by external wind invasion. Used primarily for common colds that linger with slight coughing and sore throat.**
Zhi Zhu Wan (immature bitter orange & atractylodes decoction) **C -** rfood	Zhi Shi 30g Bai Zhu 60g	• **Tonifies the Spleen, reduces distension.** Loss of appetite, distension in epigastrium and abdomen, indigestion, acid regurgitation. *Tongue:* yellow, greasy coat. *Pulse:* slippery. • **Mild formula for strengthening Stomach Qi.**
Zhi Zhuo Gu Ben Wan (hoelen & polyporus formula) **C -** clht	Lian Xu 4.00 Huang Lian 4.00 Sha Ren 2.00 Huang Bai 2.00 Fu Ling 2.00 Ban Xia 2.00 Zhu Ling 5.00 Zhi Gan Cao 6.00 Yi Zhi Ren 2.00	• **Clears heat, reduces inflammation.** • **Dispels dampness, clears turbidity.** Heat and dampness in stomach and urinary bladder, polyuria, spermatorrhea, chronic prostatitis, chronic cystitis, and chronic urethritis.
Zhu Ling Tang (polyporus decoction) **A -** edamp	Zhu Ling * 3g Fu Ling * 3g Ze Xie ** 3g Hua Shi 3g E Jiao 3g	• **Dispels dampness, promotes urination.** • **Clears heat, nourishes the Yin.** Difficult urination, fever, thirst, nausea, irritability, insomnia. *Tongue:* red body, thick white or yellow coat. *Pulse:* rapid, slippery. • **Formula for wind-damp attack penetrating the interior and transforming into heat, with fever, thirst, difficult urination.**

Formula	Herbs / Dosage	Indications / Functions
Zhu Sha An Shen Wan (cinnabar pill to calm spirit) **B -** ashen	Zhu Sha * 15g Huang Lian ** 18g Dang Gui 7.5g Sheng Di Huang 7.5g Zhi Gan Cao 16.5g	• **Settles the Heart, calms the Spirit.** • **Clears heat.** • **Nourishes Heart Yin and Heart Blood.** Insomnia, disturbed dreams, irritability, palpitations, sensation of heat in the chest, nausea, desire to vomit but without results. *Tongue:* red body. *Pulse:* thin, rapid. • **Formula for calming the Spirit and delirium due to fire rising injuring blood and yin.**
Zhu Ye Shi Gao Tang (lophatherus & gypsum decoction) **B -** clht	Dan Zhu Ye 9-15g Shi Gao 30g Ren Shen 6g Mai Men Dong 9-18g Ban Xia 9g Geng Mi 12-15g Gan Cao 3-6g	• **Clears heat and generates fluids.** • **Tonifies the Qi, harmonizes the Stomach.** Post febrile disease with lingering heat, low-grade fever with sweat, irritability, insomnia, fatigue, thirst, dry throat, fullness of the chest, vomiting, listlessness, dry cough, insomnia, bronchitis, influenza, and measles. *Tongue:* dry, red body, no coat. *Pulse:* thin, rapid. • **Sedates low-grade fevers with Qi and fluid deficiency, perhaps depleted by long-term fever. Usually used for mild fevers during recovery from excess heat and high fever.**
Zi Xue Dan (purple snow special pill) **C -** open	Pill	• **Clears heat, opens orifices.** • **Controls spasms and convulsions.** Fever, difficult speech, impaired consciousness, spasms, convulsions, thirst, constipation, dark urine. *Tongue:* dark-red, no coat. *Pulse:* rapid, forceful. • **Formula for excess heat in Pericardium generating internal Liver-wind.**
Zuo Gui Yin (restore left kidney decoction) **B -** tyin	Shu Di Huang * 6-60g Shan Zhu Yu 3-6g Gou Qi Zi ** 6g Fu Ling 6g Shan Yao 6g Zhi Gan Cao 3g	• **Nourishes the Yin and Essence.** • **Strengthens the Kidneys.** Low back soreness and pain, dizziness, tinnitus, thirst and dry throat, night sweats, seminal emissions, weak knees. *Tongue:* red, peeled, shiny coat. *Pulse:* thin, rapid. • **Kidney Yin deficiency with injury to the essence and marrow without heat signs.**
Zuo Jin Wan (coptis & evodia pill) **B -** clht	Huang Lian 180g Wu Zhu Yu 30g	• **Clears Liver fire and Stomach fire.** • **Descends Stomach Qi.** Acid regurgitation, hypochondriac pain, belching, nausea, vomiting, bitter taste, dry mouth. *Tongue:* red body, yellow coat. *Pulse:* wiry, rapid. • **Formula for Liver attacking the Stomach. This formula tonifies the mother and sedates the son.**

FORMULA INDEX

Formulas	Translations	Formula Category	Formulas	Translations	Formula Category
Ai Fu Nuan Gong Wan	mugwort & prepared aconite warming the womb pill	tblood	Dao Chi San	guide out red powder	clht
An Gong Niu Huang Wan	calm palace with cattle gallstone pill	open	Dao Shui Fu Ling Tang	hoelen atractylodes. & areca combination	edamp
An Zhong San	calm the middle powder	wint	Dao Tan Tang	guide out phlegm dect.	rphlegm
Ba Xian Chang Shou Wan	longevity pill	tyin	Di Dang Tang	rhubarb & leech combination	tblood
Ba Zhen Tang	eight corrections powder	tqiblood	Di Huang Yin Zi	rehmannia dect.	ewind
Ba Zheng San	eight corrections powder	edamp	Ding Chuan Tang	stop wheezing dect.	rqi
Bai Du San	ginseng powder to overcome pathogenic influences	rext	Ding Xiang Shi Di Tang	clove & persimmon calyx dect.	rqi
Bai He Gu Jin Tang	lily bulb to consolidate lung dect.	dry	Du Huo Ji Sheng Tang	angelica & sangjisheng dect.	edamp
Bai Hu Jia Gui Zhi Tang	white tiger dect. plus cinnamon	clht	Dun Sou Tang	morus & platycodon combination	clht
Bai Hu Jia Ren Shen Tang	white tiger plus ginseng dect.	clht	E Jiao Ji Zi Huang Tang	ass-hide gelatin & egg yolk dect.	ewind
Bai Hu Tang	white tiger dect.	clht	Er Chen Tang	two aged dect.	rphlegm
Bai Tou Weng Tang	pulsatilla dect.	clht	Er Long Zuo Ci Wan	pills for the deaf	tyin
Ban Xia Bai Zhu Tian Ma Tang	pinellia, atractylodes & gastrodia dect.	rphlegm	Er Miao San	two-marvel powder	edamp
Ban Xia Hou Po Tang	pinellia & magnolia dect.	rqi	Er Xian Tang	two immortal dect.	tyang
Ban Xia Xie Xin Tang	pinellia drain epigastrium dect.	harm	Er Zhi Wan	two-ultimate pill	tyin
Bao An Shen	polyporus & pinellia combination	rqi	Er Zhu Tang	atractylodes & arisaema combination	edamp
Bao Can Wu Yu Fang	dang gui & artemisia combination	sab	Fang Feng Tong Sheng San	ledebouriella powder sagely unblocks	rext
Bao He Wan	preserve harmony pill	rfood	Fang Ji Huang Qi Tang	stephania & astragalus dect.	edamp
Bao Yuan Chai Hu Qing Gan San	bupleurum & moutan formula	clht	Fen Xiao Tang	hoelen & alisma combination	edamp
Bei Mu Gua Lou San	fritillary & trichosantes powder	rphlegm	Fu Ling Yin	hoelen combination	edamp
Bei Xie Fen Qing Yin	dioscorea hypoglauca to separate clear dect.	edamp	Fu Tu Dan	hoelen & cuscuta formula	sab
Bu Fei E Jiao Tang	tonify lung with ass-hide gelatin dect.	tyin	Fu Yuan Huo Xue Tang	revive health by invigorating blood dect.	movexue
Bu Yang Huan Wu Tang	tonify yang to restore five-tenths dect.	movexue	Fu Zi Li Zhong Wan	prepared aconite pill to regulate the middle	wint
Bu Zhong Yi Qi Tang	tonify middle & increase qi dect.	tqi	Gan Lu Xiao Du Dan	sweet dew eliminate toxin pill	edamp
Cang Er Zi San	xanthium powder	rext	Gan Mai Da Zao Tang	licorice, wheat & jujube dect.	ashen
Chai Ge Jie Ji Tang	bupleurum & kudzu release muscle layer dect.	rext	Ge Gen Huang Lian Huang Qin Tang	kudzu, scutellaria, & coptis dect.	rext
Chai Hu Jia Long Gu Mu Li Tang	bupleurum, dragon bone & oyster shell dect.	ashen	Ge Gen Tang	kudzu dect.	rext
Chai Hu Shu Gan San	bupleurum powder to spread liver	harm	Ge Xia Zhu Yu Tang	drive out blood stasis below diaphragm dect.	movexue
Chai Ling Tang	bupleurum & hoelen combination	edamp	Gu Chong Tang	stabilize flooding dect.	astringe
Chai Xian Tang	bupleurum & scute combination	rphlegm	Gu Jing Wan	stabilize menses pill	astringe
Chuan Xiong Cha Tiao San	ligusticum powder w/ green tea	rext	Gu Yin Jian	stabilize yin dect.	tyin
Ci Zhu Wan	magnetite & cinnabar pill	ashen	Gua Lou Xie Bai Bai Jiu Tang	trichosantes, chive & wine dect.	rqi
Cong Chi Tang	scallion & prepared soybean dect.	rext	Gui Lu Er Xian Jiao	turtle shell & deer antler syrup	tyang
Da Bu Yin Wan	great tonify yin pill	tyin	Gui Pi Tang	restore spleen dect.	tqiblood
Da Chai Hu Tang	major bupleurum dect.	harm	Gui Zhi Fu Ling Wan	cinnamon & poria pill	movexue
Da Cheng Qi Tang	major order qi dect.	purg	Gui Zhi Jia Long Gu Mu Li Tang	cinnamon twig dect. plus dragon bone & oyster shell	harm
Da Ding Feng Zhu	big pearl for endogenous wind	ewind	Gui Zhi Shao Yao Zhi Mu Tang	cinnamon twig, peony & anemarrhena dect.	edamp
Da Huang Fu Zi Tang	rhubarb & aconite dect.	purg	Gui Zhi Tang	cinnamon dect.	rext
Da Huang Mu Dan Pi Tang	rhubarb & eupolypaga pill	edamp	Gun Tan Wan	vaporize phlegm pill	open
Da Huang Zhe Chong Wan	rhubarb & eupolypaga pill	movexue	Hai Zao Yu Hu Tang	seaweed dect.	rphlegm
Da Jian Zhong Tang	major strengthen middle dect.	wint	Hao Qin Qing Dan Tang	artemisia annua & scutellaria dect.	harm
Da Qin Jiao Tang	major gentiana qinjiao combination	ewind	Hei Xi Dan	lead special pill	wint
Da Qing Long Tang	major bluegrass dragon dect.	rext	Hong Hua Tao Ren Jian	safflower & peach kernel dect.	movexue
Da Xian Xiong Tang	major sinking chest dect.	purg	Hu Qian Wan	hidden tiger pill	tyin
Da Yuan Yin	reach membrane source	harm	Huai Hua San	sophora powder	stopxue
Dai Zhe Xuan Fu Tang	Inula & Hematite Combination	rphlegm	Huang Lian E Jiao Tang	coptis & ass-hide gelatin dect.	ashen
Dan Shen Yin	salvia dect.	movexue	Huang Lian Jie Du Tang	coptis dect. relieve toxicity	clht
Dang Gui Bu Xue Tang	tangkuei tonify blood dect.	tqiblood	Huang Lian Wen Dan Tang	coptis warm the gallbladder dect.	clht
Dang Gui Liu Huang Tang	angelica & six yellow dect.	clht	Huang Long Tang	yellow dragon dect.	purg
Dang Gui Nian Tong Tang	dang gui & anemarrhena combination	edamp	Huang Qi Jian Zhong Tang	astragalus dect. to construct the middle	wint
Dang Gui San	dang gui powder	tblood	Huang Tu Tang	yellow earth dect.	stopxue
Dang Gui Shao Yao San	tangkuei & peony powder	harm	Huo Luo Xiao Ling Dan	invigorate collaterals wonder pill	movexue
Dang Gui Si Ni Tang	tangkuei frigid extremity dect.	wint	Huo Po Wen Zhong Tang	magnolia warm middle dect.	rqi

Formulas	Translations	Formula Category
Huo Xiang Zheng Qi Tang	agastache correct qi powder	edamp
Ji Chuan Jian	benefit river flow dect.	purg
Ji Ming San	cock's crow powder	edamp
Jia Jian Fu Mai Tang	modified baked licorice dect.	tyin
Jia Jian Wei Rui Tang	modified polygonatum dect.	rext
Jian Er Wan	atractylodes & pogostemonis combination	clht
Jian Pi Wan	strengthen spleen pill	rfood
Jian Ying San	inphantrans formula	clht
Jiao Ai Tang	ass-hide gelatin & mugwort dect.	stopxue
Jie Geng Tang	platycodon combination	clht
Jin Fei Cao San	schizonepeta & pinellia formula	rphlegm
Jin Gui Shen Qi Wan	golden-cabinet kidney qi pill	tyin
Jin Ling Zi San	melia powder	rqi
Jin Suo Gu Jing Wan	metal lock stabilize essence pill	astringe
Jing Fang Bai Du San	schizonepeta & ledebouriella powder to overcome pathogenic influences	rext
Jing Jei Lian Qiao Tang	schizonepeta & forsythia combination	clht
Jiu Wei Qiang Huo Tang	nine-herb notopterygium dect.	rext
Jiu Xian San	nine-immortal pill	astringe
Ju He Wan	tangerine seed pill	rqi
Ju Pi Zhu Ru Tang	tangerine peel & bamboo shavings dect.	rqi
Juan Bi Tang	remove painful obstruction dect.	edamp
Ke Xue Fang	coughing blood formula	stopxue
Li Zhong Wan	regulate middle pill	wint
Liang Fu Wan	galangal & cypress pill	rqi
Liang Ge San	cools diaphragm powder	purg
Ling Gan Wu Wei Jiang Xin Tang	poria, licorice, schisandra, ginger & asarum dect.	rphlegm
Ling Gui Zhu Gan Tang	poria, cinnamon, atractylodes & licorice dect.	rphlegm
Liu Jun Zi Tang	six-ingredient rehmannia pill	tqi
Liu Shen Wan	six miracle pill	rext
Liu Wei Di Huang Wan	six-ingredient rehmannia pill	tyin
Liu Yi San	six-to-one powder	clht
Long Dan Xie Gan Tang	drain liver dect.	clht
Ma Huang Tang	ephedra dect.	rext
Ma Huang Xi Xin Fu Zi Tang	ephedra, asarum & aconite dect.	rext
Ma Xin Yi Gan Tang	ma huang & coix combination	rext
Ma Xing Shi Gan Tang	ephedra, apricot, gypsum & licorice dect.	clht
Ma Zi Ren Wan	hemp seed pill	purg
Mai Men Dong Tang	Ophiopogonis Dect.	tyin
Ming Mu Di Huang Wan	improve vision pill with rehmannia	tyin
Mu Li San	oyster shell powder	astringe
Mu Xiang Bing Lang Wan	aucklandia & betel nut pill	rfood
Niu Ke Bai Zi Ren Wan	biota & achyranthes formula	movexue
Nuan Gan Jian	warm liver dect.	rqi
Pai Nong San	platycodon & aurantium formula	movexue
Ping Wei San	calm stomach powder	edamp
Pu Ji Xiao Du Yin	universal benefit to eliminate toxin dect.	clht
Qi Ju Di Huang Wan	lycium, chrysanthemum & rehmannia pill	tyin
Qi Li San	seven-thousandths teal powder	movexue
Qi Pi Tang	lotus & citrus combination	edamp
Qian Zheng San	restore symmetry powder	ewind
Qiang Huo Sheng Shi Tang	notopterygium to overcome dampness dect.	edamp
Qin Jiao Bie Jia San	gentiana macrophlla & turtle shell formula	clht
Qing Fei Yin	platycodon & citrus formula	rphlegm

Formulas	Translations	Formula Category
Qing Gu San	cool bones powder	clht
Qing Hao Bie Jia Tang	artemisia annua & soft shelled turtle dect.	clht
Qing Luo Yin	clear collaterals dect.	clht
Qing Qi Hua Tan Wan	clear qi & resolve phlegm	rphlegm
Qing Re Zhi Beng Tang	clears heat & stop excess bleeding dect.	stopxue
Qing Shang Fang Feng Tang	ledebouriella combination	clht
Qing Shu Yi Qi Tang	clear summer-heat & augment qi dect.	clht
Qing Wei San	clear stomach powder	clht
Qing Xin Lian Zi Yin	lotus seed combination	clht
Qing Yan Li Ge Tang	arctium combination	clht
Qing Ying Tang	clear nutritive level dect.	clht
Qing Zao Jiu Fei Tang	eliminate dryness & rescue lung dect.	dry
Ren Shen Bai Du San	ginseng powder to overcome pathogenic influences powder	rext
Ren Shen Xie Fei Tang	ginseng & platycodon combination	clht
Ren Shen Yang Rong Tang	ginseng nourish nutritive qi dect.	tqi
Ren Shen Yang Ying Tang	ginseng dect. to nourish nutritive qi	tblood
Run Chang Wan	moisten intestine pill from master shen's book	purg
San Ao Tang	three-unbinding dect.	rext
San Bi Tang	three painful obstruction dect.	edamp
San Huang Shi Gao Tang	coptis & scute combination	rext
San Huang Xie Xin Tang	coptis & rhubarb combination	clht
San Jia Fu Mai Tang	three shells to restore the pulse dect.	clht
San Miao Wan	three marvel pill	clht
San Ren Tang	three-nut dect.	edamp
San Wu Bei Ji Wan	three substance emergency pill	purg
San Zhong Kui Jian Tang	forsythia & laminaria combination	clht
San Zi Yang Qing Tang	three-seed nourish parents dect.	rphlegm
Sang Ju Yin	mulberry leaf & chrysanthemum dect.	rext
Sang Piao Xiao San	mantis egg-case powder	astringe
Sang Xing Tang	mulberry leaf & apricot kernel dect.	dry
Sha Shen Mai Dong Tang	glehnia & ophiopogonis dect.	dry
Shao Fu Zhu Yu Tang	drive out blood stasis in lower abdomen dect.	movexue
Shao Yao Tang	peony dect.	clht
She Gan Ma Huang Tang	belamcanda & ephedra dect.	rext
Shen Fu Tang	ginseng & prepared aconite dect.	wint
Shen Ling Bai Zhu San	ginseng, poria & atractylodes powder	tqi
Shen Su Yin	ginseng & perilla combination	rext
Shen Tong Zhu Yu Tang	drive out blood stasis from painful body dect.	movexue
Shen Zhuo Tang	hoelen, atractylodes, combination	edamp
Sheng Hua Tang	generation & transformation dect.	movexue
Sheng Ma Ge Gen Tang	cimicifuga & kudzu dect.	rext
Sheng Mai San	generate pulse powder	tqi
Sheng Tie Luo Yin	iron fillings dect.	ashen
Sheng Yu Tang	dang gui four plus combination	tblood
Shi Hui San	ten-ingredient partially charred powder	stopxue
Shi Liu Wei Liu Qi Yin	dang gui sixteen herb combination	tqi
Shi Pi Yin	bolster spleen dect.	edamp
Shi Quan Da Bu Tang	ten complete great tonic dect.	tblood
Shi Shen Tang	ma huang & cimicifuga combination	rext
Shi Wei Bai Du San	bupleurum & schizonepeta formula	ewind
Shi Wei Xiang Ru Yin	elsholtzia ten combination	rext

FORMULA INDEX

Formulas	Translations	Formula Category
Shi Xiao San	sudden smile powder	movexue
Shi Zao Tang	ten jujube dect.	purg
Shu Gan Tang	bupleurum & evodia combination	movexue
Shu Jing Huo Xue Tan	relax channels & invigorate blood	movexue
Shu Jing Li An San	clematis & carthamus formula	edamp
Shung Jie San	modified ledebouriella & platycodon formula	edamp
Si Jun Zi Tang	four gentlemen dect.	tqi
Si Miao Wan	four-marvel pill	edamp
Si Miao Yong An Tang	four valiant for well-being dect.	clht
Si Mo Tang	four milled-herb dect.	rqi
Si Ni San	frigid extremities powder	harm
Si Ni Tang	frigid extremities dect.	wint
Si Shen Wan	four miracle pill	astringe
Si Sheng Wang	four fresh pill	stopxue
Si Wu Tang	four-substances dect.	tblood
Su Zi Jiang Qi Tang	perilla descend qi dect.	rqi
Suan Zao Ren Tang	sour jujube dect.	ashen
Suo Quan Wan	enuresis pills	astringe
Tai Shan Pan Shi San	powder that gives stability to mount tai	tblood
Tao He Cheng Qi Tang	peach pit order qi dect.	movexue
Tao Hong Si Wu Tang	four substance w/ safflower & peach pit dect.	tblood
Tao Hua Tang	peach blossom dect.	wint
Teng Long Tang	moutan & persica combination	clht
Tian Ma Gou Teng Yin	gastrodia & uncaria dect.	ewind
Tian Tai Wu Yao San	top quality lindera powder	rqi
Tian Wang Bu Xin Dan	heavenly emperor's heart tonic pill	ashen
Tiao Wei Cheng Qi Tang	regulate stomach & order qi dect.	purg
Tong Qiao Huo Xue Tang	invigorate blood circulation & open orifices dect.	movexue
Tong Xie Yao Fang	painful diarrhea formula	harm
Wan Dai Tang	end discharge dect.	astringe
Wei Jing Tang	reed dect.	clht
Wei Ling Tang	calm the stomach & poria dect.	edamp
Wei Su Ning	galanga & pinellia formula	edamp
Wen Dan Tang	warm gallbladder dect.	rphlegm
Wen Jing Tang	warm menses dect.	movexue
Wen Pi Tang	warm spleen dect.	purg
Wen Qing Yin	warming & clearing dect.	tblood
Wu Ji San	five accumulation powder	rext
Wu Ling San	five fungus powder	edamp
Wu Mei Wan	mume formula	rfood
Wu Pi San	five peel powder	edamp
Wu Tou Tang	aconite dect.	ewind
Wu Wei Xiao Du Yin	five ingredient eliminate toxin dect.	clht
Wu Yao Shun Qi San	lindera formula	ewind
Wu Zhu Yu Tang	evodia dect.	wint
Xi Jiao Di Huang Tang	rhinoceros horn & rehmannia dect.	clht
Xian Fang Huo Ming Yin	sublime formula for sustaining life	clht
Xiang Ru San	elsholtzia powder	rext
Xiang Sha Liu Jun Zi Tang	six gentlemen w/ aucklandia & amomum dect.	tqi
Xiang Sha Yang Wei Tang	cyperus & cluster combination	harm
Xiang Su San	cyperus & perilla leaf powder	rext
Xiao Chai Hu Tang	minor bupleurum dect.	harm
Xiao Cheng Qi Tang	minor order qi dect.	purg
Xiao Feng San	eliminate wind powder	ewind
Xiao Huo Luo Dan	minor invigorate collaterals pill	ewind
Xiao Ji Yin Zi	cephanoplos dect.	stopxue
Xiao Jian Zhong Tang	minor strengthen middle dect.	wint
Xiao Luo Wan	reduce scrofula pill	rphlegm

Formulas	Translations	Formula Category
Xiao Qing Long Tang	minor bluegrass dragon dect.	rext
Xiao Xian Xiong Tang	minor sinking chest dect.	rphlegm
Xiao Xu Ming Tang	minor prolong life dect.	ewind
Xiao Yao San	rambling powder	harm
Xie Bai San	drain white powder	clht
Xie Huang San	drain yellow powder	clht
Xie Xin Tang	drain epigastrium dect.	clht
Xin Jia Huang Long Tang	newly augmented yellow dragon dect.	purg
Xin Jia Xiang Ru Yin	newly-augmented elsholtzia dect.	rext
Xing Su San	apricot kernel & perilla Leaf	dry
Xuan Bi Tang	disband painful obstruction dect.	edamp
Xuan Fu Dai Zhe Tang	inula & hematite dect.	rqi
Xue Fu Zhu Yu Tang	blood mansion eliminate stasis dect.	movexue
Yang He Tang	yang heartening dect.	wint
Yang Yin Qing Fei Tang*	nourish the yin & clear lungs dect.	dry
Yi Guan Jian	one link dect.	tyin
Yi Huang Tang	change yellow discharge dect.	astringe
Yi Qi Cong Ming Tang	augment qi & increase acuity dect.	tqi
Yi Yi Ren Tang	enlightened physician coicis dect.	edamp
Yi Zi Tang	cimicifuga combination	clht
Yin Chen Hao Tang	artemisia dect.	edamp
Yin Chen Wu Ling San	capillaris & hoelen formula	edamp
Yin Qiao San	honeysuckle & forsythia powder	rext
You Gui Wan	restore right kidney pill	tyang
Yu Nu Jian	jade woman dect.	clht
Yu Ping Feng San	jade windscreen powder	astringe
Yu Ye Tang	jade fluid dect.	dry
Yu Zhen San	true jade powder	ewind
Yue Bi Jia Zhu Tang	atractylodes combination	edamp
Yue Ju Wan	escape restraint pill	rqi
Zai Zao San	renewal powder	rext
Zeng Ye Cheng Qi Tang	increase fluids & order qi dect.	purg
Zhe Cong Yin	cinnamon & persica combination	tblood
Zhen Gan Xi Feng Tang	sedate liver & extinguish wind dect.	ewind
Zhen Wu Tang	true warrior dect.	edamp
Zhi Bai Di Huang Wan	anemarrhena, phellodendron & rehmannia pill	tyin
Zhi Bao Dan	greatest treasure special pill	open
Zhi Gan Cao Tang	honey fried licorice dect.	tqiblood
Zhi Sou San	stop cough powder	rphlegm
Zhi Zhu Wan	immature bitter orange & atractylodes pill	rfood
Zhi Zhuo Gu Ben Wan	hoelen & polyporus formula	clht
Zhu Ling Tang	polyporus dect.	edamp
Zhu Sha An Shen Wan	cinnabar pill to calm spirit	ashen
Zhu Ye Shi Gao Tang	lophatherus & gypsum dect.	clht
Zi Xue Dan	purple snow special pill	open
Zuo Gui Yin	restore left kidney dect.	tyin
Zuo Jin Wan	coptis & evodia pill	clht

CONDITIONS & FORMULAS

Conditions	Formulas w/ TCM Diagnosis
Abdominal Distension	Xiang Sha Liu Jun Zi Tang - Spleen qi def. with qi stag. & damp; Ping Wei San - phlegm damp; Xiang Sha Yang Wei Wan - qi & damp stag.; Li Zhong Wan - yang def.; Bao He Wan - food stag.; Qing Gan Li Dan Tablets - Gallbladder damp heat, gallstones; Huo Hsiang Cheng Chi Pien - summer damp; Niu Huang Qing Huo Wan - heat in yang ming
Abdominal Masses	Xue Fu Zhu Yu Tang - qi & blood stag.; Ge Xia Zhu Yu Wan - Liver blood stag.; Huo Luo Xiao Ling Wan - blood stag.; Woo Garm Yuen Medical Pills - cold & blood stag.; Nei Xiao Luo Li Wan - phlegm & blood stag.; Shu Gan Wan - Liver qi stag.; Bao He Wan - food stag.; Gui Zhi Fu Ling Tang - blood stag. in the uterus
Abdominal Pain	Si Ni San - Liver qi stag.; Shu Gan Wan - Liver invading Spleen; Chai Hu Shu Gan Wan - Liver invading Spleen; Tong Xie Yao Fang Wan - Liver invading Spleen; Huo Hsiang Cheng Chi Pien - summer damp; Xiao Jian Zhong Wan - Spleen yang def.; Bao He Wan - food stag.; Xue Fu Zhu Yu Tang - blood stag.; Wei Tong Ding, Liang Fu Wan, Tong Mai Si Ni Tang - cold, yang def.; Dang Gui Si Ni Tang - cold, blood stag.; Da Cheng Qi Tang - heat
Abscess	Acute, superficial: Huang Lian Jie Du Tang - toxic & damp heat; Wu Wei Xiao Du Wan - toxic heat; Peking Niu Huang Jie Du Pian - toxic heat; Fu Fang Nan Ban Lan Gen - toxic heat; Chuan Xin Lian Antiphlogistic Tablets - toxic heat; Lien Chiao Pai Tu Pien - wind heat, toxic heat; Niu Huang Zing Huo Wan - toxic heat, yang ming heat; Fang Feng Tong Sheng Wan - recurrent; Yunnan Paiyao; Chuan Xin Lian Cream - topical
Acid Reflux	Xiang Lian Wan - Stomach heat; Wei Te Ling; hyperacidity; Xiang Sha Yang Wei Wan - qi stag.; Chai Hu Shu Gan Wan - Liver qi stag.; Shu Gan Wan - Liver qi stag.; Yi Guan Jian Wan - yin def., qi stag.; Wei Tong Ding - cold, yang def.; Bao He Wan - food stag.; Ping Wei San - phlegm damp; Jian Pi Wan - pregnancy; Bo Ying Compound - infants; Qi Xing Tea - infants
Acne	Qing Re An Chuang Pian - toxic heat & hot blood; Zhen Zhu An Chuang Tablet - toxic & damp heat; Huang Lian Jie Du Tang - toxic heat; Wu Wei Xiao Du Yin - toxic heat; Lien Chiao Pai Tu Pien - wind heat, toxic heat; Chuan Xin Lian Cream - topical
ADD/ADHD	Bu Zhong Yi Qi Tang - hyperactive Spleen qi def.; Chai Hu Long Gu Mu Li Tang - Heart & Liver fire, phlegm heat; Autoimmune disorders: Reishi Mushroom immune regulator; Xue Fu Zhu Yu Tang - blood stag.; Ge Xia Zhu Yu Wan - blood stag.; Dan Shen Huo Xue Wan - blood stag. with heat; Dang Gui Si Ni Tang - cold & blood stag.
Addison's Disease	Da Bu Yin Wan, Liu Wei Di Huang Wan, Zuo Gui Wan, Zuo Gui Yin - Kid. def.
Adrenal Insufficiency or Disorders	Liu Wei Di Huang Wan - Kid. yin def.; Fu Gui Ba Wei Wan - Kid. yang def.; Panax Ginseng Extractum - qi def.
AIDS	Sheng Mai San, Zhi Bai Di Huang Wan - yin def.; Da Ding Feng Zhu - yin def. fire
Alcohol	Headache and Dizziness Reliever; Po Chai Pills - damp heat; Bao Ji Pills - damp heat. Liver Cirrhosis: Shu Gan Wan - qi stag.; Xiao Yao Wan - qi stag., blood def., early; Xue Fu Zhu Yu Tang - blood stag.; Sunho Multi Ginseng Tablets - blood stag., qi def.; Yi Guan Jian Wan - Liver yin def., qi stag.; Ge Xia Zhu Yu Wan - blood stag., severe; Huo Luo Xiao Ling Wan - blood stag., severe
Allergy	Yu Ping Feng San, Xin Yi San - wei qi def.; Reishi Mushroom immune regulator; Bi Ye Ning Capsule - phlegm heat; Pe Min Kan Wan - wind; Xiang Sha Liu Jun Zi Tang - Spleen qi def. with phlegm damp; Ba Ji Yin Yang Wan - Lung & Kid. yang def.
Alopecia	Yang Xue Sheng Fa Capsules - blood & yin def., postpartum; Qi Bao Mei Ran Dan - blood & yin def., postpartum; Tangkwei Essence of Chicken - blood def., postpartum; Deer Velvet - jing def.; Shou Wu Chih, He Shou Wu Wan, Gui Pi Tang - blood & yin def.; Shou Wu Pian - blood def.; You Gui Wan - yang def.; Zuo Gui Wan - yin def.; Tong Qiao Huo Xue Wan - blood stag.
Alzheimer's	Huan Shao Dan - Heart & Kid. def.
Amenorrhea	Ba Zhen Tang - qi & blood def.; Si Wu Tang - blood def.; Ba Zhen Yi Mu Wan - qi & blood def. with mild blood stag.; Gui Pi Tang - Heart & Spleen def.; Shi Quan Da Bu Tang - qi & blood def. with cold; Woo Garm Yuen Medical Pills - cold & blood stag.; Wen Jing Tang - cold, def. and blood stag.; Tong Jing Wan - blood stag.; Yunnan Paiyao - blood stag. with cold, severe; Shao Fu Zhu Yu Tang - blood stag. with blood def.; Liu Wei Di Huang Wan - Kid. yin def.; Zuo Gui Wan - Kid. yin def.; Fu Gui Ba Wei Wan - Kid. yang def.; Tiao Jing Cu Yun Wan - Kid. yang def.
Anemia	Ba Zhen Tang - qi & blood def.; Si Wu Tang - blood def.; Tangkwei Essence of Chicken - qi & blood def., postpartum; Dang Gui Jing qi & blood def.; Dang Gui Su - blood def.; Wu Ji Bai Feng Wan - refractory; Bai Feng Wan - postpartum; Bu Zhong Yi Qi Tang - Spleen qi def.; Xiao Jian Zhong Wan - Spleen yang def.; You Gui Wan - Kid. yang def.; Xiao Yao Wan - qi stag., Spleen & blood def.

ACUPUNCTURE DESK REFERENCE 65

CONDITIONS & FORMULAS

Conditions	Formulas w/ TCM Diagnosis
Angina	Xue Fu Zhu Yu Tang - qi & blood stag.; Dan Shen Pill - blood & phlegm stag.; Dan Shen Yin - qi & blood stag.; Xin Mai Ling - blood stag.; Raw Tienchi Tablets - blood stag.; Tao Hong Si Wu Tang - blood stag. with blood def., mild; Guan Xin An Kou Fu Ye - blood stag.; Huo Luo Xiao Ling Wan - blood stag.; Sunho Multi Ginseng Tablets - blood stag. & qi def.
Ankle Pain	Jian Bu Qiang Shen Wan - Kid. def.
Anorexia	Bao He Wan - food stag.; Xiang Sha Liu Jun Zi Tang - Spleen & Stomach def.; Yi Wei Tang - Stomach yin def.
Anxiety	Tian Wang Bu Xin Dan - Heart & Kid. yin def.; Gui Pi Tang - Heart & Spleen qi def.; Bai Zi Yang Xin Wan - blood & yin def.; An Shen Ding Zhi Wan - yin def. with phlegm; An Shen Bu Xin Wan - yin def., yang rising; Wen Dan Tang - phlegm heat; Chai Hu Long Gu Mu Li Tang - qi stag., phlegm heat, yang rising; Ban Xia Hou Po Tang - qi & phlegm stag.; Po Lung Yuen Medical Pills - phlegm heat
Appendicitis (Acute)	Acute, uncomplicated: Huang Lian Jie Du Tang - damp & toxic heat; Wu Wei Xiao Du Yin - toxic heat; Ching Fei Yi Huo Pien - yang ming organ syndrome; Niu Huang Qing Huo Wan - yang ming organ syndrome; Liang Ge Wan - yang ming organ syndrome
Appendicitis (Chronic)	Chronic: Nei Xiao Luo Li Wan - phlegm & blood stag.; Huo Luo Xiao Ling Wan - blood stag.
Appetite	Poor: Si Jun Zi Tang - Spleen qi def.; Xiang Sha Liu Jun Zi Tang - Spleen qi def. with phlegm damp; Li Zhong Wan - yang def.; Ping Wei San - phlegm damp; Bao He Wan - food stag.; Bu Zhong Yi Qi Tang - Spleen qi def.; Huan Shao Dan - yang def.; Bo Ying Compound - infants; Healthy Child Tea - Spleen def., infants; Qi Xing Tea - food intolerance, infants
Arteriosclerosis	Dan Shen Pill - blood & phlegm stag.; Dan Shen Yin Wan - qi & blood stag.; Raw Tienchi Tablets - blood stag.; Guan Xin An Kou Fu Ye - blood stag.; Sunho Multi Ginseng Tablets - blood stag.; Xue Fu Zhu Yu Tang - blood stag.; Liu Wei Di Huang Wan - yin def.; Zhen Gan Xi Feng Wan - yang rising
Arthritis	Juan Bi Tang - wind cold damp; Qu Feng Zhen Tong Capsule - wind cold damp; Xuan Bi Tang - damp heat; Guan Jie Yan Wan - damp heat; Shu Jin Huo Xue Wan - blood & phlegm stag.; Shen Tong Zhu Yu Wan - blood stag.; Xiao Huo Luo Dan - severe cold; Du Huo Ji Sheng Tang - wind damp with Kid. def.; Jian Bu Qiang Shen Wan - Kid. def.; Fu Gui Ba Wei Wan - Kid. yang def.; Trans Wood Lock Liniment - topical; Porous Capsicum Plaster topical; Gou Pi Gao topical
Ascites	Zhen Wu Tang Wan - yang def.; Li Chung Yuen Medical Pills - Spleen yang def.; Wu Ling San - Spleen def. with fluid accumulation; Chai Hu Shu Gan Wan - qi stag.; Mu Xiang Shun Qi Wan - qi & damp stag.; Ge Xia Zhu Yu Wan - blood stag.
Asthma	Ma Huang Tang, Gui Zhi Jia Hou Po Xing Ren Tang - wind cold; Ma Xing Shi Gan Tang, Bai Hu Jia Ren Shen Tang - wind heat; Su Zi Jiang Zi Tang - cold phlegm; Xiao Qing Long Wan - wind cold with congested fluids; Ding Chuan Tang - phlegm heat; Zing Zi Hua Tan Wan - phlegm heat; Mai Wei Di Huang Wan - Lung & Kid. yin def.; Sheng Mai San, Bu Zhong Yi Qi Tang - qi & yin def.; Bu Fei Wan - Lung qi def.; Yulin Bu Shen Wan - Kid not grasping qi, yang def.; Cordyceps Essence of Chicken - Lung & Kid. def.; Jin Gui Shen Qi Wan, Shen Jie San - Kid. def.
Atherosclerosis	Dan Shen Pill - blood & phlegm stag.; Keep Fit Capsule - phlegm & blood stag.; Raw Tienqi Tablets - blood stag.; Dan Shen Yin - qi & blood stag.; Guan Xin An Kou Fu Ye - blood stag.; Sunho Multi Ginseng Tablets - blood stag.; Xue Fu Zhu Yu Tang - blood stag.
Athlete's Foot	Tujin Liniment; Hua Tuo Gao
Attention Deficit	Bu Zhong Yi Qi Tang - hyperactive Spleen qi def.; Chai Hu Long Gu Mu Li Tang - Heart & Liver fire, phlegm heat; Autoimmune disorders: Reishi Mushroom immune regulator; Xue Fu Zhu Yu Tang - blood stag.; Ge Xia Zhu Yu Wan - blood Stag.; Dan Shen Huo Xue Wan - blood stag. with heat; Dang Gui Si Ni Tang - cold & blood stag.
Back Pain	Back pain: Zhuang Yao Jian Shen - Kid. def.; Liu Wei Di Huang Wan - yin def.; Zuo Gui Wan - yin def.; Fu Gui Ba Wei Wan - Kid. yang def.; You Gui Wan - yang def.; Jian Bu Qing Shen Wan - Kid. def.; San Bi Wan - wind damp with Kid. def.; Kang Gu Zeng Sheng Pian - spondylosis; Shu Jin Huo Xue Wan - wind damp with blood stag.; Shi Lin Tong - renal calculi; Bi Xie Sheng Shi Wan - damp heat; Die Da Zhi Tong Capsules - acute blood stag.; Plaster for Bruise and Analgesic - topical; Porous Capsicum Plaster topical; Gou Pi Gao topical. Back weakness: Jian Bu Qiang Shen Wan - Kid. def.; Hua Tuo Zai Zao Wan - qi & yin def., wind damp; Ba Ji Yin Yang Wan - Kid. yang def.; Zhuang Yao Jian Shen Tablets - Kid. yang def.; Si Jun Zi Tang - Spleen qi def.

Conditions	Formulas w/ TCM Diagnosis
Bacterial Infection	Systemic: Huang Lian Jie Du Tang - damp & toxic heat; Wu Wei Xiao Du Wan - toxic heat; Chuan Xin Lian - toxic heat; Chuan Xin Lian Antiphlogistic Tablets - toxic heat; Bai Hu Tang Wan - yang ming channel syndrome; Liang Ge Wan - yang ming organ syndrome
Bad Breath	Qing Wei San - Stomach heat; Bao He Wan - food stag.; Qi Xing Tea - infants
Belching	Xiang Lian Wan - Stomach heat; Bao He Wan - food stag.; Ping Wei San - phlegm damp; Xiang Sha Yang Wei Wan - qi & damp stag.; Chai Hu Shu Gan Wan - Liver qi stag.; Mu Xiang Shun Qi Wan - qi & damp stag.; Chen Xiang Hua Zi Wan - qi def. with qi blockage
Bells Palsy	Chuan Xiong Cha Tiao Wan - wind cold, acute; Hua Tuo Zai Zao Wan - qi & yin def.; Bu Yang Huan Wu Wan - qi def. with blood stag.; Xiao Shuan Zai Zao Wan; Da Huo Luo Dan; Kang Wei Ling Wan - blood stag., wind; Tong Luo Zhi Tong Tablet - blood def.; Niu Huang Qing Xin Wan - phlegm heat
Bi-Syndrome	Wu Tou Tang, Fu Zi Tang - painful; Gui Zhi Shao Yao Zhi Mu Tang - moving; Juan Bi Tang - fixed; Bai Hu Jia Gui Zhi Tang, Er Miao San - heat; Du Huo Ji Sheng Tang - chronic
Bleeding	General, to stop: Yunnan Paiyao - hemostatic; Raw Tienchi Tablets - hemostatic
Blood in Stool	Huang Tu Tang, Huai Hua San - blood heat
Boils	Pu Ju Xiao Du Yin, Tou Nong San, Wu Wei Xiao Du Yin - toxic heat
Bone Fracture	Chin Gu Tie Shang Wan - blood stag.; Die Da Zhi Tong Capsule - blood stag.; Zheng Gu Shui - topical; Plaster for Bruise and Analgesic - topical
Borborygmi	Ban Xia Xie Xin Tang, Huo Xiang Zheng Qi San, Tong Xie Yao Fang - Spleen def.
Bowel Movement	Run Chang Wan - blood & fluid def.; Wu Ren Wan - blood & fluid def.; Cong Rong Bu Shen Wan - yang def., atonic; Mu Xiang Shun Qi Wan - qi stag., habitual; Chen Xiang Hua Zi Wan - qi stag., qi def.; Da Huang Jiang Zhi Wan - excess; Ching Fei Yi Huo Pien - yang ming syndrome, Lung fire; Da Chai Hu Tang - shao yang/yang ming syndrome; Yang Yin Qing Fei Wan - yin def., dry post febrile
Bronchitis / Bronchiectiasis	Acute: Ching Fei Yi Huo Pien - Lung fire; Sang Ju Yin - wind heat; Sang Xin Tang, Qing Zao Jui Fei Tang - heat & dryness; Qing Qi Hua Tan Wan - phlegm heat; Niu Huang Qing Huo Wan - toxic heat; Huang Lian Jie Du Tang - toxic & damp heat; Xiao Chai Hu Tang - post acute
Bruises	Die Da Zhi Tong Capsule; Chin Gu Tie Shang Wan; Huo Luo Xiao Ling Wan; Yunnan Paiyao; Raw Tienchi Tablets; Zheng Gu Shui; Die Da Tian Qi Yao Jiu - topical
Bruxism (teeth grinding)	Xiao Yao Wan - Liver qi stag.; Jia Wei Xiao Yao San - Liver qi stag.; Chai Hu Shu Gan Wan - Liver qi stag.; An Shen Jie Yu Capsule - qi stag. with shen disturbance
Burns	Ching Wan Hung - topical; Xiao Yan Tang Shang Cream - topical; Sanjin Watermelon Frost - topical
Bursitis	Juan Bi Tang - wind cold damp; Jian Bu Qiang Shen Wan - with Kid. def.; Zheng Gu Shui - topical; Trans Wood Lock Liniment - topical
Cancer Pain	Reishi Mushroom immune regulator; American Ginseng Essence of Chicken; Cordyceps Essence of Chicken; Bu Zhong Yi Qi Tang
Cancer Prevention	Reishi Mushroom immune regulator; American Ginseng Essence of Chicken; Cordyceps Essence of Chicken; Bu Zhong Yi Qi Tang
Candidiasis	Bi Xie Sheng Shi Wan - damp heat; Yu Dai Wan - damp heat, blood def.; Chien Chin Chih Tai Wan - damp heat, blood def.; Bi Xie Fen Zing Wan - damp; Ping Wei San - phlegm damp
Carpal Tunnel Syndrome (CTS)	Wu Yah Shu Qi San - blood stag.; Ge Gen Tang - blood stag.
Cataract	Ming Mu Di Huang Wan - Liver yin def.; Ming Mu Shang Ching Pien - Liver heat, fire; Fu Gui Ba Wei Wan - Kid. yang def.; Pearl Powder
Celiac Disease	Shen Ling Bai Zhu Wan - Spleen qi def.
Cellulitis	Huang Lien Shang Ching Pien - wind heat, toxic heat; Ming Mu Shang Ching Pien - Liver heat, fire; Lien Chiao Pai Tu Pien - wind heat, toxic heat; Wu Wei Xiao Du Wan - toxic heat; Chuan Xin Lian Cream - topical

CONDITIONS & FORMULAS

Conditions	Formulas w/ TCM Diagnosis
Chemotherapy	Weakness following: Cordyceps Essence of Chicken; Shi Quan Da Bu Tang. Hair loss following: Yang Xue Sheng Fa Capsule; Qi Bao Mei Ran Dan; Tangkwei Essence of Chicken. Nausea, vomiting from: Wen Dan Tang; Er Chen Tang; Xiang Sha Liu Jun Zi Tang. Oral following: American Ginseng Essence of Chicken; Yang Yin Qing Fei Wan. To protect bone marrow during: Wu Ji Bai Feng Wan; Cordyceps Essence of Chicken; Reishi Mushroom immune regulator. Weakness following: Cordyceps Essence of Chicken; Shi Quan Da Bu Tang
Chest Pain	Dan Shen Pill - blood stag.; Xin Mai Ling - blood stag.; Guan Xin An Kou Fu Ye - blood stag.; Xue Fu Zhu Yu Tang - blood & qi stag.; Sunho Multi Ginseng Tablets - mild blood stag.; Xiao Xian Xiong Tang, Wei Jing Tang - heat & phlegm
Chlamydia	Fu Yan Qing Tablet - toxic heat; Bi Xie Sheng Shi Wan - damp heat; Chuan Xin Lian Antiphlogistic Tablets - toxic heat
Cholecystitis	Acute: Da Chai Hu Tang - shao yang/yang ming syndrome; Long Dan Xie Gan Tang - Liver fire; Li Dan Tablets - damp heat; Ching Fei Yi Huo Pien - fire; Huang Lian Jie Du Tang - damp & toxic heat; Niu Huang Qing Huo Wan - yang ming syndrome. Chronic: Chai Hu Shu Gan Wan - Liver qi stag.; Shu Gan Wan - Liver qi stag.; Da Chai Hu Tang - shao yang/yang ming syndrome; Qing Gan Li Dan Tablets - damp heat; Li Dan Tablets - damp heat; Jigucao Wan - damp heat
Cholesterol / Triglycerides High	Keep Fit Capsule - phlegm & blood stag.; Bojenmi Chinese Tea; Dan Shen Pill - blood stag.; Raw Tienchi Tablets - blood stag.; Sunho Multi Ginseng Tablets - blood stag.; Reishi Mushroom immune regulator
Chrohn's Disease	Shu Gan Wan - Liver qi stag.; Chai Hu Shu Gan Wan - Liver invading the Spleen; Jia Wei Xiao Yao San - qi stag. with heat; Mu Xiang Shun Qi Wan - qi & damp stag.; Shen Ling Bai Zhu Wan - Spleen qi def.; Xiang Lian Wan - damp heat; Hua Zhi Ling Tablet - damp heat; Zi Sheng Wan - Spleen def. with food stag.; Li Zhong Wan - Spleen yang def.
Chronic Fatigue Syndrome	Xiao Chai Hu Tang - shao yang; Bu Zhong Yi Qi Tang - Spleen qi def.; Gui Pi Tang - Heart & Spleen def.; Xiang Sha Liu Jun Zi Tang - Spleen qi def. with phlegm damp
Circulation (Poor)	Si Ni San - Liver qi stag.; Sunho Multi Ginseng Tablets - qi def., blood stag.; Xin Mai Ling - blood stag.; Dang Gui Si Ni Tang - cold stag. in the channels; Xiao Huo Luo Dan - severe cold stag. in the channels; Bu Yang Huan Wu Wan - qi def., blood stag.; Li Chung Yuen Medical Pills - Spleen yang def.; Fu Gui Ba Wei Wan - Kid. yang def.
Colitis	Acute: Xing Jun San – summer damp; Huo Hsiang Cheng Chi Pien - wind cold with damp; Fu Ke An - damp heat; Tong Xie Yao Fang Wan - Liver Spleen disharmony; Huang Lian Jie Du Tang - damp heat
Common Cold	Gan Mao Ling - general; Ma Huang Tang - wind cold, wheezing; Gui Zhi Tang - wind, postpartum; Ge Gen Tang - wind cold - neck pain; Chuan Xiong Cha Tiao Wan - wind cold, headache; Jing Fang Bai Du Wan, Chong Chi Tang - wind cold/heat; Yin Chiao Chieh Tu Pien, Yin Qiao San, Sang Xing Tang - wind heat; Gan Mao Zhi Ke Chong Ji - tai yang/shao yang; Gan Mao Qing Re Chong Ji - wind heat; Shih San Tai Pao Wan - during pregnancy; Ren Shen Bai Du San - wind cold with qi def.; Xiao Chai Hu Tang - lingering; Jia Jian Wei Rui Tang - yin def.
Conjunctivitis	Yin Qiao San, Yin Chiao Chieh Tu Pien, Xie Ban San, Sang Ju Yin - wind heat; Xie Fe San - Lung & Spleen heat; Ming Mu Shang Ching Pien, Long Dan Xie Gan Tang - Liver fire; Peking Niu Huang Jie Du Pian - toxic heat; Huang Lien Shang Ching Pien - wind heat, toxic heat; Xiao Er Gan Mao Chong Ji - infants; Gan Mao Tea - infants
Constipation	Run Chang Wan, Ji Chuan Jian - blood & fluid def.; Wu Ren Wan - blood & fluid def.; Cong Rong Bu Shen Wan - yang def., atonic; Mu Xiang Shun Qi Wan - qi stag.; Chen Xiang Hua Zi Wan - qi stag., qi def.; Da Huang Jiang Zhi Wan, Ma Zi Ren Wan - excess; Ching Fei Yi Huo Pien - yang ming syndrome, Lung fire; Da Chai Hu Tang - shao yang/yang ming syndrome; Yang Yin Qing Fei Wan - yin def., dry post febrile
Convulsion	Po Lung Yuen Medical Pills - phlegm heat; Wen Dan Tang - phlegm heat; King Fung Powder - phlegm, wind; Li Zhong Wan - yang def., chronic childhood
Coronary Heart Disease (CHD)	Gua Lou Xie Bai Ban Xia Tang - yang obstruction; Dan Shen Yin, Tao Hong Si Wu Tang - blood stag.; Sheng Mai San - qi & yin, fluid def.; Jia Jian Fu Mai Tang, Zhi Gan Cao Tang - blood & yin def.; Su He Xiang Wan - resuscitation
Cough	Acute: Ma Huang Tang - wind cold; Xiao Qing Long Wan - wind cold with congested fluids; Gan Mao Zhi Ke Chong Ji - wind heat; Sang Ju Wan - wind heat; Ching Fei Yi Huo Pien - Lung heat/fire; Qing Qi Hua Tan Wan - phlegm heat; Pi Pa Cough Tea - phlegm heat; Su Zi Jiang Qi Tang - cold phlegm

Conditions	Formulas w/ TCM Diagnosis
Cystitis	Acute: Ba Zheng San, Shi Wei San - damp heat; Qing Re Qu Shi Tea - damp heat; Long Dan Xie Gan Tang - Liver fire, damp heat; Ming Mu Shang Ching Pien - damp heat; Tao Chih Pien - Heart fire; DBD Capsule - severe toxic heat; Chuan Xin Lian Antiphlogistic Tablets - toxic heat; Huang Lian Jie Du Tang - damp & toxic heat
Delirium	Niu Huang Qing Xin Wan - phlegm heat; Niu Huang Qing Huo Wan - yang ming heat; Huang Lian Jie Du Tang - toxic heat
Depression	Chai Hu Shu Gan Tang - Liver qi stag.; Xiao Yao San - qi stag. & blood def.; Tao Hong Si Wu Tang - blood stag., blood def.; Xue Fu Zhu Yu Tang - chronic, blood stag.; Wen Dan Tang - phlegm heat; Xiang Sha Yang Wei Tang - qi & damp stag.
Dermatitis	Acute: Lien Chiao Pai Tu Pien - wind heat, toxic heat; Huang Lian Shang Ching Pien - wind heat, toxic heat; Ming Mu Shang Ching Pien - Liver fire; Xiao Feng Wan - wind damp; Xiao Yan Tang Shang Cream - topical. Chronic: Bi Xie Sheng Shi Wan - damp heat; Dang Gui Yin Zi Wan - blood def. with wind in the skin; Jia Wei Xiao Yao San - qi stag. with heat; Fang Feng Tong Sheng Wan - internal & external heat; Huo Luo Xiao Ling Wan - blood stag.; Pearl Powder - topical; Fu Yin Tai Liniment topical; Xiao Yan Tang Shang Cream - topical
Diabetes	D. Insipidus: Sang Piao Xiao San - Heart & Kid. yang qi def.: D. Mellitus: Yu Quan Wan; Sugarid; Liu Wei Di Huang Wan; Shen Ling Bai Zhu San; Gu Ben Wan; Fu Gui Ba Wei Wan. D. Mellitus: Yu Quan Wan - qi & yin def.; Sugarid; Liu Wei Di Huang Wan - Kid. yin def.; Shen Ling Bai Zhu San - Spleen qi def.; Gu Ben Wan - Stomach & Kid. yin def.; Fu Gui Ba Wei Wan - Kid. yang def.
Diarrhea	Acute: Po Chai Pills - damp heat; Xing Jun San - summer damp; Huo Hsiang Cheng Chi Pien, Wei Ling Tang - wind cold with damp; Ge Gen Tang - wind cold; Bao He Wan - Food stag.; Huang Lian Jie Du Tang - damp or toxic heat; Bo Ying Compound - infantile. Chronic: Shen Ling Bai Zhu San - Spleen qi def.; Tong Xie Yao Fang Wan - Liver invading Spleen; Li Zhong Wan - Spleen yang def.; Zi Sheng Wan - Spleen def. with food stag.; Ba Ji Yin Yang Wan - Spleen & Kid. yang def., cockcrow; Yulin Da Bu Wan - yang def., cockcrow; Healthy Child Tea - infantile
Diverticulitis	Huang Lian Jie Du Tang - damp & toxic heat; Huang Lian Su Tablets - damp heat; Niu Huang Qing Huo Wan - yang ming organ syndrome; Ching Fei Yi Huo Pien - yang ming organ syndrome; Wu Wei Xiao Du Wan - toxic heat; Liang Ge Wan - yang ming organ syndrome; Chuan Xin Lian Antiphlogistic Tablets - toxic heat
Dizziness	Postural, lightheadedness: Ba Zhen Tang - qi & blood def.; Gui Pi Tang - qi & blood def.; Tangkwei Essence of Chicken - qi & blood def., postpartum; Gu Ju Di Huang Wan - Liver Kid. yin def.; Ming Mu Di Huang Wan - Liver & Kid. yin def.; Xiao Chai Hu Tang - shao yang syndrome; Er Xian Wan - Kid. yin & yang def.
Dysentery	Amoebic: Huang Lian Jie Du Tang - damp heat; Huang Lian Su Tablets, Shao Yao Tang, Jing Fang Bai Du San, Ge Gen Qin Lian Tang - damp heat; Chuan Xin Lian Antiphlogistic Tablets - toxic heat; Baby Fat Powder; Wei Ling Tang - Cold & damp; Li Zhong Tang, Tao Hua Tang, Zhen Ren Yang Zang Tang - Cold def. Bacterial: Huang Lian Jie Du Tang - damp heat; Huang Lian Su Tablets - damp heat; Ching Fei Yi Huo Pien - yang ming heat; Chuan Xin Lian Antiphlogistic Tablets - toxic heat
Dysmenorrhea	Gui Zhi Fu Ling Tang - mild blood stag., masses; Tao Hong Si Wu Tang - mild blood stag. with blood def.; Tong Jing Wan - severe blood stag.; Shao Fu Zhu Yu Tang - cold & blood stag., severe; Woo Garm Yuen Medical Pills - blood stag. with cold; Dang Gui Si Ni Tang - cold; Tong Luo Zhi Tong Tablet - blood stag., cold; Xiao Yao San - Liver qi stag.; Tian Tai Wu Yao Wan - cold in Liver channel; Ba Zhen Yi Mu Wan - mild blood def.; Yi Mu Tiao Jing Tablet - blood def. with blood stag.; Shi Xiao San - blood stag.; Shi Quan Da Bu Tang - qi & blood def. with cold; Ba Zhen Tang - qi & blood def.
Dysphagia	Hua Tuo Zai Zao Wan - qi & yin def.; Da Huo Luo Dan; Gu Ben Wan - Stomach & Lung dryness; Ban Xia Hou Po Wan - qi & phlegm stag.
Dysuria	Tong Jing Wan - blood stag.; Yunnan Paiyao - blood stag.; Qian Lie Xian Capsules - damp heat; Tian Tai Wu Yao Wan - cold in Liver channel
Ear Pain	Qing Gan Li Dan Tablets - damp heat; Long Dan Xie Gan Tang - Liver damp heat; Xiao Chai Hu Tang - shao yang; Tong Qiao Huo Xue Tang - blood stag.

CONDITIONS & FORMULAS

FORMULA

Conditions	Formulas w/ TCM Diagnosis
Eczema	General: Lien Chiao Pai Tu Pien - wind, toxic heat; Xiao Feng Wan - wind damp; Bi Xie Sheng Shi Wan - damp heat; Gui Zhi Tang - wind, worse in cold; Dang Gui Yin Zi Wan - blood def. with wind in the skin; Jia Wei Xiao Yao San - qi stag. with heat; Fang Feng Tong Sheng Wan - internal & external heat; Dan Shen Huo Xue Wan - blood stag. with hot blood; Huo Luo Xiao Ling Wan - blood stag.; Eczema Herbal Formula; Chuan Xin Lian Cream - topical; Xiao Yan Tang Shang Cream - topical; Fu Yin Tai Liniment topical; Pearl Powder - topical; Si Wu Tang - blood def. Genital: Long Dan Xie Gan Tang - Liver damp heat; Bi Xie Sheng Shi Wan - damp heat; Zing Re Qu Shi Tea - damp heat; Ke Yin Wan - damp heat; Fu Yin Tai Liniment topical; Xiao Yan Tang Shang Cream - topical
Edema	Ma Huang Tang - wind cold, acute facial; Wu Ling San - Spleen def. with congested fluids; Wu Pi Yin generalized, pregnancy, menopause; Fang Ji Huang Qi Wan - wind; Zhen Wu Tang - Heart & Kid. yang def.; Fu Gui Ba Wei Wan - Kid. yang def.; Bojenmi Chinese Tea - Spleen def.
Ejaculatory Pain	Ba Ji Yin Yang Wan - yang def.; Zhuang Yao Jian Shen - yang def.; Wu Zi Yan Zong Wan - jing def.; Gu Ben Fu Zheng Capsules - yang def; Nan Bao Capsules - yang def.; Zuo Gui Wan - yin def.
Elbow Pain	Fang Feng Tang - excess wind/cold; Shen Tong Zhu Yu Tang - blood stag.
Emphysema	Su Zi Jiang Qi Tang - phlegm damp; Xiao Qing Long Wan - wind cold with congested fluids; Ding Chuan Wan - phlegm heat; Zi Guan Yan Ke Sou Tan Chuan Wan - phlegm damp; Yulin Bu Shen Wan - Lung & Kid. yang def.; Cordyceps Essence of Chicken - yin & yang def.
Endometriosis	Woo Garm Yuen Medical Pills - blood stag., cold; Wen Jing Tang - cold, def., blood stag.; Tong Jing Wan - blood stag., severe; Tao Hong Si Wu Tang - blood stag. with blood def.; Gui Zhi Fu Ling Tang, Shi Xiao San - mild blood stag.; Shao Fu Zhu Yu Tang - blood stag. & cold; Nei Xiao Luo Li Wan - phlegm & blood stag.; Ru Jie Xiao Tablet - qi, blood & phlegm; Xue Fu Zhu Yu Wan - qi & blood stag.; Huo Luo Xiao Ling Wan - blood stag.; Cu Yun Yu Tai Capsules - Kid. yang def.; Ba Zhen Yi Mu Wan - qi & blood def.; Shi Quan Da Bu Tang - qi & blood def. with cold
Energy (Tiredness, Fatigue)	Bu Zhong Yi Qi Tang - Spleen & Lung qi def.; Bu Fei Wan - Lung qi def.; Shi Quan Da Bu Tang - qi & blood def.; Fu Gui Ba Wei Wan - yang def.; Liu Wei Di Huang Wan - yin def.; Panax Ginseng Extractum - qi def.; Sheng Mai San - qi & yin def.; American Ginseng Essence of Chicken - qi & yin def.; Xiao Chai Hu Tang - shao yang syndrome; Ping Wei San - phlegm damp; Wen Dan Tang - phlegm heat
Enuresis	Sang Piao Xiao Wan - Heart & Kid. qi def.; Chin So Ku Ching Wan; San Yuen Medical Pills - Kid. qi def.
Epigastric Pain	Shu Gan Wan - qi stag.; Wei Tong Ding - cold, yang def.; Chai Hu Shu Gan Wan - qi stag.; Dan Shen Yin Wan - blood stag.; Shi Xiao Wan - blood stag.; Qing Wei San - Stomach heat; Xiang Sha Yang Wei Wan - qi & damp stag.; Li Zhong Wan - yang def.; Wei Te Ling - hyperacidity; Bao He Wan - food stag.
Epilepsy	Po Lung Yuen Medical Pills - phlegm heat; Wen Dan Tang, Long Dan Xie Gan Tang - phlegm heat; Chai Hu Long Gu Mu Li Tang - qi stag., phlegm heat, Liver fire; Tian Ma Gou Teng Wan - Liver yang; Tong Qiao Huo Xue Wan - blood stag.; Zuo Gui Wan, He Che Da Zao Wan - Liver & Kidney yin def.
Eye	Weakness of vision: Ming Mu Di Huang Wan - Liver & Kid. yin def.; Ming Mu Capsules - yin & blood def.; Qi Ju Di Huang Wan - Liver & Kid. yin def.; Wu Zi Yan Zong Wan - jing def.; Shou Wu Pian - yin & blood def.; San Yuen Medical Pills - Kid. yang def. Strain from overuse: Ming Mu Di Huang Wan - Liver yin def.; Ming Mu Capsules - yin & blood def.; Qi Ju Di Huang Wan - Liver yin def. Red and sore: Huang Lian Shang Ching Pien - wind heat, toxic heat; Ming Mu Shang Ching Pien - damp heat; Long Dan Xie Gan Tang - Liver fire; Jia Wei Xiao Yao San - qi stag. with heat. Floaters & spots before: Ba Zhen Tang - qi & blood def.; Shi Quan Da Bu Wan - qi & blood def.; Ming Mu Di Huang Wan - Liver yin def.; Ming Mu Capsules - yin & blood def.; Dry, itchy, photophobic: Ming Mu Di Huang Wan - Liver yin def.; Qi Ju Di Huang Wan - Liver yin def.; Si Wu Tang - blood def.
Facial Pain	Chuan Xiong Cha Tiao Wan - wind cold; Xiao Huo Luo Dan - severe cold stag. in channels; Hua Tuo Zai Zao Wan - qi & yin def., wind damp; Kang Wei Ling Wan - blood stag., neuralgic; Tong Luo Zhi Tong Tablets - blood def.; Qing Wei San - Stomach heat

70

FORMULA

Conditions	Formulas w/ TCM Diagnosis
Fatigue	Bu Zhong Yi Qi Tang - Spleen & Lung qi def.; Bu Fei Wan - Lung qi def.; Shi Quan Da Bu Tang, Ba Zhen Tang - qi & blood def.; Fu Gui Ba Wei Wan - yang def.; Dang Gui Bu Xue Tang - blood def.; Liu Wei Di Huang Wan - yin def.; Panax Ginseng Extractum - qi def.; Sheng Mai San - qi & yin def.; American Ginseng Essence of Chicken - qi & yin def.; Xiao Chai Hu Tang - shao yang syndrome; Ping Wei San - phlegm damp; Wen Dan Tang - phlegm heat; Zhi Gan Cao Tang, Tian Wang Bu Xin Dan - Heart yin def.
Fever	Acute excess, high: Ma Huang Tang - wind cold; Yin Qiao San, Yin Chiao Chieh Tu Pien - wind heat; Lien Chiao Pai Tu Pien - wind heat, Warm disease; Huang Lian Jie Du Tang - damp heat, toxic heat; Long Dan Xie Gan Tang - Liver fire; Ching Fei Yi Huo Pien - Lung fire; Bai Hu Tang - yang ming channel syndrome; Niu Huang Qing Huo Wan - yang ming organ syndrome; Pu Ji Xiao Du Wan - Warm disease; King Fung Powder - phlegm heat, infants
Fibroids	Woo Garm Yuen Medical Pills - blood & cold stag.; Gui Zhi Fu Ling Tang - mild blood stag.; Tao Hong Si Wu Tang - blood stag. & blood def.; Tong Jing Wan - blood stag.; Shao Fu Zhu Yu Tang - cold & blood stag.; Xue Fu Zhu Yu Tang - qi & blood stag.; Nei Xiao Luo Li Wan - hard phlegm stag.; Hai Zao Jing Wan - phlegm stag.; Ru Jie Xiao Tablets - qi, phlegm & blood stag.; Ji Sheng Ju He Wan - qi & phlegm stag.; Shi Quan Da Bu Tang - qi & blood def. with cold
Fibromyalgia	Shu Gan Wan - qi stag.; Chai Hu Shu Gan Tang - qi stag.; Xiao Yao San - qi stag.; Shen Tong Zhu Yu Wan - blood stag.; Xue Fu Zhu Yu Tang - qi & blood stag.; Hua Tuo Zai Zao Wan - qi & yin def.; Juan Bi Tang - wind damp; Qu Feng Zhen Tong Capsules - wind cold damp
Flatulence	Bao He Wan - food stag.; Xiang Sha Yang Wei Wan - qi & damp stag. with Spleen def.; Mu Xiang Shun Qi Wan - qi & damp stag.
Flu	Gan Mao Ling - general; Ma Huang Tang - wind cold, wheezing; Gui Zhi Tang - wind, postpartum; Ge Gen Tang - wind cold, neck pain; Chuan Xiong Cha Tiao Wan - wind cold, headache; Jing Fang Bai Du Wan - wind cold/heat; Yin Qiao San, Yin Chiao Chieh Tu Pien - wind heat; Gan Mao Zhi Ke Chong Ji - tai yang/shao yang; Gan Mao Qing Re Chong Ji - wind heat; Shih San Tai Pao Wan - during pregnancy; Ren Shen Bai Du San - wind cold with qi def.; Xiao Chai Hu Tang - lingering
Focus	Concentration: Jian Nao Yi Zhi Capsule - qi def. with blood stag.; Xiang Sha Liu Jun Zi Tang - Spleen def. with phlegm damp; Gui Pi Tang - Heart blood & Spleen qi def.; Ping Wei San - phlegm damp; Wen Dan Tang - phlegm heat; Tian Wang Bu Xin Dan - Heart & Kid. yin def.; Cerebral Tonic Pills - phlegm & Kid. def. Poor memory: Jian Nao Yi Zhi Capsules - qi def., blood stag.; Cerebral Tonic Pills - blood def. & phlegm heat; Gui Pi Tang - qi & blood def.; Tian Wang Bu Xin Dan - Heart & Kid. yin def.; Huan Shao Dan - Heart & Kid. def.; Zhi Gan Cao Tang - Heart qi & blood def.; Bai Zi Yang Xin Wan - general; Wen Dan Tang - phlegm heat; Tong Qiao Huo Xue Tang - blood stag., post traumatic
Food Allergies	Xiang Sha Liu Jun Zi Tang - Spleen def. with phlegm damp; Bao He Wan - food stag.; Xiang Sha Yang Wei Wan - qi & damp stag. with Spleen def.; Shen Ling Bai Zhu Wan - Spleen def.; Li Zhong Wan - Spleen yang def.; Jian Pi Wan - food stag. with Spleen def.; Qi Ju Tea - infants
Food Poisoning	Xing Jun San - summer damp; Huo Hsiang Cheng Chi Pien - damp; Po Chai Pills - damp heat; Shen Chu Cha - damp
Forgetfulness	Gui Pi Tang - blood def.; Jian Nao Yi Zhi Capsules - qi def., blood & phlegm stag.; Bai Zi Yang Xin Wan - blood & yin def.; Cerebral Tonic Pills - phlegm & Kid. def.; Tian Wang Bu Xin Dan - Heart & Kid. yin def.; Liu Wei Di Huang Wan - Kid. yin def.
Fracture	Die Da Zhi Tong Capsules - blood stag.; Huo Luo Xiao Ling Wan - blood stag.; Zheng Gu Shui - topical; Plaster for Bruise and Analgesic - topical
Frostbite	Dang Gui Si Ni Tang - cold in the channels; Gui Zhi Tang - ying wei disharmony; Hua Tuo Zai Zao Wan - qi & yin def.
Fungal Infection	Skin: Bi Xie Sheng Shi Wan - damp heat; Xiao Feng Wan - wind, damp; Xiao Yan Tang Shang Cream - topical; Fu Yin Tai Liniment topical; Hua Tuo Gao topical; Tujin Liniment topical. Intestines: Da Huang Jiang Zhi Wan - damp heat; Huang Lian Jie Du Tang - damp heat. Toes: Hua Tuo Gao topical; Tujin Liniment topical; Xiao Yan Tang Shang Cream - topical
Gall Bladder	Damp heat: Da Chai Hu Tang; Li Dan Tablets; Jigucao Wan; Qing Gan Li Dan Tablets
Gall Stones	Da Chai Hu Tang - damp heat; Qing Gan Li Dan Tablets - damp heat; Li Dan Tablets - damp heat; Mu Xiang Shu Qi Wan - qi & damp stag.; Chai Hu Shu Gan Wan - Liver qi stag.

CONDITIONS & FORMULAS

FORMULA

Conditions	Formulas w/ TCM Diagnosis
Gastritis	Acute: Huang Lian Jie Du Tang - damp heat; Qing Wei San - Stomach heat; Xiang Lian Wan - Stomach heat; Wen Dan Tang - phlegm heat; Xiang Sha Yang Wei Wan - qi & damp stag.; Bao He Wan - food stag.
Gastroenteritis	Acute: Xing Jun San - summer damp; Huo Hsiang Cheng Chi Pien - wind cold with damp; Fu Ke An - damp heat; Po Chai Pills - damp heat; Ping Wei San - phlegm damp; Wu Ling San - Spleen damp; Qi Xing Tea - infants; Ban Xia Xie Xin Tang - cold & heat; San Ren Tang - heat & damp
Gastroesophageal Reflux Disease (GERD)	Xiang Lian Wan - Stomach heat; Wei Te Ling - hyperacidity; Xiang Sha Yang Wei Tang - qi stag.; Chai Hu Shu Gan Tang - Liver qi stag.; Shu Gan Wan - Liver qi stag.; Yi Guan Jian Wan - yin def., qi stag.; Wei Tong Ding - cold, yang def.; Bao He Wan - food stag.; Ping Wei San - phlegm damp; Bo Ying Compound - infants; Qi Xing Tea - infants
Genital Itching	Long Dan Xie Gan Tang - Liver damp heat; Bi Xie Sheng Shi Wan - damp heat; Fu Yan Zing Tablets - toxic & damp heat; Qing Re Qu Shi Tea - toxic & damp heat; Fu Yin Tai Liniment topical; Xiao Yan Tang Shang Cream - topical
Genital Pain	Tian Tai Wu Yao Wan - cold in the Liver channel; Hua Tuo Zai Zao Wan - qi & yin def., wind damp; Long Dan Xie Gan Tang - damp heat; Chai Hu Shu Gan Wan - Liver qi stag.; Ji Sheng Ju He Wan - qi, blood, phlegm stag.; Gui Zhi Fu Ling Tang - blood stag., post surgical
Glaucoma	Acute: Ming Mu Shang Ching Pien - Liver fire; Long Dan Xie Gan Tang - Liver fire. Non-acute: Ming Mu Di Huang Wan - Liver yin def.; Qi Ju Di Huang Wan - Liver yin def.
Goiter	Hai Zao Jing Wan, Dao Tan Tang - phlegm; Nei Xiao Luo Li Wan - hard phlegm
Gonorrhea	Er Miao San, Bi Xie Fen Qing Yin - damp heat
Gout	Huang Lian Jie Du Tang - damp heat; Xuan Bi Tang - damp heat; Fang Feng Tong Sheng Wan - internal & external excess heat; Tiger Balm - topical
Gums	Bleeding Gums: Qing Wei San - Stomach heat; Huang Lien Shang Ching Pien - wind heat, toxic heat; Xue Fu Zhu Yu Tang - blood stag.; Da Bu Yin Wan - yin def.; Gui Pi Tang - qi def.; Superior Sore Throat Powder - topical
Hair Loss	Yang Xue Sheng Fa Capsules - blood & yin def., postpartum; Qi Bao Mei Ran Dan - blood & yin def., postpartum; Tangkwei Essence of Chicken - blood & yin def., postpartum; Deer Velvet - jing def.; Shou Wu Chih - blood & yin def.; Shou Wu Pian - blood def.; You Gui Wan - yang def.; Zuo Gui Wan - yin def.; Tong Qiao Huo Xue Wan - blood stag.
Halitosis	Qing Wei San - Stomach heat; Bao He Wan - food stag.; Qi Xing Tea - infants
Hangover	Bao Ji Pills - damp heat; Po Chai Pills - damp heat; Headache and Dizziness Reliever; Shen Chu Cha; Huang Lian Jie Du Tang - damp heat
Headache	Acute: Tian Ma Tou Tong Capsules - cold wind, yang rising; Chuan Xiong Cha Tiao Wan, Wu Zhu Yu Tang - wind cold; Zhen Gan Xi Feng Wan - Liver yang rising, Liver wind; Tian Ma Gou Teng Yin - Liver yang rising; Qu Feng Zhen Tong Capsules - wind cold damp; Tong Luo Zhi Tong Tablets - blood def., blood stag.; Long Dan Xie Gan Tang - Liver fire; Jia Wei Xiao Yao San - Liver qi stag. with heat; Yan Hu Suo Zhi Tong Wan - analgesic; Ju Hua Cha Tiao San, Huang Lian Shang Qing Wan - wind heat; Da Bu Yuan Jian, You Gui Wan - Kidney def.; Ba Zhen Tang - qi & blood def.; Ban Xia Ba Zhu Tian Ma Tang - phlegm; Tong Qiao Huo Xue Tang - blood stag.
Hearing Loss	Er Long Zuo Ci Wan - Kid. yin def.; Zuo Gui Wan - Kid. yin def.; Fu Gui Ba Wei Wan - Kid. yang def.; You Gui Wan - Kid. yang def.; Deer Velvet - jing def.; Huan Shao Dan - Heart & Kid. qi yang def.; Tong Qiao Huo Xue Wan - blood stag.
Heel pain	Heel spur: Kang Gu Zeng Sheng Pian
Hemiplegia	Bu Yang Huan Wu Wan - qi def., blood stag.; Xiao Shuan Zai Zao Wan; Raw Tienchi Tablets - blood stag.; Sunho Multi Ginseng Tablets - blood stag.; Hua Tuo Zai Zao Wan - qi & yin def.; Xiao Huo Luo Dan - cold, phlegm & blood stag. in the channels; Da Huo Luo Dan - Kid. def.
Hemorrhoids	Hua Zhi Ling Tablets - damp heat, blood stag.; Fargelin for Piles damp heat; Huai Jiao Wan - Intestinal wind; Bu Zhong Yi Qi Tang - sinking Spleen qi; Gui Pi Tang - Spleen qi def.; Hemorrhoids Ointment topical; Ching Wan Hung - topical; Xiao Yan Tang Shang Cream - topical

FORMULA

Conditions	Formulas w/ TCM Diagnosis
Hepatitis	Acute: Long Dan Xie Gan Tang - Liver damp heat; Li Dan Tablets - damp, damp heat; Ban Lan Gen Chong Ji - toxic heat; Chuan Xin Lian Antiphlogistic Tablets - toxic heat; Herba Abri Fruticulosi Beverage damp heat; Xi Huang Cao damp heat. Chronic: Xiao Chai Hu Tang - plus Jigucao Wan; Da Chai Hu Tang - damp heat; Chai Hu Shu Gan Wan - Liver qi stag.; Shu Gan Wan - Liver qi stag.; Yi Guan Jian Wan - Liver yin def. with qi stag.; Qing Gan Li Dan Tablets - damp heat; Xue Fu Zhu Yu Tang - blood stag.; Sunho Multi Ginseng Tablets - blood stag.; Herba Abri Fruticulosi Beverage; Xi Huang Cao; Reishi Mushroom immune regulator. Hepatitis C: Xiao Chai Hu Tang - plus Jigucao Wan; Bu Zhong Yi Qi Tang - Spleen qi def.; Yang Ying Wan - qi & blood def.; Yi Guan Jian Wan - Liver yin def. with qi stag.; Qi Ju Di Huang Wan - Liver yin def.; Reishi Mushroom immune regulator
Hernia	Hiatus: Bu Zhong Yi Qi Tang - Spleen qi def.; Li Zhong Wan - Spleen yang def. Inguinal: Bu Zhong Yi Qi Tang - Spleen qi def.; Tian Tai Wu Yao Wan - cold in Liver channel
Herpes (Genital)	Acute: Bi Xie Sheng Shi Wan - damp heat; Long Dan Xie Gan Tang - Liver damp heat; Chuan Xin Lian Antiphlogistic Tablets - toxic heat; Chuan Xin Lian toxic heat; Fu Yan Qing Tablets - toxic & damp heat. Recurrent: Bi Xie Sheng Shi Wan - damp heat; Bi Xie Fen Qing Wan - damp; Chuan Xin Lian Antiphlogistic Tablets - toxic heat; Chuan Xin Lian - toxic heat
Herpes (Oral)	Lien Chiao Pai Tu Pien - wind heat, toxic heat; Peking Niu Huang Jie Du Pian - toxic heat; Huang Lien Shang Ching Pien - wind heat, toxic heat; Ban Lan Gen Chong Ji - toxic heat; Chuan Xin Lian Antiphlogistic Tablets - toxic heat; Chuan Xin Lian - toxic heat
Herpes Zoster	Lien Chiao Pai Tu Pien - wind heat, toxic heat; Long Dan Xie Gan Tang - damp heat, Liver fire; Chuan Xin Lian Antiphlogistic Tablets - toxic heat; Chuan Xin Lian - toxic heat; Bi Xie Sheng Shi Wan - damp heat; Ban Lan Gen Chong Ji - toxic heat; Superior Sore Throat Powder - topical
Hiccup	Wei Tong Ding - cold, yang def.; Bao He Wan - food stag.; Xiang Sha Yang Wei Wan - qi & damp stag.
Hip pain	Qing Gan Li Dan Tablets - Gallbladder channel dysfunction; Zhuang Yao Jian Shen - yang def.; Juan Bi Tang - wind cold damp; Shen Tong Zhu Yu Wan - blood stag.; Xuan Bi Tang - damp heat
HIV	Cordyceps Essence of Chicken - Lung & Kid. yang qi & yin def.; Reishi Mushroom
Hordeolum (Sty)	Huang Lien Shang Ching Pien - wind heat, toxic heat; Ming Mu Shang Ching Pien - Liver fire; Peking Niu Huang Jie Du Pian - toxic heat; Huang Lien Shang Ching Pien - wind heat, toxic heat
Hot Flushes/Flashes	Er Xian Wan - Kid. yin & yang def.; Da Bu Yin Wan - Kid. yin def.; Zhi Bai Ba Wei Wan - Kid. yin def.; Geng Nian Ling yin & yang def.; Jia Wei Xiao Yao San - qi stag. with heat; Kun Bao Wan - yin def. with yang rising; Tong Ren Wu Ji Bai Feng Wan - blood def., postpartum
Hyperglycemia	Sugarid; Yu Quan Wan - qi & yin def.; Liu Wei Di Huang Wan - Kid. yin def.; Panax Ginseng Extractum - qi & yin def.; American Ginseng Essence of Chicken - qi & yin def.
Hypertension	General: Zhen Gan Xi Feng Wan - Liver yang rising, Liver wind; Tian Ma Gou Teng Yin - Liver yang rising; Tian Ma Wan - yin def., yang rising; Yang Yin Jiang Ya Wan - yang rising; Fu Fang Jiang Ya Capsules - yang rising; Qi Ju Di Huang Wan - Liver yin def.; Chai Hu Long Gu Mu Li Tang, Long Dan Xie Gan Tang - Liver fire, phlegm heat; Ban Xia Bai Zhu Tian Ma Tang - wind phlegm; Huang Lian Jie Du Tang - damp heat; Xue Fu Zhu Yu Tang - qi & blood stag.; Da Chai Hu Tang - shao yang/yang ming syndrome; Er Xian Tang - yin & yang def.
Hyperthyroidism	Tian Wang Bu Xin Dan - Heart yin def.; Zhi Bai Ba Wei Wan - Kid. yin def.; Er Xian Wan - yin & yang def.; Da Bu Yin Wan - yin def. with heat; Zhi Gan Cao Tang - Heart qi & yin def.; Chai Hu Long Gu Mu Li Tang - Liver fire, phlegm heat; Long Dan Xie Gan Tang - Liver fire; Nei Xiao Luo Li Wan - phlegm heat
Hypochondriac Pain	Shu Gan Wan - qi & blood stag.; Xiao Chai Hu Tang - shao yang; Chai Hu Shu Gan Tang, Zuo Jin Wan - Liver qi stag.; Xue Fu Zhu Yu Tang, Xuan Fu Hua Tang - blood stag.; Long Dan Xie Gan Tang - damp heat; Li Dan Tablets - damp heat; Jigucao Wan - chronic hepatitis
Hypoglycemia	Si Jun Zi Tang - Spleen qi def.; Xiang Sha Liu Jun Zi Tang - Spleen qi def. with damp; Shen Ling Bai Zhu Wan - Spleen qi def.; Bu Zhong Yi Qi Tang - Spleen qi def.
Hypotension	Bu Zhong Yi Qi Tang - Spleen qi def.
Hypothyroidism	Fu Gui Ba Wei Wan, Jin Gui Shen Qi Wan - Kid. yang def.; You Gui Wan - Kid. yang def.; Zhen Wu Tang - Heart & Kid. yang def.
Hysteria	Chai Hu Long Gu Mu Li Tang - Liver fire, phlegm heat; Gan Mai Da Zao Tang

CONDITIONS & FORMULAS

Conditions	Formulas w/ TCM Diagnosis
Immunodeficiency	Bu Zhong Yi Qi Tang - Spleen & Lung qi def.; Reishi Mushroom immune regulator; Tong Luo Zhi Tong Tablets - blood def.; Deer Antler and Ginseng qi & jing def.; Yu Ping Feng San - wei qi def.; Sheng Mai San - qi & yin def.; Cordyceps Essence of Chicken - qi & yang def.; American Ginseng Essence of Chicken - qi & yin def.; Panax Ginseng Extractum - qi def.
Impotence	Gu Ben FGu Ben Fu Zheng Capsules - Kid. yang def.; Kang Wei Ling Wan - blood stag.; Zi Shen Da Bu Capsules - Kid. yang def.; Nan Bao Capsules - yang def.; Fu Gui Ba Wei Wan - Kid. yang def.; Gui Pi Tang - Heart & Spleen def.; Chai Hu Shu Gan Tang - Liver qi stag.; Wu Zi Yan Zong Wan - jing def.; Deer Velvet - jing def.; Deer Antler and Ginseng qi & jing def.
Incontinence	Excessive/frequent/nocturnal/incontinence of: Ba Ji Yin Yang Wan - yang def.; Zi Shen Da Bu Capsules - Kid. yang def.; Fu Gui Ba Wei Wan - yang def.; Yulin Da Bu Wan - Kid. yang def.; Zhuang Yao Jian Shen - yang def.; Chin So Ku Ching Wan - astringent; San - Yuen Medical Pills - Kid. def. & astringent; Bu Zhong Yi Qi Tang - sinking qi, bladder prolapse, postpartum; Bu Yang Huan Wu Wan - qi def., blood stag., post stroke. Scanty (anuria): Wu Ling San - tai yang fu syndrome; Fu Gui Ba Wei Wan - Kid. yang def.; Zhen Wu Tang - Heart & Kid. yang def. Difficult: Fu Gui Ba Wei Wan - yang def.; Ba Zheng San - damp heat; Xue Fu Zhu Yu Tang - blood stag.; Prostate Gland Pills - damp heat; Qian Lie Xian Capsules - damp heat
Indigestion	Bao He Wan - food stag.; Jian Pi Wan - food stag. during pregnancy; Ping Wei San - cold damp; Zi Sheng Wan - food stag. with Spleen def.; Mu Xiang Shun Qi Wan - qi & damp stag.; Li Zhong Wan - Spleen yang def.; Wei Tong Ding - cold; Xiang Lian Wan - Stomach heat; Xiang Sha Yang Wei Tang - qi & damp stag.; Shu Gan Wan - Liver Spleen disharmony; Wei Te Ling antacid
Infertility - All	Female: Tiao Jing Cu Yun Wan - yang def., weak progesterone phase; Cu Yun Yu Tai Capsules - yang def., weak progesterone phase; Wu Ji Bai Feng Wan - blood & yang def.; Ba Zhen Tang - qi & blood def.; Shi Quan Da Bu Tang - qi & blood def. with cold; Gui Pi Tang - Heart & Spleen def.; Wen Jing Tang - cold & def., blood stag.; You Gui Wan - Kid. yang def.; Zuo Gui Wan - Kid. yin def.; Deer Velvet - jing def.; Lu Rong Jiao - jing def.; Gui Zhi Fu Ling Tang - blood stag., masses; Tao Hong Si Wu Tang - blood def., blood stag., masses; Hai Zao Jing Wan - polycystic ovaries; Shao Yao Gan Cao Wan - polycystic ovaries
Infertility - Male	Male: Wu Zi Yan Zong Wan - jing def.; Gu Ben Fu Zheng Capsules - yang def.; Zi Shen Da Bu Capsules - yang def.; Gui Zhi Fu Ling Tang - blood stag.
Influenza	Gan Mao Ling - wind; Yin Qiao San, Yin Chiao Chieh Tu Pien - wind heat; Ma Huang Tang - wind cold; Jing Fang Bai Du Wan - wind cold damp; Chuan Xiong Cha Tiao Wan - wind cold damp; Gan Mao Qing Re Chong Ji - wind heat; Gan Mao Zhi Ke Chong Ji - tai yang/shao yang syndrome; Gui Zhi Tang - persistent, postpartum; Shih San Tai Pao Wan - during pregnancy
Insomnia	Gui Pi Tang - Heart & Spleen def.; Tian Wang Bu Xin Dan - Heart yin def.; Wen Dan Tang - phlegm heat; An Shen Bu Xin Wan - yang rising; Tao Chih Pien - Heart fire; Xue Fu Zhu Yu Tang - qi & blood stag., chronic refractory; An Shen Jie Yu Capsules - qi stag., premenstrual; Bao He Wan - food stag.; Qi Xing Tea - children; Long Dan Xie Gan Tang - Liver fire
Irritability	Chai Hu Shu Gan Tang - qi stag.; Chai Hu Long Gu Mu Li Tang - Liver fire, phlegm heat; Jia Wei Xiao Yao San - qi stag. with heat; Long Dan Xie Gan Tang - Liver fire; Fu Gui Ba Wei Wan - Kid. yang def.; Kun Bao Wan - Kid. yin def.
Irritable Bowel Syndrome (IBS)	Diarrhea predominant: Tong Xie Yao Fang Wan - Liver invading Spleen; Chai Hu Shu Gan Tang - Liver invading Spleen; Xiao Yao San - Liver qi stag.; Zi Sheng Wan - qi def. & food stag. Constipation predominant: Mu Xiang Shun Qi Wan - qi & food stag.
Jaundice	Long Dan Xie Gan Tang - damp heat; Qing Gan Li Dan Tablets - damp heat; Da Chai Hu Tang - damp heat; Li Dan Tablets - damp heat, blood stag.; Jigucao Wan - damp heat, blood stag.; Ge Xia Zhu Yu Wan - blood stag.
Jet Lag	Xiao Chai Hu Tang
Jock Itch	Hua Tuo Gao; Tujin Liniment; Bi Xie Sheng Shi Wan - damp heat; Bi Xie Fen Qing Wan - Spleen damp
Knee pain	Fang Ji Huang Qi Wan, Fu Yuan Huo Xue Tang - wind damp, qi def.; Jian Bu Qing Shen Wan - Kid. def.; Zhuang Yao Jian Shen Tablets - Kid. yang def.; Du Huo Ji Sheng Tang - wind damp with Kid. def.; Xiao Huo Luo Dan - severe cold; Fu Gui Ba Wei Wan - Kid. yang def.; Zuo Gui Wan - Kid. yin def.; Xuan Bi Tang - damp heat; Tiger Balm topical; Plaster for Bruise and Analgesic - topical; Porous Capsicum Plaster topical; Gou Pi Gao
Labor Difficult	Bu Zhong Yi Qi Tang - qi def.; Ba Zhen Yi Mu Wan - qi & blood def.; Tao Hong Si Wu Tang - blood def., blood stag.

FORMULA

Conditions	Formulas w/ TCM Diagnosis
Labor Induced	Ping Wei San - dispersing
Lactation Insufficiency	Tangkwei Essence of Chicken - qi & blood def.; Bai Feng Wan - qi & blood def.; Shi Quan Da Bu Wan - qi & blood def. with cold
Lactose Intolerance	Tangkwei Essence of Chicken qi & blood def.; Bai Feng Wan - qi & blood def.; Shi Quan Da Bu Wan - qi & blood def. with cold
Leaky Gut Syndrome	Shen Ling Bai Zhu Wan - Spleen qi def.; Xiang Sha Yang Wei Wan - Spleen qi def. with qi stag.; Xiang Sha Liu Jun Zi Tang - Spleen qi def. with phlegm damp; So Hup Yuen Medical Pills - gu syndrome; Li Zhong Wan - Spleen yang def.
Leukorrhea	White mucoid watery: Shen Ling Bai Zhu Wan - Spleen damp; Xiang Sha Liu Jun Zi Tang - Spleen def. with phlegm damp; Cu Yun Yu Tai Capsules - yang def., cold; Bi Xie Fen Qing Wan - Kid. def., damp; Ba Ji Yin Yang Wan - Kid. yang def.; Bai Feng Wan - qi & blood def. Yellow malodorous: Yu Dai Wan - damp heat; Bi Xie Sheng Shi Wan, Er Miao San, Jia Wei Er Miao San - damp heat; Long Dan Xie Gan Tang - Liver damp heat; Fu Yan Qing Tablets - toxic heat; Chien Chin Chih Tai Wan - damp heat with def.
Libido	Cu Yun Yu Tai Capsules - yang def., cold; Tiao Jing Cu Yun Wan - yang def., cold; You Gui Wan - Kid. yang def.; Gu Ben Fu Zheng Capsules - yang def.; Qian Lie Xian Capsules - damp heat
Lin (Dysuria) Syndrome	UTI: Ba Zheng San - damp heat; Long Dan Xie Gan Tang - Liver fire, damp heat; Bi Xie Sheng Shi Wan - damp heat; Qing Re Qu Shi Tea - damp heat; Ming Mu Shang Ching Pien - damp heat; Huang Lian Su Tablets - toxic heat, damp heat; Fu Yan Qing Tablets - damp heat; Tao Chih Pien - Heart fire; DBD Capsules - severe toxic heat; Ke Yin Wan - damp; Chuan Xin Lian Antiphlogistic Tablets - toxic heat; Qi Xing Tea - children
Liver Cirrhosis	Shu Gan Wan - qi stag.; Xiao Yao Wan - qi stag., blood def., early; Xue Fu Zhu Yu Tang - blood stag.; Sunho Multi Ginseng Tablets - blood stag., qi def.; Yi Guan Jian Wan - Liver yin def., qi stag.; Ge Xia Zhu Yu Wan - blood stag., severe; Huo Luo Xiao Ling Wan - blood stag., severe
Lockjaw	Su He Xiang Wan, Yu Zhen San - wind & phlegm
Low back pain	Lower back pain: Zhuang Yao Jian Shen - Kid. def.; Liu Wei Di Huang Wan - yin def.; Zuo Gui Wan - yin def.; Fu Gui Ba Wei Wan - Kid. yang def.; You Gui Wan - yang def.; Jian Bu Qing Shen Wan - Kid. def.; San Bi Wan - wind damp with Kid. def.; Kang Gu Zeng Sheng Pian - spondylosis; Shu Jin Huo Xue Wan - wind damp with blood stag.; Shi Lin Tong - renal calculi; Bi Xie Sheng Shi Wan - damp heat; Die Da Zhi Tong Capsules - acute blood stag.; Plaster for Bruise and Analgesic - topical; Porous Capsicum Plaster topical; Gou Pi Gao topical. Back weakness: Jian Bu Qiang Shen Wan - Kid. def.; Hua Tuo Zai Zao Wan - qi & yin def., wind damp; Ba Ji Yin Yang Wan - Kid. yang def.; Zhuang Yao Jian Shen Tablets - Kid. yang def.; Si Jun Zi Tang - Spleen qi def
Lymphadenitis	Acute: Pu Ji Xiao Du Wan - Lung & Stomach heat; Peking Niu Huang Jie Du Pian - toxic heat; Lien Chiao Pai Tu Pien - wind heat, toxic heat; Chuan Xin Lian Antiphlogistic Tablets - toxic heat. Chronic: Nei Xiao Luo Li Wan - hard phlegm; Hai Zao Jing Wan - phlegm accumulation; Xiao Chai Hu Tang - lingering pathogen in shao yang; Xiang Sha Liu Jun Zi Tang - chronic with Spleen def. & phlegm; Bo Ying Compound - infants
Malaria	Xiao Chai Hu Tang - shao yang; Da Chai Hu Tang - shao yang/yang ming; Ping Wei San - phlegm damp; Ge Xia Zhu Yu Wan - blood stag.
Malignancy	Reishi Mushroom immune regulator; American Ginseng Essence of Chicken; Cordyceps Essence of Chicken; Bu Zhong Yi Qi Tang
Malnutrition/ Malabsorption	Shen Ling Bai Zhu Wan - Spleen qi def.; Li Zhong Wan - Spleen yang def.; Xiang Sha Liu Jun Zi Tang - Spleen qi def. with damp; Xiang Sha Yang Wei Wan - Spleen qi def. with qi stag.; Ping Wei San - phlegm damp
Mania	An Gong Niu Huang Wan, Chai Hu Long Gu Mu Li Tang - Liver fire, phlegm heat; Xue Fu Zhu Yu Tang - yin & fire
Manic Depressive Illness	Chai Hu Long Gu Mu Li Tang - Liver fire, phlegm heat, qi stag.
Masses	Woo Garm Yuen Medical Pills - blood & cold stag.; Gui Zhi Fu Ling Tang - mild blood stag.; Tao Hong Si Wu Tang - blood stag. & blood def.; Tong Jing Wan - blood stag.; Shao Fu Zhu Yu Tang - cold & blood stag.; Xue Fu Zhu Yu Tang - qi & blood stag.; Nei Xiao Luo Li Wan - hard phlegm stag.; Hai Zao Jing Wan - phlegm stag.; Ru Jie Xiao Tablets - qi, phlegm & blood stag.; Ji Sheng Ju He Wan - qi & phlegm stag.; Shi Quan Da Bu Tang - qi & blood def. with cold

CONDITIONS & FORMULAS

Conditions	Formulas w/ TCM Diagnosis
Mastitis	Acute: Xiao Chai Hu Tang + Chuan Xin Lian Antiphlogistic Tablets; Xiao Chai Hu Tang + Wu Wei Xiao Du Yin; Lien Chiao Pai Tu Pien - toxic heat. Chronic or recurrent after antibiotics: Xiang Sha Liu Jun Zi Tang - Spleen def. with phlegm; Li Zhong Wan - Spleen yang def.
Measles	Ge Gen Tang - wind cold, early stage of; Yin Qiao San, Yin Chiao Chieh Tu Pien - wind heat, toxic heat; Lien Chiao Pai Tu Pien - wind heat, toxic heat; Ban Lan Gen Chong Ji - toxic heat; Bai Hu Tang Wan - yang ming syndrome, high fever; Liang Ge Wan - Lung & Stomach heat; Xiao Er Gan Mao Chong Ji
Memory	Concentration: Jian Nao Yi Zhi Capsule - qi def. with blood stag.; Xiang Sha Liu Jun Zi Tang - Spleen def. with phlegm damp; Gui Pi Tang - Heart blood & Spleen qi def.; Ping Wei San - phlegm damp; Wen Dan Tang - phlegm heat; Tian Wang Bu Xin Dan - Heart & Kid. yin def.; Cerebral Tonic Pills - phlegm & Kid. def. Poor memory: Jian Nao Yi Zhi Capsules - qi def., blood stag.; Cerebral Tonic Pills - blood def. & phlegm heat; Gui Pi Tang - qi & blood def.; Tian Wang Bu Xin Dan - Heart & Kid. yin def.; Huan Shao Dan - Heart & Kid. def.; Zhi Gan Cao Tang - Heart qi & blood def.; Bai Zi Yang Xin Wan - general; Wen Dan Tang - phlegm heat; Tong Qiao Huo Xue Wan - blood stag., post traumatic
Meniere's Disease	Ban Xia Bai Zhu Tian Ma Tang - wind phlegm; Zhen Wu Tang Wan - yang def.; Er Long Zuo Ci Wan - Liver & Kid. yin def.; Wen Dan Tang - phlegm heat
Menopausal Syndrome	Kun Bao Wan - Kid. yin def.; Er Xian Wan - yin & yang def.; Geng Nian Ling yin & yang def.; Zhi Bai Ba Wei Wan - Kid. yin def.; Tian Wang Bu Xin Dan - Heart & Kid. yin def.; Da Bu Yin Wan - yin def., severe heat; Gan Mai Da Zao Tang
Menorrhagia	Yunnan Paiyao - hemostatic; Raw Tienchi Tablets - hemostatic; Gui Pi Tang - Spleen qi def.; Tao Hong Si Wu Tang - blood stag., blood def.; Si Wu Tang + Huang Lian Jie Du Tang - hot blood with blood def.; Jia Wei Xiao Yao San - Liver qi stag. with heat; Li Zhong Wan - Spleen yang def.
Menstrual Amount	Scanty: Ba Zhen Tang - qi & blood def.; Shi Quan Da Bu Tang - qi & blood def.; Bai Feng Wan - qi & blood def.; Tao Hong Si Wu Tang - blood stag. with blood def.; Shao Fu Zhu Yu Tang - blood stag., cold. Prolonged: Cu Yun Yu Tai Capsules - yang def.; Tiao Jing Cu Yun Wan - yang def.; Woo Garm Yuen Medical Pills - blood stag. with cold & blood def.; Tao Hong Si Wu Tang - blood stag. with blood def.; Ba Zhen Tang - qi & blood def.; Shi Quan Da Bu Tang - qi & blood def., with cold
Menstrual Duration - Menorrhagia	Prolonged: Cu Yun Yu Tai Capsules - yang def.; Tiao Jing Cu Yun Wan - yang def.; Woo Garm Yuen Medical Pills - blood stag. with cold & def.; Tao Hong Si Wu Tang - blood stag. with blood def.; Ba Zhen Tang - qi & blood def.; Shi Quan Da Bu Wan - qi & blood def., with cold
Menstrual Irregularity	Irregular: Si Wu Tang - blood def.; Xiao Yao San - Liver qi stag.; Jia Wei Xiao Yao San - Liver qi stag. with heat; Ba Zhen Tang - qi & blood def.; Bai Feng Wan - qi & blood def.; Wu Ji Bai Feng Wan - qi, blood & yang def.; Shen Ling Bai Zhu San - Liver & Spleen disharmony
Menstruation (Disorder During Periods)	Early: Dan Zhi Xaio Yao San - blood heat; Gui Pi Tang, Bu Zhong Qi Yi Tang - qi def.; Delayed: Wen Jing Tang - cold & blood stag.; Ren Shen Yang Ying Tang - blood def.; Jia Wei Wu Yao Tang - qi stag.; Tao Hong Si Wu Tang - blood stag.; Prolonged: Gui Pi Tang - qi def.; Gu Jing Wan - blood heat
Miscarriage	Habitual: You Gui Wan - Kid. yang def.; Zuo Gui Wan - Kid. yin def.; Cu Yun Yu Tai Capsules - yang def.; Tiao Jing Cu Yun Wan - yang def.; Ba Zhen Tang - qi & blood def.; Bu Zhong Yi Qi Tang - sinking Spleen qi. Threatened: Shih San Tai Pao Wan
Mood Swing	Gan Mai Da Zao Tang; Chai Hu Shu Gan Wan - qi stag.; Xiao Yao Wan - qi stag., blood def.; Xue Fu Zhu Yu Tang - qi & blood stag.; Kun Bao Wan - yang def.
Morning Sickness	Zi Sheng Wan - Spleen def., food & damp stag.; Liu Jun Zi Wan - Spleen def. with phlegm damp; Xiang Sha Liu Jun Zi Tang - Spleen def. with phlegm damp & Qi stag.; Er Chen Tang - phlegm damp; Wen Dan Tang - phlegm heat; Shih San Tai Pao Wan
Motion Sickness	Xing Jun San - damp; Huo Hsiang Cheng Chi Pien - damp; Er Chen Tang - phlegm; White Flower Embrocation
Mucous	Er Chen Tang - phlegm damp; Wen Dan Tang - phlegm heat; Liu Jun Zi Wan - Spleen def. with phlegm damp; Xiang Sha Lu Jun Wan - Spleen def. with phlegm damp & qi stag.; Orange Peel Powder - phlegm
Multiple Sclerosis	Bu Zhong Yi Qi Tang - Spleen qi def.; Hua Tuo Zai Zao Wan - qi & yin def.; Bu Yang Huan Wu Wan - qi def., blood stag.; You Gui Wan - Kid. yang def.; Niu Huang Qing Xin Wan - phlegm heat

Conditions	Formulas w/ TCM Diagnosis
Muscle Tension	Strain: Die Da Zhi Tong Capsules - blood stag. acute; Zheng Gu Shui - topical; Trans Wood Lock Liniment topical. Muscular pain: Shao Yao Gan Cao Wan - antispasmodic; Jing Fang Bai Du Wan - wind cold; Xiao Yao San - Liver qi stag., blood def.; Shu Gan Wan - Liver qi stag.; Xing Jun San - summer damp, acute; Huo Hsiang Cheng Chi Pien - wind cold with damp, acute; Trans Wood Lock Liniment - topical; Po Sum On Medicated Oil - topical
Myasthenia Gravis	Bu Zhong Yi Qi Tang - Spleen qi def.; Huao Tuo Zai Zao Wan - qi & yin def.; Bu Yang Huan Wu Wan - qi def., blood stag.; Xiao Huo Luo Dan - severe cold in the channels; You Gui Wan - Kid. yang def.
Myopia	Ming Mu Di Huang Wan - Liver & Kid. yin def.; Ming Mu Capsules - yin & blood def.; Qi Ju Di Huang Wan - Liver & Kid. yin def.
Nasal Bleeding	Yunnan Paiyao - hemostatic; Niu Huang Qing Huo Wan - toxic heat; Huang Lian Jie Du Tang - Stomach heat
Nausea	Er Chen Tang - phlegm damp; Wen Dan Tang - phlegm heat; Ping Wei San - phlegm damp; Wen Tong Ding - yang def., cold; Xiao Chai Hu Tang - shao yang syndrome; Xing Chai Hu Tang Wan - shao yang syndrome; Xing Jun San - summer damp; Huo Hsiang Cheng Chi Pien - wind cold with damp
Neck Pain	Neck & upper back: Ge Gen Tang - wind cold; Headache and Dizziness Reliever; Chuan Xiong Cha Tiao Wan - wind cold; Xiao Yao San - Liver qi stag.; Ba Zhen Tang - qi & blood def.; Hua Tuo Zai Zao Wan - qi & yin def., wind damp
Nephritis (Acute)	Acute: Ma Huang Tang - wind cold; Fang Ji Huang Qi Wan - wind, qi def.; Ba Zheng San - damp heat; Qing Re Qu Shi Tea - damp heat
Nephritis (Chronic)	Chronic: Zhi Bai Ba Wei Wan - Kid. yin def. with heat; Liu Wei Di Huang Wan - Kid. yin def.; Fu Gui Ba Wei Wan - Kid. yang def.; Zhen Wu Tang Wan - Heart yang def.; Bi Xie Fen Qing Wan - Kid. def. with damp
Neuralgia	Facial, trigeminal: Chuan Xiong Cha Tiao Wan - wind cold; Kang Wei Ling Wan - wind, blood stag.; Xue Fu Zhu Yu Wan - qi & blood stag.; Huo Luo Xiao Ling Wan - blood stag.; Hua Tuo Zai Zao Wan - qi & yin def., wind damp; Qing Wei San - Stomach heat; Xiao Huo Luo Dan - severe cold; Tong Luo Zhi Tong Tablets - blood stag., def.; Yan Hu Suo Zhi Tong Wan - blood stag.; Shao Yao Gan Cao Wan - antispasmodic. Intercostal: Shu Gan Wan - Liver qi stag.; Xiao Chai Hu Tang - shao yang syndrome; Xue Fu Zhu Yu Wan - qi & blood stag.; Long Dan Xie Gan Tang - damp heat, Liver fire; Yi Guan Jian Wan - Liver yin def., qi stag.; Tong Luo Zhi Tong Tablets - blood stag., def.; Yan Hu Suo Zhi Tong Wan - blood stag.; Shao Yao Gan Cao Wan - antispasmodic. Postherpetic: Shu Gan Wan - Liver qi stag.; Xue Fu Zhu Yu Wan - qi & blood stag.; Huo Luo Xiao Ling Wan - blood stag.; Shen Tong Zhu Yu Wan - blood stag.; Yan Hu Suo Zhi Tong Wan - blood stag.
Neuropathy	Diabetic, peripheral: Hua Tuo Zai Zao Wan - qi & yin def.; Bu Yang Huan Wu Wan - qi def., blood stag.; Sunho Multi Ginseng Tablets - blood stag.; Xue Fu Zhu Yu Tang - blood stag.; Dang Gui Si Ni Tang - cold in the channels; Xiao Huo Luo Dan - severe cold in the channels; Xin Mai Ling blood stag. with heat; Shi Quan Da Bu Wan - qi & blood stag. with cold
Neurosis	Gui Pi Tang - Heart & Spleen def.; Tian Wang Bu Xin Dan - Heart & Kid. yin def.; Bai Zi Yang Xin Wan - blood & yin def.; Gan Mai Da Zao Tang; Wen Dan Tang - phlegm heat; Chai Hu Long Gu Mu Li Tang - Liver fire, phlegm heat; Ban Xia Hou Po Wan - qi & phlegm stag.
Night Blindness	Ming Mu Di Huang Wan - Liver & Kid. yin def.; Qi Ju Di Huang Wan - Liver & Kid. yin def.; Ming Mu Capsules - yin & blood def.
Night Sweat	Ba Xian Chang Shou Wan, Da Bu Yin Wan - yin def.
Nocturnal Emission	Jin Suo Gu Jing Wan, Gui Lu Er Xin Jiao, Da Bu Yin Wan - Kid def.
Nosebleed	Yunnan Paiyao - hemostatic; Niu Huang Qing Huo Wan - toxic heat; Huang Lian Jie Du Tang - Stomach heat
Obesity	Fang Feng Tong Sheng Wan, Dao Tan Tang - excess constitutions; Bojenmi Chinese Tea; Keep Fit Capsule - qi & blood stag., phlegm; Ping Wei San - phlegm damp
Obsessive-Compulsive Disorder	Gui Pi Tang - Heart & Spleen def.; Wen Dan Tang - phlegm heat
Osteoarthritis	Deer Velvet jing def.; Juan Bi Tang - wind cold damp; Qu Feng Zhen Tong Wan - wind cold damp; Xiao Huo Luo Dan - severe cold; Xuan Bi Tang - damp heat; Guan Jie Yan Wan - damp heat; Du Huo Ji Sheng Tang - wind damp with Kid. def.; San Bi Wan - wind damp with Kid. def.; Shu Jin Huo Xue Wan - wind damp with blood stag.; Fu Gui Ba Wei Wan - Kid. yang def.; Trans Wood Lock Liniment topical; Porous Capsicum Plaster topical
Osteoporosis	Bu Gai Zhuang Gu Capsules - yang def.

CONDITIONS & FORMULAS

Conditions	Formulas w/ TCM Diagnosis
Otitis	Otitis external: Long Dan Xie Gan Tang - Liver fire; Superior Sore Throat Powder - topical; Chuan Xin Lian Cream - topical; Tujin Liniment topical for fungal infection. Otitis media: Xiao Chai Hu Tang - shao yang; Long Dan Xie Gan Tang - Liver fire; Peking Niu Huang Jie Du Pian - toxic heat; Huang Lien Shang Ching Pien - wind heat, toxic heat; Chuan Xin Lian Antiphlogistic Tablets - toxic heat; Huang Lian Jie Du Tang - damp heat, toxic heat; Wu Wei Xiao Du Wan - toxic heat; Fang Feng Tong Sheng Wan - internal & external excess pattern; Xiao Er Gan Mao Chong Ji - infants
Ovarian Cancer	Ovarian cysts: Hai Zao Jing Wan - phlegm; Nei Xiao Luo Li Wan - hard phlegm; Ji Sheng Ju He Wan - phlegm & qi stag.; Ru Jie Xiao Tablets - qi & blood stag. with phlegm; Woo Garm Yuen Medical Pills - cold & blood stag.; Gui Zhi Fu Ling Tang - blood def. with blood stag.; Tao Hong Si Wu Tang - blood def.; Shao Fu Zhu Yu Wan - blood stag. severe; Tong Jing Wan - blood stag.; Chai Hu Shu Gan Wan - Liver qi stag.; Shi Quan Da Bu Wan - qi & blood def.
Pain	Generalized: Yan Hu Suo Zhi Tong Wan - analgesic; Shao Yao Gan Cao Wan - antispasmodic; Du Huo Ji Sheng Tang - wind damp with Kid. def.; Xiao Huo Luo Dan - severe cold; Xing Jun San - summer damp, acute; Huo Hsiang Cheng Chi Pien - wind cold with damp, acute; Xiao Yao San - Liver qi stag.; Po Sum On Medicated Oil muscle tension, qi stag.; Shu Jin Huo Xue Wan - chronic blood stag.; Zhuang Yao Jian Shen - Kid. def.
Palpitation	Tian Wang Bu Xin Dan - Heart yin def.; Gui Pi Tang - Heart blood def.; Zhi Gan Cao Tang - Heart qi, yin, blood def.; Chai Hu Long Gu Mu Li Tang - Liver fire, phlegm heat; Wen Dan Tang - phlegm heat; Dan Shen Pill - blood & phlegm stag.; Sheng Mai San - qi & yin def.; Zhen Wu Tang - Heart yang def.
Pancreas	Ching Fei Yi Huo Pien - yang ming heat; Da Chai Hu Tang - damp heat; Niu Huang Qing Huo Wan - yang ming organ syndrome; Shu Gan Wan - qi stag., chronic
Paralysis	Hua Tuo Zai Zao Wan - qi & yin def.; Bu Yang Huan Wu Wan - qi def. with blood stag.; Xiao Shuan Zai Zao Wan; Da Huo Luo Dan; Kang Wei Ling Wan - blood stag., wind; Tong Luo Zhi Tong Tablets - blood def.; Niu Huang Qing Xin Wan - phlegm heat; Xiao Huo Luo Dan - chronic, cold, severe
Paranoia	Tian Wang Bu Xin Dan - Heart & Kid. yin def.; Chai Hu Long Gu Mu Li Tang - Liver fire, phlegm heat
Parasitic disorder	Baby Fat Powder - antiparasitic; Hua Ji Xiao Zhi Oral Liquid - infants; Xiao Chai Hu Tang - shao yang; So Hup Yuen Medical Pills - cold damp; Da Huang Jiang Zhi Wan - damp heat
Parkinson's Disease	Hua Tuo Zai Zao Wan - qi & yin def.; San Bi Wan - Kid. def., wind damp; Niu Huang Qing Xin Wan - phlegm heat
Pelvic Inflammatory Disease (PID)	Acute: Fu Yan Qing Tablets - toxic & damp heat; Bi Xie Sheng Shi Wan - damp heat; Long Dan Xie Gan Tang - Liver damp heat; Wu Wei Xiao Du Yin - toxic heat; Huang Lian Jie Du Tang - toxic heat; Huang Lian Su Tablets - toxic heat; Chuan Xin Lian Antiphlogistic Tablets - toxic heat. Chronic: Woo Garm Yuen Medical Pills - cold & blood stag.; Wen Jing Tang - blood def., cold stag.; Yu Dai Wan - damp heat def.; Chien Chin Chih Tai Wan - smoldering damp heat with qi, blood & Kid. yang def.; Gui Zhi Fu Ling Tang - blood stag.; Zhi Bai Ba Wei Wan - Kid. yin def.
PMS (Premenstrual Syndrome)	Syndrome, general: Xiao Yao San - Liver qi stag., blood def.; Gui Pi Tang - Heart & Spleen def.; Chai Hu Shu Gan Tang - Liver qi stag.; Tong Luo Zhi Tong Tablets - blood def. Dizziness: Xiao Yao San - Liver qi stag., blood def.; Jia Wei Xiao Yao San - Liver qi stag. with heat. Edema: Ba Zhen Yi Mu Wan - qi & blood def., blood stag.; Si Wu Tang - + Xiao Yao San. Fever: Jia Wei Xiao Yao San - Liver qi stag. with heat. Edema: Ba Zhen Yi Mu Wan - qi & blood def., blood stag.; Si Wu Tang + Xiao Yao San. Lower backache: Wen Jing Tang - cold, def. blood stag.; Shao Fu Zhu Yu Tang - cold, blood def.; Yang Rong Wan - blood and Kid. def.; You Gui Wan - yang def. Fever: Jia Wei Xiao Yao San - Liver qi stag. with heat
Pneumonia	Ching Fei Yi Huo Pien - Lung fire; Qing Qi Hua Tan Wan - phlegm heat; Niu Huang Qing Huo Wan - toxic heat; Huang Lian Jie Du Tang - toxic heat, damp heat; Chuan Xin Lian Antiphlogistic Tablets - toxic heat; Chuan Xin Lian - toxic heat; Liang Ge Wan - Lung & Stomach heat; Xiao Chai Hu Tang - post acute
Poison Oak/Ivy	Lien Chiao Pai Tu Pien - wind heat, toxic heat
Polycystic Ovarian Syndrome	Shao Yao Gan Cao Wan; Woo Garm Yuen Medical Pills - cold & blood stag.; Liu Wei Di Huang Wan - Kid. yin def.; Zuo Gui Wan - Kid. yin def.; Hai Zao Jing Wan - phlegm; Ji Sheng Ju He Wan - phlegm qi stag.
Post-Nasal Drip	Xin Yi San - wind cold; Cang Er Zi San - heat; Bi Ye Ning Capsules - heat; Liu Jun Zi Wan - Spleen def. with phlegm damp; Er Chen Tang - phlegm; Wen Dan Tang - phlegm heat; Bo Ying Compound - infants

CONDITIONS & FORMULAS

Conditions	Formulas w/ TCM Diagnosis
Post-Partum Care	Weakness and fatigue: Tangkwei Essence of Chicken - qi & blood def.; Ba Zhen Tang - qi & blood def.; Shi Quan Da Bu Wan - qi & blood def.
Prolapse	Bu Zhong Yi Qi Tang - sinking Spleen qi; Zi Shen Da Bu Capsules - Kid. yang def.
Prostate	Acute: Ba Zheng San - damp heat; Long Dan Xie Gan Tang - Liver damp heat; Ming Mu Shang Ching Pien - Liver fire; Fu Yan Qing Tablet - damp & toxic heat; Bi Xie Sheng Shi Wan - damp heat; Chuan Xin Lian Antiphlogistic Tablets - toxic heat; Fu Fang Nan Ban Lan Gen - toxic heat
Psoriasis	Ke Yin Wan - damp; Dan Shen Huo Xue Wan - qi & blood stag. with heat; Dang Gui Yin Zi Wan - blood def. with wind in the skin; Huo Luo Xiao Ling Wan - blood stag.; Si Wu Tang + Huang Lian Jie Du Tang - stubborn; Jia Wei Xiao Yao San - qi stag.; Lien Chiao Pai Tu Pien - wind heat; Reishi Mushroom immune regulator
Psychosis	Depression: Dao Tan Tang - qi & phlegm stag.; Yang Xin Tang - Heart & Spleen def.; Mania: An Gong Niu Huan Wan, Dang Gui Long Hui Wan - fire & phlegm; Xue Fu Zhu Yu Tang - yin def.
Radiation Therapy	Weakness following: Cordyceps Essence of Chicken; Shi Quan Da Bu Wan. Nausea, vomiting from: Wen Dan Tang - phlegm heat; Er Chen Tang - phlegm damp; Xiang Sha Liu Jun Zi Tang - Spleen def. with damp. Fever following: Da Bu Yin Wan - yin def. Hair loss following: Yang Xue Sheng Fa Capsules - blood def.; Qi Bao Mei Ran Dan Liver, Kid. & blood def.; Tangkwei Essence of Chicken - qi & blood def. Oral dryness following: Gu Ben Wan - Stomach yin def.; Qing Yin Wan - dryness & heat; American Ginseng Essence of Chicken; Yang Yin Qing Fei Wan - yin def., dryness. To protect bone marrow during: Wu Ji Bai Feng Wan - blood def.; Cordyceps Essence of Chicken; Reishi Mushroom immune regulator
Raynaud's Syndrome	Dang Gui Si Ni Tang - cold in the channels; Xiao Huo Luo Dan - severe cold in the channels; Xue Fu Zhu Yu Tang - qi & blood stag.; Sunho Multi Ginseng Tablets - blood stag.; Hua Tuo Zai Zao Wan - qi & yin def.
Respiratory Disorders	Yu Ping Feng San - wei qi def.; Bu Fei Wan - Lung qi def.; Yulin Bu Shen Wan - Lung & Kid. yang qi def.; Bu Zhong Yi Qi Tang - Lung & Spleen def.; American Ginseng Essence of Chicken - qi & yin def.; Cordyceps Essence of Chicken - yin & yang def.; Sheng Mai San - qi & yin def.
Restless Leg Syndrome	Ba Zhen Tang - blood & yin def.; Liu Wei Di Huang Wan - Kid. yin def.; Zhi Bai Ba Wei Wan - Kid. yin def.; Tian Wang Bu Xin Dan - Heart & Kid. yin def.; Shao Yao Gan Cao Wan - antispasmodic
Rheumatoid Arthritis	Arthritis: Juan Bi Tang - wind cold damp; Qu Feng Zhen Tong Capsule - wind cold damp; Xuan Bi Tang - damp heat; Guan Jie Yan Wan - damp heat; Shu Jin Huo Xue Wan - blood & phlegm stag.; Shen Tong Zhu Yu Wan - blood stag.; Xiao Huo Luo Dan - severe cold; Du Huo Ji Sheng Tang - wind damp with Kid. def.; Jian Bu Qiang Shen Wan - Kid. def.; Fu Gui Ba Wei Wan - Kid. yang def.; Trans Wood Lock Liniment topical; Porous Capsicum Plaster topical; Gou Pi Gao topical. RA: Reishi Mushroom immune regulator; Xue Fu Zhu Yu Tang - qi & blood stag.
Rhinitis	Allergic: Xin Yi San - wind cold; Cang Er Zi San, Sang Ju Yin - wind heat; Xiao Qing Long Wan - wind cold with congested fluids; Hayfever Relieving Tea - phlegm heat; Qian Bai Bi Yan Pian - heat & pain; Gui Zhi Tang - ying wei disharmony. Chronic: Qian Bai Bi Yan Pian - heat & pain; Bi Yen Ning Capsules - phlegm heat; Pe Min Kan Wan - clear nasal; Cang Er Zi San - wind & phlegm heat; Yu Ping Feng San - wei qi def.; Xu Han Ting - wei qi def.; Ba Ji Yin Yang Wan - Kid. yang def.
Rosacea	Dan Shen Huo Xue Wan - blood stag. with heat; Huo Luo Xiao Ling Wan - blood stag.; Si Wu Tang - blood def.
Scabies	Tujiin Liniment - topical; Hua Tuo Gao - topical
Schizophrenia	Xue Fu Zhu Yu Tang - qi & blood stag.; Chai Hu Long Gu Mu Li Tang - Liver fire, phlegm heat; Wen Dan Tang - phlegm heat; Yang Xin Tang, Gan Mai Da Zao Tang - Heart & Spleen def.; Dao Tan Tang - qi & phlegm stag.
Sciatica	Dang Gui Si Ni Tang - cold in the channels; Xiao Huo Luo Dan - severe cold in the channels; Huo Luo Xiao Ling Wan - blood stag.; Juan Bi Tang - wind cold damp; Qu Feng Zhen Tong Capsules - wind cold damp; Shu Jin Huo Xue Wan - blood stag., wind damp; Du Huo Ji Sheng Tang - Kid. def. with wind damp; Tong Luo Zhi Tong Tablet - blood def., blood stag.; Kang Wei Ling Wan - neuralgic pain; Yan Hu Suo Zhi Tong Wan - analgesic; Shao Yao Gan Cao Wan - antispasmodic
Seizure	Po Lung Yuen Medical Pills - phlegm heat; Chai Hu Long Gu Mu Li Tang - Liver fire, phlegm heat; Niu Huang Qing Xin Wan - phlegm heat; Tong Qiao Huo Xue Wan - blood stag., post traumatic; King Fung Powder - infants, febrile
Shortness of Breath	Bu Zhong Yi Qi Tang - Lung & Spleen def.; Yu Ping Feng San - wei qi def.; Si Jun Zi Tang - Spleen qi def.; Panax Ginseng Extractum - qi def.; Yulin Bu Shen Wan - Lung & Kid. def.

CONDITIONS & FORMULAS

Conditions	Formulas w/ TCM Diagnosis
Shoulder Pain	Xiao Yao San - qi stag.; Ba Zhen Tang - blood def.; Huo Luo Xiao Ling Wan - blood stag.; Die Da Zhi Tong Capsules - blood stag., traumatic; Zheng Gu Shui - topical; Po Sum On Medicated Oil - topical
Sinusitis	Acute: Ching Fei Yi Huo Pien - Lung heat; Chuan Xin Lian Antiphlogistic Tablets - toxic heat; Peking Niu Huang Jie Du Pian - toxic heat; Qian Bai Bi Yan Pian - heat; Cang Er Zi San - wind heat; Xin Yi San - wind cold. Chronic: Bi Yen Ning Capsules - heat; Qing Qi Hua Tan Wan - phlegm heat; Jia Wei Xiao Yao San - Liver qi stag. with heat
Skin	Dry: Jing An Oral Liquid - blood & yin def.; Lady Oral Liquid - blood & yin def.; Ba Zhen San - blood def.; Si Wu Tang - blood def.; Shou Wu Chih - yin & blood def.; Yang Yin Qing Fei Wan - Lung yin def. Itch in cold weather: Xiao Feng Wan + Si Wu Tang; Gui Zhi Tang - wind cold
Smoking	Withdrawal from: Chai Hu Long Gu Mu Li Tang - phlegm heat, Liver fire. Cough from: Yang Yin Qing Fei Wan - Lung dryness; Qing Yin Wan - dryness & heat; African Sea Coconut Cough Syrup
Somnolence	Xiang Sha Liu Jun Zi Tang - Spleen qi def. with phlegm damp; Ping Wei San - phlegm damp; Ban Xia Bai Zhu Tian Ma Tang - wind phlegm; Fu Gui Ba Wei Wan - Kid. yang def.; Tong Qiao Huo Xue Wan - blood stag., post traumatic; Jian Nao Yi Zhi Capsules - qi def., blood & phlegm stag.; Cerebral Tonic Pills - phlegm heat
Sore Throat	Acute: Yin Qiao San, Yin Chiao Chieh Tu Pien - wind heat; Peking Niu Huang Jie Du Pian - toxic heat; Chuan Xin Lian Antiphlogistic Tablets - toxic heat; Ban Lan Gen Chong Ji - toxic heat; Ching Fei Yi Huo Pien - Lung fire; Superior Sore Throat Powder - topical; Gan Mao Tea - children. Chronic: Tung Hsuan Li Fei Pien - heat & dryness; Yang Yin Qing Fei Wan - Lung yin def.; Zhi Bai Ba Wei Wan - yin def.; Mai Wei Di Huang Wan - yin def.; Qing Yin Wan - Lung dryness
Sperm Count (Low)	Low count: Wu Zi Yan Zong Wan - jing def.; Fu Gui Ba Wei Wan - Kid. yang def.; You Gui Wan - Kid. yang def.; San Yuen Medical Pills - Kid. yang qi def.; Deer Velvet - jing def.; Lu Rong Jiao - jing def.; Zhuang Yao Jian Shen - Kid. yang def.; Gu Ben Fu Zheng Capsules - yang def.
Sperm Count (Motility)	Motility disorder: Fu Gui Ba Wei Wan - Kid. yang def.; You Gui Wan - Kid. yang def.; Wu Zi Yan Zong Wan - jing def.; Deer Velvet - jing def.; San Yuen Medical Pills - Kid. yang qi def.
Spermatorrhea	Zhi Bai Di Huang Wan, Zuo Gui Wan - excess fire; Jin Suo Gu Jing Wan, You Gui Wan - Kid. yang def.; Bi Xie Fen Qing Yin - heat & damp; Sang Piao Xiao San - Heart & Kid. disharmony
Sprain	Die Da Zhi Tong Capsules - blood stag.; Zheng Gu Shui - topical; Die Da Tian Qi Yao Jiu - topical
Spur (Bone)	Kang Gu Zeng Sheng Pian; Qu Feng Zhen Tong Capsules - wind cold damp
Stool	Alternating constipation and diarrhea: Tong Xie Yao Fang Wan - Liver Spleen disharmony; Mu Xiang Shun Qi Wan - qi & damp stag.; Chai Hu Shu Gan Wan - Liver qi stag.; Xiao Yao Wan - Liver qi stag.; Bao He Wan - food stag. Dry: Run Chang Wan - blood def.; Ching Fei Yi Huo Pien - yang ming syndrome, Lung fire; Niu Huang Qing Huo Wan - toxic heat; Yang Yin Qing Fei Wan - yin def. Loose: Shen Ling Bai Zhu Wan - Spleen qi def.; Zi Sheng Wan - Spleen qi def. with food stag.; Po Chai Pills - damp heat; Huo Hsiang Cheng Chi Pien - acute damp invasion
Strep Throat	Peking Niu Huang Jie Du Pian - toxic heat; Pu Ji Xiao Du Wan - toxic heat; Huang Lian Su Tablets - toxic heat; Chuan Xin Lian Antiphlogistic Tablets - toxic heat; Superior Sore Throat Powder - topical
Stress	Chai Hu Shu Gan Tang - qi stag.; Xiao Yao San - qi stag.; American Ginseng Essence of Chicken - general; Panax Ginseng Extractum - general
Stroke	Prevention of: Raw Tienchi Tablets - blood stag.; Zhen Gan Xi Feng Wan - yin def., yang rising & wind. Recovery from: Bu Yang Huan Wu Wan - qi def., blood stag.; Xiao Shuan Zai Zao Wan; Hua Tuo Zai Zao Wan - qi & yin def.
Sweat	Night: Zhi Bai Ba Wei Wan - Kid. yin def.; Da Bu Yin Wan - Kid. yin def.; Mai Wei Di Huang Wan - Lung & Kid. yin def.; Cordyceps Essence of Chicken - consumptive disease; Tong Ren Wu Ji Bai Feng Wan - blood def.; Kun Bao Wan - yin def.; Sheng Mai San - qi & yin def.
Systemic Lupus Erythematosus (SLE)	Xue Fu Zhu Yu Tang - qi & blood stag.; Ge Xia Zhu Yu Wan - blood stag.; Dan Shen Huo Xue Wan - blood stag.; Reishi Mushroom immune regulator; Xuan Bi Tang Wan - damp heat in the joints; Guan Jie Yan Wan - damp heat in the joints
Tachycardia	Tian Wang Bu Xin Dan - Heart yin def.; Zhi Gan Cao Tang - Heart qi, blood, yin def.; Gui Pi Tang - Heart qi def.; Dan Shen Pill - blood & phlegm stag.; Sheng Mai San - qi & yin def.

Conditions	Formulas w/ TCM Diagnosis
Tendonitis	Qu Feng Zhen Tong Wan - wind cold damp; Shen Tong Zhu Yu Wan - blood stag.
Thrombocytopenic	Cordyceps Essence of Chicken - yin, yang, blood def.; Tangkwei Essence of Chicken - qi & blood def.; Wu Ji Bai Feng Wan - blood & jing def.; Shi Quan Da Bu Wan - qi & blood def. with cold
Thyroid Gland	Nodules: Hai Zao Jing Wan - phlegm; Nei Xiao Luo Li Wan - Hard phlegm; Ji Sheng Ju He Wan - qi, phlegm, blood stag. Nei Xiao Luo Li Wan; Tian Wang Bu Xin Dan. Thyroiditis: Nei Xiao Luo Li Wan - phlegm heat; Tian Wang Bu Xin Dan - Heart yin def.
Tinnitus	Er Long Zuo Ci Wan, Ci Zhu Wan - Kid. yin def.; Tian Ma Gou Teng Yin - Liver yang rising; Long Dan Xie Gan Tang - Liver fire; Fang Feng Tong Sheng Wan - wind heat; Tong Qiao Huo Xue Wan - blood stag.; Ban Xia Bai Zhu Tian Ma Tang - wind phlegm; Xiang Sha Liu Jun Zi Tang - Spleen def. with phlegm damp in the ear; Wen Dan Tang - phlegm heat; Tinnitus Herbal Treatment Kid. yin def.; Zuo Gui Wan - Kid. yin def.; Shi Quan Da Bu Tang - qi & blood def.
TMJ	TMJ pain: Qing Gan Li Dan Tablets - Gallbladder channel dysfunction; Xiao Yao San - Liver qi stag., blood def.
Tonsillitis	Bacterial: Pu Ji Xiao Du Wan - Lung & Stomach fire; Peking Niu Huang Jie Du Pian - toxic heat; Wu Wei Xiao Du Wan - toxic heat; Niu Huang Qing Huo Wan - Lung & Stomach heat; Huang Lien Shang Ching Pien - wind heat, toxic heat; Huang Lian Jie Du Tang - toxic heat; Huang Lian Su Tablets - toxic heat; Chuan Xin Lian Antiphlogistic Tablets - toxic heat; Superior Sore Throat Powder - topical. Viral: Yin Qiao San, Yin Chiao Chieh Tu Pien - wind heat; Chuan Xin Lian Antiphlogistic Tablets - toxic heat; Chuan Xin Lian - toxic heat; Ban Lan Gen Chong Ji - toxic heat; Superior Sore Throat Powder - topical; Gan Mao Tea - children
Toothache	Qing Wei San - Stomach heat; Huan Lian Jie Du Tang - damp or toxic heat; Peking Niu Huang Jie Du Pian - toxic heat; Chuan Xiong Cha Tiao Wan - wind cold; Sanjin Watermelon Frost - topical
Traumatic Acute	Die Da Zhi Tong Capsules - blood stag.; Chin Gu Tie Shang Wan - blood stag.; Huo Luo Xiao Ling Wan - blood stag.; Xue Fu Zhu Yu Tang - qi & blood stag.; Zheng Gu Shui - topical; Die Da Tian Qi Yao Jiu - topical; Plaster for Bruise and Analgesic - topical
Traumatic Injuries	Die Da Zhi Tong Capsules - blood stag.; Chin Gu Tie Shang Wan - blood stag.; Huo Luo Xiao Ling Wan - blood stag.; Xue Fu Zhu Yu Tang - qi & blood stag.; Zheng Gu Shui - topical; Die Da Tian Qi Yao Jiu - topical; Plaster for Bruise and Analgesic - topical
Traveler's Diarrhea	Po Chai Pills - damp heat; Bao Ji Pills - damp heat; Fu Ke An - damp heat; Huang Lian Su Tablets - toxic heat; Xing Jun San - summerdamp; Huo Hsiang Cheng Chi Pien - wind cold with damp
Tremors	Po Lung Yuen Medical Pills - phlegm heat; Niu Huang Qing Xin Wan - phlegm heat; Zhen Gan Xi Feng Wan - yin def. with yang rising & wind; Tian Ma Gou Teng Wan - Liver yang rising, wind; Chai Hu Long Gu Mu Li Tang - Liver fire, phlegm heat; Tian Wang Bu Xin Dan - Heart & Kid. yin def.; San Bi Wan - wind damp with Kid. def.; Hua Tuo Zai Zao Wan - yin & blood def.; Shi Quan Da Bu Wan - qi & blood def.
Triglycerides	Keep Fit Capsule blood & phlegm stag.; Dan Shen Pills - blood stag.; Raw Tienchi Tablets - blood stag.
Tuberculosis	Debility in: Zhi Gan Cao Tang - Heart qi, yin, blood def. Sweating, fevers: Cordyceps Essence of Chicken - yin & yang def.; Da Bu Yin Wan - Kid. yin def.; Zhi Bai Ba Wei Wan - yin def.
Ulcer	Acute: Peking Niu Huang Jie Du Pian - Heart or Stomach fire; Huang Lien Shang Ching Pien - wind heat, toxic heat; Qing Wei San - Stomach heat; Tao Chih Pien - Heart fire; Niu Huang Qing Huo Wan - yang ming organ syndrome; Liang Ge Wan - yang ming organ syndrome; Qi Xing Tea - infants; Sanjin Watermelon Frost - topical; Superior Sore Throat Powder - topical
Ulcerative Colitis (UC)	Shu Gan Wan - Liver qi stag.; Chai Hu Shu Gan Wan - Liver invading the Spleen; Jia Wei Xiao Yao San - qi stag. with heat; Xiang Lian Wan - damp heat; Hua Zhi Ling Tablet - damp heat; Zi Sheng Wan - qi def. with food stag.; Mu Xiang Shun Qi Wan - qi & damp stag.
Upper respiratory infection	Jing Fang Bai Du San, Ma Xing Shi Gan Tang - wind & cold; Yin Qiao San, Qiang Lan Tang - wind & heat; Xiang Ru San - summer damp heat; Sang Xing Tang - wind heat attack
Urinary Incontinence	Difficult: Fu Gui Ba Wei Wan - yang def.; Ba Zheng San - damp heat; Xue Fu Zhu Yu Tang - blood stag.; Prostate Gland Pills - damp heat; Qian Lie Xian Capsules - damp heat
Urinary Stones	Calculi in: Shi Lin Tong

Conditions	Formulas w/ TCM Diagnosis
Urinary Tract Infection (UTI)	Ba Zheng San - damp heat; Long Dan Xie Gan Tang - Liver fire, damp heat; Bi Xie Sheng Shi Wan - damp heat; Qing Re Qu Shi Tea - damp heat; Ming Mu Shang Ching Pien - damp heat; Huang Lian Su Tablets - toxic heat, damp heat; Fu Yan Qing Tablets - damp heat; Tao Chih Pien - Heart fire; DBD Capsules - severe toxic heat; Ke Yin Wan - damp; Chuan Xin Lian Antiphlogistic Tablets - toxic heat; Qi Xing Tea - children
Urine	Excessive/frequent/nocturnal/incontinence of: Ba Ji Yin Yang Wan - yang def.; Zi Shen Da Bu Capsules - Kid. yang def.; Fu Gui Ba Wei Wan - yang def.; Yulin Da Bu Wan - Kid. yang def.; Zhuang Yao Jian Shen - yang def.; Chin So Ku Ching Wan - astringent; San Yuen Medical Pills - Kid. def. & astringent; Bu Zhong Yi Qi Tang - sinking qi, bladder prolapse, postpartum; Bu Yang Huan Wu Wan - qi def., blood stag., post stroke
Urolithiasis	San Jin Tang, Ba Zheng San, Shi Wei San - damp heat
Urticaria	Gui Zhi Tang - with exposure to cold; Xiao Feng Wan - wind damp; Yin Qiao San, Yin Chiao Chieh Tu Pien - wind heat; Lien Chiao Pai Tu Pien - wind, toxic heat; Ming Mu Shang Ching Pien - damp heat; Shi Du Qing - pruritus; Tian Wang Bu Xin Dan - Heart yin def., chronic; Xiao Yan Tang Shang Cream - topical
Varicose Veins	Tao Hong Si Wu Tang - mild blood stag.; Xue Fu Zhu Yu Tang - qi & blood stag.; Sunho Multi Ginseng Tablets - blood stag.; Bu Zhong Yi Qi Tang - qi def.
Vertigo	Ban Xia Bai Zhu Tian Ma Tang - wind phlegm; Zhen Gan Xi Feng Wan - Liver yin def., yang rising & wind; Tian Ma Gou Teng Yin - Liver wind; Yang Yin Jiang Ya Wan - hypertension, yang rising; Wen Dan Tang - phlegm heat; Xue Fu Zhu Yu Tang - qi & blood stag.; Tong Qiao Huo Xue Wan - blood stag.
Viral Infection	Acute: Chuan Xin Lian Antiphlogistic Tablets - toxic heat; Chuan Xin Lian - toxic heat; Fu Fang Nan Ban Lan Gen - toxic heat; Ban Lan Gen Chong Ji - toxic heat
Vitilgio	Tong Qiao Huo Xue Wan - blood stag.
Voice Loss	Loss of: Qing Yin Wan - Lung heat & dryness; Luo Han Kuo Beverage - Lung dryness; Nin Jiom Pei Pa Kao - phlegm heat
Vomiting	Xing Jun San - summer damp, acute; Huo Hsiang Cheng Chi Pien - wind cold with damp, acute; Xiang Sha Liu Jun Zi Tang - Spleen def. with qi and damp stag.; Wei Tong Ding - cold in the Stomach; Li Zhong Wan - Spleen yang def; Xiao Chai Hu Tang - shao yang syndrome; Er Chen Tang - phlegm damp; Wen Dan Tang - phlegm heat; Huang Lian Jie Du Tang - Stomach heat
Vulvitis	Bi Xie Sheng Shi Wan - damp heat; Yu Dai Wan - damp heat, blood def.; Long Dan Xie Gan Tang - damp heat; Jia Wei Xiao Yao San - Liver qi stag. with heat; Chien Chin Chih Tai Wan - damp heat with def.; Zhi Bai Ba Wei Wan - Kid. yin def., chronic; Ke Yin Wan - damp; Shi Du Qing pruritus; Fu Yin Tai Liniment topical
Warts Common	General: Chuan Xin Lian Antiphlogistic Tablets; Ban Lan Gen Chong Ji
Weakness, weakened immune system	Generalized: Bu Zhong Yi Qi Tang - Spleen qi def.; Shi Quan Da Bu Wan - qi & blood def.; Tangkwei Essence of Chicken - qi & blood def.; American Ginseng Essence of Chicken - qi & yin def.; Cordyceps Essence of Chicken - yin & yang def. Immune: Bu Zhong Yi Qi Tang - Spleen & Lung qi def.; Reishi Mushroom immune regulator; Tong Luo Zhi Tong Tablet - blood def.; Deer Antler and Ginseng qi & jing def.; Yu Ping Feng San - wei qi def.; Sheng Mai San - qi & yin def.; Cordyceps Essence of Chicken - qi & yang def.; American Ginseng Essence of Chicken - qi & yin def.; Panax Ginseng Extractum - qi def.
Weight Control	Fang Feng Tong Sheng Wan - excess constitutions; Bojenmi Chinese Tea; Keep Fit Capsule - qi & blood stag., phlegm; Ping Wei San - phlegm damp
Wheezing	Ma Huang Tang - wind cold; Xiao Qing Long Wan - wind cold with congested fluids; Su Zi Jiang Qi Tang - cold phlegm; Ding Chuan Wan - phlegm heat; Yulin Bu Shen Wan - Lung & Kid. def.; Mai Wei Di Huang Wan - chronic Lung & Kid. yin def.; Sheng Mai San - qi & yin def.; Bu Fei Wan - Lung qi def.
Worms	Baby Fat Powder; Hua Ji Xiao Zhi Oral Liquid - infants
Yeast Infection	Bi Xie Sheng Shi Wan - damp heat; Yu Dai Wan - damp heat, blood def.; Chien Chin Chih Tai Wan - damp heat, def.; Bi Xie Fen Zing Wan - damp; Ping Wei San - phlegm damp

Source: *The Clinical Manual of Chinese Herbal Patent Medicines, 2nd Edition*
Reproduced with the permission of Will Maclean and Kathryn Taylor; Pangolin Press (2003)

LUNG

Clears Heat & Transform Phlegm
- Jia Wei Cang Er San

Redirects Lung Qi
- Ding Chuan Tang

Release Heat from the Lung
- Gan Mao Ling
- Yin Qiao San
- Di Ding Qing Huo Pian
- Zhong Gan Ling Pian

Supplements Lung Qi
- Shen Mai San
- Liu Jin Zi Tang
- Bu Zhong Yi Qi Tang

Supplements Lung Yin
- Sheng Mai San
- Ba Xian Chang Shou Wan
- Bai He Gu Jin Tang

Supplements Lung Qi & Stabilizes the Exterior
- Yu Ping Feng San

Transform Phlegm-Heat
- Chuan Be Ban Xia Gao
- Transform Phlegm-Damp

Transform Phlegm-Damp
- Er Chen Tang

Warms the Lungs & Releases the Exterior
- Xiao Qing Long Tang

LARGE INTESTINE

Clears Damp Heat
- Huang Lian Jie Du Tang
- Wu Hua Tang
- Chang Mei Jun Fang
- Bai Tou Weng Li Chang Fang

Moistens & Unblocks
- Tao Ren Cong Rong Wan

Moves Stagnant Qi in the Large Intestine
- Shan Zha Xiao Hui Xiang Fang
- Shi Wu Wei Fu Ling Pian

STOMACH

Clears Fire from the Stomach
- Huang Lian Jie Du Tang
- Wu Hua Tang

Harmonizes the Stomach & Liver
- He Tu Pian

Move Stagnant Qi of the Stomach
- Kang Ning Wan
- Jia Jian Bao He Wan

Regulates the Stomach & Soothes the liver
- Shu Gan Wan

Supplements Stomach Yin
- Ba Xian Chang Shou Wan

SPLEEN

Dispels Dampness
- Er Chen Tang
- Xia Ku Huan Tan Pian

Supplements Spleen Qi
- Xiao Yao San
- Bu Zhong Yi Qi Tang
- Gui Pi Tang
- Shi Quan Da Bu Tang
- Liu Jun Zi Tang
- Ren Shen Yan Ying Wan
- Huang QI Dong Qing Wan
- Dan Shen Jia Si Jun Zi Tang

Supplements & Warms Spleen Qi
- Huang Qi Jiang Zhong Tang

Supplements Spleen Yang
- Bu Zhong Yi Qi Tang
- Qiang Lie Xian Fang

HEART

Clears Heat from the Heart
- Chai Hu Jia Long Gu Mu Li Tang

Harmonizes Heart & Kidneys
- Gui Zhi Jia Long Gu Mu Li Tang

Moves Heart Blood
- Xue Fu Zhu Yu Tang

Moves Heart Blood & Tonifies Heart Blood
- Jia Wei Si Wu Tang

Supplements Heart Blood
- Suan Zao Ren Tang

Supplements Heart Qi & Blood
- Gui Pi Tang
- An Xin Pian
- Yang Xin Ning Shen Wan
- Ren Shen Yang Ying Wan

Supplements Heart Yin
- Tian Wang Bu Xin Dan

SMALL INTESTINE

Pain along the Channel
- Ge Gen Tang
- Zhui Feng Tou Gu Wan

URINARY BLADDER

Dispels Dampness
- Wu Ling San

Drains Damp-Heat
- Long Dan Xie Gan Tang
- Zhu Ling Qu Mai Tang
- Dong Ling Cao Fang

Expels Stones & Drains Damp-Heat
- Hu Po Hua Shi Pian

KIDNEY

Harmonizes the Kidneys & Heart
- Gui Zhi Jia Long Gu Mu Li Tang

Supplements Kidney Yang
- Jia Jian Jin Gui Shen Qi Wan
- Zhen Bao Fang
- Jia Jian Er Xian Fang
- Qi Hai Yao Fang
- **Zhen Gu Xu Jin Fang**

Supplements Kidney Yin
- Zhu Gui Jia Er Zhi Tang
- Zhi Bai Di Huang Wan
- Ming Mu Di Huang Wan
- Jiang Qi Pian
- Ba Xian Chang Shou Wan

Supplements Kidney Yin & Yang
- Liu Wei Di Huang Wan

Expels Stones
Hu Po Hua Shi Pian

LIVER

Calms the Liver & Extinguishes Internal Wind
- Tian Ma Gou Teng Yin

Drains Fire
- Long Dan Xie Gan Tang

Moves Stagnant Liver Blood
- Gui Zhi Fu Ling Wan

Moves Stagnant Liver Qi
- Xiao Yao San
- Ban Xia Hou Po Tang
- Jia Wei Xiao Yao San

Supplements Liver Blood
- Suan Zao Ren Tang
- Ba Zhen Tang
- Jia Wei Si Wu Tang
- Shou Wu Pian
- Huang Qi Ji Xue Wan
- Jin Huan Mei Ran Wan

Spreads Liver Qi
- Dang Gui Shao Yao San

Supplements Liver Yin
- Zuo Jug Jia Er Zhi Wan
- Ming Mu Di Huang Wan

GALLBLADDER

Drains Fire from The Gallbladder
- Long Dan Xie Gan Tang

Harmonizes & Releases Shaoyang Disorders
- Chai Hu Gui Zhi Tang
- Xiao Chan Hu Tang

Expels Stones
- Xiao Cha Hu Jia Jin Qian Cao Pian

RELEASES THE EXTERIOR

Release Exterior Wind-Cold
- Gui Zhi Tang
- Xiao Qing Long Tang
- Gan Mao Ling

Release Exterior Wind-heat
- Gan Mao Ling
- Yin Qiao San
- Zhong Gan Ling

Release Exterior Disorders with Head & Neck
- Ge Gen Tang
- Tou Tong Pian
- Yu Ping Feng Jia Cang Er San
- Jia Wei Cang Er San

CLEARS HEAT

Clears Heat from the Nutritive Level & Cool the Blood
- Tu Fu Ling Shen Di Huang Wan

Clear Heat & Relieve Toxicity
- Jia Wei Cang Er San
- Huang Lian Jie Du Tang
- Dong Ling Cao Fang
- Di Ding Qing Huo Pian
- Hai Er Fang
- Wu Hua Tang

Clear Heat form the Organs
- Long Dan Xie Gan Tang
- Chang Me Jun Fang
- Bai Tou Wen Li Chang Fang

Clear Deficiency Heat
- Zhi Bai Di Huang Wan

DRAIN DOWNWARD

Drive out Excess Water & Unblock the Bowels
- Shan Zha Xiao Hui Xiang Fang
- Shi Wu Wei Fu Ling Pian

Moisten the Intestine & Unblock the Bowels
- Tao Ren Cong Rong Wan

HARMONIZE

Harmonizes Lesser Yang Stage
- Chai Hu Gui Zhi Tang
- Xiao Chai Hu Tang

Regulate & Harmonize the Liver & Spleen
- Xiao Yao San
- Hue Tu Pian
- Jia Wei Xiao Yao San

Regulate & Harmonize the Liver & Stomach
- He Tu Pian
- Shu Gan Wan
- Jia Jia Bao He Wan

FORMULA

TREAT DRYNESS
Enrich the Yin & Moisten Dryness
- Ba Xian Chang Shou Wan
- Ba He Gu Jin Tang
- Shou Wu Pian
Enrich the Yin, Generate Fluids, & Clear Heat
- Jia Jian Quan Wan

EXPEL DAMPNESS
Promote Urination & Leach out Dampness
- Shan Zha Xiao Hui Xiang Fang
- Zhu Ling Wu Mai Tang
- Wu Ling San
- Shi Wu We Fu Ling Tang
Clear Damp-Heat & Expel Stones
- Xiao Cha Hu Jia Jin Qian Cao Tang
Dispel-Wind-Damp
- Juan Bi Tang
- Kang Ning Wan
- Du Huo Sheng Ji Sheng Tang
- Zhui Feng Tou Gu Wan
- Zheng Gu XU Jin Fang

WARM INTERIOR COLD
Warm the Middle & Dispel Cold
- Qi Hao Yao Fang
- Huang Qi Jiang Zhong Tang

SUPPLEMENTING FORMULAS
Supplement the Qi
- Liu Jun Zi Tang
- Sheng Mai San
- Ren Shen Pian
- Bu Zhong Yi Qi Tang
- Wu Jia Shen Pian
- Qi Hai Yao Fang
Supplement the Blood
- Dang Gui Shao Yao San
- Huang Qi Ji Xue Wan
- Show Wu Pian
- Jin Hua Mei Ran Wan
Supplement the Qi & Blood
- Gui Pi Tang
- Ba Zhen Tang
- Yang Xue Zhuang Jin Jian Bu Wan
- Si Quan Da Bu Tang
- Huang Qi Dong Qing Tang
Nourish Qi & Yin
- Sheng Mai San
- Jing Qi Tang
Nourish & Supplement the Yin
- Zhi Bai Di Huang Wan
- Zuo Gui Jia Er Zhi wan
- Ming Mu Di Huang Wan
- Ba Xian Chang Shou Wan
- Jin Hua Mei Ran Wan
Nourish Yin & Yang
- Liu Wei Di Huang Wan
Warm & Supplement the Yang
- Jia Jian Jig Gui Shen Qi Wan
- Zhen Bao Fang
- Jia Jian Er Xian Tang

REGULATE THE QI
Promote the Movement of Qi
- Ban Xia Hou Po Tang
Direct Rebellious Qi Downward
- Ding Chuang Tang
- Jia Jian Bao He Wan

MOVE THE BLOOD
Transform Blood Stagnation
- Xue Fu Zhu Yu Tang
- San Qi Wan
  San Qi Pian
- Shu Jing Huo Xue Tang
- Dan Shen Hua Yu Pian
Warm the Menses & Dispels Blood Stagnation
- Gui Zhi Fu Ling Wan
Move the Blood for Traumatic Injury
- Shao Yao Gan Cao Jia Yan Hu Tang
- Di Da Wan

STOP THE BLEEDING
- San Qi Wan
- San Qi Pian

STABILIZE AND BIND
Stabilize the Exterior & the Lungs
- Yu Ping Feng Jia Can Er San
- You Ping Feng San
Stabilize the Kidneys
- Gui Zhi Jia Long Gu Mu Li Tang
- Qiang Lie Xian Fang

CALM THE SPIRIT
Nourish the Heart & Calm the Spirit
- Tian Wang Bu Xin Dan
- An Xin Pian
- Suan Zao Ren Tang
- Yin Gui Ye Wang
- Yang Xin Ning Shen Wan
Sedate & Calm the Spirit
- Chai Hu Jia Long Gu Mu Li Tang
- Dan Shen Jia Si Jun Zi Tang

EXPEL WIND
Extinguish Internal Wind
- Tian Ma Gou Teng Yin

TREAT PHLEGM
Dry Dampness & Expel Phlegm
- Er Chen Tang
Clear Heat & Transform Phlegm
- Chuan Bei Ban Xia Gao
Moisten Dryness & transform Phlegm
- Bai He Gu Jin Tang
Transform Phlegm & Dissipate Nodules
- Xia Ku Hua Tan Pian

REDUCE FOOD STAGNATION
- Shi Wu Wei Fu Ling Tang
- Jia Jian Bao He Wan
- Shan Zha Xia Hui Xiang Fang

EXPEL PARASITES
- Wu Hua Tang
- Jia We Tu Yin Chen You Jian Nan

FORMULA

Common Herbal Patents by Usage

Patents	Usage
An Shen Bu Xin Wan	For disturbed shen marked by anxiety and insomnia.
An Mian Pian	Calming formula for insomnia and anxiety.
Aplotaxis Amomi Pills	General digestive and spleen tonic for long-term digestive weakness marked by loose stool.
Armadillo Counter Poison Pill	Removes toxins and reduces itching, great for insect bites and mild to medium cases of poison oak or ivy.
Bao He Wan	For digestive harmony.
Bao Zhen Gao Plasters	Applied directly to the skin for bruises, sprains, and minor aches and pains.
Bi Yan Pian	Used to clear stuffy or runny nose.
Bojenmi Tea Bags	Pleasant diet tea for weight loss, half herbs and half tea.
Cataract Vision Improving Pill (Shi Hu Ye Guang Wan)	For cataracts caused by diabetes or other collapse of yin disease.
Cerebral Tonic Pills - Bu Nao Wan	Used for poor concentration and memory, restlessness, and insomnia. Nourishes the heart, and brain, calms the spirit.
Chi Kwan Yen Wan	Excellent formula for a variety of coughs.
Chien Chin Chih Tai Wan	For damp heat in the lower burner marked by vaginal itching or pain with abnormal discharge, also known as fungal or yeast infection.
Chili and Musk Plasters	For superficial injury and related pain.
Ching Chun Bao - Anti-Aging Pills	Reputed to increase mental capacity and counter fatigue. It strengthens kidney yang, tonifies qi and blood, promotes blood circulation, benefits the heart, and enriches sexual function.
Ching Fei Yi Huo Pian	For cough or breathing difficulties caused by liver heat scorching the lungs. Often diagnosed as asthma.
Ching Koo Tieh Shang Wan	For fresh bruises and other acute external injuries. Reduces swelling and alleviates pain.
Chuan Xin Lian (Antiphlogistic Tablets)	For viral infections, sore throat, particularly with pus.
Chuan Xiong Chai Ta Wan	For wind cold caused headache or dampness in the head.
Chuang Yao Tonic	Builds kidney yang, benefits tendons and bone. For lower back pain, weak waist and legs. Also used for problems due to excessive sexual activity, including fatigue, poor memory and lower backache.
Citrus Seed Pills (Ji Sheng Ju He Wan)	For cold in the liver channel resulting in hernia-like pain or testicular pain or swelling.
Compound Cortex Eucommiae For Hypertension	For hypertension caused by liver & kidney deficiency.
Curing Pill	Alleviates indigestion. For nausea and related headache, motion and morning sickness.
Dan Shen Tablets	For angina. Best used under the care of a licensed health care provider.
Er Long Zuo Ci Wan	Used to nourish yin and reduce liver yang. Beneficial for ringing in the ears, dizziness or poor vision due to deficient kidney yin and excess yang.
Er Yan Ling Oil	For acute ear infections.
Extractum Astragali	Astragalus has shown some benefit to strengthening immunity.
Fargelin Extra- Strength For Hemorrhoids	Amazing results, for hemorrhoids including bleeding hemorrhoids.
Fritillaria Extract Pills	For thick, difficult to expectorate phlegm on the chest, or cough with yellow phlegm.
Gan Mao Ling	Popular cold and flu remedy useful at any stage of a cold.
Gan Mao Tui Re Chong Ji (Ban Lan Gen Tea)	Sweetened isatis beverage, great for sore throat, colds, flu.
Ge Jie Da Bu Wan	Strengthens the kidney and the lung and is used to treat weakness associated with chronic illnesses, particularly when kidney deficiency has left the lung unable to grasp the qi. Often used by older people to maintain good health. Good for people with chronic lung conditions such as asthma.
Ge Lie Bu Shen Wan - Nourish Kidney Gecko Formula	For kidney yang. Good for general weakness, impotence, poor circulation, cold extremities, and frequent urination.
Ginseng & Royal Jelly - Ren Shen Feng Wang Jiang	Promotes qi, and aids in absorption. Believed to enhance immunity.
Hai Ma Bu Shen Wan/ Sea Horse Genital	Nourishes kidney yin and reinforces yang, strengthen the lumbar area and benefits the heart and brain. It is a good tonic for men and those with symptoms of kidney yin and yang deficiency.
Hawthorn Fat Reducing Pill	Extracted from hawthorn berries and used in reducing cholesterol and high triglyceride rate for hypertension due to hyperlipemia.
Huang Lian Su	For acute dysenteric diarrhea.
Jiang Ya Pian Hypertension Tablets	For high blood pressure caused by excessive liver yang.

FORMULA

Patents	Usage
Jiao Gu Lan	An anti-aging, longevity tonic herb. Chemically similar to ginseng, it is thought to be reinforcing to overall health and has a strong anti-fatigue effect. Strengthens the immune system. Used for a variety of health complaints including cholesterol reduction.
Jing Wan Hong / Ching Wan Hong	Topical ointment for burns and scalds. Stops pain, promotes tissue growth, reduces swelling and blistering.
Kai Kit Pills - Prostate Gland Pills	For acute prostatitis.
Li Dan Pian	To dissolve and remove gallstones.
Lien Chiao Pai Tu Pian Lian Qiao Bai Du Pian	For suppurative (with pus) and inflammatory skin conditions such as boils, carbuncles, acne.
Lifei Tangyi Pian	Very effective for dry or nearly dry cough caused by dryness or deficiency of lung yin. For persistent coughs following cold or flu.
Liu Shen Wan (Lu Shen Wan/ Six Spirits Pill)	Used for toxic heat in the throat such as strep throat or sore throat with swelling.
Lo Han Kuo Infusion	For phlegm in the throat or for productive cough.
Ma Hsing Chih Ke Pian	For cough due to cold. Helpful when head cold invades the lungs, or for asthma sufferers who catch cold.
Mao Dung Ching Capsules	Used for chest pain caused by poor circulation or accumulation of fat in the blood. Used in congestive heart disease. Research has shown it to break down accumulations of blood lipids and reduce hardening of the arteries. It is considered a safe preventative against heart disease.
Margarite Acne Pill	Pearl-based formula for acne.
Ming Mu Shang Ching Pian	Clears heat from the eyes. Used for conjunctivitis, painful or itchy eyes from allergy or liver heat.
Musk Hemorrhoid Ointment	Cooling topical relief for hemorrhoids.
Nan Bao Capsules	Male potency tonic. Can be used for erectile dysfunction caused by kidney yang depletion.
Nu Ke Ba Zhen Wan	Tonifies qi and blood. Excellent as a women's daily supplement. Used together with other herbs for fatigue, dizziness, irregular menstruation, deficient menses, and recovery from childbirth and illness.
Ou Jie Di Huang Wan	For liver and kidney yin and blood deficiency resulting in dry, red and itchy eyes, poor eyesight, and excessive tearing.
Panax Ginseng Extract	A liquid extract of 6 year old red ginseng roots. Said to increase endurance.
Pe Min Kan Wan	For sinus problems and allergies. Contains pharmaceutical drug chlorpheniramine.
Peach Kernel Pills	An herbal laxative for constipation. These are used to moisten the intestines.
Peking Ling Chih (Reishi) & Royal Jelly	A combination of ling chih (ganoderma, reishi) mushroom and royal jelly. Strengthens the lungs, spleen and liver and is said to promote long life.
Ping Chuan Pill	For coughs and shortness of breath caused by deficient lung qi and yin (sometimes worse in the evening, or after over-exertion.) This condition is often diagnosed as asthma.
Placenta Restorative Compound	Tonic for blood and qi depletion after childbirth, miscarriage, abortion, or depleting illness.
Po Sum On	Medicated oil for aches and pains in joints or muscles.
Ren Shen Zai Zao Wan	Stroke recovery and prevention; also used for bell's palsy.
Shi Lin Tong	Effective in large doses for dissolving and preventing kidney stones.
Shih Chuan Da Pu Wan	Boosts energy (qi) and blood, strengthens and nourishes spleen (general tonic)
Shou Wu Pian	Taken regularly it is said to nourish the hair, increase vigor, preserve youthfulness, strengthen the sexual function and lengthen life. Commonly used in China for alopecia, and to prevent hair from graying.
Tienchi Ginseng Tablets	Good geriatric tonic uses pseudo ginseng for vascular system. Promotes circulation, yet restrains bleeding.
Tung Shueh Pills	For painful arthritis like conditions known as bi-syndrome. Sometimes useful for fibromyalgia when combined with liver tonics.
Wu Cha Seng	High-grade extract said to have adaptogen properties and is sometimes used to reduce jet lag. Also used to "brighten the mind" before examinations, performances, and other mentally challenging events.
Wu Chi Pai Feng Wan Tablets	Tonifies blood and qi, warms the uterus, and resolves stagnation of liver blood. Used for menstrual disorders due to deficiency or cold, including lack of menstruation, painful menstruation, or infertility.
Yang Rong Wan/ Ginseng Tonic Pills	All purpose tonic for longevity.
Zhi Sou Ding Chuan Wan	For acute cough with labored breathing related to asthma or bronchial phlegm.
Zi Sheng Wan	Used for a variety of digestive disturbances, particularly poor appetite, food stagnation, and malnutrition.

1. Tonics
- Ba Zhen Wan
- Ge Jie Da Bu Wan
- Jin Gui Shen Qi Wan
- Ling Zhi 100% Chinese Lucid Ganoderma
- Oral Liquid of Ginseng and Royal Jelly
- Qing Chun Bao
- Rengseng Yang Rong Wan
- Shen Qi Da Bu Wan
- Shi Quan Da Bu Wan
- You Gui Wan
- Zuo Gui Wan

2. Herbs for the Prevention and Treatment of Cold and Flu
- Bo Ji Wan
- Chun Xiong Chao Tiao Wan
- Ban Lan Gen Chong Ji
- Sang Ju Pian
- Xiao Chai Hu Tang Wan
- Yin Qiao Pills

3. Herbs for Heat Clearing and Detoxification
- Chuan Xin Lian Pian
- Niu Huang Jie Du Pian

4. Herbs for Dispelling Wind & Fire
- Huang Lian Shang Qiang Pian
- Long Dan Xie Gan Wan
- Qing Fei Ye Huo Pian

5. Antitussive, Expectorants & Anti-Asthmatics
- Er Chen Wan
- Luo Han Guo Zhi Ke Chong Ji
- Ping Chuan Wan
- Qing Qi Hua Tan Wan
- Xiao Ke Wan

6. Herbs for Antiarrythmics
- An Shen Bu Xin Wan
- Bai Zi Yang Xin Wan
- Dong Chong Xia Cao Jiao Nang

7. Herbs for Hypertension, Cholesterol and Weight Loss
- Du Zhong Jiang Yao Pian
- Fat Reducing Slimming Tea
- Lower Cholesterol Capsules
- Natural Slimming Capsules
- San Zha Jiang Zhi Wan
- Shou Fu Jiang Zhi Jian Fei Wan
- Xiao Ke Wan
- Yu Quan Wan

8. Herbs for Gastrointestinal Disease
- Xiang Sha Yang Wei Wan
- Yuan Hu Zhi Tong Jiao Nang

9 Herbs for Soothing the Liver & Invigorating the Spleen & Regulating the Stomach
- Shu Gan Wan
- Xiao Yao Wan

10. Herbs for Digestive Systems
- Bu Zhong Yi Qi Wan
- Fu Zi Li Zhong Wan
- Gui Pi Wan
- Huo Xiang Zheng Qi Wan
- Jian Pi Wan
- Xiang Sha Liu Jun Zi Wan
- Bao He Wan
- Mu Xiang Shun Qi Wan

11. Herbs for Hepatopathy, Cholecystitis and Cholelithiasis
- Li Dan Pian
- Li Gan Pian

12. Herbs for Urinary Diseases and Stool
- Liu Wei Di Huang Wan
- Qian Lie Xian
- Run Chang Wan
- Shi Lin Tong

13. Herbs for Wind-Cold Dampness, Arthritis, Arthralgia
- Du Huo Ji Sheng Wan
- Guan Jie Wan
- Zuo Gu Shen Jing Tong Pian
- Hua Tuo Die Da Feng Shi Gao
- Kang Gu Zeng Sheng Pian
- Te Xiao Yao Tong Ling
- Tian Qui Du Zong Wan
- Xiao Huo Luo Dan

14. Herbs for Blood Disorder
- Dang Gui Wan
- Dan Shen Pian

15. Herbs for Stroke, Hemiplegia
- Rengshen Zai Zao Wan
- Tian Ma Wan

16. Herbs for Insomnia, Neurasthenia
- An Shen Bu Xin Wan
- Bu Nao Wan
- Tian Wan Bu Xin Dan

17. Herbs for Diabetes
- Jin Gui Shen Qi Wan
- Yu Quan Wan

18. Herbs for Trauma
- Yun Nan Bai Yao Caps
- Yun Nan Bai Yao Powder

19. Herbs for Women
- Da Bu Yin Wan
- Geng Nian Ling
- Nuan Gong Yun Zi Wan
- Wu Ji Bai Feng Wan
- Yu Dai Wan
- Wu Ji Bai Feng Wan

20. Herbs for Allergy, Ears and Eyes
- Bi Yan Wan
- Cai Feng Zhen Zhu
- Qing Re An Chuang Wan
- Er Ming Zuo Ci Wan
- Ming Mu Di Huang Wan
- Qi Jue Di Huang Wan

21. Herbs for Alopecia, Hair Loss
- Shou Wu Chih
- Shou Wu Pian

22. Herbs for Insomnia, Sleeping
- An Mian Pian
- Suan Zao Ren Tang Pian

TOPICAL APPLICATIONS

Product	Indication	Notes
ABC Plaster	Injuries, aches and pains	Hot
Anti-Rheumatic Plaster (Tientsin Drug)	Re-injured joints or other tissues	Aromatic
Axe brand oil	Injuries, aches and pains	Warm
Bao Zhen Gao/ Shang Yao Plasters	Injuries, aches and pains	Warm
Chili Plasters	Injuries, aches and pains	Hot
Ching Wan Hung (Great Wall)	Abrasions, cuts, and open wounds	Best burn cream, heals tissue, can be applied to open wounds to reduce scarring, and heals bleeding hemorrhoids
Compound Prescribed Watermelon Frost (Guilin)	Abrasions, cuts, and open wounds	For non-healing or infected open wounds with redness and swelling
Dit Dat Jow	Tissue damage from trauma, strains, tears, contusions, and bruises	Good at tissue repair and healing burns, stopping bleeding, reducing pain and swelling as well as long term wound care. Based on formula Qi Li San, or Die Da Wan
Die Da Wan Hua (Jingxiutang Pharm.)	Tissue damage from trauma, strains, tears, contusions, and bruises	Good on burns
Die-Da Analgesic Essence (China National)	Tissue damage from trauma, strains, tears, contusions, and bruises	
Dr. Bob's Medicated oil (Blue Poppy)	Injuries, aches and pains	Warm to neutral
Dr. Shir's Liniment (Spring Wind brand)	Joint strain or sprain	
Dragon Fire Liniment (Oriental Herb Co.)	Injuries, aches and pains	Hot
Dragon's Blood Liniment (Blue Poppy)	Tissue damage from trauma, strains, tears, contusions, and bruises	For swelling and pain when there is no redness or heat
E Mei Shan Plasters	Injuries, aches and pains	Warm
Eagle oil	Over-worked, exhausted muscles, general after-workout soreness and pain	Strong pain reliever
Essential Balm	Over-worked, exhausted muscles, general after-workout soreness and pain	
Fast Patch (Wei Labs)	Tissue damage from trauma, strains, tears, contusions, and bruises	Long term use plaster for healing injuries
Felursa Plaster For Bruise (Zhanjiang)	Tissue damage from trauma, strains, tears, contusions, and bruises	
Feng Liu Sing Tincture	Tissue damage from trauma, strains, tears, contusions, and bruises	Warm
Flower oil (Shanghai medicines)	Injuries, aches and pains	Warm to neutral
Golden sunshine patches/ spray cream	Over-worked, exhausted muscles, general after-workout soreness and pain	Cool
Green Willow liniment (Blue Poppy)	Injuries, aches and pains	Hot
Hua To's Eight Immortal's Iron Palm (Oriental Herb Co.)	Tissue damage from trauma, strains, tears, contusions, and bruises	Designed for training as well as injury
Hua To's Eight Immortals Dit Da Jow (Oriental herb Co.)	Tissue damage from trauma, strains, tears, contusions, and bruises	For post trauma healing
Hua Tuo Plasters (Kwang Chow United)	Injuries, aches and pains	
Huo Lu Medicated Oil (East West USA)	Tissue damage from trauma, strains, tears, contusions, and bruises	
Huo Tuo Plasters (Jingxiutang Pharm.)	Injuries, aches and pains	Warm
Imperial Phoenix (Oriental Herb Co.)	Tissue damage from trauma, strains, tears, contusions, and bruises	Training formula, hot
Iron Fist Liniment (Oriental Herb Co.)	Tissue damage from trauma, strains, tears, contusions, and bruises	Designed for training as well as injury

FORMULA

Product	Indication	Notes
Iron Hand Liniment (East Earth)	Tissue damage from trauma, strains, tears, contusions, and bruises	Designed for training as well as injury
Jade Goddess (Oriental Herb Co.)	Tissue damage from trauma, strains, tears, contusions, and bruises	Training formula, tissue repair, cooling
Joseph's Si Chi Pain relieving oil	Over-worked, exhausted muscles, general after-workout soreness and pain	
King Care Arthritis Pain Formula	Injuries, aches and pains	Warm
King Care Original Formula	Over-worked, exhausted muscles, general after-workout soreness and pain	
King Care Sports Pain Formula	Over-worked, exhausted muscles, general after-workout soreness and pain	
Kou Pi Analgesic Plasters (Tientsin Drug)	Injuries, aches and pains	Warm
Kou Pi Analgesic Plasters (Beijing Tung Jen Tang)	Injuries, aches and pains	Warm
Kupico Plaster (Great Wall Brand)	Re-injured joints or other tissues	Aromatic
Kwan Loong	Injuries, aches and pains	Warm to neutral, also indicated for itching
Mao She Xiang San Xiong Dan Rheumatic oil (Kwangchow)	Injuries, aches and pains	Warm
Mopiko	Over-worked, exhausted muscles, general after-workout soreness and pain	Indicated for pain as well as itch from insect bites and eczema
Musk Anti-Contusion Plasters (Tianjin Drug)	Re-injured joints or other tissues	Aromatic
Musk plaster (Jingxiutang Pharm)	Re-injured joints or other tissues	Aromatic
Musk Rheumatic oil (Guangdong Medicines)	1. Re-injured joints or other tissues 2. Injuries, aches and pains	Aromatic and warm
Musk Rheumatism-Expelling Plasters (Guilin Fourth Pharm.)	Re-injured joints or other tissues	Aromatic
Ni Tian/Yee Tin Tong Oil	Joint strain or sprain	
Notoginseng Herbal Analgesic Liniment	Over-worked, exhausted muscles, general after-workout soreness and pain	Camphor free
Notoginseng Herbal Analgesic Liniment (Guangxi Med.)	Injuries, aches and pains	Warm to neutral
Po Sum On	Injuries, aches and pains	Warm to neutral, good massage oil for sore muscles
Porous Capsicum Plaster	Injuries, aches and pains	Hot
Red Dragon Balm	Injuries, aches and pains	Warm
Salonpas Plasters	Injuries, aches and pains	Warm to neutral, focused on pain
San qi powder	Bleeding, external and internal, severe bruising	
Shang Shi Bao Zhen Medicated Plaster (Shanghai Med. Works)	Re-injured joints or other tissues	Aromatic and warm
Shaolin Dee Dat Jow (Blue Poppy)	Tissue damage from trauma, strains, tears, contusions, and bruises	For acute injury with redness and swelling
Sprain Ointment (Blue Poppy)	Joint strain or sprain	
Spring Wind Herbal Muscle and Joint rub (Spring Wind)	Joint strain or sprain	
Stop Pain (Blue Poppy)	Over-worked, exhausted muscles, general after-workout soreness and pain	
Three Angels Liniment (Blue Poppy)	Red painful muscles and joints due to chronic injury, rheumatoid arthritis, gout	Cool - red painful muscles & joints due to chronic Injury, rheumatoid arthritis, gout
Tie Bi (Oriental Herb Co.)	Tissue damage from trauma, strains, tears, contusions, and bruises	Training formula, cooling

TOPICAL APPLICATIONS

Product	Indication	Notes
Tieh Ta Yao Gin (Chu Kiang Brand)	Tissue damage from trauma, strains, tears, contusions, and bruises	Great on severe bruises
Tieh Ta Yao Gin (United Pharm.)	Tissue damage from trauma, strains, tears, contusions, and bruises	
Tieh Ta Yao Jiu (Five Photos brand)	1. Abrasions, cuts, and open wounds 2. Tissue damage from trauma, strains, tears, contusions, and bruises	Great on "Qi burn" and abrasions
Tien chi powder	Bleeding, external and internal, severe bruising	
Tiger Balm Red	1. Injuries, aches and pains 2. Over-worked, exhausted muscles, general after-workout soreness and pain	Warm
Tiger balm white	Over-worked, exhausted muscles, general after-workout soreness and pain	
Tokhuon Plasters	Injuries, aches and pains	Warm
Wan Hua Oil (United Pharm)	1. Tissue damage from trauma, strains, tears, contusions, and bruises 2. Abrasions, cuts, and open wounds	Good for hard swellings, burns, necrotic wounds
White Dragon Balm	Over-worked, exhausted muscles, general after-workout soreness and pain	
White Flower oil	Over-worked, exhausted muscles, general after-workout soreness and pain	Cool
White Tiger Liniment (Oriental Herb Co.)	Red painful muscles and joints due to chronic injury, rheumatoid arthritis, gout	Cool - red painful muscles & joints due to chronic Injury, rheumatoid arthritis, gout
White Patch (Wei Labs)	Injuries, aches and pains	Warm
Wood lock oil	Over-worked, exhausted muscles, general after-workout soreness and pain	
Wu yang Plaster for bruise	Tissue damage from trauma, strains, tears, contusions, and bruises	Better than ice on acute injuries
Xi Shang Le Ding (Pham. Factory of TCM)	Joint strain or sprain	
Xin Fang Shang Shi Bao Zhen Gao Plasters (Shanghai Med. Works)	Injuries, aches and pains	Warm
Yang Cheng Medicated Herbal Plaster	Tissue damage from trauma, strains, tears, contusions, and bruises	Similar to Wu Yang brand
Yun Xiang Jin	Injuries, aches and pains	Warm
Yun Xiang Jing liniment (Yulin)	Injuries, aches and pains	Hot
Yunnan Baiyao liniment	Over-worked, exhausted muscles, general after-workout soreness and pain	
Yunnan Baiyao Plasters	Over-worked, exhausted muscles, general after-workout soreness and pain	
Yunnan Baiyao Powder,	1. Bleeding, external and internal, severe bruising 2. Abrasions, cuts, and open wounds	The stop-bleeding formula, open wounds
Zheng Gu Shui (Yulin Drug)	1. Joint strain or sprain 2. Re-injured joints or other tissues	Aromatic. "Heal bone water". Great on any joint pain including carpel tunnel, overuse soreness and tennis elbow. Apply to feet before standing for hours.
Zhitong Gao/ Shang Yao Plasters	Injuries, aches and pains	Warm

U.S. HERBAL MANUFACTURERS

Key Table for Herbal Manufacturers

Manufacturer	Key
Blue Poppy	BP
China Herb Company	CHC
Chinese Modular Solutions	CMS
East Tao Pharmacy	ETHP
Evergreen Herbs	EVG
Far East Summit	FES
Golden Flower Chinese Herbs	GFCH

Manufacturer	Key
Health Concerns	HC
Kan Herbals	Kan
Metagenics	MG
ProBotanixx	Pro
The Three Treasure	TTT
Women's Treasure Formula	WT

A listing of manufacturers contact can be found on page 391.

Syndrome	Types	US Formula and Manufacturer
Abdominal Pain	Accumulation of cold in the abdomen	1. Purge Cold (CMS); 2. Balance Cold (EVG)
	Milk and food retention	1. Meal Mover (CMS); 2. Purge Qi (CMS); 3. Morning Glory (ETHP); 4. Chzyme (HC); 5. Quiet Digestion (HC); 6. GI Harmony (EVG)
	Middle jiao deficient cold	1. Purge Cold (CMS); 2. Astragalus Formula (GFCH); 3. GI Tonic (EVG)
	Qi and blood stagnation	1. Corydalis Formula (GFCH); 2. Purge Blood (CMS); 3. Invigorate the Collaterals (Kan); 4. San Qi Tablets (GFCH); 5. Resolve Lower (EVG); 6. Meridian Passage (Kan); 7. Channel Flow (HC)
Acne	Stomach and spleen damp heat	1. Skin Balance + Coptis Purge Fire (HC); 2. CoptiDetox (Kan); 3. Coptis Relieve Toxicity Formula (GFCH); 4. Detox Compound (CHC); 5. Purge Heat + Phlogisticlean (CMS); 6. LD-477 (Pro); 7. Flavor 21 (ETHP); 8. Dematrol PS + Herbal ENT (EVG); 9. Colorful Phoenix Pearl Combo (Kan)
	Disharmony between the Chong and Ren	1. Smooth Passage + Break Into a Smile (TTT); 2. Woman's Balance + Two Immortals (HC); 3. Heavenly Water (HC) – heart and spleen deficiency; 4. Jade Shining + Er Xian Tang Plus (ETHP); 5. Women's Journey (Kan); 6. Wise Woman's Well (CMS); 7. PM-637 + ME-523 (Pro); 8. Free and Easy Wanderer Plus (GFCH); 9. Calm (EVG)
Amenorrhea	Liver and kidney deficiency	1. Unicorn Pearl (WT) - Yin xu; 2. Ease Journey-Yin (WT); 3. Quiet Contemplative (Kan) - Yang xu; 4. Ease Journey-Yang (WT); 5. Warm the Mansion (WT); 6. Balance Cold (EVG); 7. Gracious Power (Kan); 8 Astra Essence (HC); 9.Nine Flavor Tea (HC)
	Qi and blood deficiency	1. Precious Sea (WT); 2. Women's Precious (Kan); 3. Eight Treasures (HC); 4. Gather Vitality (Kan); 5. Imperial Tonic (EVG); 6. Marrow Plus (HC)
	Qi and blood stagnation	1. Women's Rhythm (Kan); 2. Women's Chamber (Kan); 3. Channel Flow (HC); 4. Cramp Bark Plus (HC); 5. Menotrol (EVG)
	Phlegm damp retention	1. Clear the Palace (WT); 2. Lucid Channel (Kan); 3. Disperse the Moisture (CMS); 4. Women's Chamber (Kan); 5. Resolve Lower (EVG)
Asthma	Dormant cold in the lung – acute stage	1. Minor Blue Dragon (HC); 2. AS-135 (Pro); 3. Minor Bluegreen Dragon Formula (GFCH); 4. Respitrol Cold (EVG); 5. Blue Green Lung Clearing Formula (Kan); 6. AllerEase (BP); Note: If external cold signs present, add CO-195 (Pro)
	Phlegm heat in the lung – acute stage	1. AS-137 (Pro); 2. Clear Air (HC); 3. Chest Relief (CMS); 4. Respitrol Heat (EVG); 5. Pinellia Phlegm Dispersing (Kan); Note: With profuse yellow sputum, add Fritillaria and Pinellia Syrup (GFCH)
	Spleen and lung qi deficiency – remission stage	1. Astra C (HC); 2. IM-401 (Pro); 3. Prosperous Farmer (Kan); 4. Six Gentlemen Formula (GFCH); 5. Strengthen Lung (CMS); 6. Six Gentlemen (HC); 7. Modified Astragalus & Ginseng (BP); 8. Immune + (EVG)
	Lung and kidney qi deficiency – remission stage	1. Ginseng and Gecko Herbal Formula (HC); 2. Dynamic Warrior (Kan); 3. Strengthen Kidney (CMS); 4. Mo Plus (ETHP); 5. Respitrol Deficient (EVG); 6. Cordyceps 3 (EVG)

U.S. HERBAL MANUFACTURERS

Syndrome	Types	US Formula and Manufacturer
Back Pain	Damp cold	1. AR-125 (Pro); 2. Mobility 2 (HC); 3. Meridian Circulation (Kan); 4. Mobility 3 (HC); 5. Impediment Magic (BP); 6. Flex CD + Back Support Acute (EVG)
	Damp heat	1. Golden Rose (ETHP); 2. Unlocking Formula + Drain Dampness (HC); 3. Dang Gui & Anemarrhena (BP); 4. Flex Heat + Back Support Acute (EVG)
	Blood stagnation	1. Meridian Passage (Kan); 2. TR-797 (Pro); 3. New Resinall K (HC); 4. Traumanex + Back Support Acute (EVG); 5. Channel Flow (HC)
	Kidney qi deficiency	Kidney yin deficiency: 1. Nine Flavor Tea (HC); Kidney yang deficiency: 1. LI-487 (Pro); 2. BO-163 (Pro); 3. Dynamic Warrior (Kan); 4. MA-511 (Pro); 5. Back Support Chronic (EVG); 6. Angelica and Eucommia (Kan); 7. Rehmannia 8 (HC); 8. Kidney Mansion (BP)
Benign Prostate Hypertrophy	Damp heat	1. Akebia Moist Heat + Unlocking Formula (HC); 2. UI-821 (Pro); 3. Unlocking the Gate (CMS); 4. Ling Syndrome Formula (ETHP); 5. P-Statin or Saw Palmetto Complex (EVG); 6. Relieving Formula (Kan); 7. Clear the Root (TTT)
	Kidney qi/yang deficiency	1. Essence Chamber + Astra Essence (HC); 2. Strengthen the Root (TTT); 3. Essential Yang Formula (GFCH); 4. Dynamic Warrior (Kan); 5. Replenish Essence (CMS); 6. MA-511 (Pro); 7. P-Statin or Saw Palmetto Complex (EVG)
	Blood stagnation	1. Unlocking Formula + Crampbark Plus (HC); 2. Stir Field of Elixir (TTT); 3. Purge Blood (CMS); 4. Cinnamon and Poria Formula (GFCH); 5. Women's Chamber (Kan); 7. Kai Tong Pian (ETHP); 8 Channel Flow (EVG); 9. Resolve Lower (EVG)
Bi Syndrome (Painful Obstruction Syndrome)	Wandering Bi	1. Chase Wind, Penetrate Bone Formula (GFCH); 2. AR-125 (Pro); 3. Flex (EVG); 4. Meridian Comfort (Kan); 5. Mobility 2 (HC)
	Painful Bi	1. Juan Bi Formula (GFCH); 2. AR-125 (Pro); 3. TCB2 Stephania Combination (MG); 4. Mobility 2 (HC); 5. Clear Channels (Kan); 6. Flex Heat (EVG)
	Fixed Bi	1. Bi Syndrome Formula (ETHP); 2. Meridian Circulation (Kan); 3. Channel Flow (HC); 4. Impediment Magic (BP); 5. Flex (EVG)
	Febrile Bi	1. Smilax Compound (ETHP); 2. Flex Heat (EVG)
	Stubborn Bi	1. Meridian Passage (Kan); 2. PA-623 (Pro); 3. AC-Q (HC); 4. Flex CD (EVG); Note: For patients with weak constitution or prolonged Bi with liver and kidney deficiency, add any of the following: Du Huo and Loranthus Formula (GFCH), Mobility 3 (HC), or AR-127 (Pro)
Candidiasis	Liver qi stagnation with damp	1. Break Into a Smile + Central Mansion (TTT); 2. Bupleurum and Tang Kuei Formula (GFCH); 3. Woman's Balance (HC); 4. Yellow Xiao Yao San (ETHP); 5. PM-637 (Pro); 6. Harmonize Liver-Spleen (CMS); 7. V-Statin (EVG); 8. Phellostatin (HC); 10. Unlocking (HC); 11. Modified Perilla & Mentha (BP); 12. Gentiana Complex (EVG)
	Damp heat disturbance	1. Aquilaria 22 + Colostroplex (HC); 2. Drain the Jade Valley (WT); 3. A.V.D. (ETHP); 4. Purge Damp Heat (CMS); 5. CY-207 (Pro); 6. Phellostatin (HC); 7. V-Statin (EVG)
	Lung and kidney qi deficiency	1. Energy E (ETHP); 2. Quiet Contemplative + Wise Judge (Kan); 3. Phellostatin (HC); 4. CY-207 + IM-401 (Pro); 5. Harmonize Spleen-Kidney (CMS)
Canker Sores	Excessive heat accumulation	1. Coptis Relieve Toxicity Formula (GFCH); 2. CoptiDetox (Kan); 3. Gardenia Complex (EVG); 4. Cool the Stomach (Kan); 5. Copticlear (Kan); 6. Coptis Purge Fire (HC)
	Deficient fire flaring up	1. Temper Fire (Kan); 2. Rehmannia and Scrophularia Formula (GFCH); 3. Nine Flavor Tea (HC); 4. Great Yin (HC); 5. Nourish (EVG)
Carpal Tunnel Syndrome	Qi and blood stagnation	1. Arm Support (EVG)
Cataract	Liver and kidney deficiency	1. Nine Flavor Tea + Fertile Garden (HC); 2. Heaven Age Tea (ETHP); 3. Replenish Essence (CMS); 4. LI-487 (Pro); 5. Brighten the Eyes + Strengthen the Root (TTT); 6. Bright Eye Rehmannia (Kan); 7. Nourish Essence Formula (GFCH); 8. Nourish (EVG)
	Spleen qi deficiency	1. Arouse Vigor (Kan); 2. Astra 8 (HC); 3. Tonify Qi and Ease the Muscles (TTT); 4. Energy K (ETHP); 5. Tonify Qi (CMS); 6. Ginseng and Astragalus Formula (GFCH); 7. Raise Qi (HC)

Syndrome	Types	US Formula and Manufacturer
	Liver heat	1. Bend Bamboo (TTT); 2. Ming Mu Formula (GFCH); 3. Clear Vision (CHC); G. Plus + Wolfberry Compound (ETHP)
Chronic Fatigue Syndrome	Qi deficiency	1. Move Mountains (CMS); 2. EN-261 (Pro); 3. Prosperous Farmer (Kan); 4. Salvia 10 Formula (GFCH); 5. Vibrant (EVG); 6. Astra 8 (HC)
	Qi and blood deficiency	1. Eight Treasures (HC); 2. Tonify Blood (CMS); 3. Ginseng Nourishing Formula (GFCH); 4. EN-261 (Pro); 5. Women's Precious (Kan); 6. Marrow Plus (HC); 7. Imperial Tonic (EVG)
	Yin deficiency	1. Fertile Garden (HC); 2. Nine Flavor Tea (HC); 3. Tonify Moisture (CMS); 4. R. Plus (ETHP); 5. Nourish Essence Formula (GFCH); 6. Quiet Contemplative (Kan); 7. Vibrant + Imperial Tonic (EVG); 8. Anti-Nue Boost the Qi (BP)
	Yang deficiency	1. Rehmannia (HC); 2. Strengthen Kidney (CMS); 3. Dynamic Warrior (Kan); 4. Energy D (ETHP); 5. Essential Yang Formula (GFCH); 6. MA-511 (Pro); 7. Virility Tabs (HC); 8. Vibrant + Kidney Yang Tonic (EVG)
	Spleen Qi and Heart blood deficiency	1. Gather Vitality (Kan); 2. Shen-Gem (HC); 3. Peaceful Spirit Formula (GFCH); 4. Energy A (ETHP); 5. Calm the Spirit (TTT); 6. Vibrant + Schisandra ZZZ (EVG)
Common Cold	Wind Cold	1. Dispel Invasion (Kan); 2. CO-195 (Pro); 3. Respitrol Cold (EVG)
	Wind Heat	1. Initial Defense (Kan); 2. CO-197 (Pro); 3. Yin Qiao (Kan); 4. Yin Chiao Formula (GFCH); 5. Zhong Gan Ling (Kan); 6. Lonicera Complex (EVG); 7. Yin Chao Jin (HC); 8. Yin Chao Junior (HC); 9. Cold Away (HC); 10. Isatis Gold (HC); 11. Cold Quell (BP)
	Wind cold with internal damp	1. Early Comfort (Kan); 2. Quiet Digestion (HC); 3. Yin Chao Junior (HC) (for children)
	Common cold with weak constitution	1. IM-401 (Pro); 2. Jade Windscreen (Kan); 3. Jade Screen (TTT); 4. Astra-C (HC); 5. Herbal Sentinel-Yang (TTT); 6. Consolidate Qi (CMS); 7. Lonicera Complex or Respitrol Cold with Immune + (EVG); 8. Yin Chao Junior (HC); 9. Cold Quell (BP)
	Half exterior and half interior pattern	1. Minor Bupleurum (Kan); 2. AL-113 (Pro); 3. Shaoyang Formula (ETHP); 4. Ease 2 (HC)
Conjunctivitis	Wind heat	1. Yin Chao Jin + New Astra 18 Diet (HC); 2. Yin Chiao Formula + Coptis Relieve Toxicity Formula (GFCH); 3. Expel Wind Heat (TTT); 4. Initial Defense (Kan); 5. Clear Lungs (CHC); 6. CO-197 (Pro); 7. Purge Heat (CMS); 8 Lonicera Complex (EVG)
	Liver/gallbladder fire	1. Coptis Purge Fire (HC); 2. Drain Fire (TTT); 3. Quell Fire (Kan); 4. R.D.Y. (ETHP); 5. Detox Compound (CHC); 6. LD-477 (Pro); 7. Gentiana Drain Fire Formula (GFCH); 8. Purge Damp Heat (CMS); 9. Gentiana Complex (EVG)
Constipation	Heat	1. Gentle Senna (HC); 2. HE 349 (Pro); 3. Gentle Lax Excess (EVG); 4. Max Lax (CMS)
	Qi stagnation	1. Disperse Qi + Purge Qi (CMS); 2. Relaxed Wanderer (Kan); 3. Gentle Lax + GI Harmony (EVG); 4. Aquilaria 22 (HC); 5. Ease the Flow (BP); Note: qi, blood, yin, and yang deficiency with qi stagnation and some blood stasis commonly seen in older patients
	Qi deficiency	1. Smooth Response (Kan); 2. Gentle Lax Deficient (EVG)
	Blood deficiency	1. Tonify Blood (CMS) + Smooth Response (Kan); 2. GI Lax + Schisandra ZZZ (EVG); 3. Marrow Plus (HC)
	Yin deficiency	1. Smooth Response (Kan) + Quiet Contemplative (Kan); 2. Nine Flavor Tea (HC); 3. GI Lax + Nourish Fluids (EVG)
	Yin cold	1. Dynamic Warrior (Kan); 2. Purge Cold (CMS); 3. Po Plus (ETHP); 4. Gentle Lax + Kidney Yang Tonic (EVG)
Cough	Phlegm heat with a liver-spleen disharmony	1. Golden Qi (BP); 2. Lung Qi Jr. (BP) pediatric formula
Depression	Liver qi stagnation	1. Free and Easy Wanderer (Kan); 2. Break Into a Smile (TTT); 3. Shine (EVG); 4. Heavenly Water (HC)
	Liver fire	1. Woman's Balance (HC) + GI-337 (Pro); 2. Coptis Purge Fire (HC); 3. Shine + Circulation SJ (EVG); Note: Add Smooth Response (Kan) if dry stool present

FORMULA

Syndrome	Types	US Formula and Manufacturer
	Stagnation of phlegm	1. Purge Phlegm (CMS); 2. Clear the Soul + Break Into a Smile (TTT); 3. Shine (EVG); 4. Peaceful Shen (Kan); 5. Escape Restraint (HC)
	Impairment of mind	1. Shen Gem (HC); 2. SL-749 (Pro); 3. Shine (EVG); Note: The above can be used in combination
	Deficiency of heart and spleen	1. SL-749 (Pro); 2. Calm Spirit (HC); 3. Shen Gem (HC); 4. Peaceful Shen (Kan); 5. Schisandra ZZZ (EVG)
	Yin deficiency	1. Nine Flavor Tea (HC) + PM-637 (Pro); 2. Woman's Balance (HC); 3. Calm ZZZ (EVG); Note: Celestial Emperor's Blend (Kan) can be combined with either of the above to strengthen the effect
Diabetes	Upper Xiao – lung heat and consumption of body fluid	1. Tonify Moisture (CMS); 2. Herbal Sentinel-Yin (TTT); 3. Wise Judge (Kan); 4. Equilibrium (EVG); 5. Myrtle Seng (HC)
	Middle Xiao – stomach fire with consumption of yin	1. Jade Spring Nourishing (Kan); 2. Chemo-Support (TTT); 3. Tonify Moisture (CMS); 4. TCB14 Trichosantes Combination (MG); 5. Equilibrium (EVG); 6. Clearing (HC); 7. DiaQuell (BP); Note: For fire in the stomach and intestines with constipation, add Smooth Response (Kan); Note: Qi & yin insufficiency with heat and possible minor blood stasis
	Lower Xiao – kidney yin deficiency	1. Nine Flavor Tea (HC); 2. TCB 7 (Cornus Combination) (MG); 3. Temper Fire (Kan); 4. Equilibrium + Nourish (EVG); Note: For profuse urination with cloudy urine, add Restore Integrity (Kan)
	Lower Xiao – deficiency of both yin and yang	1. Dynamic Warrior (Kan); 2. Rehmannia 8 (HC); 3. Astra Essence (HC); 4. Equilibrium + Imperial Tonic (EVG); Note: The above can be combined with Restore Integrity (Kan)
Diarrhea	Damp cold (wind cold)	1. Early Comfort (Kan)
	Damp heat (summer heat)	1. Copticlear (Kan); 2. CoptiDetox (Kan); 3. Phellostatin (HC); 4. GI Care II (EVG); 5. Coptis Purge Fire (HC)
	Retention of food	1. Meal Mover (CMS); 2. Quiet Digestion (HC); 3. Purge Qi (CMS); 4. Chzyme (HC); 5. GI Harmony (EVG)
	Disharmony between the liver and spleen	1. Harmonize Liver and Spleen (CMS); 2. Irritease (Kan); 3. Ease 2 (HC); Note: Strengthen Spleen (CMS) may be added; 4. Modified Perilla & Mentha (BP); 5. Calm (EVG)
	Spleen and stomach deficiency	1. Source Qi (HC); 2. GI Tonic (EVG)
	Kidney yang deficiency	1. Purge Cold (CMS) + Consolidate Qi (CMS); 2. Virility Tabs (HC); 3. Kidney Tonic Yang (EVG)
Dysmenorrhea	Qi and blood stagnation	1. Stir-Field of Elixir (WT); 2. Purge Blood (CMS); 3. Women's Rhythm (Kan); 4. Crampbark Plus (HC); 5. Women's Chamber (Kan); 6. Mense Ease (EVG); 7. Phoenix Rising (BP)
	Damp cold	1. Women's Journey (Kan); 2. Warm the Menses (WT); 3. Warm the Mansion (WT); 4. Cramp Bark Plus (HC); 5. Balance Cold (EVG)
	Damp heat	1. Drain Redness (WT); 2. Quell Fire (Kan); 3. Gentiana Drain Fire Formula (GFCH); 4. Unlocking (HC); 5. V-Statin (EVG)
	Qi and blood deficiency	1. Women's Precious (Kan); 2. Precious Sea (WT); 3. Eight Treasures (HC); 4. Marrow Plus (HC); 5. Imperial Tonic (EVG)
	Liver and kidney deficiency	1. Unicorn Pearl (WT); 2. Astra Essence (HC)
Ear Infection	Acute type from wind heat or gallbladder damp heat	1. Yin Chao Jin + Isatis Gold (HC); 2. Initial Defense + Quell Fire (Kan); 3. Children's Herbal Sentinal + Expel Wind Heat (TTT) (initial stage); 4. Expel Wind Heat + Drain Fire (TTT) (severe cases); 5. Isatis Compound (ETHP); 6. Purge Damp Heat (CMS); 7. Herbal ENT (EVG)
	Chronic type – yin fluid deficiency	1. Nine Flavor Tea + Astra C (HC); 2. Ease the Journey – Yin (TTT); 3. Strengthen Kidney (CMS); 4. Energy L + Sheng Mai San Plus (ETHP); 5. Rehmannia and Scrophularia Formula (GFCH); 6. Temper Fire (Kan)
Early Menstrual Cycle	Qi deficiency	1. Arouse Vigor (Kan); 2. Source Qi (HC); 3. Ginseng and Astragalus Formula (GFCH); 4. Gather Vitality (Kan); 5. Imperial Tonic (EVG); 6. Raise Qi (HC); 7. Added Flavors Supplement the Center and Boost the Qi (BP)

Syndrome	Types	US Formula and Manufacturer
	Blood heat – yang heat	1. Cool the Menses (WT); 2. Clear Empty Heat and Cool the Menses (WT); 3. Unlocking (HC); 4. Gardenia Complex (EVG)
	Blood heat – liver qi stagnation	1. Woman's Balance (HC); 2. PM-637 (Pro); 3. Free Flow (WT); 4. Free and Easy Wanderer Plus (GFCH); 5. Calm (EVG); Note: Above products may be used in combination with Cool the Menses (WT)
	Blood heat – deficient heat	1. Temper Fire (Kan); 2. Calm + Nourish (EVG); 3. Great Yin (HC)
Eczema	Acute stage – damp heat	1. Skin Balance (HC); 2. ZiCao Compound (ETHP); 3. Golden Balm (ETHP) (topical use); 4. Coptis Relieve Toxicity Formula (GFCH); 5. Clear Lustre (TTT); 6. Clear Skin (CHC); 7. Phlogisticlean (CMS); 8. Quell Fire (Kan); 9. CY-207 (Pro); 10. Silerex + Gentiana Complex (EVG)
	Chronic stage – blood/fluid deficiency	1. Eight Treasures (HC); 2. Glorious Sea (TTT); 3. Energy C (ETHP); 4. Tonify Moisture (CMS); 5. Eight Immortals Formula (GFCH); 6. Luminescence (Kan); 7. Marrow Plus (HC); 8. Dermatrol PS + Nourish (EVG)
Gastric Pain (Stomachache)	Stomach cold	1. Purge Cold (CMS); 2. GI Tonic (EVG)
	Retention of food	1. Meal Mover (CMS); 2. Purge Qi (CMS); 3. Quiet Digestion (HC); 4. Chzyme (HC)
	Liver qi attacking the stomach	1. Break Into a Smile (TTT); 2. Disperse Qi (CMS); 3. Shu Gan (HC); 4. GI Harmony (EVG)
	Stomach fire	1. GI-335 (Pro); 2. GI-337 (Pro); 3. Cool the Stomach (Kan); 4. Coptis Purge Fire (HC); 5. GI Care (EVG); Note: The above can be used with PM-637 (Pro), Woman's Balance (HC), or Relaxed Wanderer (Kan)
	Stagnation of blood	1. VA-841 (Pro) + Break Into a Smile (TTT); 2. Purge Blood (BOP); 3. Invigorate the Collaterals (Kan); 4. Channel Flow (HC); 5. Circulation SJ (EVG)
	Stomach yin deficiency	1. Jade Spring (TTT); 2. Tonify Moisture (CMS); 3. Wise Judge (Kan); 4. Clearing (HC); 5. Nourish Fluids (EVG)
	Deficient cold of the spleen and stomach	1. Purge Cold (CMS); 2. New Astra 8 (HC); 3. GI Tonic (EVG)
Glaucoma	Liver qi stagnation with liver fire	1. G. Plus (ETHP); 2. Smooth Passage (TTT); 3. Woman's Balance (HC); 4. Relaxed Wanderer (Kan); 5. Free and Easy Wanderer Plus (GFCH); 6. PM-637 (Pro); 7. Bright Eye Rehmannia (Kan); 8. Gardenia Complex (EVG)
	Phlegm fire rising	1. Clear Phlegm (HC); 2. CR-201 (Pro); 3. PhL-II (ETHP); 4. Lucid Channel (Kan); 5. Purge Phlegm (CMS); 6. Gentiana Complex (EVG)
	Liver and kidney yin deficiency with empty fire	1. Ming Mu Formula (GFCH); 2. Wolfberry Compound (ETHP); 3. Replenish Essence (CMS); 4. Brighten the Eyes (TTT); 5. Astra Essence + Nine Flavor Tea (HC); 6. Nourish (EVG)
Headache	Wind cold	1. HA-341 (Pro); 2. Head-Q (HC); 3. Corydalin (EVG); Note: Combine with Dispel Invasion (Kan) or CO-195 (Pro) to increase dispersing of wind cold. Combine with PA-621 (Pro) for rigidity and pain in the nape and the back
	Wind heat	1. Initial Defense (Kan); 2. Corydalin + Lonicera Complex (EVG); 3. Yin Chao Jin (HC); Note: Add Angelica Dahuricae (Bai Zhi) to strengthen the action of stopping pain
	Wind damp	1. HA-341 (Pro); 2. Head-Q (HC)
	Liver yang hyperactivity	1. New Gastrodia Relieve Wind Formula (HC); 2. HB-345 (Pro); 3. Purge Internal Wind (CMS); 4. Corydalin + Gastrodia Complex (EVG); 5. Timely Assertion (Kan); Note: Add U.S. equivalents of Liu Wei Di Huang Wan for presence of kidney yin deficiency
	Kidney yin deficiency	1. Quiet Contemplative (Kan); 2. Strengthen Kidney (CMS); 3. Nine Flavor Tea (HC); 4. Corydalin + Kidney Yin Tonic (EVG); Note: For kidney yang deficiency use Rehmannia 8 (HC)
	Blood deficiency	1. Women's Precious (Kan); 2. Tonify Blood (CMS); 3. Eight Treasures (HC); 4. Migratrol (EVG); 5. Marrow Plus (HC)
	Damp phlegm stagnation	1. Ascending Clarity (Kan); 2. Purge Phlegm (CMS); 3. Clear the Soul (TTT); 4. Clear Phlegm (HC); 5. Corydalin + Herbal DRX (EVG)

FORMULA

Syndrome	Types	US Formula and Manufacturer
	Blood stagnation	1. Blood's Mansion (Kan); 2. Channel Flow (HC); 3. Celestial Mansion (BP); 4. Corydalin + Circulation SJ (EVG)
Heart Disease	Heart qi and blood stagnation	1. Red Stirring (TTT); 2. Invigorate the Collaterals (Kan); 3. Q.B.A. (ETHP); 4. VA-841 (Pro); 5. Disperse Blood (CMS); 6. Cinnamon and Poria Formula (GFCH); 7. Invigorate QB (CHC); 8. Circulation + Herbal Analgesic (EVG); 9. Cool Salvia Formula (Kan); 10. Flavonex (HC); 11. Cir-Q (HC)
	Damp phlegm obstruction	1. Clear Phlegm (HC); 2. Limpid Sea (TTT); 3. Salvia 10 Formula (GFCH); 4. Lucid Channel (Kan); 5. PhL II (ETHP); 6. Purge Phlegm (CMS); 7. Circulation + Herbal DRX (EVG)
	Cold accumulation	1. Virility Tablets (HC); 2. Energy D (ETHP); 3. Purge Cold (CMS); 4. Strengthen the Root (TTT); 5. Dynamic Warrior (Kan); 6. Circulation + Kidney Tonic Yang (EVG)
	Qi and yin deficiency	1. Wise Judge (Kan); 2. Sheng Mai San Plus (ETHP); 3. Strengthen Heart + Harmonize Heart-Lung (CMS); 4. Herbal Sentinel-Yin (HC); 5. Heavenly Emperor's Formula (GFCH); 6. Marrow Plus (HC); 7. Calm Spirit (HC); 8. Circulation + Imperial Tonic (EVG)
Hemorrhoids	Spleen qi deficiency and sinking	1. Source Qi (HC); 2. Energy K (ETHP); 3. Soothe the Center (TTT); 4. Prosperous Farmer (Kan); 5. Ginseng and Astragalus Formula (GFCH); 6. Tonify Qi (CMS); 7. EN-261 (Pro); 8. Hemorrease (Kan); 9. GI Care HMR (EVG)
	Large intestine damp heat	1. Formula H (HC); 2. Wu Hua Formula (GFCH); 3. D.U. Compound (ETHP); 4. GI Care HMR + Gentle Lax (EVG)
	Liver qi and blood stagnation	1. Bupleurum Entangled Qi Formula (HC); 2. Freeing the Moon (TTT); 3. Free and Easy Wanderer Plus (GFCH); 4. Relaxed Wanderer (Kan); 5. GI Care HMR + Calm (EVG)
Herpes Simplex and Herpes Zoster	Liver qi stagnation with damp heat	1. Coptis Purge Fire (HC); 2. Lotus Balm (ETHP) (topical application); 3. Gentiana Drain Fire Formula (GFCH); 4. Purge Damp Heat (CMS); 5. LD-477 (Pro); 6. Quell Fire (Kan)
	Dai meridian damp heat	1. Drain Dampness + Phellostatin (HC); 2. Coptis Relieve Toxicity Formula (GFCH); 3. Jade Shining (ETHP); 4. Gentiana Complex (EVG)
	Wind fire with qi deficiency	1. Isatis Gold + Clearing (HC); 2. Mountain Sophora (ETHP); 3. Viola Clear Fire Formula (GFCH); 4. Initial Defense (Kan); 5. Gentiana Complex + Immune + (EVG)
HIV/AIDS	Lung heat with defensive qi deficiency	1. Enhance + Astra Isatis (HC); 2. Enhance + Clear Heat (HC); 3. Strengthen Lung + Purge Heat (CMS); 4. Resilience (CMS); 5. Jade Screen + B. Plus (ETHP); 6. IM-401 + CO-197 (Pro); 7. Immune + Herbal ABX (EVG)
	Blood and yin deficiency with empty heat	1. Tremella and American Ginseng + Clear Heat (HC); 2. Harmonize Kidney-Heart + Phlogisticlean (CMS); 3. Q.B.R. + A.V.B. (ETHP); 4. Temper Fire (Kan); 5. Nourish the Root (TTT); 6. Nourish + Immune + (EVG)
	Heat toxin accumulation	1. Phellostatin + Coptis Purge Fire Formula (HC); 2. Akebia Moist Heat Formula + Clear Heat (HC); 3. A.V.A. + Q.B.S. (ETHP); 4. Purge Damp Heat + Purge Heat (CMS); 5. Quell Fire (Kan); 6. LD-477 (Pro); 7. Rehmannia and Scrophularia Formula + Coptis Relieve Toxicity Formula (GFCH); 8. Herbal ABX (EVG)
	Spleen qi deficiency or sinking	1. Source Qi + Six Gentlemen (HC); 2. Energy K + SLB (ETHP); 3. Wu Mei Wan Plus (ETHP); 4. Soothe the Center (TTT); 5. Astragalus Formula + Ginseng and Astragalus Formula (GFCH); 6. Tonify Qi (CMS); 7. Arouse Vigor (Kan); 8. Raise Qi (HC); 9. GI Tonic (EVG)
	Liver qi stagnation/ heart shen disturbance	1. Ease Plus + Bupleurum Entangled Formula (HC); 2. Calm Dragon (Kan); 3. Shu Xie Tea (ETHP); 4. Free and Easy Wanderer Plus (GFCH); 5. Relaxed Wanderer + Compassionate Sage (Kan); 6. Freeing the Moon (TTT); 7. RE-699 (Pro); 8. Ease Strain + Strengthen Heart (CMS); 9. Comfort Shen (CMS); 10. Calm Spirit + Nourish Heart (FE); 11. Calm ZZZ (EVG)
Hypertension	Liver yang/fire rising	1. Coptis Purge Fire Formula + Ease Plus (HC); 2. Drain Fire (TTT); 3. Anchor the Yang (Kan); 4. R.D.Y. + Gentiana Compound (ETHP); 5. LD-477 (Pro); 6. Gentiana Drain Fire Formula (GFCH); 7. Purge Damp Heat (CMS); 8. Gastrodia Complex (EVG)

FORMULA

Syndrome	Types	US Formula and Manufacturer
	Damp phlegm	1. Clear Yang (TTT); 2. Pinellia Phlegm Dispersing Formula (Kan); 3. Purge Phlegm (CMS); 4. HB-345(Pro); 5. Clear Phlegm (HC); 6. Gastrodia Complex + Cholisma (EVG)
	Liver yang excess with yin deficiency	1. Peaceful Sunset (TTT); 2. Bend Bamboo (TTT); 3. Wolfberry Compound + Lo Bu Ma Compound (Kan); 4. Ascending Clarity (Kan); 5. Anchor the Yang (Kan); 6. Gastrodia Complex + Nourish (EVG)
	Liver wind	1. Gastrodia Relieve Wind (HC); 2. Gastrodia and Uncaria Formula (GFCH); 3. Purge Internal Wind (CMS); 4. G. Plus (ETHP); 5. Gastrodia and Uncaria Wind Relief (Kan); 6. Gastrodia Complex (EVG)
	Qi, blood, and yin deficiency	1. Hyperquell (BP)
Hyperthyroidism	Qi stagnation with phlegm obstruction	1. Pinellia Phlegm Dispersing Formula (Kan); 2. Bupleurum D Formula (GFCH); 3. Cluster Dissolving (CMS); 4. Thyrodex (EVG)
	Liver fire	1. Coptis Purge Fire (HC); 2. Drain Fire + Smooth Passage (TTT); 3. Quell Fire (Kan) + Pinellia Phlegm Dispersing Formula (Kan); 4. R.D.Y. + Green Xiao Yao San (ETHP); 5. Detox Compound (CHC); 6. LD-477 (Pro); 7. Gentiana Drain Fire Formula (GFCH); 8. Purge Damp Heat (CMS); 9. Thyrodex (EVG)
	Heart and liver yin deficiency	1. Heavenly Emperor's Formula (GFCH); 2. Ming Mu Formula (GFCH); 3. Calm Spirit + Schisandra Dreams (HC); 4. Fertile Garden (HC); 5. Energy S (ETHP); 6. Strengthen Liver + Strengthen Heart (CMS); 7. Clear the Soul + Root the Spirit (TTT); 8. Thyrodex + Nourish (EVG)
Hypochondriac Pain	Liver qi stagnation	1. Break Into a Smile (TTT); 2. Chai Hu Shu Gan San Plus (ETHP); 3. Escape Restraint (HC); 4. Calm (EVG)
	Liver blood stasis	1. Disperse Blood (CMS); 2. Tang Kuei and Saliva Formula (GFCH); 3. Q.B.A. (ETHP); 4. Shu Gan (HC); 5. Circulation SJ (EVG)
	Liver and gallbladder damp heat	1. Quell Fire (Kan); 2. Gentiana Drain Fire Formula (GFCH); 3. Coptis Purge Fire Formula (HC); 4. Dissolve GS (EVG)
	Liver yin deficiency	1. Strengthen Liver (CMS); 2. Radio-Support (TTT); 3. Nine Flavor Tea (HC)
Hypomenorrhea	Blood deficiency	1. Precious Sea (WT); 2. Women's Precious (Kan); 3. Eight Treasures (HC); 4. Tonify Blood (CMS); 5. Marrow Plus (HC); 6 Schisandra ZZZ (EVG)
	Kidney deficiency	1. Unicorn Pearl (WT); 2. Virility Tabs (HC); 3. Kidney Tonic Yin (EVG); Note: For kidney yin deficiency, add Ease Journey-Yin (WT). For kidney yang deficiency, add Ease Journey-Yang (WT)
	Blood stasis	1. Women's Rhythm (Kan); 2. Women's Chamber (Kan); 3. Channel Flow (HC); 4. Resolve Lower (EVG); Note: For blood stasis with cold stagnation, combine with Women's Journey (Kan) or Warm the Menses (WT)
	Phlegm damp	1. Clear the Palace (WT); 2. Lucid Channel (Kan); 3. Disperse Moisture (CMS); 4. Clear Phlegm (HC)
Impotence	Kidney deficiency	1. MA-511 (Pro); 2. TCB4 Eucommia Combination (MG); 3. Essential Yang Formula (GFCH); 4. Tian Kui T-M (ETHP); 5. Dynamic Warrior (Kan); 6. Replenish Essence (CMS); 7. Strengthen the Root (TTT); 8. Restore Integrity (HC); 9. Virility Tabs (HC); 10. Vitality (EVG)
	Impairment of heart and spleen	1. Gather Vitality (Kan); 2. Ginseng Nourishing Formula (GFCH); 3. General Tonic Formula (GFCH); 4. Passion Potion (CMS); 5. Shen-Gem (HC); 6. Schisandra ZZZ (EVG)
	Downward flowing of damp heat	1. Quell Fire (Kan); 2. Temper Fire (Kan); 3. Clear the Root (TTT); 4. Gentiana Compound (ETHP); 5. Gentiana Drain Fire Formula (GFCH); 6. Coptis Purge Fire (HC); 7. V-Statin (EVG)
Infantile Cough	Wind cold	1. AS-135 (Pro); 2. Jade Windscreen (Kan); 3. Chill Chaser (CMS); 4. Respitrol Cold (EVG)
	Wind heat	1. Initial Defense (Kan); 2. Bug Beater (CMS); 3. Yin Chao Junior (HC); 4. Lonicera Complex (EVG); Note: For severe cases, add Clear Air (HC) or AS-137 (Pro)
	Phlegm heat	1. AS-137 (Pro); 2. Clear Air (HC); 3. Chest Relief (CMS); 4. Lung Qi Jr. (BP); 5. Poria XPT + Respitrol Heat (EVG)

U.S. HERBAL MANUFACTURERS

Syndrome	Types	US Formula and Manufacturer
	Phlegm dampness	1. Lucid Channel (Kan); 2. Poria XPT (EVG); Note: For spleen deficiency symptoms, add Prosperous Farmer (Kan)
	Yin deficiency	1. Wise Judge (Kan); 2. Lily Preserve Metal Formula (GFCH); 3. Tremella + American Ginseng (HC); 4. Lily Bulb (HC); 5. Nourish Fluids (EVG)
	Lung qi deficiency	1. Six Gentlemen Formula (GFCH); 2. Prosperous Farmer (Kan); 3. Ginseng and Gecko Herbal Formula (HC); 4. Astra 8 (HC)
Infantile Diarrhea	Overfeeding	1. Meal Mover (CMS); 2. Quiet Digestion (HC); 3. Purge Qi (CMS); 4. Digest Aid (CMS); 5. Belly Binder (CMS); 6. Chzyme (HC); 7. Cordyceps 3 (EVG); 8. GI Harmony (EVG)
	Cold damp	1. Early Comfort (Kan); 2. Ease Digestion Formula (GFCH); 3. Drain Dampness (HC); 4. GI Tonic (EVG); Note: For watery diarrhea, add Water Way (Kan)
	Damp heat	1. Copticlear (Kan); 2. Phellostatin (HC); 3. GI Care II (EVG)
	Spleen deficiency	1. Source Qi (HC); 2. Prosperous Farmer (Kan); 3. Arouse Vigor (Kan); 4. Raise Qi (HC); 5. GI Tonic (EVG)
	Spleen and kidney yang deficiency	1. Purge Cold (CMS) + Consolidate Qi (CMS); 2. GI Tonic + Kidney Yang Tonic (EVG)
Infertility	Kidney yang deficiency	1. Unicorn Pearl (WT); 2. Warm the Mansion (WT); 3. Virility Tabs (HC) + Backbone (HC); 4, Vitality (EVG)
	Kidney yin deficiency	1. Growing Jade (WT); 2. Replenish Essence (CMS); 3. Strengthen the Root (TTT); 4. Fertile Garden (HC); 5. Nine Flavor Tea (HC); 6. Blossom Phase 1 + Kidney Tonic (EVG); Note: To strengthen the action of tonifying kidney yin, add Ease Journey-Yin (WT). With yin deficiency with deficient heat, use together with Temper Fire (Kan)
	Liver qi stagnation	1. Free and Easy Wanderer (Kan); 2. Woman's Balance (HC); 3. Freeing the Moon (WT); 4. Bupleurum and Tang Kuei Formula (GFCH); 5. Heavenly Water (HC); 6. Blossom Phase 4 (EVG); Note: For heat transformation of liver qi, add Free Flow (WT)
	Phlegm damp	1. Clear the Palace (WT); 2. Lucid Channel (Kan); 3. Drain the Jade Valley (WT); 4. Clear Phlegm (HC); 5. Resolve Lower (EVG)
	Blood stagnation	1. Women's Rhythm (Kan); 2. Women's Chamber (Kan); 3. Stir the Field of Elixir (WT); 4. Harmonizing the Moon (WT); 5. Channel Flow (HC); 6. Blossom Phase 1 (EVG); Note: For blood stasis with cold, add either Women's Journey (Kan) or Warm the Menses (WT)
	Spleen-kidney yang deficiency with liver qi plus heat and blood stasis	1. Added Flavors Supplement the Center & Boost the Qi
Insomnia	Deficiency of the heart and spleen	1. Gather Vitality (Kan); 2. Compassionate Sage: Heart Spirit (Kan); 3. Shen-Gem (HC); 4. Calm Spirit (HC); 5. Women's Precious (Kan); 6. Schisandra ZZZ (EVG)
	Disharmony between the heart and kidney	1. Celestial Emperor's Blend (Kan); 2. Compassionate Sage: Heart Spirit + Temper Fire (Kan); 3. Quiet Contemplative: Kidney Yin (Kan) + Compassionate Sage (Kan); 4. Comfort Shen (CMS); 5. Replenish Essence (CMS); 6. Clear mind (EVG); 7. Enhance Memory (EVG)
	Upward attack of liver fire	1. PM-637 (Pro); 2. Woman's Balance (HC); 3. Quell Fire: Liver Fire and Damp Heat (Kan); 4. HB-345 (Pro); 5. New Gastrodia Relieve Wind Formula (HC); 6. Calm Dragon (Kan); 7. Calm ES (EVG)
	Dysfunction of the stomach	1. Quiet Digestion (HC); 2. Meal Mover (CMS); 3. Purge Qi (CMS); 4. GI-337 (Pro); 5. Lucid Channel (Kan); 6. Chzyme (HC); 7. GI Care or GI Harmony (EVG)
	Gallbladder and heart qi deficiency	1. SL-749 (Pro); 2. Clear Phlegm (HC); 3. Modified 11 Flavors Warm the Gallbladder (BP)
	Qi and blood stagnation	1. Resolve Depression & Stabilize Sleep (BP)
Insufficient Lactation	Qi and blood deficiency	1. General Tonic Formula (GFCH); 2. Women's Precious (Kan); 3. 10 Treasures (Kan); 4. Postpartum (HC) + Marrow Plus (HC); 5. Venus (EVG)
	Liver qi stagnation	1. Bupleurum Entangled Qi Formula (HC); 2. Yellow Xiao Yao San (ETHP); 3. Freeing the Moon (TTT); 4. Free and Easy Wanderer Plus (GFCH); 5. Calm (EVG)

FORMULA

Syndrome	Types	US Formula and Manufacturer
Irregular Menstruation	Liver qi stagnation	1. Relaxed Wanderer (Kan); 2. Woman's Balance (HC); 3. Bupleurum and Tang Kuei Formula (GFCH); 4. Heavenly Water (HC); 5 Calm (EVG)
	Kidney deficiency	1. Unicorn Pearl (TTT); 2. Astra Essence (HC); 3. Blossom (EVG)
Late Menstrual Cycle	Blood cold – excess	1. Women's Journey (Kan); 2. Warm the Menses (WT); 3. Backbone (HC); 4. Menotrol (EVG); 5. Balance Cold + Kidney Tonic Yang (EVG); Note: If blood stasis is present, add Women's Chamber (Kan)
	Cold - excess	1. Purge Cold (TTT)
	Blood cold – deficient	1. Warm the Palace (WT) to strengthen the effect of tonifying kidney yang; 2. Marrow Plus (HC)
	Blood deficiency	1. Women's Precious (Kan); 2. Eight Treasures (HC); 3. Ginseng Nourishing Formula (GFCH); 4. Gather Vitality (Kan); 5. 10 Treasures (Kan); 6. Tonify Blood (CMS); 7. Replenish Essence (CMS); 8. Marrow Plus (HC); 9. Schisandra ZZZ (EVG)
	Qi stagnation	1. Relaxed Wanderer (Kan); 2. Bupleurum and Tang Kuei Formula (GFCH); 3. Shu Gan (HC); 4. Calm (EVG)
Leukorrhea	Spleen deficiency	1. Golden Rose (ETHP); 2. Clear Palace (WT); 3. Six Gentlemen (HC)
	Kidney deficiency	1. Harmonize Spleen and Kidney + Consolidate Qi (CMS); 2. Astra Essence (HC)
	Damp heat (toxic damp) retention	1. Quell Fire (Kan); 2. Drain the Jade Valley (WT); 3. Temper Fire (Kan); 4. Purge Damp Heat (CMS); 5. Isatis Cooling (HC); 6. V-Statin (EVG)
Menopausal Syndrome	Kidney yin deficiency	1. Ease Journey-Yin (WT); 2. Female Treasure (WT); 3. Nine Flavor Tea (HC); 4. Energy L (ETHP); 5. Two Immortals (Kan); 6. Temper Fire (Kan); 7. Nine Flavor Tea (HC) + Great Yin (HC); 8. Supplement Yin (BP); 9. Ultimate Immortals (BP); 10. Balance Heat (EVG); Note: For disharmony between heart and kidney, add Celestial Emperor's Blend (Kan) or Heavenly Empress (WT). For presence of liver qi stagnation, add Relaxed Wanderer (Kan) or other Xiao Yao Wan equivalent
	Kidney yang deficiency	1. Ease Journey-Yang (WT) + Purge Cold (TTT); 2. Energy D (ETHP); 3. Astra Essence (HC); 4. Three Immortals (HC); 5. Kidney Yang Tonic (EVG); Note: For damp cold, add Dynamic Warrior (Kan) and Water Way (Kan)
Morning Sickness	Spleen and stomach deficiency	1. Six Gentlemen (HC); 2. Ping Wei San Plus (ETHP); 3. Six Gentlemen Formula (GFCH); 4. GI-335 (Pro); 5. Strengthen Spleen (CMS)
	Disharmony between liver and stomach	1. Shu Gan (HC); 2. Women's Relaxing (ETHP); 3. Break Into a Smile (TTT); 4. Ping Wei San Plus (ETHP); 5. PM-637 (Pro); 6. Harmonize Liver-Spleen (CMS)
Mumps	Wind heat	1. Yin Chiao Formula (GFCH); 2. Initial Defense (Kan); 3. Expel Wind-Heat (TTT); 4. CO-197 (Pro); 5. Phlogisticlean (CMS); 6. Yin Chao Jin (HC); 7. Clear Heat (HC); 8. Herbal ENT + Resolve AI (EVG)
	Toxic heat	1. Purge Heat (CMS); 2. Viola Clear Fire Formula (GFCH); 3. CoptiDetox (Kan); 4. Clear Heat (HC); 5. Herbal ENT + Resolve AI (EVG)
Neck Pain	Qi and blood stagnation	1. Meridian Passage, Meridian Comfort, Meridian Circulation, or Invigorate the Collaterals (Kan); 2. Channel Flow (HC); 3. SPZM (HC); 4. Impediment Magic (BP); 5. Neck & Shoulder (EVG)
	Kidney yin and essence deficiency	1. Osteo 8 + Neck & Shoulder (EVG)
Obesity	Middle jiao hyperactivity	1. Gentle Senna (HC); 2. Copticlear (Kan); 3. Morning Glory (ETHP); 4. Weight Manager (CMS); 5. Herbalite (EVG)
	Damp phlegm accumulation	1. Astra 18 Diet (HC); 2. Prosperous Farmer (Kan); 3. Purge Phlegm (CMS); 4. Green Xiao Yao San (ETHP); 5. Black Dragon (BP); 6. Herbalite + Cholisma (EVG)
	Blood stasis in meridians	1. Crampbark Plus (HC); 2. Red Stirring (TTT); 3. Circulation SJ (EVG)
	Constitutional	1. DI-221 (Pro); 2. Drain Dampness (HC)

FORMULA

Syndrome	Types	US Formula and Manufacturer
Premenstrual Syndrome	Liver qi stagnation	1. Relaxed Wanderer (Kan); 2. Woman's Balance (HC); 3. Smooth Passage (TTT) (with more GI symptoms); 4. Freeing Constraint (WT); (if much pain present); 5. Disperse Qi (CMS); 6. Shu Xie Tea (ETHP); 7. Smooth Cycle (CHC); 8. Xiao Yao Wan Plus (GFCH) (if heat present); 9. Bupleurum and Tang Kuei Formula (GFCH); 10. Freeing the Moon (WT); 11. Heavenly Water (HC); 12 Calm (EVG)
	Liver and kidney yin deficiency	1. Fertile Garden + Nine Flavor Tea (HC); 2. Tonify Moisture (CMS); 3. Nourish the Root (TTT); 4. Nourish Essence Formula (GFCH); 5. Quiet Contemplative (Kan); 6. Energy L (ETHP); 7. Wise Women's Well (Kan); 8. Replenish Essence (CMS); 9. Nourish (EVG)
Rhinitis and Sinusitis	Wind cold	1. Xanthium Relieve Surface (HC); 2. AL-113 (Pro); 3. Purge External Wind (CMS); 4. Jade Screen and Xanthium Formula (GFCH); 5. X. Plus (ETHP); 6. Bi Yan Pian (Kan), 7. Jade Screen (TTT); 8. Jade Windscreen (Kan); 9. Strengthen Lung (CMS); 10. Magnolia Clear Sinus (EVG)
	Wind dry heat	1. Astra C + Yin Chiao Jin (HC); 2. CO-197 + HA-341 (Pro); 3. Yin Chiao Formula (GFCH) + Light Clearing (ETHP); 4. B. Plus + Isatis Compound (ETHP); 5. Purge Heat (CMS); 6. Initial Defense (Kan); 7. Welcome Fragrance (TTT); 8. Strengthen Lung (CMS); 9. Pueraria Clear Sinus (EVG)
	Liver/gallbladder heat	1. Coptis Purge Fire (HC); 2. Quell Fire (Kan); 3. Purge Internal Wind (CMS); 4. Q.B.Y. (ETHP); 5. Gentiana Drain Fire Formula (GFCH); 6. Gentiana Complex (EVG)
	Liver-spleen disharmony with heat & toxins	1. Fragrant Passage (BP)
Smoking Addiction	Heart and lung qi deficiency	1. Ginseng and Gecko Herbal Formula (HC); 2. Energy A (ETHP); 3. Open the Heart (TTT); 4. Ginseng and Astragalus Formula (GFCH); 5. Calm Dragon (Kan); 6. Astra 8 (HC); 7. Respitrol Deficient (EVG)
	Liver and kidney yin deficiency with empty heat	1. Nine Flavor Tea (HC); 2. Energy L (ETHP); 3. Nourish the Root (TTT); 4. Quiet Contemplative (Kan); 5. Nourish Essence Formula (GFCH); 6. Temper Fire (Kan); 7. Great Yin (HC); 8. Nourish Fluids (EVG)
	Spleen and stomach deficiency	1. Six Gentlemen (HC); 2. Source Qi (HC); 3. Energy K (ETHP); 4. Soothe the Center (TTT); 5. Prosperous Farmer (Kan); 6. Astragalus Formula (GFCH); 7. GI Tonic (EVG)
	Stomach damp heat	1. Gentle Senna (HC); 2. Copticlear (Kan); 3. V-Statin (EVG)
Sore Throat	Wind heat	1. Yin Chao Jin + Clear Heat (HC); 2. Light Clearing (ETHP); 3. Initial Defense (Kan); 4. Expel Wind Heat (TTT); 5. CO-197 (Pro); 6. Yin Chiao Formula (GFCH); 7. Cold Quell (BP); 8. Lonicera Complex (EVG)
	Accumulated stomach and lung heat	1. Isatis Gold + Coptis Purge Fire Formula (HC); 2. Mountain Sophora (ETHP); 3. Detox Compound (CHC); 4. Phlogisticlean (CMS); 5. Viola Clear Fire Formula (GFCH); 6. Herbal ENT(EVG)
	Kidney yin deficiency with heat	1. Nine Flavor Tea (HC); 2. Energy L + Pang Da Hai Compound (ETHP); 3. Nourish the Root (TTT); 4. Quiet Contemplative (Kan); 5. Nourish Essence Formula (GFCH); 6. Tonify Moisture (CMS); 7. Full Circle (CHC); 8. Nourish (EVG)
Tinnitus and Deafness	Deficient type	1. Astra Essence (HC); 2. Quiet Contemplative (Kan); 3. Eight Immortals Formula (GFCH); 4. Energy L (ETHP) (yin essence deficiency); 5. Nourish the Root (TTT) (yin essence deficiency); 6. Strengthen the Root (TTT) (yang qi deficiency); 7. Energy D (ETHP) (yang qi deficiency); 8. Flavonex (HC); 9. Cordyceps 3 + Nourish (EVG)
	Excess type	1. Coptis Purge Fire (HC); 2. Release Constraint + Drain Fire (TTT); 3. Quell Fire (Kan); 4. R.D.Y. (ETHP); 5. Detox Compound (CHC); 6. LD-477 (Pro); 7. Gentiana Drain Fire Formula (GFCH); 8. Purge Damp Heat (CMS); 9. Pinellia Phlegm Dispersing Formula (Kan); 10. Quell Fire (Kan); 11. Purge Damp Heat (CMS); 12. Gentiana Complex (EVG)

FORMULA

Syndrome	Types	US Formula and Manufacturer
Urinary Tract Infection	Retention of damp heat in the bladder	1. UI-821 (Pro); 2. Relieving Formula (Kan); 3. Jin Qian Cao Stone Formula (HC); 4. Akebia Moist Heat Formula (HC); 5. V-Statin (EVG); Note: For pathogen in the shaoyang with chills, fever, bitter taste in the mouth, nausea, or vomiting, add AL-113 (Pro), or Minor Bupleurum (Kan)
	Spleen deficiency	1. Arouse Vigor (Kan); 2. Source Qi (HC); 3. EN-261 (Pro); 4. Raise Qi (HC); 5. V-Statin + GI Tonic (EVG)
	Liver qi stagnation	1. PM-637 (Pro) + Jin Qian Cao Stone Formula (HC); 2. Woman's Balance (Kan) + Jin Qian Cao Stone Formula (HC); 3. Coptis Purge Fire Formula (HC) + Jin Qian Cao Stone Formula (HC); 4. Quell Fire (Kan) + Jin Qian Cao Stone Formula (HC); 5. CY-207 (Pro) + Jin Qian Cao Stone Formula (HC); 6. V-Stain + Calm (EVG)
	Kidney deficiency	Kidney yin deficiency: 1. Temper Fire (Kan) or Quiet Contemplative (Kan); 2. V-Statin + Nourish (EVG); Kidney yang deficiency: 1. Dynamic Warrior (Kan) or Rehmannia 8 (HC); Kidney qi deficiency: 1. R.D.K. (ETHP); 2. Nine Flavor Tea (HC)
Urticaria	Wind heat	1. Clear Heat + Yin Chao San (HC); 2. Glorious Sea + Expel Wind Heat (TTT); 3. Clear Lungs (CHC); 4. Purge External Wind (CMS); 5. Initial Defense + Dispel Invasion (Kan); 6. CO-197 (Pro); 7. Colorful Phoenix Pearl Combo (Kan); 8. Silarex (EVG)
	Wind damp	1. Early Comfort (Kan); 2. Drain Fields (TTT); 3. R.D.A. (ETHP); 4. Derma Wind Release (Kan); 5. Silerex + Herbal ABX (EVG)
	Damp heat toxin	1. Coptis Purge Fire Formula + Skin Balance (HC); 2. Flavor 21 (ETHP); 3. Coptis Relieve Toxicity Formula (GFCH); 4. Clear Lustre (TTT); 5. Clear Skin (CHC); 6. Purge Heat + Purge Damp Heat (CMS); 7. LD-477 (Pro); 8. CoptiDetox (Kan); 9. Dermatrol PS + Gardenia Complex (EVG)
Uterine Bleeding	Spleen qi deficiency	1. Restrain the Flow (WT); 2. Gather Vitality (Kan); 3. Energy A (ETHP); 4. Shen-Gem (HC); 5. Schisandra ZZZ + Notoginseng 9 (EVG)
	Kidney yang deficiency	1. Ease the Journey-Yang (WT); 2. Planting Seeds (WT); 3. Energy D (ETHP); 4. Virility Tabs (HC); 5. Added Flavors Supplement the Center and Boost the Qi (BP); 6. Kidney Yang Tonic + Notoginseng 9 (EVG)
	Kidney yin deficiency	1. Nourish Yin and Restrain the Flow (WT); 2. Temper Fire (Kan); 3. Rehmannia and Scrophularia Formula (GFCH); 4. Great Yin (HC) + Nine Flavor Tea (HC); 5. Kidney Yin Tonic + Notoginseng 9 (EVG); Note: Use any of the above in combination with Clear Empty-Heat and Cool the Menses (WT) to increase the action of cooling blood
	Blood heat	1. Cool the Menses (WT); 2. Notoginseng 9 (EVG); 3. Clear Heat (HC); 4. Gardenia Complex + Notoginseng 9 (EVG); Note: for presence of liver fire, combine with Free and Easy Wanderer Plus (GFCH)
	Damp heat	1. Quell Fire (Kan); 2. Gentiana Drain Fire Formula (GFCH); 3. Unlocking (HC); 4. V-Statin + Notoginseng 9 (EVG)
	Blood stasis	1. Invigorate Blood and Stem the Flow (WT); 2. Resolve Lower + Notoginseng 9 (EVG)
Uterine Prolapse	Qi deficiency	1. Arouse Vigor (Kan); 2. Ginseng and Astragalus Formula (GFCH); 3. Energy K (ETHP); 4. Consolidate Qi (CMS); 5. Astra 8 (HC); 6. Raise Qi (HC); 7. C/R Support (EVG)
	Kidney deficiency	1. Unicorn Pearl (WT); 2. Astra Essence (HC); 3. Raise Qi (HC); 4. Kidney Yang Tonic (EVG); Note: Use either of the above together with Arouse Vigor (Kan) or Ginseng and Astragalus Formula (GFCH)
	Damp heat	1. Quell Fire (Kan); 2. Gentiana Drain Fire Formula (GFCH); 3. Coptis Purge Fire (HC); 4. Gentiana Compound (ETHP); 5. V-Statin (EVG)
Vaginitis	Damp heat	1. Drain the Jade Valley (WT); 2. Quell Fire (Kan); 3. Gentiana Drain Fire Formula (GFCH); 4. Purge Damp Heat (CMS); 5. Akebia Moist Heat (HC); 6. V-Statin (EVG)
	Liver and kidney yin xu	1. Temper Fire (Kan); 2. Rehmannia and Scrophularia (GFCH); 3. Q.B.Y. (ETHP); 4. Clearing (HC); 5. V-Statin + Nourish (EVG)
	Heart and liver stagnated fire	1. Free Flow (WT); 2. Free and Easy Wanderer Plus (GFCH); 3. Woman's Balance (HC); 4. Clear Heat (HC); 5. V-Statin + Calm (EVG)

FORMULA

Dosing Guidelines

The standard dose of herbal extracts for an average adult is 6 to 10 grams per day. In treating acute or severe cases, the dosage may be increased up to 20 grams per day. Since not everybody is an "average adult," the fundamental concept in dosing is to realize that one size does not fit all. Every person is unique and must be treated individually.

The principle behind the Age-To-Dose Dosing Guideline is assessment of the maturity of the organs' ability to metabolize, utilize and eliminate herbs. This detailed chart is especially useful for adjusting dosages for infants and younger children. The recommendations are taken from *Herbology*, published by Nanjing College of Traditional Chinese Medicine.

The principle underlying the Weight-To-Dose Dosing Guideline is based on gauging the effective concentration of the herb after it is distributed throughout the body. This dosing strategy is especially useful for patients whose body weight falls outside of the normal range. All calculations are based on *Clark's Rule in Pharmaceutical Calculations*, by Mitchell Stoklosa and Howard Ansel.

These two charts provide the herbal practitioner with a handy reference for calculating dosages for those patients who fall outside the definition of an 'average adult.' It is still important to keep in mind, however, that these charts serve only as a guidelines - not absolute rules. Every person is unique and must be treated as such. One must always remember to treat each patient as an individual, not as a chart!

Table I. Age-to-Dose Dosing Guideline

Age	Recommended Daily Dosage	Fine Granules	Capsules
0 - 1 month	1/18 - 1/14 of adult dose	0.3 - 0.4 grams	N/R*
1 - 6 month	1/14 - 1/7 of adult dose	0.4 - 0.9 grams	N/R*
6 - 12 month	1/7 - 1/5 of adult dose	0.9 – 1.2 grams	N/R*
1 - 2 years	1/5 - 1/4 of adult dose	1.2 -1.5 grams	N/R*
2 - 4 years	1/4 - 1/3 of adult dose	1.5 - 2.0 grams	N/R*
4 - 6 years	1/3 - 2/5 of adult dose	2.0 - 2.4 grams	N/R*
6 - 9 years	2/5 - 1/2 of adult dose	2.4 - 3.0 grams	5 - 6 capsules**
9 - 14 years	1/2 - 2/3 of adult dose	3.0 - 4.0 grams	6 - 8 capsules**
14 - 18 years	2/3 - full adult dose	4.0 - 6.0 grams	8 - 12 capsules**
18 - 60 years	**adult dose**	**adult dose**	**12**
60 years and over	3/4 or less of adult dos	4.5 - 6.0 grams	9 - 12 capsules**

Table II. Weight-to-Dose Dosing Guideline

Weight	Recommended Daily Dosage	Fine Granules	Capsules
30 - 40 lbs	20% - 27% of adult dose	1.2 - 1.6 grams	N/R*
40 - 50 lbs	27% - 33% of adult dose	1.6 - 1.9 grams	N/R*
50 - 60 lbs	33% - 40% of adult dose	1.9 - 2.4 grams	N/R*
60 - 70 lbs	40% - 47% of adult dose	2.4 - 2.8 grams	N/R*
70 - 80 lbs	47% - 53% of adult dose	2.4 - 2.8 grams	5 - 6 capsules**
80 - 100 lbs	53% - 67% of adult dose	3.2 - 4.0 grams	6 - 8 capsules**
100 - 120 lbs	67% - 80% of adult dose	4.0 - 4.8 grams	8 - 10 capsules**
120 - 150 lbs	80% - 100% of adult dose	4.8 - 6.0 grams	10 - 12 capsules**
150 lbs	**adult dose**	**6.0 grams**	**12**
150 – 200 lbs	100% - 133% of adult dose	6.0 – 7.9 grams	12 - 16 capsules**
150 – 200 lbs	100% - 133% of adult dose	6.0 – 7.9 grams	12 - 16 capsules**
200 - 250 lbs	133% - 167% of adult dose	7.9 - 10.0 gram	16 - 20 capsules**
250 - 300 lbs	167% - 200% of adult dose	10.0 - 12.0 grams	20 - 24 capsules**

*   N/R: Not Recommend for infants and young children since they may have difficulty swallowing.

** Each capsule weighs 500 mg or 0.5 gram.

Source: *Clinical Manual of Oriental Medicine*, 2nd Edition, 2006.
Reproduced with the permission of Lotus Institute of Integrative Medicine; www.elotus.org

FORMULA

BRAND NAME	GENERIC NAME	TYPE OF DRUGS	EFFECT OF INTERACTION	COMMENT
	**Recognition of Drugs with Higher Risk of Interaction**				
Amphotericin	*Amphotericin*	antifungal	may reduce elimination of herbs	decrease dose of herbs if necessary
Axid	*Nizatidine*	acid-reducer	may interfere with absorption of herbs	adjust herb doses accordingly
Carafate	*Sucralfate*	anti-ulcer	may interfere with absorption of herbs	separate taking herbs and drugs by two hours
Cholestid	*Colestipol*	antihyperlipidemic	may interfere with absorption of herbs	separate taking herbs and drugs by two hours
Coumadin	*Warfarin*	anticoagulant	this effect may change with herbs	monitor Coumadin effectiveness closely
Diflucan	*Fluconazole*	antifungal	may slow the metabolism of herbs	decrease dose of herbs if necessary
Dilantin	*Phenytoin*	anticonvulsant	may increase the metabolism of herbs	increase dose of herbs if necessary
E-Mycin	*Erythromycin*	antibiotic	may slow the metabolism of herbs	decrease dose of herbs if necessary
EES	*Erythromycin*	antibiotic	may slow the metabolism of herbs	decrease dose of herbs if necessary
Eryc	*Erythromycin*	antibiotic	may slow the metabolism of herbs	decrease dose of herbs if necessary
Ethanol	*Alcohol*	alcohol	may slow the metabolism of herbs	decrease dose of herbs if necessary
Haldol	*Haloperidol*	antipsychotic	may interfere with absorption of herbs	decrease dose of herbs if necessary
Maalax	*Antacid*	antacid	may interfere with absorption of herbs	separate taking herbs and drugs by two hours
Methotrexate	*Methotrexate*	antineoplastic	may reduce elimination of herbs	decrease dose of herbs if necessary
Mylanta	*Antacid*	antacid	may interfere with absorption of herbs	separate taking herbs and drugs by two hours
Nexium	*Esomeprazole*	acid-reducer	may interfere with absorption of herbs	adjust herb doses accordingly
Nizoral	*Ketoconazole*	antifungal	may slow the metabolism of herbs	decrease dose of herbs if necessary
Pepcid	*Famotidine*	acid-reducer	may interfere with absorption of herbs	adjust herb doses accordingly
Phenobarbital	*Phenobarbital*	anticonvulsant	may increase the metabolism of herbs	increase dose of herbs if necessary
Prevacid	*Lansoprazole*	acid-reducer	may interfere with absorption of herbs	adjust herb doses accordingly
Prilosec	*Omeprazole*	acid-reducer	may interfere with absorption of herbs	adjust herb doses accordingly
Propulsid	*Cisapride*	GI stimulant	may interfere with absorption of herbs	increase dose of herbs if necessary
Protonix	*Pantoprazole*	GI stimulant	may interfere with absorption of herbs	increase dose of herbs if necessary
Questran	*Cholestyramine*	antihyperlipidemic	may decrease absorption of herbs	separate taking herbs and drugs by two hours
Reglan	*Metoclopramide*	GI stimulant	may interfere with absorption of herbs	increase dose of herbs if necessary
Rifadin	*Rifampin*	antibiotic	may increase the metabolism of herbs	increase dose of herbs if necessary
Sporonox	*Itraconazole*	antifungal	may slow the metabolism of herbs	decrease dose of herbs if necessary
Tagamet	*Cimetidine*	acid-reducer	may interfere with absorption of herbs	adjust herb doses accordingly
Tegretol	*Carbamazepine*	anticonvulsant	may increase the metabolism of herbs	increase dose of herbs if necessary
Tums	*Antacid*	antacid	may interfere with absorption of herbs	separate taking herbs and drugs by two hours
Zantac	*Ranitidine*	acid-reducer	may interfere with absorption of herbs	adjust herb doses accordingly

Source: *Clinical Manual of Oriental Medicine*, 2nd Edition, 2006. Reproduced with the permission of Lotus Institute of Integrative Medicine and Dr. John Chen; www.elotus.org

HERB

HERB

Cathartics - *cath*
Ba Dou
Gan Sui
Jing Da Ji
Qian Niu Zi
Shang Lu
Yuan Hua

Clear Heat & Phlegm - *clht phlegm*
Chuan Bei Mu
Fu Hai Shi
Gua Lou
Gua Lou Ren
Hai Ge Ke
Hai Zao
Kun Bu
Meng Shi
Pang Da Hai
Qian Hu
Tian Hua Fen
Tian Zhu Huang
Wa Leng Zi
Zhi Bei Mu
Zhu Li
Zhu Ru

Clear Heat & Damp - *clht-damp*
Hu Huang Lian
Huang Bai
Huang Lian
Huang Qin
Ku Shen
Long Dan Cao
Qin Pi

Clear Heat & Detoxify - *clht-detox*
Bai Hua She She Cao
Bai Jiang Cao
Bai Tou Weng
Bai Xian Pi
Ban Lan Gen
Chuan Xin Lian
Da Qing Ye
Guan Zhong
Jin Yin Hua
Lian Qiao
Lou Lu
Ma Bo
Ma Chi Xian
Pu Gong Ying
Qing Dai
Shan Dou Gen
She Gan
Tu Fu Ling
Ye Ju Hua
Yu Xing Cao
Zi Hua Di Ding

Clear Heat & Drain Fire - *clht-fire*
Dan Zhu Ye
Han Shui Shi
Jue Ming Zi
Lian Zi Xin
Lu Gen
Mi Meng Hua
Qing Xiang Zi
Shi Gao
Xia Ku Cao
Xiong Dan
Zhi Mu
Zhi Zi

Clear Heat & Relieve Summerheat - *clht-sumr*
Bai Bian Dou
Chang Shan
Dou Juan
He Ye
Lian Geng
Lu Dou
Qing Hao
Xi Gua
Ya Dan Zi

Transform Cold Phlegm - *cold-phlegm*
Bai Fu Zi
Bai Jie Zi
Bai Qian
Ban Xia
Dan Nan Xing
Jie Geng
Tian Nan Xing
Xuan Fu Hua
Zao Jiao

Cool Blood - *coolxue*
Bai Wei
Di Gu Pi
Mu Dan Pi
Sheng Di Huang
Shui Niu Jiao
Xi Jiao
Xuan Shen
Yin Chai Hu
Zi Cao

Stop Cough - *cough*
Bai Bu
Kuan Dong Hua
Ma Dou Ling
Pi Pa Ye
Sang Bai Pi
Su Zi
Ting Li Zi
Xing Ren
Zi Wan

Calm Shen - *cshen*
Bai Zi Ren
Ci Shi
Dai Zhe Shi
He Huan Pi
Hu Po
Ling Zhi
Long Gu
Mu Li
Sheng Tie Luo
Suan Zao Ren
Ye Jiao Teng
Yuan Zhi
Zhen Zhu
Zhu Sha
Zi Shi Ying

Dispel Wind & Damp - *d-w-damp*
Bai Hua She
Can Sha
Cang Er Zi
Du Huo
Hai Feng Teng
Hai Tong Pi
Hu Gu
Luo Shi Teng
Mu Gua
Qin Jiao
Sang Zhi
Shen Jin Cao
Wei Ling Xian
Wu Jia Pi

Expel Parasites - *ebugs*
Bing Lang
Fei Zi
Shi Jun Zi

Expel Damp - *edamp*
Bei Xie
Bian Xu
Che Qian Zi
Chi Xiao Dou
Deng Xin Cao
Di Fu Zi
Dong Gua Pi
Dong Gua Ren
Dong Kui Zi
Fu Ling
Fu Ling Pi
Fu Shen
Hai Jin Sha
Han Fang Ji
Hua Shi
Jin Qian Cao
Mu Tong
Qu Mai
Sheng Jiang Pi
Shi Wei
Yi Yi Ren
Yin Chen Hao
Yu Mi Xu
Ze Xie
Zhu Ling

External Application - *etop*
Chan Su
Er Cha
Liu Huang
Qing Fen
She Chuang Zi
Xiong Huang

Expel Wind - *ewind*
Bai Ji Li
Di Long
Gou Teng
Jiang Can
Ling Yang Jiao
Quan Xie
Shi Jue Ming
Tian Ma
Wu Gong

Laxative - *lax*
Huo Ma Ren
Yu Li Ren

Move Blood - *movexue*
Chi Shao
Chuan Niu Xi
Chuan Shan Jia
Chuan Xiong
Dan Shen
E Zhu
Feng Mi
He Shou Wu
Hong Hua
Hu Zhang
Ji Xue Teng
Jiang Huang
Liu Ji Nu
Lu Lu Tong
Mo Yao
Niu Xi
Ru Xiang
San Leng
Si Gua Luo
Tao Ren
Wang Bu Liu Xing
Wu Ling Zhi
Xue Jie
Yan Hu Suo
Yi Mu Cao
Yu Jin
Yue Ji Hua
Ze Lan
Zi Ran Tong

Open Orifices - *open*
An Xi Xiang
Bing Pian
Niu Huang
She Xiang
Shi Chang Pu
Su He Xiang
Zhang Nao

Herb   Herb Category

Purgative - *purg*
Da Huang
Fan Xie Ye
Lu Hui
Mang Xiao

Release Exterior Wind-Cold - *rext w-c*
Bai Zhi
Cong Bai
Fang Feng
Gao Ben
Geng Mi
Gui Zhi
Jing Jie
Ma Huang
Qiang Huo
Sheng Jiang
Xi Xin
Xiang Ru
Xin Yi Hua
Zi Su Ye

Release Exterior Wind-Heat - *rext w-h*
Bo He
Chai Hu
Chan Tui
Dan Dou Chi
Fu Ping
Ge Gen
Ju Hua
Man Jing Zi
Mu Zei
Niu Bang Zi
Sang Ye
Sheng Ma

Food Stagnation - *rfood*
Gu Ya
Ji Nei Jin
Lai Fu Zi
Mai Ya
Shan Zha
Shen Qu

Regulate Qi - *rqi*
Chen Pi
Chen Xiang
Chuan Lian Zi
Da Fu Pi
Fo Shou
Ju Hong
Li Zhi He
Mu Xiang
Qing Pi
Shi Di
Tan Xiang
Wu Yao
Xiang Fu
Xie Bai
Zhi Ke
Zhi Shi

Stabilize & Bind - *sab*
Bai Guo
Chi Shi Zhi
Chun Pi
Fu Pen Zi
Fu Xiao Mai
Hai Piao Xiao
He Zi
Jin Yin Zi
Lian Zi
Qian Shi
Rou Dou Kou
Shan Zhu Yu
Wu Mei
Wu Wei Zi
Xue Yu Tan
Ying Su Ke

Stop Bleeding - *stopxue*
Ai Ye
Bai Ji
Bai Mao Gen
Ce Bai Ye
Da Ji
Di Yu
Fu Long Gan
Huai Hua Mi
Ou Jie
Pu Huang
Qian Cao Gen
San Qi
Xian He Cao
Xiao Ji
Zong Lu Pi

Tonify Blood - *tblood*
Bai Shao
Dang Gui
E Jiao
Gou Qi Zi
Long Yan Rou
Sang Shen
Shu Di Huang

Tonify Qi - *tqi*
Bai Zhu
Da Zao
Dang Shen
Gan Cao
Huang Jing
Huang Qi
Ren Shen
Shan Yao
Tai Zi Shen
Yi Tang

Aromatic Damp - *movedamp*
Bai Dou Kou
Cang Zhu
Cao Dou Kou
Cao Guo
Hou Po
Huo Xiang
Pei Lan
Sha Ren

Tonify Yang - *tyang*
Ba Ji Tian
Bu Gu Zhi
Du Zhong
Ge Jie
Gou Ji
Gu Sui Bu
Hai Shen
Hu Lu Ba
Hu Tao Ren
Lu Rong
Rou Cong Rong
Suo Yang
Tu Si Zi
Xian Mao
Xu Duan
Yi Zhi Ren
Yin Yang Huo
Zi He Che

Tonify Yin - *tyin*
Bai He
Bai Mu Er
Bie Jia
Gui Ban
Han Lian Cao
Hei Zhi Ma
Mai Men Dong
Nu Zhen Zi
Sang Ji Sheng
Sha Shen
Shi Hu
Tian Men Dong
Xi Yang Shen
Yu Zhu

Warm Interior - *wint*
Bi Ba
Cao Wu
Chuan Jiao
Chuan Wu
Ding Xiang
Fu Zi
Gan Jiang
Gao Liang Jiang
Hu Jiao
Rou Gui
Wu Zhu Yu
Xiao Hui Xiang

HERB

Herbs	Channels / Properties	Indications / Actions
Ai Ye *(ai-yeh)* stopxue	LIV, SP, KID bitter acrid warm	• **Warms the womb, stops bleeding**: Used to treat menorrhagia or uterine bleeding from deficiency cold. • **Quiets the fetus**: Used to treat a restless fetus including lower abdominal pain, and flooding or spotting during pregnancy that threatens miscarriage. Used for infertility due to a cold womb. • **Warms the channels, dispels cold, and stops pain**: Used to treat abdominal pain including dysmenorrhea.
An Xi Xiang *(an-his-hsiang)* open	HT, SP, LIV acrid bitter neutral	• **Opens the orifices, moves Qi and Blood**: Used to treat sudden stroke, pain in the abdomen and chest, postpartum dizziness, child fright epilepsy, and wind painful obstruction of the lumbar region.
Ba Dou *(pa-tou)* cath	LU, ST, LI acrid toxic hot	• **Drains cold accumulations**: Severely treats constipation, abdominal fullness, distention, and pain associated with cold accumulation in the interior. • **Drains water & reduces edema:** Used to treat edema. • **Breaks Phlegm:** Used to treat wheezing and severe fullness and distention in the chest and diaphragm obstructing the throat. • **Promotes healing:** Used to treat abscesses and ulcerations.
Ba Ji Tian *(pa-chi-tien)* tyang	KID, LIV sweet pungent warm	• **Tonifies the Kidney Yang:** Used to treat premature ejaculation, frequent urination, urinary incontinence, impotence, infertility, and irregular menstruation, associated with cold from deficiency. • **Strengthens the sinews and bones:** Used to treat lumbar and knee pain or muscle atrophy. • **Dispels Wind-Damp-Cold:** Used to treat wind-damp-cold painful obstruction in the lower back and wind-cold-damp leg qi with pain in the legs.
Bai Bian Dou *(pai-pian-tou)* clht-sumr	SP, ST sweet neutral	• **Clears Summerheat:** Used to treat diarrhea or vomiting associated with summerheat. • **Fortifies Qi, harmonizes the Center:** Used to treat chronic vaginal discharge, chronic diarrhea, and poor appetite associated with spleen deficiency.
Bai Bu *(pai-pu)* cough	LU sweet bitter sl warm	• **Warms and moistens Lung Qi and suppresses cough**: Used to treat for both acute and chronic cough. • **Expels parasites:** Used to kill parasites including pinworms and head lice.
Bai Dou Kou *(pai-tou-kou)* movedamp	SP, ST, LU acrid warm	• **Warms the Center, transforms Dampness:** Used to treat nausea and vomiting associated with internal dampness, usually from spleen deficiency. • **Moves Qi:** Used to treat feelings of fullness and distention in the chest or epigastrium, and poor appetite associated with stagnant qi; and nausea or vomiting associated with food stagnation.
Bai Fu Zi *(pai-fu-tsu)* cold-phlegm	LIV, LU, SP acrid sweet warm toxic	• **Dries Dampness, transforms Phlegm, dispels Wind-Damp**: Used to treat wind-stroke, deviation of the face and mouth, hemiplegia, or migraine headaches associated with phlegm obstruction and wnd-damp obstructing the orifices. • **Relieves toxicity and dissipates nodules:** for snakebite, scrofula, or other nodules due to phlegm and toxicity.
Bai Guo *(pai-kou)* *AKA yin xing* sab	KID, LIV, LU sweet bitter astringent neutral sl toxic	• **Constrains Lung Qi and calms wheezing:** Used to treat wheezing and coughing with copious sputum. • **Retains Dampness and stops discharge**: Used to treat vaginal discharge or turbid urine. • **Reduces urine flow:** Used to treat urinary frequency, incontinence, or spermatorrhea.

Herbs	Channels / Properties	Indications / Actions
Bai He *(pai-ho)* tyin	HT, LU sweet sl bitter sl cold	• **Moistens the Lung, suppresses cough:** Used to treat Lung dryness, dry coughing, coughing with blood-tinged sputum. • **Clears the Heart and quiets the Spirit**: Used to treat fright palpitations, restlessness, irritability, and insomnia associated with yin not nourishing the Heart.
Bai Hua She *(pai-hua-sheh)* d-w-damp	SP, LIV salty sweet toxic warm	• **Dispels Wind-Damp, penetrates the sinews and bones, calms fright spasm:** Used to treat wind-damp paralysis and joint pain, numbness, child fright wind, lockjaw, scrofula, and sores.
Bai Hua She She Cao *(pai-hua-sheh-cao)* clht-detox	LIV, ST, LI bitter sweet cold	• **Clears Heat, resolves toxicity:** Used to treat Lung heat panting and cough, tonsillitis, pharyngitis, appendicitis, dysentery, swollen welling abscesses and sores. • **Clears heat and resolves Dampness**: Used to treat pelvic inflammatory disease with hot painful urinary dysfunction and damp-heat jaundice. • **Removes toxins:** Used to treat poisonous snake bites.
Bai Ji *(pai-chi)* stopxue	LIV, ST, LU bitter sweet cool	• **Stops bleeding, treats blood ejection:** Used to treat epistaxis, hemoptysis, or vomiting blood. • **Relieves swelling and aids in regeneration of flesh:** Applied topically to treat abscesses or ulcerations and is used in general for trauma.
Bai Ji Li *(pai-chi-li)* ewind	LIV, LU pungent bitter warm	• **Pacifies the Liver and subdues the Yang:** Used to treat headache, vertigo, or dizziness due to ascendant Liver yang. • **Dispels Wind, brightens the eyes, stops itching**: Used to treat red, swollen, and painful eyes. • **Regulates Qi:** Used to treat pain and distention in the chest or hypochondrium and insufficient lactation associated with stagnant Liver qi
Bai Jiang Cao *(pai-chiang-tsao)* clht-detox	LIV, ST, LI acrid bitter sl cold	• **Clears Heat, resolves toxins, and eliminates pus:** Used to treat swelling abscesses, intestinal abscess, diarrhea, red and white vaginal discharge, red, painful, swollen eyes, sores and swellings. • **Breaks Blood stasis:** Used to treat pain in the chest and abdomen and post partum stagnation pain associated with heat-induced blood stasis.
Bai Jie Zi *(pai-cheih-tsu)* cold-phlegm	LU acrid warm	• **Warms the Center, regulates the Qi, and transforms Phlegm:** Used to treat coughing with copious sputum, chest and hypochondrial pain and distention, and vomiting or reflux due to obstruction caused by accumulation of phlegm-cold. • **Softens Hardness, relieves swelling, and stops pain**: Used to treat painful, swollen joints or sores and eczema due to phlegm obstruction.
Bai Mao Gen *(pai-mao-ken)* stopxue	LU, ST, SI, UB sweet cold	• **Cools the Blood and stops bleeding**: Used to treat hematuria, vomiting of blood, epistaxis or hemoptysis. • **Clears heat and promotes urination:** Used to treat painful urinary dysfunction associated with heat in the bladder such as hematuria, dysuria. • **Treats heat disease with vexation and heat:** Used to treat hiccough or thirst due to Stomach heat, or wheezing due to Lung heat.
Bai Mu Er *(pai-mu-erh)* tyin	LU, ST sweet bland neutral	• **Supplements the Stomach yin, moistens the Lungs:** Used to treat yin deficiency with yang ascending. • **Nourishes Lung yin.**
Bai Qian *(pai-chien)* cold-phlegm	LU acrid sweet sl warm	• **Descends rebellious Qi and dispels Phlegm:** Used to treat coughing with copious sputum, panting and fullness.

HERB

Herbs	Channels / Properties	Indications / Actions
Bai Shao *(pai-shao-yao)* tblood	LIV, SP — bitter sour cool	• **Supplements the Blood and regulates menstruation**: Used to treat vaginal discharge, uterine bleeding, and other menstrual irregularities that are related to blood deficiency. • **Calms the Liver yang and stops pain and spasms**: Used to treat pain in the flank, chest, or abdomen, due to Liver qi stagnation or disharmony between the Liver and Spleen, and headaches from Liver yang rising. • **Benefits the Yin and harmonizes Ying and Wei:** Used to treat continuous sweating, spontaneous sweating or night sweats, and vaginal discharge or spermatorrhea caused by yin deficiency or disharmony between ying and wei.
Bai Tou Weng *(pai-tou-weng)* clht-detox	ST, LIV, LI — bitter cold	• **Clears Heat, cools the Blood and relieves toxins**: Used to treat bloody dysentery, malaria with fever and chills, epistaxis, and bleeding hemorrhoids.
Bai Wei *(pai-wei)* coolxue	LU, ST, KID — bitter salty cold	• **Clears Heat and cools the Blood:** Used to treat coughing of blood and other symptoms of heat entering the blood, and from fever due to yin deficiency, malaria, or post partum fever. • **Cools the Blood and promotes urination:** Used to treat dysuria and hematuria associated with heat. • **Expels Wind-Damp:** Used to treat painful obstruction caused by wind-damp. • **Relieves inflammation and toxins:** Used to treat toxic sores, swollen and painful throat, and snakebites.
Bai Xian Pi *(pai-hsien-pi)* clht-detox	SP, ST — bitter cold	• **Clears Heat, resolves toxins, dispels Wind, and dries Dampness:** Used to treat wind-heat sores and other itchy skin lesions, and wind-damp-impediment painful obstruction.
Bai Zhi *(pai-chih)* rext w-c	LU, ST — pungent warm	• **Dispels Wind and alleviates pain:** Used to treat headache, pain around the eyes, nasal congestion, and toothache or pain along the Stomach channel in the head. • **Reduces swelling:** Used to treat early stage sores • **Opens the nose**: Used to treat sinus congestion and nasal discharge. • **Dries Dampness:** Used to treat vaginal discharge.
Bai Zhu *(pai-chu)* tqi	SP, ST — bitter sweet warm	• **Supplements the Spleen, Strengthens the Center and Boosts the Qi:** Used to treat vomiting, diarrhea, fatigue, nausea or poor appetite due to Spleen and Stomach qi deficiency. • **Improves Spleen Function and dries dampness:** Used to treat diarrhea, edema, reduced urination caused by reduced Spleen function of transportation and transformation of fluids. • **Stops sweating:** Used to treat spontaneous sweating. • **Quiets the fetus:** Used to treat a restless fetus due to Spleen qi deficiency.
Bai Zi Ren *(pai-tzu-jen)* cshen	HT, SP, KID, LI — sweet neutral	• **Nourishes the Heart and quiets the Spirit:** Used to treat fright palpitations, anxiety, irritability, insomnia, poor memory associated with Heart blood deficiency. • **Moistens the Intestines:** Used to treat constipation associated with qi and blood deficiency. • **Stops sweating:** Used to treat night sweats associated with yin deficiency.
Ban Lan Gen *(pan-lang-ken)* clht-detox	HT, LU, ST — bitter cold	• **Drains Heat, resolves toxins, cools the Blood, and benefits the throat:** Used to treat flu, epidemic encephalitis, encephalitis B, pneumonia, maculopapular eruptions, mumps, sore throat, damp-heat jaundice.

Herbs	Channels / Properties	Indications / Actions
Ban Xia *(pan-hsia)* cold-phlegm	LU, SP, ST — acrid warm toxic	• **Dries Dampness, transforms Phlegm, descends rebellious Qi:** Used to treat coughing with copious sputum associated with ascendant Lung qi, and nausea and vomiting associated with phlegm-dampness due to Spleen not transforming or transporting, causing Stomach qi to rebel upwards. • **Dissipates nodules and reduces distention:** Used to treat hard and soft nodules, and distention or pain in the chest, hypochondrium, or abdomen associated with qi stagnation.
Bei Xie *(pieh-hsieh)* edamp	UB, LIV, ST — bitter neutral	• **Separates the pure from the turbid:** Used to treat turbid and cloudy urine or vaginal discharge resulting from interior dampness. **Expels Wind and unblocks Dampness:** Used to treat painful obstruction of the lower back with pain, numbness or stiffness of the lower extremities or muscle aches associated with wind-dampness or damp-heat. • **Clears damp-heat from the skin:** Used to treat eczema and other damp-heat skin lesions.
Bi Ba *(pi-pa)* wint	ST, LI — pungent hot sl toxic	• **Warms middle, dissipates cold, descends Qi, and alleviates pain:** Used to treat cold pain in the abdomen and heart, vomiting, acid regurgitation, borborygmus, diarrhea, cold dysentery, headache, nasal congestion, and toothache.
Bian Xu *(pian-shu)* edamp	UB — bitter sl cold	• **Clears damp-heat, promotes urination, and unblocks painful urinary dysfunction:** Used to treat dysuria, urinary obstruction, hematuria, jaundice, vaginal discharge, swollen hemorrhoids and damp sores associated with damp heat in the lower burner. • **Kills parasites and stops itching:** Used to treat tinea, or for tapeworm, hookworm, and pinworm infestations.
Bie Jia *(pieh-chia)* tyin	LIV, SP — salty sl cold	• **Nourishes the yin and extinguishes wind:** Used to treat steaming bone disorder, night sweats due to yin deficiency, and dizziness, tinnitus, spasms and tremors associated with internal movement of Liver wind associated with deficiency of Liver and Kidney yin. • **Activates the blood, unblocks menstruation, and softens hardness:** Used to treat accumulations in the chest and flank causing pain, and amenorrhea, and menorrhagia associated with heat in the blood.
Bing Lang *(pin-lang)* ebugs	LI, ST — acrid bitter warm	• **Kills parasites:** Used to treat abdominal pain and distention due to roundworms. • **Breaks accumulation and descends Qi:** Used to treat food stagnation, diarrhea with rectal heaviness, and phlegm obstruction causing qi to rebel. • **Reduces edema:** Used to treat edema and leg qi. Treats malaria.
Bing Pian *(pin-pian)* open	ST, LU, SP — pungent bitter cool	• **Opens the orifices, clears Heat, brightens the eyes, disperses swelling and relieves pain:** Used to treat wind stroke with clenched jaw, clouded spirit in febrile disease, fright, epilepsy, deafness, mouth sores, otitis media, swollen abscesses, hemorrhoids, and eye screens.
Bo He *(po-he)* rext w-h	LU, LIV — pungent aromatic cool	• **Releases the exterior, disperses Wind-Heat:** Used to treat flu and colds causing fever, headache, and cough, sore throat, and red eyes. • **Vents rashes:** Used in the early stages of rashes with dormant papules such as measles. • **Soothes the Liver qi:** Used to treat constrained Liver qi with pressure or fullness in the chest or flanks, depression or angers easily, and menstrual irregularities including dysmenorrhea.

HERB

Herbs	Channels / Properties	Indications / Actions
Bu Gu Zhi *(pu-ku-chih)* tyang	KID, SP bitter pungent very warm	• **Tonifies the Kidney Yang, retains the Essence:** Used to treat spermatorrhea, incontinence of urine, enuresis, and frequent urination associated with Kidney deficiency not retaining essence, and impotence, premature ejaculation, painful lower back associated with cold from deficiency. • **Warms the Spleen Yang:** Used to treat diarrhea, borborygmus, and abdominal pain associated with cold from Spleen yang deficiency. Most appropriate for both Spleen and Kidney deficiency. • **Benefits coughing and wheezing:** Used to treat wheezing associated with Kidney qi deficiency. • **Clears Wind or Wind-Damp:** Used topically to treat skin lesions such as alopecia, psoriasis, and vitiligo.
Can Sha *(can-sha)* d-w-damp	SP, LIV, ST acrid sweet warm	• **Dispels Wind-Dampness:** Used to treat painful obstruction or itchy, skin rashes due to wind-damp. • **Harmonizes the Stomach and dries Dampness:** Used to treat vomiting, diarrhea, cramps, abdominal pain, borborygmus and spasms in the lower leg associated with dampness.
Cang Er Zi *(tsang-erh-tzu)* d-w-damp	LU sweet sl bitter warm toxic	• **Disperses Wind and dispels Dampness:** Used to treat wind-damp painful obstruction or hypertonicity of the limbs. • **Expels exterior Wind:** Used to treat headache due to wind-damp. • **Opens the nasal passages:** Used to treat sinus congestion and obstruction.
Cang Zhu *(tsang-chu)* movedamp	SP, ST acrid bitter warm	• **Dries Dampness and fortifies the Spleen:** Used to treat nausea and vomiting, diarrhea, poor appetite, epigastric distention, fatigue, lassitude, somnolence, vaginal discharge, or swollen joints associated with dampness caused by poor Spleen transportation and transformation function and can be either hot or cold natured. • **Dispels Wind-Dampness:** Used to treat wei (weakness) of the legs and painful obstruction of the arms and legs due to wind-cold-dampness. • **Diaphoresis, releases the exterior:** Used to treat colds and flu with symptoms of headache and body ache. Improves vision: Used to treat night blindness or poor vision.
Cao Dou Kou *(tsao-tou-kou)* movedamp	SP, ST acrid warm	• **Warms the Center, dispels Cold, moves Qi and dries Dampness:** Used to treat cold pain in the chest and abdomen, distention and fullness in the chest and abdomen, cold-damp diarrhea and vomiting, and phlegm obstructing.
Cao Guo *(tsao-kuo)* movedamp	SP, ST acrid warm	• **Dries dampness and dispels Cold:** Used to treat distention and fullness in the epigastrium, vomiting is associated with turbid damp-cold obstruction. • **Interrupts malaria:** Used to treat alternating fever and chills associated with malaria. • **Disperses food stagnation and transforms accumulation:** Used to treat indigestion and focal distention associated with food stagnation.
Cao Wu *(tsa-woo)* *See fu zi* wint	HT, LIV, SP pungent bitter warm very toxic	• **Expels wind-dampness, disperses cold, and alleviates pain:** Used to treat wind, cold, and damp painful obstruction, wind stroke paralysis, lockjaw, headache, pain in the stomach, scrofula and phlegm obstructions.

Herbs	Channels / Properties	Indications / Actions
Ce Bai Ye *(che-pei-yeh)* stopxue	LIV, HT, LI bitter astringent sl cold	• **Cools the Blood and stops bleeding:** Used to treat excess or deficiency heat entering the blood causing vomiting of blood, hemoptysis, bleeding gums, hematuria or blood in the stool, dysentery with blood and mucus in the stool, and uterine bleeding. • **Stops coughing:** Used to treat heat in the Lungs causing coughing due to accumulation of phlegm or with blood-streaked sputum.
Chai Hu *(chai-hu)* rext w-h	LIV, GB, PC, SJ bitter pungent cool	• **Harmonizes the exterior and interior:** Used to treat alternating chills and fever accompanied by a bitter taste in the mouth, flank pain, irritability, vomiting, and a stifling sensation in the chest associated with the Shaoyang stage disease. • **Soothes the Liver qi:** Used to treat distention and fullness in the chest and abdomen, dizziness, vertigo, chest and flank pain, emotional instability, a stifling sensation in the chest, abdominal bloating, nausea, and indigestion, or menstrual irregularities including dysmenorrhea and amenorrhea, associated with constrained Liver qi and disharmonies between the Liver and the Spleen. • **Raises the Yang:** Used to treat gastroptosis, hemorrhoids, anal or uterine prolapse, and diarrhea due to Spleen qi not holding the organs in place.
Chan Su *(chan-su)* etop	KID, ST sweet pungent warm toxic	• **Resolves toxins, disperses swelling, strengthens the Heart, and relieves pain:** Used to treat sores, abscesses, scrofula, chronic osteomyelitis, sore and swollen throat, cardiac failure, toothache.
Chan Tui *(chan-tui)* rext w-h	LU, LIV sweet salty sl cold	• **Releases the exterior, disperses Wind-Heat:** Used to treat flu and colds causing sore, swollen throat, loss of voice, nasal discharge, headache, and red, painful, and swollen eyes, or blurry vision. • **Vents rashes:** Used in the early stages of rashes with dormant papules such as measles. • **Stops spasms and extinguishes Wind:** Used to treat tetanus, convulsions, spasms, delirium, or night fright epilepsy caused by interior wind.
Chang Shan *(chong shan)* clht-sumr	HT, LU, LIV acrid bitter toxic cold	• **Malarial conditions:** Used as a prophylactic for malaria. • **Eliminates Phlegm.**
Che Qian Zi *(che-chien-tzu)* edamp	UB, LU, LIV, KID sweet cold	• **Promotes urination and clears Heat:** Used to treat diarrhea, dysuria, hematuria, summerheat-damp diarrhea, and urinary obstruction. • **Brightens the eyes:** Used to treat red, sore and painful eyes, and visual obstructions. • **Expels Phlegm and stops cough:** Used to treat with copious sputum due to phlegm obstructing the Lung qi.
Chen Pi *(chen-pee)* rqi	SP, ST, LU pungent bitter aromatic warm	• **Regulates the Qi, rectifies the center:** Used to treat distention and fullness in the epigastrium and abdomen, hiccough, bloating, belching, nausea and vomiting associated with Spleen not transforming and transporting fluids effectively. • **Dries Dampness and transforms Phlegm:** Used to treat phlegm and dampness obstructing the middle and upper burners causing coughing with copious, viscous sputum, a stifling sensation in the chest, abdominal distention, little appetite, fatigue, diarrhea or loose stools.

Herbs	Channels / Properties		Indications / Actions
Chen Xiang (shen-hsiang) rqi	SP, ST, KID	pungent bitter warm	• **Descends Qi and alleviates pain:** Used to treat distention and pain in the epigastrium and abdomen, wheezing, vomiting, belching, or hiccups due to cold from deficiency. • **Warms the Kidneys and absorbs Qi:** Used to treat asthma with wheezing due to Kidney deficiency.
Chi Shao (chih-shao-yao) movexue	LIV, SP	sour bitter sl cold	• **Activates the Blood and disperses Blood stasis:** Used to treat menstrual irregularities including dysmenorrhea, amenorrhea, and blood stasis causing abdominal pain, immobile abdominal masses, swelling and pain caused by trauma. • **Clears Heat and cools the Blood:** Used to treat spontaneous external bleeding, bloody dysentery, and bleeding from internal wind. • **Clears Fire:** for red, swollen, painful eyes associated with Liver fire.
Chi Shi Zhi (chih-shi-chih) sab	SP, ST, LI	sweet sour astringent warm	• **Astringes the Intestines and stops diarrhea:** Used to treat chronic diarrhea or dysentery. • **Stops bleeding:** Used to treat uterine bleeding, excessive menstruation, and blood in the stool. • **Promotes healing of wounds.**
Chi Xiao Dou (chih-hsiao-tou) edamp	HT, SI	sweet sour neutral	• **Clears Heat and promotes urination:** Used to treat edema, dysuria, leg qi, or jaundice due to damp-heat. • **Disperses blood stasis, reduces swelling & relieves toxins:** Used to treat sores, carbuncles, and abscesses.
Chuan Bei Mu (chuan-pei-mu) clht-phlegm	LU, HT	bitter sweet sl cold	• **Moistens the Lung, transforms Phlegm, stops cough:** Used to treat cough with sputum that is difficult to expectorate, or with blood-tinged sputum, associated with Lung heat due to Lung yin deficiency, phlegm-heat obstruction, or constrained qi causing heat. • **Dissipates nodules, relieves toxins:** Used to treat phlegm-fire nodules including scrofula, pulmonary abscesses, throat obstructions, sores and toxins.
Chuan Jiao (chuan-chiao) wint	KID, SP, ST	pungent hot sl toxic	• **Warms the center, disperses cold, and alleviates pain:** Used to treat cold and pain in the abdomen, vomiting and diarrhea associated with deficiency cold. • **Kills parasites:** Used to treat abdominal pain from roundworms.
Chuan Lian Zi (chuan-lien-tzu) rqi	UB, LIV, SI, ST	bitter sl cold toxic	• **Regulates qi and stops pain:** Used to treat pain in the hypochondrium and abdomen, and for hernia pain due to constrained Liver qi or Liver-Stomach disharmony. • **Clears Heat, dries dampness:** Used to treat fullness and distention in the abdomen due to damp-heat. • **Kills parasites and stops pain:** Used to treat distention and pain due to roundworms and tapeworms.
Chuan Niu Xi (chuan-niu-tzu) See niu xi movexue	LIV, KID	bitter sweet neutral	• **Activates the Blood, dispels Wind, dries dampness:** Used to treat wind-damp lumbar and knee pain, weakness of the lower extremities and ligaments. • **Relieves Urination, benefits menstruation:** Used to treat dysuria, hematuria, amenorrhea and dysmenorrhea.
Chuan Shan Jia (chuan-shan-chia) movexue	LIV, ST	salty cool	• **Dispels blood stasis, frees menstruation, promotes lactation:** Used to treat amenorrhea, dysmenorrhea, and insufficient lactation associated with blood stasis. • **Reduces inflammation:** Used to treat toxins, abscesses, boils. • **Expels Wind-Damp, unblocks the channels:** Used to treat damp impediment Bi causing stiffness or spasms in the limbs or joints.

Herbs	Channels / Properties	Indications / Actions
Chuan Wu *(chuan-wu)* *See Fu zi* wint	HT, SP, LIV pungent bitter warm toxic	• **Expels cold-damp, dissipates Wind, warms the channels, and relieves pain:** Used to treat wind, cold, and damp painful obstruction, hypertonicity of the limbs, hemiplegia, headache, pain in the abdomen and chest.
Chuan Xin Lian *(chuan-hsin-lian)* clht-detox	LI, LU, SI, ST bitter cold	• **Clears Heat and relieves toxins:** Used to treat acute bacillary dysentery, gastroenteritis, colds, epidemic encephalitis, tracheitis, pneumonia, whooping cough, pulmonary tuberculosis, cholecystitis, and snakebites. • **Clears Heat, cools the Blood:** Used to treat epistaxis. • **Relieves hypertension:** Used to treat elevated blood pressure.
Chuan Xiong *(chuan-chiang)* movexue	LIV, GB, PC acrid warm	• **Activates the Blood, moves Qi, alleviates pain:** Used to treat dysmenorrhea, amenorrhea, difficult labor, post-partum stasis, pain in the hypochondrium and headache pain. • **Expels wind and relieves pain:** Used to treat headache and dizziness associated with exterior wind attack.
Chun Pi *(chun-pi)* sab	LI, ST bitter astringent cold	• **Clears Heat, dries dampness, and astringes the Intestines:** Used to treat chronic diarrhea or dysentery and chronic vaginal discharge. • **Kills parasites:** Used to treat pain and distention in the abdomen due to roundworms.
Ci Shi *(tsi-chi)* cshen	KID, LIV acrid salty cold	• **Subdues the Yang, quiets the Spirit:** Used to treat restlessness, palpitations, insomnia, or tremors, dizziness or vertigo associated with ascendant yang. • **Benefits hearing and vision:** Used to treat impaired hearing or deafness, tinnitus, or floaters and poor vision associated with Liver and Kidney yin deficiency. • **Benefits wheezing and coughing:** Used to treat chronic asthma associated with the Kidney failing to grasp qi.
Cong Bai *(chung-pai)* rext w-c	LU, ST pungent warm	• **Releases the exterior:** Used to treat early stage exterior wind-cold attack. • **Disperses cold and frees the Yang:** Used to treat pain and distention in the abdomen or nasal congestion due to deficiency cold obstruction. • **Relieves toxins:** Treats sores and abscesses.
Da Fu Pi *(ta-fu-pi)* rqi	SP, ST, LI, SI pungent sl warm	• **Descends Qi and relieves stagnation:** Used to treat epigastric and abdominal distention, vomiting, belching, acid regurgitation, and constipation. • **Expels dampness:** Used to treat damp stagnation in the Stomach and Intestines. • **Promotes urination and reduces edema:** Used to treat edema and damp leg qi.
Da Huang *(ta-huang)* *AKA chuan jun* purg	HT, LI, LIV, ST bitter cold	• **Drains heat and breaks accumulations:** Used to treat intestinal heat excess and Yangming patterns with high fever, profuse sweating, extreme thirst, constipation, abdominal distention and pain, and in extreme cases, delirium. • **Clears Heat and dries dampness:** Used to treat dysentery and damp-heat diarrhea. • **Cools the Blood:** Used to treat vomiting blood, epistaxis, hemoptysis, blood in the stool and hemorrhoids. • **Activates the Blood:** Used to treat amenorrhea, immobile abdominal masses, or fixed pain due to blood stasis. • **Clears heat obstructing the blood level:** Used to treat fever, swollen and painful eyes, or sores due to heat in the blood.
Da Ji *(ta-chi)* stopxue	LIV, SP sweet cool	• **Stops bleeding, treats blood ejection:** Used to treat epistaxis, hemoptysis, vomiting blood, flooding or spotting. • **Relieves swelling and aids in the regeneration of flesh.**

HERB

Herbs	Channels / Properties	Indications / Actions
Da Qing Ye *(ta-ching-yeh)* clht-detox	HT, LU, ST bitter very cold	• **Clears Heat and relieves toxins:** Used to treat warm febrile diseases with fever, thirst, bacillary dysentery, acute gastroenteritis, acute pneumonia, acute infectious hepatitis, jaundice, dysentery, swellings, and abscesses. • **Cools the Blood and stops bleeding:** Used to treat spontaneous external bleeding and for blotches or other skin eruptions due to heat in the blood.
Da Zao *(ta-tsao)* tqi	SP, ST sweet neutral	• **Supplements the Spleen and reinforces the Qi:** Used to treat fatigue, weakness, shortness of breath, poor appetite, nausea, and loose stools caused by qi deficiency. • **Nourishes the Blood and quiets the Spirit:** Used to treat irritability, agitation, depression and other emotional disorders. Moderates the properties of other herbs.
Dai Zhe Shi *(tai-che-shi)* cshen	HT, LIV, PC bitter cold	• **Calms the Liver, subdues Yang:** Used to treat tinnitus, dizziness, vertigo, headache, and pain or pressure around the eyes associated with Liver yang rising. • **Descends rebellious Qi:** Used to treat hiccough, vomiting, belching, and wheezing associated with qi failing to descend. • **Cools the Blood, stops bleeding:** Used to treat epistaxis, spontaneous external bleeding, flooding and spotting, and vomiting blood.
Dan Dou Chi *(tan-tou-shi)* rext w-h	LU, ST sweet sl bitter acrid cold	• **Releases the exterior:** Used to treat flu and colds causing fever, chills, and headache. • **Relieves restlessness:** Used to treat restlessness and irritability, fullness or oppressed sensations in the chest, and insomnia following febrile disease.
Dan Nan Xing *(tan-nan-hsiang)* cold-phlegm	LIV, LU, SP bitter cool	• **Clears Fire, transforms Phlegm, dispels internal Wind**: Used to treat convulsions, spasms, stroke, seizures, and lockjaw.
Dan Shen *(tan-shen)* movexue	HT, PC, LIV bitter sl cold	• **Activates the blood and breaks up blood stasis:** Used to treat pain in the chest and abdomen, epigastric pain, pain in the hypochondrium, dysmenorrhea, amenorrhea, and palpable masses associated with blood stasis and qi constraint. • **Quiets the Heart and the Spirit:** Used to treat restlessness, irritability, palpitations, and insomnia associated with heat in the blood or heat in the nutritive level.
Dan Zhu Ye *(tan-chu-yeh)* clht-fire	HT, SI, ST sweet bland cold	• **Clears Heart Fire:** Used to treat mouth sores and swollen, painful gums, irritability, and thirst due to heat in the Heart or Stomach channels. • **Promotes urination and clears Damp-Heat:** Used to treat dysuria associated with heat in the Small Intestine channel due to Heart fire pouring downward.
Dang Gui *(tang-kuei)* tblood	LIV, HT, SP sweet pungent bitter warm	• **Supplements the Blood and regulates menstruation:** Used to treat irregular menstruation, amenorrhea, dysmenorrhea and other symptoms related to blood deficiency including a pale, white complexion, blurred vision, dry or brittle nails, dry hair, and heart palpitations. • **Invigorates the Blood:** Used to treat pain due to blood stagnation including abdominal pain and traumatic injury. • **Moistens the Intestines:** Used to treat dry Intestines due to blood deficiency. • **Relieves swelling:** Used to treat sores and abscesses, helping to regenerate flesh.

Herbs	Channels / Properties	Indications / Actions
Dang Shen *(tang-shen)* tqi	SP, LU / sweet neutral	• **Tonifies the Center and reinforces the Qi:** Used to treat fatigue, poor appetite, nausea, diarrhea, vomiting, prolapse of the uterus, stomach, or rectum due to sinking Spleen qi. • **Strengthens qi and nourishes fluids:** thirst due to injury of fluids or wasting and thirsting disorder. • **Tonifies the Lung Qi:** Used to treat Lung deficiency causing chronic cough and shortness of breath, or cough with copious sputum due to Spleen qi deficiency.
Deng Xin Cao *(teng-hsin-tsao)* edamp	HT, SI, LU / sweet bland sl cold	• **Promotes urination and dries dampness:** Used to treat dysuria, edema, obstructed urination, and damp-heat jaundice. • **Clears Heat from the Heart channel:** Used to treat insomnia and irritability accompanying urinary distress and associated with heart fire or with kidney yin deficiency.
Di Fu Zi *(ti-fu-tzu)* edamp	UB / sweet bitter cold	• **Clears damp-heat and promotes urination:** Used to treat dysuria, urinary obstruction, and vaginal discharge. • **Expels dampness and stops itching:** Used to treat genital damp itching and damp heat skin lesions such as eczema and scabies.
Di Gu Pi *(ti-ku-pi)* coolxue	LU, LIV, KID / sweet cold	• **Drains Fire from Yin deficiency:** Used to treat tidal fever, night sweats, steaming bone disorder, irritability, toothache, and thirst associated with fire from deficiency flaring up. • **Clears Heat and stops coughing:** Used to treat coughing and panting associated with Lung heat. • **Clears Heat and cools the blood:** Used to treat hematuria, epistaxis, vomiting blood with heat in the blood. • **Lowers Blood Pressure:** Used to treat hypertension.
Di Long *(ti-lung)* ewind	LIV, LU, SP, UB / salty cold	• **Drains Heat and relieves spasms:** Used to treat spasms and convulsion, manic agitation and fright wind associated with high fevers resulting from movement of internal wind in the blood or channels. • **Suppresses wheezing:** Used to treat panting and wheezing due to Lung heat. • **Clears Heat and frees the channels:** Used to treat wind stroke and hemiplegia, joint pain and painful obstruction. • **Clears Heat and promotes urination:** Used to treat dysuria due to heat in the Bladder. • **Calms the Liver:** Used to treat headache, painful red eyes and hypertension associated with Liver yang rising.
Di Yu *(ti-yu)* stopxue	LIV, ST, LI / bitter sour sl cold	• **Cools the Blood and stops bleeding:** Used to treat epistaxis, hemoptysis, blood in the stool, bleeding hemorrhoids and bloody dysentery due to damp-heat, and profuse uterine bleeding. • **Clears Heat and aids in regeneration of flesh:** Applied topically to treat trauma or other types of sores.
Ding Xiang *(ting-hsiang)* wint	KID, SP, ST / pungent warm	• **Warms the center and descends rebellious Qi:** Used to treat abdominal pain, vomiting and diarrhea, hiccough, stomach reflux, poor appetite associated with interior cold. • **Warms the Kidneys:** Used to treat impotence or clear vaginal discharge due to yang deficiency.
Dong Gua Pi *(tung-kua-pee)* edamp	LU, SI / sweet sl cold	• **Unblocks urination, disperses swelling, clears heat and resolves summerheat:** Used to treat edema, urinary obstruction, and summerheat.

HERB

Herbs	Channels / Properties	Indications / Actions
Dong Gua Ren *(tung-kua-ren)* edamp	LU, ST, LI, SI — sweet cold	• **Clears Heat, moistens the Lung, transforms phlegm:** Used to treat phlegm-heat cough with dry thick sputum and Lung or intestinal abscess. • **Clears Heat and dries dampness:** Used to treat edema, dysuria and vaginal discharge due to damp-heat.
Dong Kui Zi *(tung-kui-tzu)* edamp	UB, LI, SI — sweet cold	• **Promotes urination:** Used to treat dysuria, edema, hematuria or cystic calculi associated with damp-heat. • **Frees lactation:** Used to treat insufficient lactation and distended and painful breasts. • **Moistens the intestines and unblocks the bowels:** Used to treat constipation.
Dou Juan *(tou-chuang)* clht-sumr	SP, ST — sweet neutral	• **Clears Summerheat & Damp heat:** Used in early stages of summerheat or warm febrile disease especially with joint pain, sensation of heaviness, minimal sweating & greasy tongue coating due to presence of dampness.
Du Huo *(tu-huo)* d-w-damp	KID, UB — bitter pungent warm	• **Dispels Wind-Dampness and relieves pain:** Used to treat aching pain in the lower back and knees, and hypertonicity of the limbs associated with wind-cold-damp painful obstruction and headache and toothache associated with penetrating dampness. • **Releases the exterior:** Used to treat exterior attack of wind-cold together with dampness.
Du Zhong *(tu-chung)* tyang	KID, LIV — sweet sl pungent warm	• **Tonifies Liver and Kidneys; Strengthens Sinews and Bones:** Used to treat painful or weak lower back and knees, frequent urination associated with Liver and Kidney deficiency. • **Quiets the Fetus:** Used to treat flooding or spotting during pregnancy and to prevent miscarriage when there is back pain associated with deficiency cold. • **Stops Dizziness:** Used to treat dizziness associated with hypertension due to ascendant Liver yang.
E Jiao *(ah-chiao)* tblood	LIV, LU, KID — sweet neutral	• **Supplements the Blood:** Used to treat irregular menstruation, amenorrhea, dysmenorrhea and other symptoms related to blood deficiency including a pale, white complexion, blurred vision, dry or brittle nails, dry hair, and heart palpitations. • **Stops bleeding:** Used to treat hemoptysis, blood in the stool, menorrhagia, or spotting. • **Enriches the yin:** Used to treat yin deficiency that causes irritability, insomnia, or coughing.
E Zhu *(o-chu)* movexue	LIV, SP — bitter acrid warm	• **Dispels Wind, clears Heat, disperses swelling, and resolves toxins:** Used to treat distention and pain in the abdomen and region of the heart, masses, food stagnation, menstrual irregularities, and trauma.
Er Cha *(erh-cha)* etop	LU — bitter astringent neutral	• **Drains dampness:** Used to treat non-healing sores. • **Stops bleeding.** • **Clears Heat, transforms Phlegm:** Used to treat cough due to Lung heat, and thirst associated with summerheat.
Fan Xie Ye *fang-hsieh-yeh)* purg	LI — bitter sweet cold	• **Drains Heat and breaks up stagnation:** Used to treat constipation, and accumulation and stagnation with abdominal distention.
Fang Feng *(fang-feng)* rext w-c	UB, LIV, SP — pungent sweet sl warm	• **Releases the exterior and dispels Wind:** Used to treat headache, chills, stiff neck and body aches due to exterior wind-cold attack. • **Expels wind-dampness, Relieves Pain:** Used to treat exterior wind-damp painful obstruction causing joint pain. • **Dispels Wind:** Used to treat migraine headache, hypertonicity of the limbs, lockjaw, trembling and spasms associated with internal wind.

Herbs	Channels / Properties	Indications / Actions
Fei Zi *(fei-tzu)* ebugs	LU, ST, LI — sweet, astringent, neutral	• **Kills parasites:** Used to treat abdominal pain and distention caused by tapeworms, hookworms, and roundworms. • **Moistens dryness:** Used to treat constipation and mild coughs due to dryness in the Lungs.
Feng Mi *(feng-mi)* movexue	SP, LU, LI — sweet, neutral	• **Supplements the Center, relieves pain, moistens the lung, resolves toxins:** Used to treat toxins of Chuan Wu Tou, cough due to lung dryness, constipation, stomach pain, nasal congestion, mouth sores and burns.
Fo Shou *(fo-shou)* rqi	LU, SP, ST, LIV — acrid, bitter, sl warm	• **Soothes and regulates the Liver Qi:** Used to treat Stomach pain, distention in the hypochondrium. • **Dries dampness & transforms phlegm:** Used to treat panting and coughing due to phlegm obstructing the Lungs.
Fu Hai Shi *(fu-hai-shi)* clht-phlegm	LU — salty, cold	• **Clears Lung Heat, transforms Phlegm, softens hardness:** Used to treat phlegm-heat panting and cough, old phlegm accumulations, goiters and tumors of the neck, scrofula, dysuria, sores and swelling.
Fu Ling *(fu-ling)* edamp	HT, SP, LU — sweet, bland, neutral	• **Promotes urination and dries out dampness:** Used to treat edema, dysuria, and diarrhea resulting from either deficiency of Spleen qi or excess interior dampness. • **Boosts the Spleen, harmonizes the Stomach, Transforms Phlegm:** Used to treat vomiting, diarrhea, epigastric distention, abdominal fullness and poor appetite associated with Spleen deficiency, and phlegm congestion obstructing and causing headache, dizziness or palpitations. • **Quiets the Heart and calms the spirit:** Used to treat palpitations, insomnia, or poor memory associated with disharmony between the Heart and Spleen.
Fu Ling Pi *(fu-ling-pee)* edamp	HT, SP, LU — sweet, bland, neutral	• **Promotes urination and dries out dampness:** Used to treat edema, dysuria, and diarrhea resulting from either deficiency of Spleen qi or excess interior dampness. • **Boosts the Spleen, harmonizes the Stomach, Transforms Phlegm:** Used to treat vomiting, diarrhea, epigastric distention, abdominal fullness and poor appetite associated with Spleen deficiency, and phlegm congestion obstructing and causing headache, dizziness or palpitations. • **Quiets the Heart and calms the spirit:** Used to treat palpitations, insomnia, or poor memory associated with disharmony between the Heart and Spleen.
Fu Long Gan *(fu-lung-kan)* stopxue	SP, ST — acrid, warm	• **Warms the Middle and stops bleeding:** Used to treat blood in the urine or stool, or vomiting of blood. • **Warms the Middle:** Used to treat Stomach patterns due to deficiency cold with vomiting, morning sickness, or chronic Spleen deficiency diarrhea.
Fu Pen Zi *(fu-pen-tzu)* sab	KID, LIV — sweet, astringent, sl warm	• **Supplements the Liver and Kidney, secures Essence:** Used to treat polyuria, enuresis, spermatorrhea, premature ejaculation, or wet dreams caused by Kidney yang deficiency. • **Assists the yang and improves vision:** Used to treat poor vision, sore low back, and impotence due to Liver and Kidney deficiency.
Fu Ping *(fu-ping)* rext w-h	UB, LU — acrid, cold	• **Diaphoretic, dispels wind, reduces edema, resolves toxins:** Used to treat seasonal febrile diseases, non-eruption of maculopapules, itching skin, edema, urinary obstruction, sores and abscesses.

Herbs	Channels / Properties	Indications / Actions
Fu Shen *(fu-sheng)* edamp	HT, SP, LU sweet bland neutral	• **Promotes urination and dries out dampness:** Used to treat edema, dysuria, and diarrhea resulting from either deficiency of Spleen qi or excess interior dampness. • **Quiets the heart and the spirit:** Used to treat fright palpitations, poor memory, insomnia, fright epilepsy.
Fu Xiao Mai *(fu-hsiao-mai)* sab	HT sweet salty cool	• **Supplements the Heart and quiets the Spirit:** Used to treat depression and emotional instability or disorientation, palpitations, insomnia, and irritability. • **Constrains sweating:** Used to treat spontaneous sweating due to qi deficiency and night sweats due to yin deficiency. • **Astringes Essence:** Used to treat bedwetting in children.
Fu Zi *(fu-tzu)* wint	HT, KID, SP pungent hot toxic	• **Restores the Yang:** Used to treat diarrhea with undigested food, chills, cold extremities, severe vomiting, diarrhea, or sweating, and loss of consciousness associated with devastated yang. • **Supplements the Fire:** Used to treat chest and abdominal pain, edema, sweating and other manifestations of interior cold due to yang deficiency. • **Disperses cold, warms the channels, alleviates pain:** Used to treat painful obstruction of the low back and sinews and tendons caused by wind-damp-cold painful obstruction.
Gan Cao *(kan-tsao)* tqi	ALL 12 sweet neutral (raw) warm (dry-fried)	• **Supplements the Spleen and reinforces Qi and Blood:** Used to treat fatigue, shortness of breath, loose stools, irregular or intermittent pulse, and palpitations. • **Nourishes the Lungs and stops coughing,** for coughing and wheezing. **Relieves spasms and stops pain:** Used to treat pain or spasms of the abdomen or legs. • **Clears Heat and resolves toxins:** Used to treat carbuncles, sores, or other conditions resulting from heat toxins. Moderates the properties of other herbs.
Gan Jiang *(kan-chiang)* wint	HT, LU, SP, ST pungent hot	• **Warms the center and expels cold:** Used to treat chest and abdominal pain and distention, and vomiting or diarrhea due to interior cold blocking the middle associated with deficiency or excess. • **Restores Yang:** Used to treat cold limbs and extreme weakness associated with devastated yang. • **Warms the lungs and transforms phlegm:** Used to treat cold phlegm coughing and panting. • **Unblocks the channels and stops bleeding:** Used to treat bleeding associated with cold obstructing the channels.
Gan Sui *(kan-sui)* cath	KID, LI, LU bitter sweet toxic cold	• **Drains water downward:** Used to treat severe accumulation of fluid in the chest and abdomen, generalized edema, facial edema, and abdominal distention. • **Relieves inflammation:** Used topically to treat swelling and painful skin lesions.
Gao Ben *(gao-pen)* rext w-c	UB pungent warm	• **Dispels Wind, Cold and Damp and alleviates pain:** Used to treat headache, vertex headache, abdominal pain, or diarrhea associated with wind-cold-damp.
Gao Liang Jiang *(gao-liang-chiang)* wint	SP, ST pungent hot	• **Warms the Stomach, dispels wind, dissipates cold, moves Qi, relieves pain:** Used to treat cold and pain in the abdomen, vomiting, diarrhea, and food stagnation.

Herbs	Channels / Properties	Indications / Actions
Ge Gen *(ke-ken)* rext w-h	SP, ST	pungent sweet cool	• **Releases the exterior, relaxes the muscles and clears Heat:** Used to treat disorders causing aching muscles, stiff neck and upper back, fever, headache. • **Nourishes the fluids and alleviates thirst:** Used to treat wasting-thirsting and thirst due to Stomach heat. • **Vents rashes:** Used in the early stages of rashes with dormant papules such as measles. • **Stops diarrhea:** Used to treat diarrhea and dysentery associated with damp-heat. • **Lowers blood pressure:** Used to treat hypertension with headache, dizziness, tinnitus, and angina pectoris.
Ge Jie *(ke-chieh)* tyang	LU, KID	salty neutral	• **Supplements the Lung and boosts the Kidneys:** Used to treat coughing or wheezing, possibly with blood-tinged sputum, associated with Kidney and Lung deficiency. • **Benefits the Kidney yang:** Used to treat impotence, daybreak diarrhea, and urinary frequency associated with Kidney yang deficiency.
Geng Mi *(jeng-mi)* rext w-c	SP, ST	sweet cool	• **Supplements the center and boosts Qi.** • **Fortifies the Spleen and harmonizes the Stomach.**
Gou Ji *(kou-chi)* tyang	KID, LIV	bitter sweet warm	• **Tonifies the Liver and Kidney and benefits the sinews and bones:** Used to treat vaginal discharge, urinary incontinence, and pain in the low back and knees. • **Eliminates Wind-Dampness:** Used to treat wind-damp painful obstruction with pain, soreness, or numbness.
Gou Qi Zi *(kou-chi-tzu)* tblood	LIV, LU, KID	sweet neutral	• **Enriches the Kidney:** Used to treat yin and blood deficiency causing sore low back and knees, impotence, nocturnal emission, and diabetes. • **Supplements the Liver, brightens the eyes**: Used to treat Liver and Kidney yin or essence deficiency causing dizziness, blurred vision, or poor vision. • **Stops Cough:** Used to treat coughing due to Lung yin deficiency.
Gou Teng *(kou-teng)* ewind	LIV, HT	sweet cool	• **Extinguishes Wind and relieves spasms:** Used to treat tremors, seizures, and eclampsia resulting from movement of internal wind in the blood or channels. • **Clears Heat and subdues the Yang:** Used to treat headache, irritability, red eyes, and dizziness due to Liver fire or Liver yang rising. • **Lowers the blood pressure:** Used to treat hypertension. • **Releases the exterior:** Used to treat exterior wind-heat attacks causing headache, fever, and red eyes or sore throat.
Gu Sui Bu *(ku-sui-pu)* tyang	KID, LIV	bitter warm	• **Tonifies the Kidneys:** Used to treat pain or weakness in the lower back and knees, diarrhea, tinnitus, deafness, deficiency heat flaring up causing bleeding around the teeth and gums. • **Benefits sinews and bones:** Used to treat trauma to ligaments, tendons and bones resulting in sprains, strains or fractures.
Gu Ya *(ku-ya)* rfood	SP, ST	sweet neutral	• **Fortifies the Spleen, opens the Stomach, harmonizes the center and disperses food stagnation:** Used to treat food retention with abdominal fullness, diarrhea, poor appetite, and poor digestion of starchy foods.
Gua Lou *(kua-lou)* clht-phlegm	LU, ST, LI	sweet cold	• **Moistens the Lung and transforms Phlegm-Heat:** Used to treat cough with thick, sticky sputum, or blood-tinged sputum. • **Dissipates nodules:** Used to treat chest impediment. • **Lubricates the Intestines:** Used to treat thirst and dryness causing constipation.

HERB

Herbs	Channels / Properties	Indications / Actions
Gua Lou Ren *(kua-lou-ren)* clht-phlegm	LU, ST, LI / sweet cold	• **Moistens the Lung and transforms Phlegm-Heat:** Used to treat cough with thick, sticky sputum, or blood-tinged sputum. • **Dissipates nodules:** Used to treat chest impediment. • **Lubricates the Intestines:** Used to treat thirst and dryness causing constipation.
Guan Zhong *(kuan-chung)* clht-detox	LIV, SP / bitter cold	• **Kills parasites:** Used to treat intestinal parasites including tapeworms, roundworms, and hookworms. • **Clears Heat and relieves toxins:** Used to treat wind-heat colds, maculopapular eruptions, or damp-heat induced sores, carbuncles, mumps, and epidemic toxins. • **Cools the Blood and stops bleeding:** Used to treat blood in the stool, bloody dysentery, profuse flooding and spotting, and vaginal discharge.
Gui Ban *(kuei-pan)* tyin	HT, KID, LIV / sweet salty cold	• **Nourishes the yin and subdues the yang:** Used to treat night sweats, dizziness, tinnitus, and spasms, and tremors associated with ascendant yang or Liver and Kidney yin deficiency generating internal wind. • **Supplements the Kidneys and fortifies the bones:** Used to treat seminal emissions, soreness and weakness of the lower back and knees, weakness in the legs, and retarded early skeletal development including non-closure of the fontanels. • **Nourishes the Blood and strengthens the Heart:** Used to treat anxiety, insomnia, poor memory associated with Heart yin deficiency. • **Cools the Blood and stops bleeding:** Used to treat flooding and spotting, spontaneous external bleeding, and menorrhagia.
Gui Zhi *(kuei-chih)* rext w-c	LU, UB, HT / pungent sweet warm	• **Releases the exterior, harmonizes Ying and Wei:** Used to treat exterior cold deficiency patterns where there is sweating with no improvement in the patient's condition. • **Warms and frees the channels and disperses cold:** Used to treat wind-cold-damp painful obstruction in the joints and limbs, and to treat dysmenorrhea caused by cold obstructing the blood. • **Warms and frees the Yang:** Used to treat edema caused by cold phlegm obstruction, and for palpitations due to obstruction to the flow of yang qi in the chest. • **Warms the blood vessels:** Used to treat dysmenorrhea due to cold in the uterus.
Hai Feng Teng *(hai-feng-teng)* d-w-damp	LIV / acrid bitter sl warm	• **Dispels wind dampness & unblocks the channels:** Used to treat wind-cold-damp painful obstruction with stiff joints, lower back pain, sore knees, cramping of the muscles and sinews and pain due to trauma. • **Regulates Qi:** Used to treat abdominal pain, panting, and coughing associated with rebellious qi.
Hai Ge Ke *(hai-ke-ke)* clht-phlegm	LU, ST, KD / bitter salty neutral	• **Clears Heat, transforms Phlegm, softens hardness:** Used to treat heat-phlegm panting and cough, edema, dysuria, goiters and tumors of the neck, accumulations, pain in the chest due to blood stasis, dysentery, hemorrhoids, flooding and spotting, and vaginal discharge.
Hai Jin Sha *(hai-chin-sha)* edamp	SI, UB / sweet cool	• **Clears Heat, resolves toxins, promotes urination:** Used to treat urinary tract infection, urinary calculus, vaginal discharge, hepatitis, nephritic edema, sore, swollen throat, mumps, enteritis, dysentery, eczema, and herpes zoster associated with damp heat.

Herbs	Channels / Properties	Indications / Actions
Hai Piao Xiao (hai-paio-chiao) sab	KID, LIV, ST / salty astringent sl warm	• **Stops bleeding and vaginal discharge:** Used to treat uterine bleeding and vaginal discharge. • **Astringes the Essence:** Used to treat nocturnal emissions, premature ejaculation, or vaginal discharge due to Kidney deficiency. • **Controls acidity and relieves pain:** Used to treat epigastric pain, belching, or acid regurgitation associated with excess production of stomach acid. • **Resolves dampness and promotes healing:** Used to treat chronic, non-healing skin ulcers or rashes associated with dampness. • **Stops diarrhea:** Used to treat chronic diarrhea or dysentery.
Hai Shen (hai-sheng) tyang	KID, HT / salty warm	• **Tonifies the Kidney Yang, benefits the Essence:** Used to treat impotence, nocturnal emission, and frequent urination.
Hai Tong Pi (hai-tung-pi) d-w-damp	SP, LIV, KID / acrid bitter neutral	• **Dispels Wind-Damp, frees the Channels**: Used to treat wind-damp painful obstruction. • **Promotes urination and reduces edema:** Used to treat edema. Relieves itching: Used to treat scabies and other skin lesions.
Hai Zao (hai-tsao) clht-phlegm	LU, LIV, ST, KID / bitter salty cold	• **Reduces Phlegm & softens hardness:** Used to treat goiters, nodules and tumors in the neck or sensation of distention and fullness in the chest associated with phlegm, hyperthyroidism and hypothyroidism. • **Promotes urination & drains Fire:** Used to treat edema, swelling and pain in the testicles, and leg qi.
Han Fang Ji (han-fang-ji) edamp	UB, SP, KID / bitter acrid cold	• **Promotes urination and reduces edema:** Used to treat damp-heat leg qi, gurgling sounds in the intestines, abdominal distention, or ascites associated with damp accumulations. • **Expels Damp-Heat:** Used to treat hypertonicity of the extremities, fever and red, swollen, hot, painful joints.
Han Lian Cao (han-lien-tsao) tyin	KID, LIV / sweet sour cool	• **Supplements the Liver and Kidney yin:** Used to treat vaginal discharge, dysuria, turbid urination, dizziness, blurred vision, vertigo, and premature graying of the hair associated with yin deficiency. • **Cools the Blood and stanches bleeding:** Used to treat hemoptysis, vomiting of blood, coughing of blood, hematuria, blood in the stool, bloody dysentery, diphtheria, and spontaneous external bleeding.
Han Shui Shi (han-xue-tzu) clht-fire	HT, ST, KID / acrid salty cold	• **Clears Heat, drains Fire:** Used to treat seasonal febrile diseases, heat accumulation with vexation and thirst, vomiting, diarrhea, and bleeding gums. • **Disperses swellings:** applied topically for sore throats, ulcers and burns.
He Huan Pi (he-huan-pi) cshen	HT, LIV / sweet neutral	• **Resolves depression, quiets the Heart:** Used to treat anger, depression, insomnia, irritability, and poor memory. • **Harmonizes the Blood, relieves pain and disperses swellings:** Used to treat pain and swelling due to trauma and abscesses and swellings.

Herbs	Channels / Properties	Indications / Actions
He Shou Wu *(he-shou-wu)* movexue	LIV, KID bitter sweet astringent sl warm	• **Supplements the Liver and boosts the Kidneys, nourishes the Blood, retains the Essence:** Used to treat dizziness, blurred vision, premature graying of the hair associated with yin and blood deficiency. • **Retains the Essence:** Used to treat nocturnal emission, spermatorrhea and vaginal discharge. • **Moistens the intestines:** Used to treat constipation associated with blood deficiency. • **Expels Wind from the skin, lowers serum cholesterol levels**. Used to treat malaria.
He Ye *(he-yen)* clht-sumr	HT, LIV, SP bitter sl sweet neutral	• **Clears Summerheat:** Used to treat fever, irritability, sweating, scanty urine, and diarrhea associated with summerheat. • **Circulates and clears the Spleen Yang:** Used to treat diarrhea associated with Spleen deficiency. • **Stops bleeding:** Used to treat blood ejection, spontaneous external bleeding, flooding and spotting, blood in the stool, and postpartum dizziness due to blood deficiency.
He Zi *(ho-tzu)* sab	LI, ST, LU bitter \sour astringent neutral	• **Astringes the Intestines and stops diarrhea:** Used to treat chronic diarrhea and dysentery. • **Constrains Lung Qi, stops coughing:** Used to treat chronic coughing and wheezing, and loss of voice. • **Astringes the Essence:** Used to treat flooding and spotting, vaginal discharge, seminal emission and polyuria.
Hei Zhi Ma *(hay-chih-ma)* tyin	KID, LIV sweet neutral	• **Supplements the Liver and Kidney Yin:** Used to treat premature graying of the hair, blurred vision, tinnitus, and dizziness. • **Extinguishes wind:** Used to treat headaches, dizziness, and numbness associated with movement of internal wind. • **Moistens the intestines:** Used to treat constipation due to deficiency of yin or blood and scanty breast milk.
Hong Hua *(hong-hua)* movexue	HT, LIV acrid warm	• **Activates the Blood and unblocks the menses:** Used to treat amenorrhea, abdominal pain, post partum dizziness, retention of lochia and abdominal masses. • **Dispels Blood stasis and stops pain:** Used to treat chest and abdominal pain associated with blood stasis including angina pectoralis. • **Relieves rashes:** Used to treat measles when rash is incomplete.
Hou Po *(hu-po)* movedamp	SP, ST, LU, LI acrid bitter warm aromatic	• **Moves Qi, dries Dampness:** Used to treat pain or distention and fullness in the chest and abdomen, poor appetite, vomiting and diarrhea associated with Damp obstruction of the middle burner. • **Warms the Center, transforms Phlegm and descends rebellious Qi:** Used to treat coughing or wheezing with a stifling or oppressed sensation in the chest associated with phlegm obstructing the normal downward movement of Lung qi.
Hu Gu *(hu-gu)* d-w-damp	LIV, KD acrid sweet warm	• **Dispels Wind Dampness and relieves pain:** Used to treat stiffness and migratory pain in the joints. • **Disperses Wind-Cold and strengthens sinews and bones:** Used to treat weak knees and legs, spasms, paralysis, stiffness and pain in the lower back, and cold pain in the bones.
Hu Huang Lian *(hu-huang-lien)* clht-damp	LIV, ST, LI bitter cold	• **Clears Damp-Heat:** Used to treat dysentery and skin lesions associated with damp-heat. • **Clears Heat and cools the Blood:** Used to treat spontaneous external bleeding. • **Clears deficiency Heat:** Used to treat night sweats, malar flush, irritability, and dryness associated with yin deficiency heat.

Herbs	Channels / Properties	Indications / Actions
Hu Jiao *(hu-chiao)* wint	ST, LI pungent hot	• **Warms the center, precipitates Qi, disperses Phlegm, and resolves toxins**: Used to treat cold phlegm, food stagnation, cold pain in the abdomen, stomach reflux, vomiting of clear fluids, diarrhea and cold dysentery.
Hu Lu Ba *(hu-lu-pa)* tyang	KID, LIV bitter warm	• **Warms the Kidney Yang, dispels cold-damp and relieves pain:** Used to treat distention and fullness in the abdomen, impotence, pain in the low back and knees, and cold-damp leg qi.
Hu Po *(hu-po)* cshen	HT, LIV, UB sweet neutral	• **Settles fright and quiets the Spirit:** Used to treat anxiety, fright palpitations, insomnia, forgetfulness, and convulsions or seizures. • **Activates the Blood:** Used to treat coronary heart disease, amenorrhea, post-partum pain in the abdomen, and immobile masses associated with blood stasis. • **Stops bleeding:** Used to treat hematuria and dysuria. • **Relieves inflammation:** Used to treat sores, carbuncles, and ulcerations of the skin.
Hu Tao Ren *(hu-tao-jen)* tyang	KID, LU, LI sweet warm	• **Tonifies the Kidneys and secures the Essence:** Used to treat pain in the lower back and knees and frequent, pale, copious urination. • **Warms the Lungs and stops cough:** Used to treat chronic cough and wheezing associated with Lung and Kidney yang deficiency. • **Moistens the Intestines:** Used to treat constipation.
Hu Zhang *(hu-chang)* movexue	LU, LIV, GB bitter cold	• **Activates the Blood and breaks up Blood Stasis**: Used to treat amenorrhea, wind dampness painful obstruction and traumatic injury. • **Clears Heat, dries dampness:** Used to treat damp-heat jaundice, and vaginal discharge. • **Drains heat downward, transforms phlegm and stops coughing:** Used to treat cough and constipation due to accumulations of heat. • **Expels Fire toxins:** Used to treat burns, carbuncles, other skin infections and snake bites.
Hua Shi *(hua-shih)* edamp	UB, ST sweet bland cold	• **Promotes urination and clears Heat:** Used to treat dysuria, hematuria, scanty urine, and diarrhea caused by damp-heat. • **Clears Heat and releases Summerheat:** Used to treat dysuria, fever, irritability, and thirst caused by summerheat.
Huai Hua Mi *(hui-hua-mi)* stopxue	LIV, LI bitter cool	• **Clears Heat, Cools the Blood, stops bleeding**: Used to treat damp heat in the Large Intestine causing bleeding hemorrhoids and bloody dysentery, and hemoptysis, epistaxis, or flooding or spotting. • **Cools Upward Stirring of Liver Wind or Wind Heat:** For red eyes and dizziness due to Liver heat or wind heat.
Huang Bai *(huang-pai)* clht-damp	KID, UB bitter cold	• **Clears Heat, dries Dampness:** Used to treat red and white vaginal discharge, diarrhea, dysentery, dysuria, hematuria, wasting thirst, jaundice, hemorrhoids, blood in the stool associated with damp-heat. • **Drains deficiency Fire:** Used to treat steaming bone taxation, fever, red, sore, swollen eyes, mouth sores, night sweats, afternoon fevers and sweating, nocturnal emissions and spermatorrhea associated with Kidney yin deficiency fire flaring up. • **Relieves toxins**: Used to treat sores, eczema and other damp skin lesions.

Herbs	Channels / Properties	Indications / Actions
Huang Jing *(huang-cho)* tqi	SP, LU, KID — sweet neutral	• **Tonifies Spleen and Stomach:** Used for fatigue, poor appetite. Nourishes vital essence of the Lung: Used for dry cough, chronic bronchitis, and pulmonary TB.
Huang Lian *(huang-lien)* clht-damp	HT, LIV, ST, LI — bitter cold	• **Drains Fire:** Used to treat vomiting, belching, acid regurgitation, foul breath, polyphagia, high fevers, insomnia, irritability, disorientation, delirium, painful red eyes and sore throat associated with Heart fire, Liver fire and Stomach fire. • **Clears Heat and dries Dampness**: Used to treat diarrhea, dysentery and jaundice. • **Clears Heat and stops bleeding:** Used to treat vomiting blood, hemoptysis, epistaxis, hematuria, and blood in the stool associated with heat in the blood. • **Clears toxins:** Used topically for abscesses, sores, red and painful eyes and ulcerations of the tongue and month.
Huang Qi *(huang-chi)* tqi	SP, LU — sweet sl warm	• **Supplements the Center and reinforces Qi:** Used to treat fatigue, poor appetite, nausea, and diarrhea caused by Spleen or Stomach qi deficiency. • **Raises the Yang Qi:** Used to treat bleeding disorders where the qi is not holding blood in the vessels, or where the qi is not raising organs as in prolapsed uterus, stomach, or rectum. • **Boosts the protective Qi and secures the exterior:** Used to treat spontaneous sweating caused by qi deficiency and is used for chronic colds and other manifestations of immune deficiency. • **Tonifies Qi and blood:** Used to treat qi and blood deficiency presenting with pallor, fatigue, palpitations. • **Reduces edema:** Used to treat edema caused by qi deficiency. • **Promotes regeneration of flesh:** Used to treat abscesses, chronic ulcerations and sores from deficiency. • **Increases white blood cell count.**
Huang Qin *(huang-qi)* clht-damp	LU, ST, GB, LI — bitter cold	• **Clears Heat and drains Fire:** Used to treat vigorous fever, irritability, thirst, cough with thick, yellow sputum associated with Lung heat, or hot sores and swellings associated with fire toxins flaring up. • **Eliminates Damp-Heat:** Used to treat diarrhea, dysentery, coughing and wheezing with a stifling sensation in the chest, thirst without the desire to drink, and dysuria or hematuria associated with damp heat. • **Clears Heat and stops bleeding:** Used to treat spontaneous external bleeding, vomiting blood, hematuria, and epistaxis. • **Clears Heat and quiets the fetus:** Quiets a restless fetus associated with threatened miscarriage. • **Subdues ascendant Liver yang**: Used to treat headache, irritability, red eyes, flushed face, and bitter taste in the mouth associated with ascendant Liver yang.
Huo Ma Ren *(huo-ma-ren)* lax	SP, ST, LI — sweet neutral	• **Moistens Dryness, lubricates the intestines:** Used to treat constipation due to intestinal dryness, nourishes the yin in wasting and thirsting disorder, treats dysentery, menstrual irregularities, and heat-related dysuria.
Huo Xiang *(huo-hsiang)* movedamp	SP, ST, LU — acrid sl warm	• **Dispels Dampness:** Used to treat pain and fullness of the epigastrium and abdomen, nausea, vomiting, poor appetite associated with dampness obstructing the center. • **Harmonizes the Center, normalizes the Qi:** Used to treat vomiting associated with disharmony in the center. • **Releases the exterior:** Used to treat summerheat and colds or flu with fever and chills, headache, oppression in the chest, vomiting, diarrhea, malaria, and dysentery.

Herbs	Channels / Properties	Indications / Actions
Ji Nei Jin *(chi-nei-chin)* rfood	SP, ST, UB, SI sweet neutral	• **Disperses food stagnation, fortifies the Spleen and Stomach:** Used to treat food stagnation with distention and fullness, vomiting, retching, stomach reflux, diarrhea and childhood nutritional impairment associated with food retention. • **Astringes the Essence:** Used to treat polyuria, nocturia, and bedwetting. • **Softens hardness and dissolves stones:** Used to treat stones in either the urinary or biliary tract.
Ji Xue Teng *(chi-hsueh-teng)* movexue	HT, SP, LIV bitter sweet warm	• **Activates the Blood, soothes the Sinews:** Used to treat lumbar and knee pain, numbness, paralysis, and menstrual irregularities.
Jiang Can *(chiang-tsan)* ewind	LIV, LU salty pungent neutral	• **Extinguishes Wind and relieves spasms:** Used to treat wind-stroke with loss of voice and facial paralysis and for childhood convulsions. • **Dispels Wind and stops pain:** Used to treat headache, red eyes, and sore throat. • **Transforms Phlegm:** Used to treat deviated mouth, hemiplegia, scrofula and phlegm nodules associated with phlegm obstruction of the orifice. • **Extinguishes wind and stops itching:** Used to treat skin rashes.
Jiang Huang *(chiang-huang)* movexue	SP, ST, LIV acrid bitter warm	• **Breaks up Blood stasis, moves Qi, frees menstruation, relieves pain:** Used to treat pain and fullness in the chest and abdomen, pain in the kidney, accumulations, amenorrhea, postpartum abdominal pain, and pain from trauma.
Jie Geng *(chieh-keng)* cold-phlegm	LU bitter acrid neutral	• **Diffuses the Lung Qi and expels Phlegm:** Used to treat cough, fullness and pain of the chest and hypochondrium associated with phlegm obstructing the qi of the chest. • **Expels pus:** Used to treat abscesses, coughing of blood and pus. • **Benefits the throat:** Used to treat sore throat associated with heat from excess or deficiency. • **Guides herbs upward.**
Jin Qian Cao *(chin-yin-tsao)* edamp	UB, GB, KD, LIV sweet bland neutral	• **Clears Heat, unblocks urination, disperses swelling, and resolves toxins:** Used to treat jaundice, edema, dysuria, urinary calculus, cough, pulmonary abscesses, malaria, vaginal discharge, wind-damp painful obstruction, fright epilepsy, and eczema.
Jin Yin Hua *(chin-yin-hua)* clht-detox	LU, ST, LI sweet cold	• **Clears Heat, expels Wind and resolves toxins:** Used to treat initial-stage warm febrile disease with heat in the upper burner, for hot, painful sores and pain and swellings of the breast, throat, or eyes, and for intestinal abscess. • **Clears damp-heat:** Used to treat dysentery and blood in the stool and hematuria associated with damp-heat in the lower burner.
Jin Yin Zi *(chin-yin-tzu)* sab	KID, UB, LI sour astringent neutral	• **Secures the Essence:** Used to treat seminal emissions, enuresis, polyuria, and spontaneous sweating. • **Astringes the Intestines:** Used to treat chronic diarrhea.
Jing Da Ji *(ching-ta-chieh)* cath	KID, LI, LU bitter cold toxic	• **Drains water downward:** Used to treat labored breathing with pain in the chest associated with accumulation of fluids in the chest and hypochondrium. • **Relieves inflammation:** Used topically for sores and inflammation.

HERB

Herbs	Channels / Properties	Indications / Actions
Jing Jie *(ching-chieh)* rext w-c	LU, LIV — pungent aromatic sl warm	• **Releases the exterior and dispels wind:** Used to treat chills and fever, headache, sore throat caused by exterior wind-cold or exterior wind-heat attacking. • **Stops rashes and itching:** Used to treat early stage measles and skin eruptions. • **Stops bleeding:** Used to treat blood in the stool or uterine bleeding.
Ju Hong *(chu-hong)* rqi	LU, ST — pungent bitter warm	• **Dries Dampness and transforms Phlegm:** Used to treat phlegm and dampness obstructing the middle and upper burners causing coughing with copious, viscous sputum, a stifling sensation in the chest, abdominal distention, little appetite, fatigue, diarrhea or loose stools. • **Regulates the Qi, rectifies the center:** Used to treat distention and fullness in the epigastrium and abdomen, hiccough, bloating, belching, nausea and vomiting associated with Spleen not transforming and transporting fluids effectively.
Ju Hua *(chu-hua)* rext w-h	LU, LIV — sweet bitter sl cold	• **Releases the exterior, disperses Wind-Heat:** Used to treat wind-heat patterns with fever and headache. • **Clears the liver and brightens the eyes**: Used to treat red, painful, dry eyes or excessive tearing, floaters, blurry vision, or dizziness due to either wind-heat attack or Liver and Kidney yin deficiency. • **Subdues the Liver and dispels wind:** Used to treat headache, red eyes, blurred vision, dizziness, headache, tinnitus and deafness caused by ascendant Liver yang.
Jue Ming Zi *(chueh-ming-tzu)* clht-fire	LIV, KID, LI — bitter sweet cool	• **Expels Wind-Heat:** Used to treat red, painful or itchy eyes with sensitivity to light associated with externally contracted wind-heat. • **Clears the Liver Fire, descends Liver Yang:** Used to treat headache, red, painful eyes, excessive tearing, or sensitivity to light associated with Liver fire and Liver yang rising. • **Moistens the Intestines and frees the stool:** Used to treat chronic constipation associated with Liver yin deficiency. • **Lowers blood pressure and serum cholesterol:** Used to treat hypertension.
Ku Shen *(ku-sheng)* clht-damp	HT, LIV, SI, LI, UB — bitter cold	• **Clears Heat and dries Dampness:** Used to treat red and white vaginal discharge, dysentery, jaundice, and heat toxins causing skin sores. • **Disperses Wind, stops itching:** Used to treat chronic itching, seepage, and bleeding associated with wind-damp-heat invasions. • **Kills parasites:** Used to treat parasite infections. • **Promotes urination:** Damp heat in Small Intestine, painful urinary dysfunction and hot edema.
Kuan Dong Hua *(kuan-tong-hua)* cough	LU — acrid sweet warm	• **Moistens the Lungs, precipitates Qi, transforms Phlegm, and suppresses cough:** Used to treat counterflow cough, panting and wheezing, and stagnation in the throat.
Kun Bu *(kun-pu)* clht-phlegm	ST, LIV, KD — salty cold	• **Softens hardness and moves water:** Used to treat scrofula, goiters and tumors of the neck, dysphagia-occlusion, edema, painful distention of the testicles, vaginal discharge.

Herbs	Channels / Properties	Indications / Actions
Lai Fu Zi (*lai-fu-tzu*) rfood	SP, acrid ST, sweet LU neutral	• **Disperses food stagnation and relieves accumulation:** Used to treat fullness and distention in the chest and abdomen, belching, acid regurgitation, abdominal pain, and diarrhea associated with food accumulation and qi stagnation. • **Descends Qi and stops coughing:** Used to treat chronic cough or wheezing due mostly to phlegm obstruction of the Lungs.
Li Zhi He (*li-chih-he*) rqi	ST, astringent LIV sweet warm	• **Regulates Qi and stops pain:** Used to treat abdominal and epigastric pain due to Liver qi constraint, premenstrual or postpartum pain due to qi stagnation and blood stasis, and hernia or testicular pain due to cold stagnation in the Liver channel.
Lian Geng (*lien-gen*) clht-sumr	HT, bitter LIV, sl sweet SP neutral	• **Clears Summerheat:** Used to treat fever, irritability, sweating, scanty urine, and diarrhea, and coughing due to summerheat.
Lian Qiao (*lien-chaio*) clht-detox	HT, bitter LIV, sl acrid GB cool	• **Clears heat and toxins, dissipates nodules, and relieves swellings:** Used to treat neck lumps, scrofula, hot toxic sores, and carbuncles. • **Expels externally-contracted Wind-Heat:** Used to treat sore throat, fever, and headache associated with externally-contracted wind-heat.
Lian Zi (*lien-hsin*) sab	KID, sweet SP, astringent HT neutral	• **Tonifies the Spleen and stops diarrhea:** Used to treat chronic diarrhea and loss of appetite due to Spleen deficiency. • **Tonifies the Kidneys and astringes the Essence:** Used to treat premature ejaculation, spermatorrhea, flooding and spotting, and vaginal discharge. • **Quiets the spirit:** Used to treat anxiety, palpitations, irritability, and insomnia associated with disharmony between the Kidneys and the Heart.
Lian Zi Xin (*lien-tzu*) clht-fire	HT, bitter PC cold	• **Clears Heat:** Used to treat red, swollen and painful eyes, insomnia, irritability and mental confusion or delirium associated with Heart fire. • **Stops bleeding and astringes the Essence:** Used to treat vomiting of blood or spermatorrhea.
Ling Yang Jiao (*ling-yang-chueh*) ewind	HT, salty LIV cold	• **Extinguishes Wind and relieves spasms:** Used to treat seizures, spasms and convulsions caused by internal movement of wind in the channels and vessels. • **Calms the Liver and subdues the yang:** Used to treat headaches, red eyes, blurred vision, dizziness, spasms and convulsions caused by ascendant Liver yang or Liver fire. • **Clears heat and relieves toxins:** Used to treat high fever, delirium, mania and loss of consciousness due to febrile diseases. • **Clears damp-heat:** Used to treat wind-damp-heat painful obstruction.
Ling Zhi (*ling-chih*) cshen	HT, sweet LU, sl warm SP, LIV KD	• **Nourishes the Heart, quiets the Spirit**: Used to treat insomnia and poor memory. Lowers blood pressure & reduces serum cholesterol.
Liu Huang (*lu-huang*) etop	KID, sour LI, hot PC toxic	• **Relieves toxins, kills parasites, and stops itching:** Used to treat scabies, ringworm, and relieves itching. • **Supports Yang:** Used to treat interior cold due to yang deficiency.
Liu Ji Nu (*lu-ji-nu*) movexue	HT, bitter SP warm	• **Breaks Blood stasis, frees menstruation, closes sores, and disperses swelling:** Used to treat amenorrhea, postpartum blood stasis, traumatic injury pain, swellings, and sores.

Herbs	Channels / Properties	Indications / Actions
Long Dan Cao *(lung-tan-tsao)* clht-damp	LIV, GB, ST / bitter cold	• **Drains Damp-Heat:** Used to treat jaundice, genital damp itching, or vaginal discharge and itching associated with damp-heat in the Liver and Gallbladder affecting the lower burner. Also used to treat sore throat and eyes, and swelling and painful ears, tinnitus or acute deafness associated with damp-heat obstructing the Gallbladder channel in the head. • **Drains Liver Fire:** Used to treat hypochondriac pain, fright epilepsy, manic agitation, headache, deafness, tinnitus, dream disturbed sleep, red eyes, and sore throat associated with Liver fire blazing upward.
Long Gu *(lung-ku)* cshen	HT, LIV, KID / sweet astringent neutral	• **Settles fright and quiets the Spirit:** Used to treat palpitations, anxiety, restlessness, insomnia, emotional distress, seizures or mania associated with a disturbed spirit. • **Calms the Liver, subdues the Yang:** Used to treat dizziness, vertigo, blurred vision, and bad temper associated with Kidney and Liver yin deficiency causing the yang to ascend. • **Constrains perspiration and secures Essence:** Used to treat nocturnal emissions, spermatorrhea, night sweats, spontaneous sweating, vaginal discharge and uterine bleeding. • **Benefits open sores**: Used topically to treat chronic, non-healing sores and ulcerations.
Long Yan Rou *(lung-yen-jou)* tblood	HT, SP / sweet warm	• **Harmonizes the Heart and Spleen, tonifies the blood, and quiets the Spirit:** Used to treat insomnia, fright palpitations, fearfulness, poor memory, or dizziness caused by deficiency of qi and blood.
Lou Lu *(lo-lu)* clht-detox	ST, LI / bitter salty cold	• **Clears Heat, relieves toxins, disperses swellings, expels pus, promotes lactation, unblocks the sinews:** Used to treat welling abscesses, swollen breasts, absence of breast milk, scrofula, sores, bloody dysentery, bleeding hemorrhoids, and Damp Impediment Bi with hypertonicity of the sinews and joint pain.
Lu Dou *(lu-tou)* clht-sumr	HT, ST / sweet cool	• **Clears Heat, resolves toxins, disperses Summerheat and resolves edema:** Used to treat summerheat, thirst, edema, diarrhea, swellings, and abscesses.
Lu Gen *(lu-gen)* clht-fire	LU, ST / sweet cold	• **Clears Heat and generates fluids:** Used to treat fever, irritability, and thirst associated with excess heat, coughing and expectoration of thick, yellow sputum or welling pulmonary abscess associated with excess heat in the Lungs and for vomiting and belching associated with excess heat in the Stomach. • **Clears Heat and promotes urination:** Used to treat hematuria and dark, scanty urine.
Lu Hui *(lu-huei)* purg	LI, LIV, ST / bitter cold	• **Clears Heat, frees the stools, and kills worms**: Used to treat constipation, amenorrhea, child fright epilepsy, hemorrhoids, fistulas, and intestinal parasites.
Lu Lu Tong *(lu-lu-tong)* movexue	ST, LIV / bitter neutral	• **Dispels wind, reduces edema and eliminates dampness:** Used to treat painful obstruction in the limbs and extremities, stomach pain, edema, distention, amenorrhea, scanty breast milk, abscesses, fistulas, and eczema.

HERB

Herbs	Channels / Properties	Indications / Actions
Lu Rong *(lu-jong)* tyang	KID, LIV — sweet, salty, warm	• **Tonifies the Kidneys and fortifies the Original Yang:** Used to treat impotence, cold extremities, fatigue, dizziness, tinnitus, deafness, soreness and weakness in the low back and knees, and frequent, copious, clear urination. • **Supplements Essence and strengthens the Sinews and Bones:** Used to treat insufficiencies of essence resulting in poor development including bed wetting, mental retardation, learning disorders, or skeletal development disorders with poor bone growth. • **Warms the Uterus:** Used to treat infertility, vaginal discharge or uterine bleeding due to cold in the Chong and Ren channels and the Uterus.
Luo Shi Teng *(luo-shi-teng)* d-w-damp	LIV — bitter, sl cold	• **Dispels Wind, frees the channels, stops bleeding, and disperses stasis:** Used to treat wind-damp impediment Bi pain, hypertonicity of the sinews, swollen abscesses, throat impediment, blood ejection, trauma, and retention of lochia.
Ma Bo *(ma-po)* clht-detox	LU — acrid, neutral	• **Clears Heat, resolves toxins:** Used to treat sore throat with swelling, and loss of voice due to heat toxins, and for cough due to Lung heat. • **Stops bleeding:** Used topically to stop bleeding.
Ma Chi Xian *(ma-chi-hsian)* clht-detox	LIV, LI — sour, cold	• **Relieves toxins and cools the Blood:** Used to treat appendicitis, carbuncles, sores, red and white vaginal discharge, and hematuria associated with hot, painful urinary dysfunctions. Snake bite and wasp stings.
Ma Dou Ling *(ma-tou-ling)* cough	LU, LI — bitter, sl acrid, cold	• **Clears Lungs, transforms Phlegm, precipitates Qi, stops coughing, and calms wheezing:** Used to treat coughing and wheezing associated with phlegm-heat obstructing the Lungs. • **Lowers blood pressure:** Used to treat hypertension accompanied by lightheadedness. Treats bleeding hemorrhoids.
Ma Huang *(ma-huang)* rext w-c	LU, UB — pungent, sl bitter, warm	• **Releases the exterior, dispels Cold:** Used to treat chills, fever, headache, absence of sweating, and a tight, floating pulse. • **Assists Lung qi and stops wheezing:** Used to treat cough and wheezing due to obstruction of Lung qi by wind and cold. • **Promotes Urination and reduces edema:** Used to treat edema due to obstruction from exterior pathogenic attack.
Mai Men Dong *(mai-men-tong)* yin	HT, LU, ST — sweet, sl bitter, sl cold	• **Nourishes the Yin, moistens the Lungs, and stops cough:** Used to treat dry cough with little or no sputum production, blood-tinged cough, hemoptysis, and pulmonary abscess associated with Lung yin deficiency. • **Boosts the Stomach yin and generates liquids:** Used to treat conditions where there is little or no appetite, empty and uncomfortable feelings in the stomach, hunger with no desire to eat, afternoon fever, constipation, dry stools, burning epigastric pain, dry mouth and throat, thirst with no desire to drink, feelings of fullness after eating, or constipation associated with Stomach yin deficiency. • **Clears the Heart and relieves irritability:** Used to treat irritability associated with yin deficiency.
Mai Ya *(mai-ya)* food	SP, ST, LIV — sweet, neutral	• **Disperses food stagnation, fortifies the Spleen and Stomach:** Used to treat vomiting and diarrhea and loss of appetite associated with food retention or Spleen deficiency. • **Regulates Qi:** Used to treat persistent breast distention, stifling sensation and distention in the epigastrium or hypochondrium, belching, or loss of appetite associated with Liver qi stagnation. • **Inhibits Lactation:** Used to treat women wishing to stop nursing.

HERB

ACUPUNCTURE DESK REFERENCE   129

HERB

Herbs	Channels / Properties	Indications / Actions
Man Jing Zi *(man-ching-tzu)* rext w-h	LIV, ST, UB pungent bitter cool	• **Releases the exterior, disperses Wind-Heat:** Used to treat headache or eye pain caused by wind-heat attack. • **Clears the head and eyes:** Used to treat red, painful, or swollen eyes, excessive tearing, or floaters associated with Liver wind-heat. • **Dries dampness and expels Wind:** Used to treat wind-dampness in the extremities causing stiffness, numbness, cramping or heaviness.
Mang Xiao *(mang-hsiao)* purg	ST, LI pungent bitter salty very cold	• **Drains Heat, moistens dryness and softens hardness:** Used to treat heat stagnation and accumulation, abdominal distention, constipation, phlegm accumulation, red eyes, and swollen welling abscesses.
Meng Shi *(meng-shi)* clht-phlegm	LU, LIV sweet salty neutral	• **Expels Phlegm, Relieves food stagnation, descends rebellious Qi, calms the Liver:** Used to treat stubborn phlegm accumulation, mania, depression, epilepsy, cough, and rapid panting breathing.
Mi Meng Hua *(mi-meng-hua)* clht-fire	LIV sweet cool	• **Benefits the eyes:** for red, swollen, painful eyes, excessive tearing, superficial visual obstruction, or sensitivity to light. Can be used in treating both excessive and deficient patterns.
Mo Yao *(mo-yao)* movexue	LIV, SP, HT bitter neutral	• **Activates the blood and dispels blood stasis, reduces inflammation, regenerates flesh:** Used to treat pain, swelling and inflammation from traumatic injury, sores, carbuncles, immovable abdominal masses, joint pain, chest and abdominal pain, dysmenorrhea and amenorrhea associated with blood stasis.
Mu Dan Pi *(mu-tan-pi)* coolxue	HT, LIV, KID acrid bitter cool	• **Clears Heat and cools the Blood:** Used to treat spontaneous external bleeding, epistaxis, vomiting blood, blood in the stool, flooding or spotting, or prolonged menstrual bleeding associated with heat in the blood. • **Clears deficiency Heat:** Used to treat steaming bone fever and heat associated with yin deficiency. • **Activates the Blood and disperses Blood stasis:** Used to treat amenorrhea and abdominal masses associated with blood stasis, or traumatic injury. • **Clears Liver Fire:** Used to treat headache, painful red eyes, hypochondriac pain, and dysmenorrhea with Liver fire. Reduces swelling: Used to treat abscesses.
Mu Gua *(mu-kua)* d-w-damp	SP, LIV sour sl warm	• **Eliminates Dampness, soothes the sinews:** Used to treat damp painful obstruction in the extremities, and weakness in the lower back and lower extremities. • **Harmonizes the Stomach, calms the Liver:** Used to treat abdominal pain, spasms, cramping of the calves, and edema due to leg qi.
Mu Li *(mu-li)* cshen	LIV, KID salty astringent cool	• **Settles and calms the spirit:** Used to treat palpitations, anxiety, restlessness, and insomnia associated with a disturbed spirit. • **Calms the Liver and subdues the Yang:** Used to treat dizziness, vertigo, blurred vision, and bad temper associated with Kidney and Liver yin deficiency causing the yang to ascend. • **Constrains perspiration and secures Essence:** Used to treat nocturnal emissions, spermatorrhea, night sweats, spontaneous sweating, vaginal discharge and uterine bleeding. • **Softens hardness:** Used to help dissipate lumps in the neck, goiters, and scrofula. • **Stops pain:** Used in calcined form to treat stomach pain associated with excess stomach acid.

Herbs	Channels / Properties	Indications / Actions
Mu Tong *(mu-tung)* edamp	UB, HT, SI	bitter cool	• **Promotes urination and drains Fire:** Used to treat dysuria, edema and leg qi due to damp-heat invading the lower burner, sores on the tongue and mouth, and irritability associated with fire from the Heart pouring down via the Small Intestine. • **Promotes lactation and frees the blood vessels:** Used to treat amenorrhea, joint pain due to blood stasis, and insufficient lactation.
Mu Xiang *(mu-hsiang)* rqi	SP, ST, GB, LI	pungent bitter warm	• **Regulates Qi, strengthens the Stomach and alleviates pain:** Used to treat pain and distention in the epigastrium and abdomen, nausea and vomiting, poor appetite, flank pain, distention, or soreness in the hypochondrium, and dysenteric disease with abdominal urgency and rectal heaviness (tenesmus)
Mu Zei *(mu-tsei)* rext w-h	LU, LIV	sweet bitter neutral	• **Releases the exterior, disperses Wind-Heat and eliminates superficial visual obstruction:** Used to treat red, swollen, painful eyes, blurred vision, or excessive tearing associated with wind-heat attack. • **Clears Heat, stops bleeding:** Used to treat bloody dysentery, and spontaneous external bleeding associated with wind-heat.
Niu Bang Zi *(niu-pang-tzu)* rext w-h	LU, ST	pungent bitter cold	• **Releases the exterior and disperses Wind-Heat:** Used to treat flu and colds causing fever, cough, and a sore, red, swollen throat. • **Clears Heat and relieves toxicity:** Used to treat maculopapular rashes including carbuncles, erythemas, and mumps. • **Vents rashes:** Used in the early stages of rashes with dormant papules such as measles. • **Moistens the Intestines:** Used to treat constipation.
Niu Huang *(niu-huang)* open	HT, LIV	bitter sweet cool	• **Clears the Heart, opens the orifices, and transforms phlegm:** Used to treat clouded spirit, delirious speech, windstroke, convulsions, seizures, or coma, caused by phlegm and heat obstructing the Pericardium. • **Clears the Liver, stops tremors:** Used to treat spasms, tremors, or convulsions with high fever due to heat in the Liver. Drains heat and relieves toxins: Used to treat sore throat.
Niu Xi *(niu-tzu)* movexue	LIV, KID	bitter sour neutral	• **Activates the Blood and expels Blood stasis:** Used to treat menstrual irregularities including dysmenorrhea and amenorrhea. • **Strengthens sinews and bones, dries dampness:** Used to treat painful low back and knee joints due to blood stasis and damp painful obstruction. • **Clears Damp-Heat:** Used to treat hematuria, dysuria, urinary incontinence, and vaginal discharge. • **Descends Heat:** Used to treat epistaxis, vomiting of blood, toothaches, bleeding gums, dizziness, headache and blurred vision associated with heat flaring up.
Nu Zhen Zi *(nu-chen-tzu)* yin	KID, LIV	sweet bitter neutral	• **Supplements the Liver and Kidney Yin:** for yin deficiency of the Liver and Kidneys with dizziness, floaters, poor vision, soreness and weakness of the low back and knees, tinnitus, deafness, premature graying of the hair. Clears deficiency heat.
Ou Jie *(ou-chieh)* topxue	LU, ST, LIV	sweet astringent neutral	• **Stops bleeding and Moves the Blood:** Used to treat bleeding due to heat in the blood mostly in the Lungs or Stomach causing vomiting or coughing of blood. Moves the blood and relieves stasis.

HERB

Herbs	Channels / Properties	Indications / Actions
Pang Da Hai *(pang-ta-hai)* clht-phlegm	LU, LI — sweet cool	• **Clears Heat, moistens the Lungs, benefits the throat, resolves toxins:** Used to treat dry cough without phlegm, sore throat, loss of voice, steaming bone disorder, spontaneous external bleeding, red eyes, toothache, hemorrhoids and fistulas.
Pei Lan *(pei-lan)* movedamp	SP, ST — acrid neutral	• **Transforms Dampness:** Used to treat externally contracted summerheat with fever, chills and headache, or dampness obstructing the center causing a stifling sensation in the chest, poor appetite with a sweet taste in the mouth, nausea and vomiting. • **Regulates menstruation:** Used to treat menstrual irregularities.
Pi Pa Ye *(pi-pa-yen)* cough	LU, ST — bitter cool	• **Transforms Phlegm, clears Lung heat, and precipitates Lung Qi:** Used to treat coughing and wheezing caused by phlegm blocking the Lung qi from descending. • **Harmonizes the Stomach:** Used to treat nausea, vomiting, hiccough, and belching due to Stomach heat.
Pu Gong Ying *(pu-kung-ying)* clht-detox	LIV, ST — bitter sweet cold	• **Clears Heat, relieves toxins, dissipates nodules:** Used to treat acute mastitis, lymphadenitis, scrofula, clove sores, swollen sores, acute inflammation, acute conjunctivitis, colds and flu with fever, acute tonsillitis or bronchitis, and gastritis. • **Promotes lactation:** Used to treat insufficient lactation due to excess heat. • **Clears Heat and dries Dampness:** Used to treat jaundice, cholecystitis and urinary tract infections.
Pu Huang *(pu-huang)* stopxue	LIV, SP, HT — sweet acrid neutral	• **Stops Bleeding:** Used to treat bleeding due to trauma. Also used to treat epistaxis, hemoptysis, uterine bleeding, and blood in the stool. • **Activates The Blood and disperses blood stasis:** Used to treat post-partum block, dysmenorrhea, or chest pain due to blood stagnation.
Qian Cao Gen *(chien-tsao-jen)* stopxue	LIV, HT — bitter cold	• **Cools the Blood and Stops Bleeding:** Used to treat profuse flooding or spotting, vomiting of blood, epistaxis, hemoptysis, blood in the stool, hematuria and other bleeding disorders due to heat penetrating the blood. • **Moves the Blood and breaks up blood stasis:** Used to treat chest and flank pain. • **Wind-Damp Impediment:** Used to treat joint pain.
Qian Hu *(chien-hu)* clht-phlegm	LU — bitter acrid sl cold	• **Descends rebellious Qi and dispels Phlegm:** Used to treat coughing and wheezing, fullness and oppression in the chest and diaphragm, and panting associated with thick, sticky sputum due to heat in the Lungs. • **Releases exterior Wind-Heat:** Used to treat externally contracted wind-heat or wind-cold patterns associated with coughing and copious sputum.
Qian Niu Zi *(chien-niu-tzu)* *See bai chou* cath	KID, LI, LU, SI — bitter acrid cold sl toxic	• **Drains water, precipitates qi and kills parasites:** Used to treat edema, fullness and distention of the chest with shortness of breath, leg qi, and food stagnation.
Qian Shi *(chien-shih)* sab	KID, SP — sweet astringent neutral	• **Strengthens the Spleen and stops diarrhea:** Used to treat chronic diarrhea caused by Spleen deficiency. • **Secures the Essence:** Used to treat nocturnal emission, premature ejaculation, spermatorrhea, and urinary frequency. • **Dispels Dampness:** Used to treat vaginal discharge.

Herbs	Channels / Properties	Indications / Actions
Qiang Huo *(chiang-huo)* rext w-c	UB, KID	pungent bitter aromatic warm	• **Releases the exterior and dispels cold:** Used to treat chills, fever, headache, body aches and pains, joint pain, a general feeling of heaviness, lassitude, or pain in the occipital region. • **Dispels Wind-Cold Damp, stops pain:** Used to treat wind-cold-damp painful obstruction of the upper limbs or back. Guides herbs in a prescription to the Taiyang and Du channels.
Qin Jiao *(chin-chiao)* d-w-damp	LIV, GB, ST	acrid bitter sl cold	• **Dispels Wind, eliminates Dampness and soothes the sinews:** Used to treat hypertonicity of the sinews and bones, wind-damp painful obstruction and cramping associated with wind-damp. • **Clears Heat from Deficiency:** Used to treat steaming bone tidal fever. • **Dries dampness:** Used to treat jaundice and heat. • **Moistens the Intestines and unblocks the bowels:** Used to treat constipation.
Qin Pi *(chin-pi)* clht-damp	LIV, GB, ST, LI	bitter cold	• **Clears Damp-Heat:** Used to treat bacillary dysentery, enteritis, vaginal discharge. • **Clears Liver Fire and benefits the Eyes:** Used to treat painful, red, swollen eyes. • **Expels Wind-Dampness:** Used to treat painful obstruction.
Qing Dai *(ching-dai)* clht-detox	LIV, LU, ST	salty cold	• **Clears Heat and relieves toxicity.** • **Cools the Blood and disperses swellings.** Used topically for inflammation of the oral cavity and throat (including mumps) and internally for bleeding due to reckless movement of blood, febrile convulsions in children, and cough due to Lung heat.
Qing Fen *(ching-fen)* etop	UB, KID, LIV	acrid cold toxic	• **Kills worms, attacks toxins, promotes urination, unblocks the stool:** Used to treat scrofula, syphilis, ulcerations of the skin, edema, urinary and fecal obstruction.
Qing Hao *(ching-hao)* clht-sumr	LIV, GB, KID	bitter cold	• **Clears Heat, relieves Summerheat:** Used to treat low grade fever, headache, dizziness, and a stifling sensation in the chest associated with summerheat. • **Relieves steaming bone fever:** Used to treat fevers associated with blood deficiency or for unremitting fever or night fever and morning coolness with an absence of sweating associated with yin deficiency. • **Cools Blood and stops bleeding:** Used to treat epistaxis and pupura associated with heat in the blood. • **Relieves malaria:** Used to treat the alternating fever and chills accompanying malaria and jaundice.
Qing Pi *(chin-pi)* rqi	GB, LIV, ST	bitter pungent warm	• **Soothes the Liver Qi and breaks up stagnation:** Used for constrained Liver qi patterns with such symptoms as distention and pain in the chest or hypochondrium, and for breast and hernia pain. • **Dissipates, binds, and reduces stagnation:** Used to treat pain, distention, or a stifling sensation in the epigastrium due to food stagnation with accumulation. • **Dries Dampness and transforms Phlegm:** Used to treat breast abscesses and malaria caused by phlegm obstruction.
Qing Xiang Zi *(ching-hsian-tzu)* clht-fire	LIV	sweet cool	• **Clears Wind-heat, clears the Liver and brightens the eyes:** Used to treat red, sore, swollen eyes, floaters and cataracts associated with wind-heat attacks or Liver fire. • **Lowers Blood Pressure:** Used to treat hypertension associated with Liver yang rising.

HERB

Herbs	Channels / Properties	Indications / Actions
Qu Mai *(chu-mai)* edamp	UB, HT, SI bitter cold	• **Clears damp-heat, promotes urination:** Used to treat urinary obstruction, dysuria, edema. • **Breaks up blood stasis, unblocks menstruation:** Used to treat amenorrhea due to blood stasis. • **Unblocks the bowels:** Used to treat constipation.
Quan Xie *(chuan-hsieh)* ewind	LIV salty pungent neutral toxic	• **Dispels Wind, frees the vessels, resolves toxins:** Used to treat fright wind, epilepsy, wind stroke with hemiplegia, hemilateral headache, wind-damp painful obstruction, lockjaw, sluggish speech, wind papules and swollen sores.
Ren Shen *(jen-sheng)* tqi	SP, LU sweet sl bitter sl warm	• **Strongly supplements the Original Qi:** Used to treat collapse of the qi causing extreme fatigue, shallow respiration, shortness of breath, cold limbs, profuse sweating, and profuse diarrhea. • **Tonifies Qi, benefits the Lungs:** Used to treat wheezing, shortness of breath, and labored breathing with exertion caused by Lung qi deficiency and usually the Kidneys failure to grasp the qi. • **Supplements the Center and reinforces Qi:** Used to treat fatigue, poor appetite, chest and abdominal distention, chronic diarrhea, and organ prolapse. • **Augments fluid:** Used to treat wasting and thirsting disorder, or acute conditions of dehydration due to febrile disease or spontaneous sweating. • **Augments the Heart Qi and quiets the Spirit:** Used to treat fright palpitations, anxiety, insomnia, poor memory, and irritability or restlessness.
Rou Cong Rong *(jou-tsung-jung)* tyang	KID, LI sweet salty warm	• **Tonifies the Kidneys, increases the Essence and Warms the Womb:** Used to treat female infertility, vaginal discharge, flooding and spotting, impotence, spermatorrhea, urinary incontinence, and painful low back and knees associated with cold from deficiency of Kidney yang or essence. • **Moistens and lubricates the Intestine:** Used to treat constipation.
Rou Dou Kou *(jou-tou-kou)* sab	LI, SP, ST acrid warm	• **Astringes Intestines and stops diarrhea:** Used to treat chronic diarrhea or daybreak diarrhea caused by cold from deficiency of the Spleen and Kidneys. • **Warms the center, precipitates food, and alleviates pain:** Used to treat pain and distention in the epigastrium and abdomen, retention of food, poor appetite, and retching and vomiting due to cold from deficiency of the Spleen and Stomach.
Rou Gui *(jou-kuei)* wint	HT, LIV, KID, SP pungent sweet hot	• **Warms the kidneys and supplements the Yang:** Used to treat impotence, frequent urination, aversion to cold, cold limbs, weak back, wheezing, abdominal pain and cold, poor appetite, and diarrhea due to deficient Kidney or Spleen yang. • **Leads the fire back to its source:** Used to treat diarrhea, spontaneous sweating, wheezing, weakness and cold in the lower extremities, dry mouth and sore throat, toothache that is worse at night and low back pain caused by yang collapse. • **Disperses cold, warms the channels:** Used to treat dysmenorrhea, damp-cold painful obstruction, and non-healing sores associated with interior cold.
Ru Xiang *(ju-hsiang)* movexue	LIV, SP, HT bitter acrid warm	• **Activates the blood, moves Qi:** Used to treat chest, epigastric or abdominal pain associated with blood stasis. • **Clears toxins:** Used to treat carbuncles and sores. • **Clears the channels:** Used to treat wind-damp Painful Obstruction in the channels causing rigidity and spasms. • **Reduces inflammation, regenerates flesh:** Used to stop pain, promote healing in sores and carbuncles for traumatic injury.

Herbs	Channels / Properties	Indications / Actions
San Leng *(sun-leng)* movexue	LIV, SP	bitter acrid neutral	• **Breaks up Blood Stasis, moves Qi, disperses accumulations, and relieves pain**: Used to treat masses, pain in the abdomen and chest pain and distention in the hypochondrium, postpartum blood stasis abdominal pain, and traumatic injury.
San Qi *(san-qi)* stopxue	LIV, ST, LI	sweet sl bitter warm	• **Stops bleeding and transforms blood stasis:** Used to treat all kinds of bleeding including vomiting of blood, blood in the stool, hematuria, epistaxis, and hemoptysis. • **Activates the Blood:** Used to treat blood stasis and related pain. • **Relieves swelling and stops pain:** Used to treat swelling and pain due to traumatic injuries.
Sang Bai Pi *(sang-pai-pi)* cough	LU, SP	sweet cold	• **Drains Heat from the Lung and stops coughing and wheezing:** Used to treat coughing and wheezing with thick, yellow sputum caused by Lung heat. • **Promotes urination and reduces edema:** Used to treat floating edema, facial edema, swelling of the extremities, fever, thirst, and dysuria.
Sang Ji Sheng *(sang-chi-sheng)* tyin	KID, LIV	bitter neutral	• **Supplements the Liver and Kidneys, strengthens the sinews and bones, and eliminates Wind-Damp**: Used to treat arthritis, soreness and pain in the low back and knees, wind-damp painful obstruction in the joints, hemiplegia, numbness, muscle and tendon weakness, and atrophy. • **Nourishes the Blood and quiets the fetus**: Used to quiet a restless fetus or for flooding and spotting during pregnancy. • **Lowers blood pressure:** Used to treat hypertension.
Sang Shen *(sang-chen)* tblood	LIV, HT, KID	sweet cold	• **Tonifies the blood, Supplements the Liver and Kidneys**: Used to treat Liver and Kidney yin depletion, wasting and thirsting, constipation, poor vision, tinnitus, scrofula and inhibited movement of the joints.
Sang Ye *(sang-yeh)* rext w-h	LU, LIV	bitter sweet cold	• **Releases the exterior and dispels Wind-Heat:** Used to treat wind-heat patterns causing fever, headache, sore throat, and coughing. • **Clears the Liver and brightens the eyes:** Used to treat red, sore, dry or painful eyes or floaters associated with Liver or wind-heat. • **Nourishes the Lungs:** Used to treat dryness associated with wind-heat or yin deficiency involving the Lungs causing thirst, or dry cough with thick, yellow sputum.
Sang Zhi *(sang-chih)* d-w-damp	LIV	bitter sweet sl cold	• **Dispels Wind-Damp, benefits the joints, reduces edema:** Used to treat wind-cold-damp painful obstruction, especially in the upper limbs, leg qi, edema, and itchy skin.
Sha Ren *(sha-jen)* movedamp	SP, ST	acrid warm	• **Transforms Dampness, moves Qi, harmonizes the Center:** Used to treat pain and discomfort in the epigastrium, nausea, vomiting and diarrhea associated with dampness obstructing the center due to Spleen not transforming and transporting. • **Quiets the fetus:** Used to treat morning sickness or a restless fetus.
Sha Shen *(sha-sheng)* tyin	LU, ST	sweet sl bitter bland cool	• **Moistens the Lungs and suppresses coughs:** Used to treat dryness in the lungs due to Lung yin deficiency, chronic cough, coughing without production of sputum, and coughing with blood-tinged sputum. • **Nourishes the Stomach, generates fluids:** Used to treat dryness in the throat and constipation associated with yin deficiency causing heat in the Lungs, Stomach, and Intestines.

HERB

Herbs	Channels / Properties	Indications / Actions
Shan Dou Gen *(shan-tou-ken)* clht-detox	LU, LI bitter cold	• **Clears Fire, relieves toxins, disperses swelling and relieves pain:** Used to treat sore throat pain and abscesses, throat wind, throat impediment, swollen gums, snake and insect bites. • **Clears the Lungs:** Used to treat cough due to Lung heat. • **Clears Damp-Heat:** Used to treat jaundice and bleeding hemorrhoids.
Shan Yao *(shan-yao)* tqi	SP, LU, KID sweet neutral	• **Supplements the Center and reinforces Qi:** Used to treat fatigue, nausea, diarrhea, poor appetite, spontaneous sweating. • **Tonifies Qi and Yin and benefits the Lung:** Used to treat chronic cough or wheezing. • **Secures the Kidneys and boosts the Essence:** Used to treat yin and yang deficiency of the Lungs and Kidneys including polyuria, polydypsia, spermatorrhea, and vaginal discharge.
Shan Zha *(shan-cha)* rfood	SP, ST, LIV sour sweet sl warm	• **Disperses food stagnation:** Used to treat abdominal distention or pain, acid regurgitation, diarrhea associated with accumulation due to meat or greasy foods, and stagnation of milk in suckling infants. • **Dissipates Blood stasis:** Used to treat persistent flow of lochia and hernia disorder associated with blood stasis. • **Reduces blood pressure and serum cholesterol:** Used to treat coronary artery disease and hypertension.
Shan Zhu Yu *(shan-shu-yu)* sab	KID, LIV sour sl warm	• **Astringes the Essence:** Used to treat spermatorrhea, polyuria, urinary incontinence, and excessive sweating due to Kidney deficiency. • **Astringes sweating:** Used to treat excessive sweating associated with yang deficiency. • **Tonifies the Liver and Kidneys:** Used to treat soreness and weakness in the lower back, dizziness, or impotence associated with Liver and Kidney deficiency. • **Stabilizes the menses and Stops Bleeding:** For deficiency patterns of excessive uterine bleeding and prolonged menstruation.
Shang Lu *(shang-lu)* cath	UB, KD, LI, SP bitter toxic cold	• **Frees urine and stool, drains water, and dissipates binds:** Used to treat swelling, distention and fullness, leg qi, throat impediment, swellings, and abscesses.
She Chuang Zi *(she-chuang-tzu)* etop	KID pungent bitter warm	• **Dries dampness, kills parasites, dispels Wind and stops itching:** Used to treat ringworm, scrotal damp itching, genital itching, vaginal discharge, and damp sores. • **Warms the Kidney, assists the Yang:** Used to treat impotence or infertility due to Kidney deficiency cold.
She Gan *(she-kan)* clht-detox	LU bitter cold	• **Clears Heat, relieves toxins, and benefits the throat:** Used to treat sore throat, sore pharynx, scrofula, toxin swelling abscesses and sores. • **Disperses Phlegm:** Used to treat cough and wheezing associated with phlegm obstruction.
She Xiang *(she-hsiang)* open	HT, SP, LIV pungent aromatic warm	• **Opens the orifices:** Used to treat heat in the Pericardium, Closed disorders, phlegm obstruction, and seizures. • **Activates the Blood:** Used to treat carbuncles, and immobile masses, and traumatic injury or painful obstruction due to blood stagnation. • **Hastens delivery:** Used to treat a stillborn fetus or retained placenta.
Shen Jin Cao *(shen-jin-tsao)* d-w-damp	LIV acrid bitter warm	• **Dispels Wind and dissipates Cold, eliminates Dampness:** Used to disperse swelling, soothe the sinews and activate the vessels, kill worms, and clear heat.

Herbs	Channels / Properties	Indications / Actions
Shen Qu *(shen-chu)* rfood	SP, ST	sweet acrid warm	• **Fortifies the Spleen and Stomach, disperses food stagnation and harmonizes the center:** Used to treat fullness and distention in the chest and abdomen, vomiting and diarrhea, postpartum stasis and abdominal pain.
Sheng Di Huang *(sheng-di-huang)* coolxue	HT, LIV, KID	sweet bitter cold	• **Clears Heat and cools the blood:** Used to treat spontaneous external bleeding, profuse flooding and spotting, and blood ejection associated with heat in the blood. • **Enriches the Yin:** Used to treat yin deficiency heat, wasting and thirsting disorder, constipation associated with yin deficiency. • **Clears Heart Fire:** Used to treat sores in the mouth and tongue, irritability, insomnia, tidal fevers and malar flush associated with Heart fire.
Sheng Jiang *(sheng-chiang)* rext w-c	LU, SP, ST	pungent warm	• **Releases the exterior and dispels cold:** Used to treat colds and flu caused by exterior cold attack. • **Warms the center, stops vomiting:** Used to treat vomiting caused by cold in the Stomach. • **Disperses Phlegm and stops coughing:** Used to treat coughing due to phlegm obstruction of the Lung. • **Reduces toxicity:** Used to treat medicinal toxicity and seafood toxicity. • **Harmonizes Ying and Wei:** Used to treat patients suffering from exterior deficiency that sweat without an improvement in their condition.
Sheng Jiang Pi *(sheng-chiang-pi)* edamp	LU, ST, SP	pungent warm	• **Promotes Urination:** Used to treat edema and urinary dysfunction. • **Reduces Edema.**
Sheng Ma *(sheng-ma)* rext w-h	LU, SP, ST, LI	sweet pungent cool	• **Releases the exterior:** Used to treat headache due to exterior wind-heat. • **Clears Heat and relieves toxicity:** Used to treat maculopapular rashes including carbuncles, erythemas, and mumps. • **Vents rashes:** Used in the early stages of rashes with dormant papules such as measles. • **Raises the yang:** Used to treat shortness of breath, fatigue, and prolapse associated with yang qi deficiency. • **Guides herbs upward.**
Sheng Tie Luo *(sheng-tie-luo)* cshen	HT, LIV	acrid cool	• **Calms the Liver and quiets the Spirit:** Used to treat mania, delirium, fright palpitations, insomnia and anger.
Shi Chang Pu *(shih-chang-pu)* open	HT, ST	pungent aromatic sl warm	• **Opens orifices, transforms Phlegm, and quiets the Spirit:** Used to treat seizures, loss of consciousness, deafness, dizziness or stupor caused by phlegm obstructing the orifices. • **Harmonizes the center, transforms dampness:** Used to treat fullness in the chest and epigastrium caused by interior dampness. • **Activates the Blood and relieves pain:** Used to treat painful obstruction due to blood or wind-cold-damp painful obstruction.
Shi Di *(shih-ti)* rqi	LU, ST	bitter sour neutral	• **Directs the qi downward:** Used to treat counterflow cough, stomach reflux and hiccups.

Herbs	Channels / Properties	Indications / Actions
Shi Gao *(shih-kao)* clht-fire	LU, ST sweet acrid very cold	• **Clears Heat:** Used to treat high fever, profuse sweating, extreme thirst, and a big pulse, without chills and irritability associated with interior excess heat in the Yangming or qi level. • **Clears Heat from the Lungs:** Used to treat coughing and wheezing with fever and thick, sticky sputum. • **Clears Stomach Fire**: Used to treat upward blazing Stomach fire causing toothache, swollen gums, or headache. Relieves sores: Used to treat eczema, burns, sores and ulcerations.
Shi Hu *(shih-ku)* tyin	KID, ST sweet sl salty bland cold	• **Clears Heat, nourishes yin, boosts the Stomach and generates fluids:** Used to treat thirst, dry mouth, Stomach pain from yin deficiency and to replenish fluids following febrile disease. • **Brightens the vision:** Used to treat poor vision associated with damage to the yin.
Shi Jue Ming *(shih-chueh-ming)* ewind	LIV, KID salty cold	• **Drains fire and subdues the Yang:** Used to treat headache, dizziness, and red eyes due to Liver fire or Liver yang rising. • **Brightens the eyes:** Used to treat red eyes and blurred vision, photophobia and other superficial visual obstructions associated with Liver heat. • **Unblocks the bowels:** Used to treat constipation. • **Lowers cholesterol:** Used to treat hypertension.
Shi Jun Zi *(shih-chun-tzu)* ebugs	SP, ST sweet warm	• **Kills parasites, disperses stagnation, fortifies the Spleen:** Used to treat abdominal pain and distention due to roundworms and pinworms, stagnation of milk and food in infants, diarrhea, tenesmus, and constipation due to qi stagnation.
Shi Wei *(shih-wei)* edamp	UB, LU bitter sweet sl cold	• **Clears damp-heat, frees urination, stops bleeding:** Used to treat hematuria, nephritis, uterine bleeding, vomiting blood, and dysentery due to damp heat. • **Clears the Lungs, dispels Phlegm, stops coughing:** Used to treat coughing and wheezing associated with heat in the Lungs.
Shu Di Huang *(shih-ti-huang)* tblood	LIV, HT, KID sweet sl warm	• **Tonifies the Blood:** Used to treat irregular menstruation, amenorrhea, dysmenorrhea, flooding and spotting, and other symptoms related to blood deficiency including a pale, white complexion, blurred vision, dry or brittle nails, dry hair, and heart palpitations. • **Benefits the Yin:** Used to treat Kidney yin deficiency causing night sweats, polyuria, nocturnal emissions, steaming bone disorder, and wasting and thirsting disorder. • **Augments the Essence:** Used to treat pain in the low back and knees, weakness of the lower extremities, dizziness, tinnitus, deafness, and poor vision.
Shui Niu Jiao *(xue-niu-chao)* coolxue	HT, LIV, ST salty cold	• **Clears Heat, resolves toxins, and cools the Blood:** Used to treat blood ejection, spontaneous external bleeding, precipitation of blood including erythema, purpura, epistaxis, and vomiting of blood, associated with heat in the blood. Also used to treat convulsions and delirium, loss of consciousness, and convulsions, or manic behavior due to heat in the blood.
Si Gua Luo *(shih-gua-lou)* movexue	LU, ST, LIV sweet neutral	• **Activates the Blood, frees menstruation, clears heat and transforms phlegm, stops bleeding:** Used to treat pain in the chest and hypochondrium, abdominal pain, lumbar pain, painful swollen testicles, lung heat phlegm cough, amenorrhea, absence of breast milk, hemorrhoids and fistulas, blood in the stools, and flooding and spotting.
Su He Xiang *(su-he-hsiang)* open	HT, SP sweet pungent aromatic warm	• **Opens orifices, frees the vessels, dissipates stasis:** Used to treat wind stroke, phlegm reversal, fright epilepsy, sores, and pain in the chest and abdomen.

Herbs	Channels / Properties	Indications / Actions
Su Zi *(su-tzu)* cough	LU, LI acrid warm	• **Stops coughing and wheezing, precipitates Qi, and disperses Phlegm:** Used to treat coughing and wheezing with copious phlegm and a stifling sensation in the chest. • **Moistens the Intestines:** Used to treat constipation due to dryness in the intestines.
Suan Zao Ren *(suan-tsao-jen)* cshen	HT, LIV, SP, GB sweet sour neutral	• **Nourishes the Heart yin, Nourishes Liver Blood, and quiets the Spirit:** Used to treat insomnia, irritability, anxiety and palpitations associated with blood or yin deficiency. • **Constrains perspiration:** Used to treat spontaneous sweating and night sweating.
Suo Yang *(suo-yang)* tyang	KID, LIV, LI sweet warm	• **Tonifies the Kidney Yang:** Used to treat frequent urination, spermatorrhea, and impotence associated with cold from deficiency. • **Boosts the Essence, and strengthens the sinews:** Used to treat weakness of the low back and knees, sinews, motor impairment, or paralysis associated with deficiency of essence or blood. • **Moistens Intestines:** Used to treat constipation associated with blood stagnation.
Tai Zi Shen *(tai-tzu-sheng)* tqi	SP, LU sl bitter sweet neutral	• **Supplements the Spleen and reinforces Qi:** Used to treat exhaustion of essence or spirit, poor appetite, nausea, vomiting and fatigue that accompany Spleen qi deficiency or spontaneous sweating due to Lung qi deficiency. • **Nourishes Fluids:** Used to treat thirst and dehydration.
Tan Xiang *(tan-hsian)* rqi	SP, ST, LU pungent aromatic warm	• **Regulates Qi and alleviates pain:** Used to treat pain in the chest and abdomen associated with qi stagnation, angina, and coronary artery disease.
Tao Ren *(tao-jen)* movexue	HT, LI, LIV, LU bitter sweet neutral	• **Breaks up Blood Stasis:** Used to treat menstrual irregularities including amenorrhea, dysmenorrhea, abdominal pain, chest pain, pain in the hypochondrium, and pain due to traumatic injury. • **Moistens dryness and lubricates the Intestines:** Used to treat constipation due to dry Intestines.
Tian Hua Fen *(tien-hua-fen)* clht-phlegm	LU, ST bitter sl sweet cold	• **Drains Fire, transforms Phlegm, moistens Lung dryness, and alleviates thirst:** Used to treat thirst, wasting thirst, jaundice, pulmonary dryness with coughing of blood associated with phlegm-heat. • **Relieves toxicity and expels pus:** Used to treat abscesses, and hemorrhoids.
Tian Ma *(tien-ma)* ewind	LIV sweet neutral	• **Extinguishes Wind, relieves spasms and stops pain:** Used to treat epilepsy, childhood convulsions, headache, dizziness, spasms, and wind stroke with numbness in the extremities caused by internal movement of wind in the vessels or channels or wind-phlegm causing painful migraine-type headaches or painful obstruction in the low back.
Tian Men Dong *(tien-men-tong)* tyin	LU, KID sweet bitter very cold	• **Enriches Kidney Yin and clears deficiency heat, moistens dryness:** Used to treat deficiency heat flaring up causing dryness and cough with blood-tinged sputum, and supplements liquids to relieve constipation due to dryness in the Intestines or wasting and thirsting disorder.
Tian Nan Xing *(tien-nan-hsiang)* cold-phlegm	LU, LIV, SP acrid warm toxic	• **Dries Dampness, transforms Phlegm:** Used to treat coughing, a stifling sensation in the chest, pain and distention in the chest associated with phlegm obstruction. • **Dispels Wind:** Used to treat dizziness, numbness, facial paralysis, spasms, hemiplegia, stroke or seizures. • **Relieves swelling and stops pain:** Used to treat scrofula, abscesses, insect bites and traumatic injury.

Herbs	Channels / Properties		Indications / Actions
Tian Zhu Huang (tien-chu-huang) clht-phlegm	HT, LIV, GB	sweet sl cold	• **Clears Heat, dissipates Phlegm, cools the Heart and calms fright:** Used to treat clouded spirit in febrile diseases, wind-stroke, loss of speech, child fright, wind and convulsion epilepsy.
Ting Li Zi (ting-li-tzu) cough	LU, UB	acrid bitter cold	• **Precipitates Qi and resolves edema:** Used to treat rapid panting breathing due to pulmonary congestion, phlegm cough, edema and distention.
Tu Fu Ling (tu-fu-ling) clht-detox	LIV, ST	sweet bland neutral	• **Relieves toxins and dries Dampness**: Used to treat joint pain, hypertonicity of the bones and sinews, turbid dysuria or jaundice associated with damp-heat and swellings, abscesses and other skin lesions associated with damp-heat.
Tu Si Zi (tu-szu-tzu) tyang	KID, LIV	pungent sweet neutral	• **Tonifies Kidney Yin and Yang, retains the Essence:** Used to treat vaginal discharge, impotence, nocturnal emission, premature ejaculation, spermatorrhea, frequent urination, wasting thirst, tinnitus, and low back ache associated with deficiency of yin, yang or essence. • **Tonifies Liver and Kidneys, Brightens the eyes, improves vision:** Used to treat blurred vision, floaters, night blindness, dizziness and tinnitus associated with Liver yin and Kidney yang deficiency. • **Warms the Spleen and Kidney:** Used to treat diarrhea associated with Spleen and Kidney yang deficiency. • **Quiets the Fetus:** Used to treat miscarriage.
Wa Leng Zi (wa-ling-tzu) clht-phlegm	LIV, SP	sweet salty neutral	• **Transforms Phlegm, softens hardness, dissipates stasis, and disperses accumulation**: Used to treat phlegm accumulation, stomach pain, and acid regurgitation.
Wang Bu Liu Xing (wang-pu-liu-hisang) movexue	LIV, ST	bitter neutral	• **Moves the Blood, frees the channels, frees lactation:** Used to treat amenorrhea, absence of breast milk, difficult delivery, dysuria, and swelling and pain in the testicles.
Wei Ling Xian (wei-ling-hsien) d-w-damp	UB	acrid salty warm	• **Dispels Wind dampness, frees the channels, disperses Phlegm and dissipates Damp accumulation:** Used to treat wind-cold-damp painful obstruction, cold, aching low back and knees, leg qi, malaria, tonsillitis, and fish bones stuck in the throat.
Wu Gong (wu-kong) ewind	LIV	acrid toxic warm	• **Dispels Wind, settles fright, attacks toxins, and dissipates binds**: Used to treat wind stroke, fright epilepsy, lockjaw, whooping cough, scrofula, nodes, swelling of sores, hemorrhoids, and fistulas.
Wu Jia Pi (wu-chia-pi) d-w-damp	KID, LIV	acrid bitter warm	• **Dispels Wind-Damp, strengthens sinews and bones, activates the Blood and stops stasis:** Used to treat wind, cold or damp obstruction Bi, hypertonicity of the sinews, lumbar pain, impotence, slow development to walk in children, edema, leg qi, toxin swelling of low abscesses and sores, trauma.
Wu Ling Zhi (wu-ling-chih) movexue	LIV, SP	bitter sweet warm	• **Disperses Blood stasis and stops pain:** Used to treat amenorrhea, dysmenorrhea, post partum abdominal pain, and epigastric pain associated with blood stasis. • **Stops bleeding:** Used to treat uterine bleeding.

Herbs	Channels / Properties	Indications / Actions
Wu Mei *(wu-mei)* sab	LI, LIV, LU, SP sour warm	• **Constrains Lung qi and stops coughing:** Used to treat chronic coughing and wheezing due to Lung and Kidney deficiency. • **Astringes the Intestines and stops diarrhea:** Used to treat chronic diarrhea or dysentery. • **Generates fluids and relieves thirst**: Used to treat thirst due to heat from deficiency of qi and yin. • **Kills Parasites:** Used to treat abdominal pain and distention caused by roundworms. • **Stops bleeding:** Used to treat flooding and spotting and blood in the stool.
Wu Wei Zi *(wu-wei-tzu)* sab	KID, HT, LU sour warm	• **Constrains Lung qi and stops coughing:** Used to treat chronic coughing and wheezing due to Lung and Kidney deficiency. • **Fortifies the Kidneys, astringes the Essence:** Used to treat diarrhea, vaginal discharge, nocturnal emission, spermatorrhea, and polyuria due to Kidney deficiency. • **Constrains sweating and generates fluids**: Used to treat excessive sweating, spontaneous sweating, thirst or a dry throat. • **Quiets the spirit and calms the Heart:** Used to treat insomnia, palpitations, dream-disturbed sleep due to Heart and Kidney deficiency. • **Improves Liver Function:** Used to treat hepatitis with reduced Liver function.
Wu Yao *(wu-yao)* rqi	SP, LU, UB, KID pungent warm	• **Regulates Qi and alleviates pain:** Used to treat pain in the epigastrium and abdomen, a stifling sensation in the chest, flank pain, lower abdominal pain, hernia or menstrual disorders. • **Warms the Kidneys, dissipates Cold:** Used to treat polyuria or urinary incontinence caused by deficiency cold.
Wu Zhu Yu *(wu-shu-yu)* wint	LIV, KID, SP, ST pungent hot sl toxic	• **Dissipates Cold, moves Qi, dries dampness and relieves pain, soothes the Liver and precipitates Qi, warms the center and checks vomiting:** Used to treat abdominal pain, leg qi, vertex headache, acid regurgitation and vomiting of clear fluids, diarrhea and dysentery, and mouth sores.
Xi Gua *(hsi-kua)* clht-sumr	UB, HT, ST sweet cold	• **Clears Summerheat, benefits thirst:** Used to treat summerheat patterns with thirst and scanty urine.
Xi Jiao *(hsi-chiao)* coolxue	HT, LIV, ST bitter salty cold	• **Clears Heat, resolves toxins, and cools the Blood:** Used to treat blood ejection, spontaneous external bleeding, precipitation of blood including erythema, purpura, epistaxis, and vomiting of blood associated with heat in the blood. Also used to treat convulsions and delirium, loss of consciousness, convulsions, or manic behavior due to heat in the blood.
Xi Xin *(hsi-hsin)* rext w-c	LU, KID pungent warm	• **Releases the exterior, dispels Wind-Cold, relieves pain:** Used to treat exterior cold causing headache, nasal congestion, toothache or painful obstruction. • **Warms the Lung and transforms Phlegm:** Used to treat coughing with copious, watery sputum associated with externally contracted wind-cold. • **Opens the nasal orifices:** Used to treat nasal congestion.
Xi Yang Shen *(hsi-yang-chen)* tyin	HT, KID, LU sweet sl bitter cold	• **Supplements the Yin, Clears Deficiency Fire:** Used to treat yin deficiency and deficiency fire.

Herbs	Channels / Properties	Indications / Actions
Xia Ku Cao *(hsia-ku-tsao)* clht-fire	LIV, GB — acrid bitter cold	• **Clears Liver Fire:** Used to treat headache, dizziness, or red, painful, and swollen eyes, hepatitis, and pulmonary tuberculosis associated with Liver fire or Liver heat ascending due to Liver yin deficiency. • **Clears Heat and dissipates nodules:** Used to treat scrofula, goiter, mammary abscesses and other glandular swellings. • **Reduces blood pressure:** Used to treat hypertension associated with Liver fire or ascendant Liver yang rising.
Xian He Cao *(hsien-ho-tsao)* stopxue	LIV, SP, LU — bitter acrid neutral	• **Stops Bleeding:** Used for hemoptysis, epistaxis, bleeding gums, hematuria, uterine bleeding, vomiting blood. • **Stops diarrhea:** for chronic diarrhea and dysentery. • **Stops Vaginal Discharge:** Used to treat vaginal discharge from damp-heat and parasites (trichomonisis vaginitis).
Xian Mao *(hsien-mao)* tyang	KID, LIV — pungent hot toxic	• **Warms the Kidney Yang and expels cold:** Used to treat infertility, impotence, urinary incontinence, nocturnal emission, and pain in the chest or abdomen associated with cold from deficiency. • **Dispels Cold-Damp:** Used to treat damp-cold painful obstruction with generalized pain, weakness in the bones and sinews, and low back and knee pain. • **Stops bleeding:** Used to treat flooding or spotting associated with deficiency cold.
Xiang Fu *(hsiang-fu)* rqi	LIV, SJ — sl bitter sl sweet neutral	• **Soothes and regulates Liver qi:** Used to treat depression, hypochondriac pain and epigastric distention caused by constrained Liver qi and the disharmony between the Liver and Spleen. • **Regulates menstruation and alleviates pain:** Used to treat menstrual irregularities, dysmenorrhea, flooding and spotting and vaginal discharge associated with stagnant Liver qi.
Xiang Ru *(hsiang-ju)* rext w-c	LU, SP, ST — pungent aromatic sl warm	• **Releases the exterior, expels summer heat, and transforms dampness:** Used to treat summerheat with absence of sweating. • **Dries Dampness and harmonizes the center.** • **Promotes urination and reduces swelling.**
Xiao Hui Xiang *(hsiao-huei-hsiang)* wint	LIV, KID, SP, ST — pungent warm	• **Warms the Kidney, dissipates cold, harmonizes the center, and regulates Qi:** Used to treat cold pain in the lower abdomen, lumbar pain, stomach pain, vomiting, dry and damp leg qi.
Xiao Ji *(hsiao-chi)* stopxue	LIV, SP — sweet cool	• **Stops bleeding:** Used for hemoptysis, epistaxis, bleeding gums, hematuria, uterine bleeding, and vomiting blood.
Xie Bai *(hsieh-pai)* rqi	LU, ST, LI, HT — acrid bitter warm	• **Frees the Yang and dispels cold:** Used to treat angina-type chest pain, damp-cold painful obstruction of the chest and dysentery.
Xin Yi Hua *(hsin-yi-hua)* rext w-c	LU, ST — pungent warm	• **Releases the exterior and unblocks the nasal passages:** Used to treat sinus congestion, sinus headaches, nasal discharge, loss of sense of smell, and toothache.
Xing Ren *(hsiung-jen)* cough	LU, LI — bitter sl warm sl toxic	• **Stops coughing and calms wheezing:** Used to treat cough, fullness and panting or wheezing. • **Moistens the intestines, unblocks the bowels:** Used to treat constipation due to dryness in the intestines.

Herbs	Channels / Properties	Indications / Actions
Xiong Dan *(hsiung-tan)* clht-fire	HT, LIV, GB bitter cold	• **Clears Heat and relieves spasms:** Used to treat Child Fright epilepsy with high fever and convulsions or delirium. • **Clears Heat, relieves inflammation and relieves toxins:** Used to treat trauma, sprains, fractures, or hemorrhoids and hot skin lesions. • **Brightens the eyes:** Used to treat red, painful, and swollen eyes and visual obstructions.
Xiong Huang *(hsiung-huang)* etop	HT, LIV, ST bitter pungent warm toxic	• **Dries dampness, dispels wind, kills worms, and resolves toxins:** Used to treat sores, abscesses, shingles, and herpes zoster.
Xu Duan *(hsu-tuan)* tyang	KID, LIV bitter pungent sl warm	• **Tonifies Liver and Kidney, strengthens sinews and bones:** Used to treat painful low back and knees, weakness in the knees, and joint stiffness. • **Stops Bleeding and quiets the fetus**: Used to treat flooding and spotting during pregnancy associated with cold in the womb and threatened miscarriage. • **Regulates Blood:** Used to treat pain due to blood stasis associated with traumatic injury.
Xuan Fu Hua *(suan-fu-hua)* cold-phlegm	LU, LIV, SP, ST bitter acrid sl warm	• **Descends the Qi downward and disperses Phlegm, stops cough, stops vomiting:** Used to treat coughing due to phlegm obstruction and hiccough, nausea or vomiting associated with Stomach cold and Stomach rebellious qi.
Xuan Shen *(suan-sheng)* coolxue	LU, ST, KID salty sweet bitter cold	• **Clears Heat and cools the blood:** Used to treat heat entering the blood causing spontaneous external bleeding or fever. • **Enriches the Yin:** Used to treat constipation and irritability associated with yin deficiency. • **Drains Fire and relieves toxins:** Used to treat maculopapular eruptions, sore throat and red, painful and swollen eyes. • **Softens hardness:** Used to treat scrofula.
Xue Jie *(hsueh-cheih)* movexue	HT, LIV sweet salty neutral	• **Dissipates stasis and relieves pain, stops bleeding and generates flesh:** Used to treat bone fractures, pain due to internal injury, and persistent bleeding from external injury.
Xue Yu Tan *(hsueh-yu-tan)* sab	HT, LIV, KD bitter neutral	• **Restrains leakage and stops bleeding:** Used to treat hematuria, and blood in the stool.
Ya Dan Zi *(ya-tan-tzu)* clht-sumr	LIV, LI bitter very toxic cold	• **Clears Heat, dries Dampness, kills parasites, resolves toxins:** Used to treat dysentery, chronic diarrhea, malaria, hemorrhoids, warts, and corns.
Yan Hu Suo *(yan-hu-suo)* movexue	HT, LIV, LU, ST acrid bitter warm	• **Activates the Blood, dispels Blood stasis, and stops pain:** Used to treat pain in the chest and abdomen, menstrual irregularities including dysmenorrhea, menorrhagia, profuse flooding and spotting, postpartum dizziness, retention of lochia and pain due to blood stasis from traumatic injury. • **Rectifies Qi and stops pain:** Used to treat chest pain, abdominal pain, epigastric pain, hypochondriac pain, headache pain, and menstrual pain associated with qi stagnation.
Ye Jiao Teng *(yeh-chiao-teng)* cshen	HT, LIV sweet sl bitter neutral	• **Nourishes the Heart Blood and quiets the Spirit:** Used to treat insomnia including dream disturbed sleep associated with Heart blood deficiency. • **Nourishes the Blood and unblocks the channels:** Used to treat generalized weakness, soreness, pain and numbness due to blood deficiency. • **Relieves itching:** Used to treat itching and skin rashes associated with wind.

HERB

Herbs	Channels / Properties	Indications / Actions
Ye Ju Hua *(yi-chih-jen)* clht-detox	LU, LIV bitter acrid sl cold	• **Clears Heat and relieves toxins:** Used to treat sore, swollen throat, carbuncles, and sores.
Yi Mu Cao *(i-mu-tsao)* movexue	HT, LIV, UB acrid bitter sl cold	• **Activates the Blood, dispels stasis, and regulates the fluids:** Used to treat menstrual irregularities, flooding and spotting in pregnancy, amenorrhea, retained placenta, postpartum dizziness, abdominal pain, scanty or profuse flooding and spotting, hematuria, and abscesses and sores associated with blood stasis.
Yi Tang *(i-tang)* tqi	SP, LU, ST sweet sl warm	• **Warms the Center and reinforces Qi:** Used to treat shortness of breath, fatigue, poor appetite, nausea, abdominal pain due to cold from qi deficiency. • **Nourishes the Lungs and stops coughs:** Used to treat dry, nonproductive coughs that accompany Lung qi deficiency.
Yi Yi Ren *(i-yi-jen)* edamp	LU, SP, KID sweet bland sl cold	• **Promotes urination and dries Damp-Heat:** Used to treat vaginal discharge, dysuria, damp leg qi, and edema. • **Fortifies the Spleen and the Lungs:** Used to treat diarrhea caused by mild Spleen qi deficiency and pulmonary abscesses or lung weakness. • **Expels Wind-Dampness:** Used to treat spasms due to wind-damp painful obstruction.
Yi Zhi Ren *(yi-chih-jen)* tyang	KID, SP pungent warm	• **Tonifies Kidneys, secures Kidney Qi, retains Essence:** Used to treat nocturia, spermatorrhea, frequent and copious urination, and urinary incontinence, or dribbling of urine associated with deficiency cold or qi deficiency. • **Warms the Spleen, stops diarrhea:** Used to treat vomiting, diarrhea, borborygmus, and abdominal pain associated with Spleen yang deficiency.
Yin Chai Hu *(yin-chai-hu)* coolxue	LIV, ST sweet cool	• **Clears Heat from deficiency:** Used to treat steaming bone fever and malaria associated with yin deficiency. • **Clears Heat and reduces childhood nutritional impairment**: Used to treat fever, thirst, and irritability associated with childhood nutritional impairment due to accumulation with heat. • **Cools the Blood and stops bleeding:** Used to treat hematuria, epistaxis, vomiting blood, and flooding and spotting associated with heat in the blood.
Yin Chen Hao *(yin-chen-hao)* edamp	LIV, SP, GB, ST bitter pungent cool	• **Clears damp-heat:** Used to treat jaundice due to either damp-heat or damp-cold. **Clears Heat in the Shaoyang Stage:** Used to treat alternating fever and chills with a bitter taste in the mouth, stifling sensation in the chest, hypochondriac pain, dizziness, nausea, and poor appetite associated with heat either in the Shaoyang stage or damp-heat in the Liver and Gallbladder channel.
Yin Yang Huo *(yin-yang-huo)* tyang	KID, LIV sweet pungent warm	• **Tonifies the Kidneys and invigorates the yang:** Used to treat poor memory, depression, and pain in the lower back and knees, impotence, spermatorrhea, and urinary incontinence or frequent urination associated with deficiency cold. • **Dispels Wind and eliminates Dampness:** Used to treat wind-damp-cold painful obstruction arthritis, hypertonicity of sinews or bones, pain and cramping of the hands and feet, hemiplegia or numbness in the extremities. • **Tonifies the Yin and Yang and descends Liver Yang:** Used to treat pain in the lower back and knees, tinnitus, dizziness, headache and irregular menstruation associated with Liver yang rising.

Herbs	Channels / Properties	Indications / Actions
Ying Su Ke (ying-su-ke) sab	KID, LI, LU — sour astringent neutral toxic	• **Constrains the Lung and suppresses cough, astringes the intestines and relieves pain:** Treats chronic cough, chronic diarrhea or dysentery, prolapse of the rectum, blood in the stool, abdominal pain, pain in the joints and tendons, copious urine, and vaginal discharge.
Yu Jin (yu-chin) movexue	HT, LU, LIV — acrid bitter cool	• **Activates the Blood, breaks up Blood stasis, Moves the Qi:** Used to treat pain in the chest, abdomen, and hypochondrium associated with blood stasis, and for menstrual pain associated with Liver qi stagnation. • **Clears the Heart and cools the Blood:** Used to treat depression, mania, withdrawal or clouded spirit associated with heat in the blood agitating the Spirit. • **Soothes the Liver and Gallbladder and reduces jaundice.**
Yu Li Ren (yu-li-ren) lax	SI, LI, SP — acrid bitter sweet neutral	• **Moistens Dryness, lubricates the intestines, precipitates Qi, and relieves edema:** Used to treat Large Intestine qi stagnation with dry stools, inhibited urination, ascites, edema, and leg qi.
Yu Mi Xu (yu-mi-shu) edamp	LIV, GB, UB — sweet neutral	• **Promotes urination, clears heat, calms the Liver, benefits the Gallbladder:** Used to treat nephritic edema, leg qi, icteric hepatitis, hypertension, cholecystitis, gallstones, diabetes mellitus, blood ejection, spontaneous external bleeding, nasal congestion, and mammillary abscesses.
Yu Xing Cao (yu-hsiang-cao) clht-detox	LI, LU — acrid cool	• **Clears Heat, resolves toxins, promotes urination, disperses swellings:** Used to treat pneumonia, suppurative sores, dysentery, malaria, edema, dysuria, vaginal discharge, abscesses, hemorrhoids, prolapse of the rectum, and eczema.
Yu Zhu (yu-chu) tyin	LU, ST — sweet sl cold	• **Nourishes yin and moistens dryness:** Used to treat damage done to yin in the aftermath of febrile diseases causing irritability, thirst, dry cough, or insatiable hunger. • **Extinguishes wind:** Used to treat pain, spasms and dizziness associated with yin deficiency causing internal movement of wind.
Yuan Hua (yuan-hua) cath	LU, LI, KD — acrid bitter toxic warm	• **Expels water and flushes Phlegm:** Used to treat panting and coughing, edema, hypochondriac pain, distention and fullness in the chest and abdomen.
Yuan Zhi (yuan-chih) cshen	HT, LU — bitter acrid sl warm	• **Quiets the Spirit:** Used to treat palpitations, anxiety, insomnia, restlessness, and disorientation. • **Dispels Phlegm and unblocks the orifices:** Used to treat depression and disorientation associated with phlegm blocking the Heart orifice. • **Dispels Phlegm, stops cough:** Used to treat coughing with copious sputum that is difficult to expectorate associated with phlegm obstructing the Lungs. • **Relieves inflammation:** Used to treat abscesses and reduce swellings and sores including breast swellings.
Yue Ji Hua (yue-chi-hua) movexue	LIV — sweet warm	• **Activates the Blood and regulates menstruation, disperses swelling and resolves toxins:** Used to treat menstrual irregularities, abdominal pain during menstruation, swelling due to trauma, and toxin swelling and abscesses.
Zao Jiao (zao-chiao) cold-phlegm	LU, LI — acrid warm sl toxic	• **Expels Wind, draws out toxins, disperses swellings, and expels pus:** Used to treat swollen abscesses, sores, and retention of placenta.
Ze Lan (tse-lan) movexue	LIV, SP — bitter acrid aromatic sl warm	• **Activates the Blood:** Used to treat menstrual pain and postpartum abdominal pain associated with blood stasis. • **Promotes urination:** Used to treat postpartum edema, postpartum painful urinary dysfunction, and systemic or facial edema.

HERB

Herbs	Channels / Properties	Indications / Actions
Ze Xie *(tse-hsieh)* edamp	UB, KID sweet bland cold	• **Promotes urination and dries dampness:** Used to treat dysuria, hematuria, edema, leg qi and diarrhea associated with damp-heat. • **Drains Kidney Fire:** Used to treat dizziness and tinnitus associated with Kidney yin deficiency.
Zhang Nao *(chang-nao)* open	HT, SP acrid toxic hot	• **Open Orifices, kills worms, relieves pain:** Used to treat painful distention in the chest and abdomen, leg qi, toothache, and trauma.
Zhen Zhu *(chen-chu)* cshen	HT, LIV sweet salty cold	• **Settles the Heart, quiets the Spirit:** Used to treat fright, palpitations, epilepsy, and childhood convulsions and seizures. • **Removes visual obstructions:** Used to treat blurred vision and other superficial disorders of the eyes. • **Relieves sores and regenerates flesh:** Used to treat chronic, non-healing ulcers and sores.
Zhi Bei Mu *(che-pei-mu)* clht-phlegm	LU, HT bitter cold	• **Clears Heat and transforms Phlegm:** Used to treat acute cough associated with phlegm-heat. • **Dissipates nodules, and relieves toxins:** Used to treat phlegm-fire nodules including scrofula, pulmonary abscesses, throat obstructions, sores and toxins.
Zhi Ke *(chih-ko)* rqi	SP, ST bitter pungent cool	• **Breaks up stagnant qi and disperses accumulation, moves Phlegm:** Used to treat phlegm stagnation in the chest and diaphragm, distention in the hypochondrium, food stagnation, belching, counterflow retching, diarrhea with pressure in the rectum, and prolapse of the rectum or uterus.
Zhi Mu *(chih-mu)* clht-fire	LU, ST, KID bitter cold	• **Clears Heat and drains Fire:** Used to treat excess heat causing fever, irritability, thirst, and cough with thick, yellow sputum. • **Enriches Yin, benefits fluids, and moistens dryness:** Used to treat spermatorrhea, nocturnal emissions, and excess sexual drive, night sweats, five palm heat, steaming bone taxation fever, irritability, and afternoon or low-grade fevers associated with yin deficiency.
Zhi Shi *(chih-shih)* rqi	SP, ST, LI bitter pungent sl cold	• **Breaks up stagnant qi and disperses accumulation:** Used to treat focal distention and fullness in the chest and abdomen with accompanying epigastric and abdominal pain or indigestion. • **Descends Qi:** Used to treat abdominal pain, diarrhea, tenesmus and constipation, gastroptosis, and prolapse of the uterus and rectum caused by stagnation. • **Transforms phlegm:** Used to treat distention and fullness in the chest and epigastrium due to phlegm obstruction.
Zhi Zi *(chih-tzu)* clht-fire	HT, LU, LIV, ST, SJ bitter cold	• **Clears Heat, drains Fire:** Used to treat insomnia, irritability, restlessness, a stifling sensation in the chest associated with excess heat. • **Clears Damp-Heat:** Used to treat painful urinary dysfunction associated with damp-heat in the Liver and Gallbladder channels. • **Cools the Blood and stops bleeding:** Used to treat epistaxis, hemoptysis, hematuria, vomiting blood or blood in the stool caused by heat in the blood. • **Reduces inflammation and activates the blood:** Used to treat skin sores caused by heat and stasis of blood.
Zhu Ling *(chu-ling)* edamp	UB, SP, KID sweet bland sl cool	• **Promotes urination and dries dampness:** Used to treat edema, dysuria, scanty urine, vaginal discharge, jaundice and diarrhea.

Herbs	Channels / Properties	Indications / Actions
Zhu Ru *(chu-ju)* clht-phlegm	LU, GB, ST	sweet sl cold	• **Clears Heat, transforms Phlegm, stops vomiting, cools the Blood:** Used to treat retching, vomiting, hiccough, phlegm-heat cough and panting with thick sputum that is difficult to expectorate, hemoptysis, epistaxis, vomiting blood, flooding and spotting, and morning sickness associated with phlegm-heat obstruction of the Lungs, Stomach or Gallbladder.
Zhu Sha *(chu-sha)* cshen	HT	sweet cool toxic	• **Calms the Heart and quiets the Spirit:** Used to treat anxiety, palpitations, restlessness, insomnia, or convulsions. • **Clears Heat, relieves toxicity:** applied topically to treat carbuncles, mouth sores, sore throat, and snakebites. • **Dispels Wind-Phlegm:** Used to treat dizziness and clouded vision due to wind-phlegm obstructing the normal movement of qi and blood.
Zi Cao *(tsu-tsao)* coolxue	HT, LIV	sweet cold	• **Clears Heat, cools the Blood, and relieves toxins:** Used to treat spontaneous external bleeding, blood ejection, hematuria, bloody dysentery and maculopapular eruptions such as measles or chickenpox that are not fully expressed. • **Clears Damp-Heat from the skin:** Used to treat eczema, cinnabar toxin, abscesses and vaginal itching with damp-heat. • **Moistens the Intestines and unblocks the bowels:** Used to treat constipation caused by heat in the blood.
Zi He Che *(tsu-ho-che)* tyang	KID, LIV, LU	sweet salty warm	• **Boosts the Essence:** Used to treat essence deficiencies including impotence, spermatorrhea, infertility, pain in the low back and knees, dizziness, deafness, and tinnitus. • **Augments Qi and nourishes the blood:** Used to treat severe qi and blood deficiency with accompanying signs of emaciation, pallor, insufficient lactation, and seizures. • **Supplements the Lung qi and benefits the Kidneys:** Used to treat wheezing, coughing or night sweats due to Lung qi deficiency or Lung and Kidney yin deficiency.
Zi Hua Di Ding *(tsu-hua-ti-tang)* clht-detox	HT, LIV	acrid bitter cold	• **Clears heat and resolves toxins, dries dampness and disperses swellings:** Used to treat sores, swollen abscesses, scrofula, jaundice, dysentery, diarrhea, red eyes, throat impediment Bi, and poisonous snake bites.
Zi Ran Tong *(tsu-ran-tong)* movexue	LIV, KID	acrid bitter neutral	• **Dissipates stasis and relieves pain, joins bone and sinews:** Used to treat torn ligaments, fractured bones, and blood stasis pain due to trauma, accumulations, goiter, and tumors.
Zi Shi Ying *(tsu-shih-ying)* cshen	HT, LIV	sweet warm	• **Settles the Heart and quiets the Spirit:** Used to treat anxiety, palpitations, disorientation, and insomnia. • **Descends the Qi:** Used to treat coughing or wheezing with copious sputum associated with Lung deficiency. • **Warms the Uterus:** Used to treat infertility and uterine bleeding.
Zi Su Ye *(tsu-su-yeh)* rext w-c	LU, SP	pungent aromatic warm	• **Releases the exterior:** Used to treat aversion to cold and fever, cough, panting and other early stages of virus and cold attack. • **Regulates Qi:** Used to treat vomiting, nausea, fullness in the chest and abdomen, and coughing and panting associated with qi stagnation. • **Calms the fetus:** Used to treat morning sickness. • **Detoxification:** Used to treat seafood toxicity.
Zi Wan *(tsu-wan)* cough	LU	bitter sl warm	• **Warms the Lung, precipitates Qi, disperses Phlegm and suppresses cough:** Used to treat coughing of various etiologies including wind-cold cough and panting, coughing of blood and pus caused by deficiency. • **Unblocks urination:** Used to treat dysuria.
Zong Lu Pi *(zong-lu-pi)* stopxue	LIV, LU, LI, SP	bitter astringent neutral	• **Stops bleeding:** Used to treat coughing or spitting of blood, epistaxis, blood in the stools, and uterine bleeding.

HERB INDEX

Herbs	Botanical Name	Common Name	Herb Category
Ai Ye	artemisiae, folium	mugwort leaf	stopxue
An Xi Xiang	benzoinum	benzion	open
Ba Dou	croton tiglii, semen	croton seed	cath
Ba Ji Tian	morinda, radix	morinda root	tyang
Bai Bian Dou	dolichoris, semen	flat bean	clht-sumr
Bai Bu	stemonae, radix	stemona root	cough
Bai Dou Kou	amomi kravanh, fructus	white cardamon	movedamp
Bai Fu Zi	aconitum, rdx coreanum	white appendage	cold-phlegm
Bai Guo	ginkgo, semen biloba	glutinous rice root	sab
Bai He	lilii, bulbus	lily bulb	tyin
Bai Hua She	agkistrodon seu bungarus	white pattern snake	d-w-damp
Bai Hua She She Cao	hedyotidis, herba	oldenlandia	clht-detox
Bai Ji	bletilla, rhizoma	bletilla rhizome	stopxue
Bai Ji Li	tribulus, fructus	caltrop fruit	ewind
Bai Jiang Cao	patrinia, hb	patrinia, thiaspi	clht-detox
Bai Jie Zi	sinapis, semen	white mustard seed	cold-phlegm
Bai Mao Gen	cylindrica, rhizome	rhz of woolly grass	stopxue
Bai Mu Er	tremella	wood ear	tyin
Bai Qian	cynanchi, rd/rhz	cynanchum	cold-phlegm
Bai Shao	paeonia, radix	white peony	tblood
Bai Tou Weng	pulsatilla chinesis, radix	chin anemone rt	clht-detox
Bai Wei	cynanchi, rd	swallowwort root	coolxue
Bai Xian Pi	cortex dictamni	chinese dittany	clht-detox
Bai Zhi	angelica dahurica, radix	angelica root	rext w-c
Bai Zhu	atractylodis, rz	white atractylodes	tqi
Bai Zi Ren	biotae orientalis, semen	arbor-viatae seed	cshen
Ban Lan Gen	lastidis, radix	woad root	clht-detox
Ban Xia	pinellia, rhizoma	half summer	cold-phlegm
Bei Xie	dioscorea	yam rhizome	edamp
Bi Ba	piperis longi, fructus	long pepper fruit	wint
Bian Xu	polygoni, herba	knotweed	edamp
Bie Jia	sinensis	chinese soft shelled turtle	tyin
Bing Lang	arecae catechu, semen	betel nut	ebugs
Bing Pian	borneol	ice slice	open
Bo He	mentha, herba	mint	rext w-h
Bu Gu Zhi	psoralae, fructus	psoralea fruit	tyang
Can Sha	excrementum bombycis mori	silkworm feces	d-w-damp
Cang Er Zi	xanthii, fructus	cocklebur fruit	d-w-damp
Cang Zhu	atractylodis, rhizoma	black atractylodes	movedamp
Cao Dou Kou	alpiniae katsumadai, semen	grass cardamon	movedamp
Cao Guo	amoni tsao-ko, fructus	grass fruit	movedamp
Cao Wu	aconiti kusnezoffii	wild aconite	wint
Ce Bai Ye	biota orientalis	flat fir leaves	stopxue
Chai Hu	bupleurum, radix	hare's ear root	rext w-h
Chan Su	secretio bufonis	toad venom	etop
Chan Tui	cicadae, periostracum	cicada moulting	rext w-h
Chang Shan	dichrae febrifugae, radix	dichroa root	clht-sumr

Herbs	Botanical Name	Common Name	Herb Category
Che Qian Zi	plantaginis, semen	plantago seeds	edamp
Chen Pi	citri, pericarpium	tangerine peel	rqi
Chen Xiang	lignum aquilariae	aloes wood	rqi
Chi Shao	paeoniae, radix rubrae	red peony root	movexue
Chi Shi Zhi	halloysitum	halloysite	sab
Chi Xiao Dou	phaseaoli, semen	aduki bean	edamp
Chuan Bei Mu	fritillaria, bulbus	fritillaria	clht phlegm
Chuan Jiao	zanthoxyli, pericarpium	fruit of szechuan pepper	wint
Chuan Lian Zi	meliae, toosendan fructus	sichuan true fruit	rqi
Chuan Niu Xi	cyathula officinali, radix	sichuan ox knee	movexue
Chuan Shan Jia	manitis, squama pentadact	anteater scales	movexue
Chuan Wu	aconiti, carmichaeli	sichuan aconite	wint
Chuan Xin Lian	andrographitis, herba	green chiretta	clht-detox
Chuan Xiong	ligustici, radix	cnidium	movexue
Chun Pi	ailanthis, cortex	ailanthus bark	sab
Ci Shi	magnetitum	magnitite	cshen
Cong Bai	allium fistulosi	scallion	rext w-c
Da Fu Pi	arecae, pericarpium	areca peel	rqi
Da Huang	rhei, radix/ rhizoma	rhubarb root	purg
Da Ji	japonicum, herba/radix	japanese thistle	stopxue
Da Qing Ye	lastidis, folium	isatis:	clht-detox
Da Zao	ziziphus, fructus	chinese dates	tqi
Dai Zhe Shi	haematitum	hematite	cshen
Dan Dou Chi	sojae praeparatum, semen	prepared soybean	rext w-h
Dan Nan Xing	ariasaema,cum felle bovis	jack in the pulpit	cold-phlegm
Dan Shen	salviae, radix miltiorrhiz	salvia root	movexue
Dan Zhu Ye	lophatherum, herba	bland bamboo leaves	clht-fire
Dang Gui	angelica sinensis, radix	chinese angelica root	tblood
Dang Shen	codonopsitis, radix	codonopsis root	tqi
Deng Xin Cao	juncus	juncus	edamp
Di Fu Zi	kochia, fructus	kochia fruit	edamp
Di Gu Pi	lycium, cortex	lycium bark	coolxue
Di Long	lumbricus	earthworms	ewind
Di Yu	sanguisorbae, radix	burnet-bloodwort rt	stopxue
Ding Xiang	caryophylli, flos	clove flower bud	wint
Dong Gua Pi	epicarpium beninccasae	winter melon peel	edamp
Dong Gua Ren	beninccasae, semen	winter melon seed	edamp
Dong Kui Zi	malvai, semen	musk mallow seeds	edamp
Dou Juan	glycines germin, semen	young soybean	clht-sumr
Du Huo	angelica, radix	pubescent angelica root	d-w-damp
Du Zhong	eucommiae, cortex	eucommia bark	tyang
E Jiao	gelatinum	geletin	tblood
E Zhu	curcuma, rhizoma	zedoria	movexue
Er Cha	arcaciae catechu	catechu	etop
Fan Xie Ye	sennae, folium	senna leaf	purg

HERB

HERB

Herbs	Botanical Name	Common Name	Herb Category	Herbs	Botanical Name	Common Name	Herb Category
Fang Feng	ledebouriellae, radix	ledebouriellae root	rext w-c	Hong Hua	carthamus, flos tinctorii	safflower flower	movexue
Fei Zi	torreyae grandis, semen	torreya seeds	ebugs	Hou Po	magnolia, cortex	magnolia bark	movedamp
Feng Mi	mel	honey	movexue	Hu Gu	os tigris	tiger bone	d-w-damp
Fo Shou	sarcodactylis, fructus citri	finger citron fruit	rqi	Hu Huang Lian	picrorhiza, rhizoma	picrorhiza rhizome	clht-damp
Fu Hai Shi	pumice	pumice	clht phlegm	Hu Jiao	piperis, fructus	barbarian pepper	wint
Fu Ling	poria	hoelen	edamp	Hu Lu Ba	trigonella, semen	fenugreek seed	tyang
Fu Ling Pi	poria, cortex	poria skin	edamp	Hu Po	succinum	amber	cshen
Fu Long Gan	terra flava usta	ignited yellow earth	stopxue	Hu Tao Ren	juglandis, semen	walnut nut	tyang
Fu Pen Zi	rubi, fructus	chinese raspberry	sab	Hu Zhang	polygoni cuspid, radix/rhizoma	bushy knotweed	movexue
Fu Ping	lemnae seu spirodel, herb	duckweed	rext w-h	Hua Shi	talcum	talcum	edamp
Fu Shen	poria, cortex cocos	fungus around root	edamp	Huai Hua Mi	sophorae japonicae, flos	pagoda tree flower	stopxue
Fu Xiao Mai	tritici, semen	wheat	sab	Huang Bai	phellodendrum, cortex	phellodendron	clht-damp
Fu Zi	aconiti, radix lateralis	aconite	wint	Huang Jing	polygonati, rhizoma	polygonatum root	tqi
Gan Cao	glycyrrhiza, radix	licorice root	tqi	Huang Lian	coptidia, rhizoma	golden thread	clht-damp
Gan Jiang	zingerberis, rhizoma	dried ginger	wint	Huang Qi	astragalus, radix	astragalus root	tqi
Gan Sui	euphorbiae kansui, radix	kan-sui root	cath	Huang Qin	scutellariae, radix	skullcap root	clht-damp
Gao Ben	ligustici, radix & rhizoma	ligusticum root	rext w-c	Huo Ma Ren	cannabis sativae, semen	hemp seeds	lax
Gao Liang Jiang	alpinia, rhizoma	lesser galangal	wint	Huo Xiang	agastache, herba	patchouli	movedamp
Ge Gen	puerariae, radix	kudzu root	rext w-h	Ji Nei Jin	endotheliuem, c. g. galli	chicken gizzard lining	rfood
Ge Jie	gecko	gecko	tyang	Ji Xue Teng	jixueteng, radix & caulis	millettia root/ vine	movexue
Geng Mi	semen, oryzae	rice	rext w-c	Jiang Can	bombyx	silkwormbody, sick	ewind
Gou Ji	cibotii, rhizoma	chain fern rhizome	tyang	Jiang Huang	curcumae, rhizoma longae	turmeric rhizome	movexue
Gou Qi Zi	lycium, fructus	lycium fruit	tblood	Jie Geng	platycodi, radix	root of ballon flwr	cold-phlegm
Gou Teng	uncariae, ramulus uncis	hook vine	ewind	Jin Qian Cao	lysimachiae, herba	gold money hb	edamp
Gu Sui Bu	drynariae, rhizome	shattered bones	tyang	Jin Yin Hua	lonicera japonica, flos	honeysuckle flower	clht-detox
Gu Ya	oryzae sativae, fructus	rice sprout	rfood	Jin Yin Zi	rosae, fructus	cherokee rosehip	sab
Gua Lou	trichosanthis, semen	trichosanthis fruit	clht phlegm	Jing Da Ji	euphorbia	peking spurge root	cath
Gua Lou Ren	trichosanthis, semen	trichosanthis seed	clht phlegm	Jing Jie	schizonepeta, herba/flos	schizonepeta stem	rext w-c
Guan Zhong	dryopteria, rhizoma	dryopoteris	clht-detox	Ju Hong	citri, erythrocarpae	tangerine peel	rqi
Gui Ban	testudinis	fresh water turtle	tyin	Ju Hua	chrysanthemi, flos	chrysanthemum flower	rext w-h
Gui Zhi	cinnamomi, ramulus	cinnamon twig	rext w-c	Jue Ming Zi	cassia, semen	cassia seeds	clht-fire
Hai Feng Teng	caulis piperis futokadsur	sea wind vine	d-w-damp	Ku Shen	sophora flavescenti, radix	bitter root	clht-damp
Hai Ge Ke	concha cyclinae sinensis	clam shell	clht phlegm	Kuan Dong Hua	farfara, flos	coltsfoot flower	cough
Hai Jin Sha	spora lygodii japonici	sea gold sand spores	edamp	Kun Bu	laminariae, herba	kelp thallus	clht phlegm
Hai Piao Xiao	sephiae, os	cuttlefish bone	sab	Lai Fu Zi	raphani sativie, semen	radish seed	rfood
Hai Shen	japonicus, strichopus	sea cucumber	tyang	Li Zhi He	litchi chinensis, semen	leechee nut	rqi
Hai Tong Pi	erythrainae, cortex	coral bean bark	d-w-damp	Lian Geng	nelumbinis, ramulus	lotus stem	clht-sumr
Hai Zao	sargassii, herba	sea weed, sargassum	clht phlegm	Lian Qiao	forsythia, fructus	forsythia fruit	clht-detox
Han Fang Ji	stephania, radix	stephania root	edamp	Lian Zi	nuciferae, semen	lotus seed	sab
Han Lian Cao	ecliptae, herba prostrata	eclipta	tyin	Lian Zi Xin	plumuia nelumbini	lotus plumule	clht-fire
Han Shui Shi	calcitum	same	clht-fire	Ling Yang Jiao	cornu antelopis	antelope horn	ewind
He Huan Pi	albizziae julibrissin, cortex	mimosa tree bark	cshen	Ling Zhi	ganoderma	reishi mushroom	cshen
He Shou Wu	polygoni, radix multiflori	fleecflower root	movexue	Liu Huang	sulphur	sulphur yellow	etop
He Ye	nelumbinis, folium	lotus leaf	clht-sumr	Liu Ji Nu	artemisiae anomalae, herb	liu's resident slave	movexue
He Zi	chebula, fructus	myrobalan fruit	sab	Long Dan Cao	gentianae, radix	chinese gentian root	clht-damp
Hei Zhi Ma	sesami, semen	sesame seeds	tyin				

HERB INDEX

Herbs	Botanical Name	Common Name	Herb Category
Long Gu	draconis, os	fossilized bones	cshen
Long Yan Rou	euphoria	dragon eye flesh	tblood
Lou Lu	rhapontici, radix	broadleaf globe thistle	clht-detox
Lu Dou	phaseoli, semen	mung bean	clht-sumr
Lu Gen	phragmiti, rhizoma	reed rhizome	clht-fire
Lu Hui	aloes, herba	juice of aloe leaf	purg
Lu Lu Tong	liquidambaris, fructus	sweetgum fruit	movexue
Lu Rong	cornu cervi	deer antler	tyang
Luo Shi Teng	caulis trachelospermi	star jasmine stem	d-w-damp
Ma Bo	lasiosphaera, fructus	puffball fruiting body	clht-detox
Ma Chi Xian	portulacae, herba	puslane	clht-detox
Ma Dou Ling	aristolochiae, fructus	aristolochia fruit	cough
Ma Huang	ephedrae, herba	ephedra stem	rext w-c
Mai Men Dong	ophiopogonis, tuber	ophiopogon tuber	tyin
Mai Ya	hordei vulgaris, fructus	barley sprout	rfood
Man Jing Zi	viticis, fructus	vitex fruit	rext w-h
Mang Xiao	mirabilitum	epson's salt	purg
Meng Shi	lapis micae seu chloriti	chlorite	clht phlegm
Mi Meng Hua	buddleiae, flos	buddleia flower bud	clht-fire
Mo Yao	myrrha, commiphora	myrrha	movexue
Mu Dan Pi	moutan cortex	tree peony root	coolxue
Mu Gua	chaenomelis, fructus	chinese quince fruit	d-w-damp
Mu Li	ostreae, concha	oyster shell	cshen
Mu Tong	mutong, caulis	akebia caulis	edamp
Mu Xiang	aucklandiae lappae, radix	saussurea	rqi
Mu Zei	equisetum, herba	scouring rush	rext w-h
Niu Bang Zi	arctii, fructum	burdock fruit	rext w-h
Niu Huang	calculus bovis	cattle gallstone	open
Niu Xi	achyranthes, radix bidentat	achyranthes root	movexue
Nu Zhen Zi	ligustrum lucidum, fructus	privet fruit	tyin
Ou Jie	nelumbinis, nodus	node of lotus rhz	stopxue
Pang Da Hai	sterculia, semen	herb	clht phlegm
Pei Lan	eupatorii fortunei, herba	ornamental orchid	movedamp
Pi Pa Ye	japonica, folium	loquat leaf	cough
Pu Gong Ying	taraxace, herba	dandelion	clht-detox
Pu Huang	typhae, pollen	cattail pollen	stopxue
Qian Cao Gen	cordifoliae, radix	madder root	stopxue
Qian Hu	peucedani, radix	hogfennel root	clht phlegm
Qian Niu Zi	pharbitidis, semen	morning glory	cath
Qian Shi	euryales, semen	euryale seeds	sab
Qiang Huo	notoptery, radix & rhizoma	notopterygium root	rext w-c
Qin Jiao	gentianae qinjiao, radix	gentiana root	d-w-damp
Qin Pi	fraxani, cortex	korean ash	clht-damp
Qing Dai	indigo pulverata levis	processed da qing ye	clht-detox
Qing Fen	calomelas	calomel	etop
Qing Hao	artemisiae, herba	wormwood	clht-sumr

Herbs	Botanical Name	Common Name	Herb Category
Qing Pi	citri, pericarpium viride	immature tangerine peel	rqi
Qing Xiang Zi	celosiae, semen	celosia seeds	clht-fire
Qu Mai	dianthi, herba	fringed pink	edamp
Quan Xie	scorpion	scorpion	ewind
Ren Shen	ginseng, radix	ginseng root	tqi
Rou Cong Rong	cistanches, herba	broomrape	tyang
Rou Dou Kou	myristicae, semen	nutmeg seeds	sab
Rou Gui	cinnamomi, cortex	cinnamon bark	wint
Ru Xiang	olibanum, gummi	frankincense	movexue
San Leng	sparganium, rhizoma stolonifer	bur-reed rhizome	movexue
San Qi	notoginseng, radix	notoginseng root	stopxue
Sang Bai Pi	mori alba, cortex	mulberry bark	cough
Sang Ji Sheng	loranthus, ramulus	mulberry mistletoe	tyin
Sang Shen	mori, fructus	morus fruit	tblood
Sang Ye	mori, follium	mulberry leaf	rext w-h
Sang Zhi	mori alba, ramulus	mulberry twig	d-w-damp
Sha Ren	amomi, fructus	sand seeds	movedamp
Sha Shen	glehnia, radix	glehnia root	tyin
Shan Dou Gen	sophorae tonk, radix	sophora root	clht-detox
Shan Yao	dioscorea, radix	chinese yam	tqi
Shan Zha	crataegi, fructus	hawthorn berry	rfood
Shan Zhu Yu	corni, fructus	asiatic cherry fruit	sab
Shang Lu	phytolaccae, radix	poke root	cath
She Chuang Zi	cnidii monniere, fructus	cnidii seeds	etop
She Gan	belamcanda, rhizoma	belamcanda rhizome	clht-detox
She Xiang	sceretio moschus	musk deer secretion	open
Shen Jin Cao	lycopodii, herba	club moss	d-w-damp
Shen Qu	massa fermenta	divine fermented mass	rfood
Sheng Di Huang	rehmannia, radix	chinese foxglove root	coolxue
Sheng Jiang	zingiberis, rhizoma	fresh ginger	rext w-c
Sheng Jiang Pi	zingiberis, cortex	ginger peel	edamp
Sheng Ma	cimicifugae, rhizoma	black cohosh	rext w-h
Sheng Tie Luo	ferri, frusta	iron fillings	cshen
Shi Chang Pu	acori graminei, rhizoma	sweetflag rhizome	open
Shi Di	diospyros	persimmon	rqi
Shi Gao	gypsum	stone paste	clht-fire
Shi Hu	dendrobium, herba	dendrobium	tyin
Shi Jue Ming	haliotidis	abalone shell	ewind
Shi Jun Zi	quisqualis indicae, fructus	envoy seeds	ebugs
Shi Wei	pyrrosia, folium	pyrrosia leaves	edamp
Shu Di Huang	rhemannia, radix	cooked rhemannia	tblood
Shui Niu Jiao	bubalus bubalis, cornu	water buffalo horn	coolxue
Si Gua Luo	fasciculus vascularis luffae	net of string melon	movexue
Su He Xiang	liquidamber styrax	resin of rose maloes	open
Su Zi	perilla, fructus	perilla seed	cough

HERB

Herbs	Botanical Name	Common Name	Herb Category	Herbs	Botanical Name	Common Name	Herb Category
Suan Zao Ren	ziziphus	sour jujube seed	cshen	Xue Yu Tan	crinis carbonisatus	charred human hair	sab
Suo Yang	cynomori, herba	cynomorium	tyang	Ya Dan Zi	brucae javanicae, fructus	java brucea fruit	clht-sumr
Tai Zi Shen	pseudostellaria, radix	pseudostellaria	tqi	Yan Hu Suo	corydalis, rhizoma yanhusuo	corydalis rhizome	movexue
Tan Xiang	lignum santali	sandalwood	rqi				
Tao Ren	persica, semen	peach kernel	movexue	Ye Jiao Teng	polygoni, caulis multiflor	polygonum vine	cshen
Tian Hua Fen	trichothansis, radix	trichosanthes root	clht phlegm	Ye Ju Hua	chrysanthemi, flos	wild chrysanthem	clht-detox
Tian Ma	gastrodiae elatae, rhizoma	gastrodia rhoizome	ewind	Yi Mu Cao	leonuri, herba heterophylli	benefit mother herb	movexue
Tian Men Dong	asparagus, tuber	asparagus tuber	tyin	Yi Tang	saccharum	barley malt sugar, maltose	tqi
Tian Nan Xing	ariasaema, rhizome	jack in the pulpit	cold-phlegm	Yi Yi Ren	coix lachryma	seeds of job's tears	edamp
Tian Zhu Huang	concretio silicea bambusa	bamboo silicea	clht phlegm	Yi Zhi Ren	alpiniae, fructus	black cardamon	tyang
Ting Li Zi	descurainiae, semen	lepidium	cough	Yin Chai Hu	stellaria, radix	stellaria root	coolxue
Tu Fu Ling	smilacia, rhizoma	simlax; greenbrier	clht-detox	Yin Chen Hao	artemisia, herba	capillaris	edamp
Tu Si Zi	cuscutae, semen	chinese dodder seeds	tyang	Yin Yang Huo	epimedium, herba	epimedium	tyang
Wa Leng Zi	concha arcae	cockle shell	clht phlegm	Ying Su Ke	papaveris, pericarpium	opium poppy husk	sab
Wang Bu Liu Xing	vaccaria, semen segetalis	vicarria seeds	movexue	Yu Jin	curcuma, tuber	turmeric tuber	movexue
Wei Ling Xian	clematidis, radix	clematis root	d-w-damp	Yu Li Ren	pruni, semen	bush cherry pit	lax
Wu Gong	scolpendra subspinipes	centipede	ewind	Yu Mi Xu	stylus zeae mays	cornsilk	edamp
Wu Jia Pi	acanthopanax, cortex	bark of 5 additions	d-w-damp	Yu Xing Cao	houttuynia, herba	heart leaf	clht-detox
Wu Ling Zhi	excrementum trogopteri	flying squirrel feces	movexue	Yu Zhu	polygonatum odoratum	jade bamboo	tyin
Wu Mei	pruni, fructus	mume fruit	sab	Yuan Hua	daphnes genkwa, flos	genkwa flower	cath
Wu Wei Zi	schizandrae, fructus	schizandra fruit	sab	Yuan Zhi	polygalaceae	ch senega root	cshen
Wu Yao	linderae, radix	lindera root	rqi	Yue Ji Hua	rosae chinensis, flos & fructus	moon season flower	movexue
Wu Zhu Yu	evodiae rutaecarpae, fructus	evodia fruit	wint	Zao Jiao	gleditsiae, fructus	chinese honey locust	cold-phlegm
Xi Gua	citrullus vulgaris	watermelon fruit	clht-sumr	Ze Lan	lycopi, herba lucidi	bugleweed	movexue
Xi Jiao	cornu rhinoceri	rhinoceros horn	coolxue	Ze Xie	alismatis, rhizoma	water plantain	edamp
Xi Xin	ascari, herba cum radix	(wild ginger)	rext w-c	Zhang Nao	camphora	camphor	open
Xi Yang Shen	panacis, radix	american ginseng	tyin	Zhen Zhu	margarita	pearl	cshen
Xia Ku Cao	spica prunella	self heal	clht-fire	Zhi Bei Mu	fritillaria, bulbus t	fritillaria bulb	clht phlegm
Xian He Cao	agrimoniae, herba	immortal crane herb	stopxue	Zhi Ke	citri aurantii, fructus	mature bitter orange	rqi
Xian Mao	curculiginis, rhizoma	curculigo	tyang	Zhi Mu	anemarrhena	anemarrhena rhizome	clht-fire
Xiang Fu	cyperus, rhizoma rotundi	cyperus	rqi	Zhi Shi	citri, fructus	immature bitter orange	rqi
Xiang Ru	elsholtzia, herba	aromatic madder	rext w-c	Zhi Zi	gardenia, fructus	gardenia fruit	clht-fire
Xiao Hui Xiang	foeniculi vulgaris, fructus	fennel fruit	wint	Zhu Li	bambusae, succus	dried bamboo sap	clht phlegm
Xiao Ji	cephalanoplos, herba	small thistle	stopxue	Zhu Ling	sclerotium polyporus umbellati	polyporus sclerotium	edamp
Xie Bai	bulbus allii	chinese chive	rqi	Zhu Ru	bambusae, caulis	bamboo shavings	clht phlegm
Xin Yi Hua	magnoliae liliflorae, flos	magnolia -pussy willow	rext w-c	Zhu Sha	cinnabaris	cinnabar	cshen
Xing Ren	armeniaca, semen	apricot seed	cough	Zi Cao	arnebiae lithospermi, radix	groomwell root	coolxue
Xiong Dan	fel ursi	bear gall bladder	clht-fire	Zi He Che	placenta hominis	human placenta	tyang
Xiong Huang	realgar	realgar male-yellow	etop	Zi Hua Di Ding	viola, herba cum radice	yedeon's violet	clht-detox
Xu Duan	dipsaci, radix	japanese teasel root	tyang	Zi Ran Tong	pyritum	natural copper	movexue
Xuan Fu Hua	inulae, flos	inula flower	cold-phlegm	Zi Shi Ying	fluoritum	fluorite	cshen
Xuan Shen	scrofularia, radix	ningpo figwort rt.	coolxue	Zi Su Ye	perrilla, frutescens	perrila leaf	rext w-c
Xue Jie	sanguis draconis	exhausted blood	movexue	Zi Wan	asteris tatarici, radix	purple aster root	cough
				Zong Lu Pi	fibra stipulae	stiple fiber	stopxue

HERB

Herbs Contraindicated during pregnancy

Ba Dou	Qu Mai
Ban Mao	Ru Xiang
Chan Su	San Leng
Che Qian Zi	Shang Lu
Chuan Niu Xi	She Gan
Da Ji	She Xiang
E Zhu	Shui Zhi
Fu Zi	Tao Ren
Gan Sui	Tian Hua Fen
Hai Long	Wu Gong
Hai Ma	Wu Tou
Hong Hua	Xiong Huang
Liu Huang	Xuan Ming Fen
Ma Chi Xian	Yan Hu Suo
Ma Qian Zi	Yi Mu Cao
Mang Xiao	Yu Li Hua
Mo Yao	Yuan Hua
Niu Huang	Zao Jiao
Qian Niu Zi	Zhang Nao
Qing Fen	

Herbs Caution during pregnancy

Bai Fu Zi	Quan Xie
Ban Xia Bing Pian	Rou Gui
Chang Shan	San Qi
Chuan Jiao	Su He Xiang
Chuan Shan Jia	Tao Ren
Da Huang	Tian Nan Xing
Dai Zhe Shi	Tong Cao
Dong Kui Zi	Wang Bu Liu Xing
Fu Zi	Xue Jie
Gan Jiang	Yi Yi Ren
Hong Hua	Yu Jin
Hou Po	Ze Lan
Hua Shi	Zhi Ke
Huai Niu Xi	Zhi Shi
Lou Lu	
Mu Tong	
Pu Huang	

Herbs containing animal products

Bai Hua She	Multibranded krait	Long Gu	Fossilized bone
Bie Jia	Tortoise shell	Lu Rong	Deer velvet and horn
Chan Tui	Cicada shell	Mu Li	Oyster shell
Di Be Chong	Field cockroach	Niu Huang	Cow gallstone
Di Long	Earthworm	Sang Piao Xiao	Praying mantis case
Dong Chong Xia Cao	Dead silkworm fungus	She Tui	Snake skin
E Jiao	Donkey skin	Shi Jue Ming	Abalone shell
Ge Jie	Gecko	Shui Niu Hiao	Water buffalo horn
Gui Ban	Turtle shell	Shui Zhi	leech
Hai Ge Ke	Clam shell	Wu Ling Zih	Flying squirrel feces
Hai Piao Xiao	Cuttlefish bone	Wu Shao She	Black tailed snake
Hou Zao	Gallstone	Xue Yu Tan	Charred human hair
Ji Nei Jin	Chicken gizzards	Yu Nao Shi	Fish bones
Jiang Can	Dried silkworms	Zhen Zhu Mu	Mother of pearl shell
Long Chi	Fossilized teeth	Zi He Che	Human placenta

Incompatibility with foods

Bo He	Sea turtle meat
Chang Shan	Chives and scallions
Feng Mi	Scallions
Fu Ling	Vinegar
Han Cai	Sea turtle meat
He Shou Wu	Garlic, chives, scallions, and turnips
Sheng Di Huang	Garlic, chives, scallions, and turnips

Eighteen incompatible herbs

Gan Cao	Gan Sui
	Da Ji
	Yuan Hua
	Hai Zao
Wu Tou	Ban Xia
	Gua Lou
	Bei Mu
	Bai Lian
	Bai Ji
Li Lu	Ren Shen
	Sha Shen
	Dan Shen
	Xuan Shen
	Ci Shao
	Ku Shen
	Bai Shao
	Xi Xin

Nineteen antagonistic herbs

Ren Shen	Wu Ling Zhi
Rou Gui	Chi Shi Zhi
Chuan Wu	Xi Jiao
Cao Wu	Xi Jiao
Ya Xiao	San Leng
Ding Xiang	Yu Jin
Ba Dou	Qian Niu Zi
Lang Du	Mi Tuo Seng
Shui Yin	Pi Shuang
Liu Huang	Po Xiao

HERB

Potential toxic effects

Herb	Safe Dose Range	Toxic effects	Antidote
Ai Ye	3-10g	Dry mouth and throat, epigastric pain, vomiting, abdominal pain, seizures, cold clammy skin, weakened vision	Zi Xue Dan for spasms
Ba Dou	0.1-0.3g in pill or powder	Gastrointestinal problems abdomen pain, nausea, vomiting, diarrhea, dehydration, jaundice, hypotension, dizziness, respiratory and circulatory problems	Egg white, milk, activated charcoal, morphine or atropine
Bai Bu	5-10g	Nausea, epigastric pain, diarrhea, respiratory problems	Fresh ginger juice or ginger decoction, rice vinegar
Bai Fu Zhi	3-5g	Mouth and tongue numbness, dizziness, spasms, vomiting	Decoction of Gan Cao 30g and ginger 30g
Bai Gui	5-10g	Headache, diarrhea, dizziness, fever, spasm, vomiting, abdominal pain	Decoction of Gan Cao 60g and mung beans 60g
Ban Xia	3-12g	Swelling, stiff tongue, throat and lips, numbness, nausea, chest pressure	Ginger juice or strong ginger decoction, vinegar, choline
Cang Er Zi	3-10g	Headache, nausea, vomiting, abdominal pain, liver damage, jaundice, bleeding, respiratory problems	Activate charcoal, vitamin C, decoction of Ban Lan Gen 120g, Gan Cao Lu Dou Tang, Zhi Bao Dan
Chan Su	0.02-0.03g	Nausea, vomiting, hyper salivation, abdominal pain, diarrhea, cyanosis, palpitations, dizziness, headache, slowed reflexes, numbness of the limbs,	Atropine, Sheng Mai San decoction, She Fu Tang decoction
Chuan Lian Zi	5-10g	Nausea, vomiting, diarrhea, palpitations, dizziness, tremors, spasms, numbness	Activated charcoal, egg white
Da Ji	0.6-1.5g	Nausea, vomiting, abdominal pain, diarrhea, dizziness, spasms respiratory problems	Decoction of Lu Gen 120g
Fu Zi (Wu Tou, Cao Wu, Chuan Wu)	3-12g	Numbness of the mouth and extremities, dizziness, headache, blurry vision, tremors, cardiac problems, hypotension, server respiratory problems, shock	Activated charcoal, atropine, decoction of Ku Shen 30g, Gan Cao 15g, Huang Lian 3g, Sheng Jiang 15g, or Jin Yin Hua 15g
Gan Sui	0.6-1.5	Nausea, vomiting, palpations, abdominal pain, dizziness, hypotension, low back pain,	
Ku Xing Ren	5-10g	Dizziness, abdominal pain, nausea, vomiting, headache, coma, numbness	Activated charcoal, fresh radish juice, decoction of Gan Cao 12g, black beans 120g
Lu Hui	1-2g	Vomiting, nausea, abdominal pain, diarrhea, low back pain, miscarriage	Activated charcoal, egg white
Ma Dou Ling	3-9g	Abdominal pain, diarrhea, rectal bleeding	Strong tea
Ma Huang	2-9g	Hypertension, vasoconstriction, sweating, dizziness, tremors, nausea, headache, urinary retention, abdominal pain	Atropine
Quan Xia	1.5-5.0g	Dizziness, headache, palpations, cyanosis, respiratory problems	Atropine, decoction of Jin Yin Hua 30g, Ban Bian Lian 10g, Fu Fu Ling 10g, Lu Dou 15g, Gan Cao 10g
Shang Lu	2-5g	Nausea vomiting, diarrhea, abdominal pain, limb spasm, hypotension, miscarriage, delirium cardiac arrest	Vitamin C, decoction of Fang Ji, Gang Feng, Gan Cao And Gui Zhi
Tian Nan Xing	3-10g	Gastrointestinal irritation, dizziness, delirium, respiratory problems, neurological symptoms	Strong black tea, egg white, ginger juice or strong ginger decoction, vinegar, tannic acid
Wei Ling Xiang	3-9g	redness and pain of the skin, abdominal pain, diarrhea, black stools, dilated pupils, stiff tongue	Egg white, garlic, decoction of Gan Cao 30g and ginger 30g
Xi Xin	1-3g	Headache, tachycardia sweating, restlessness, hypertension, stiff new and jaw, confusion, respiratory problems	Decoction of Ren Shen, Mai Dong and Wu Wei Zi
Yua Hua	0.6-1.5g	Vomiting, diarrhea, dehydration, muscle spasms	Vitamin C, fluid replacement

Source: Will Maclean & Jane Lyttleton, *Clinical Handbook of Internal Medicine, Volume 1 & 2*, 2002, University of Western Sydney, Campleton Australia.

HERB

Organ Systems	Herbal Support	Nutritional Support
Adrenal Glands	Ashwagandha: 450 mg daily Cordyceps: 1,000 mg tid Ginseng: 200 mg daily Licorice: 250 mg tid Schisandra: 100 mg bid	Adrenal extract: 200 mg bid B Complex: 25 mg daily Vitamin C: 500 to 1,000 mg bid
Brain	Ginkgo: 50 mg tid Gotu Kola: 100 mg tid Vinpocetine: 10 mg bid	Acetyl-L-carnitine: 500 mg tid
Eyes	Bilberry: 80 mg bid Eyebright: 250 mg bid	Beta-carotene: 10,000 IU daily Vitamin C: 1,000 mg daily Lutein: 2 mg daily
Heart	Cayenne: 400 mg tid Garlic: 400 mg bid or 600 mg daily for extract Grape seed: 100 mg daily Green tea: 500 mg daily Hawthorn: 250 mg daily	Aortic extract: 100 mg daily CoQ10: 30 mg daily Fish oils: 1,000 daily Flaxseed oil: 1 tbsp daily Magnesium: 400 mg daily Vitamin E: 400 IU daily
Immune System	Astragalus: 250 mg bid Cordyceps: 1,000 mg bid Echinacea: 250 mg daily, 3 weeks on and 1 week off Ginseng: 200 mg daily, 2 weeks on and 1 week off Reishi: 250 mg daily Schisandra: 100 mg daily	Vitamin A: 5,000 IU daily Vitamin C: 1,000 mg daily Selenium: 200 mcg daily Thymus extract: 250 mg daily Zinc: 50 mg daily
Kidney	Cordyceps: 1,000 mg bid Cranberry: 300 mg daily Dandelion leaf: 250 mg daily	Vitamin C: 1,000 mg daily Vitamin E: 400 IU daily
Liver/ Gallbladder	Artichoke: 250 mg daily Milk thistle: 150 mg daily Schisandra: 100 mg daily	Liver extract: 500 mg daily L-Carnitine: 250 mg daily N-Acetyl cysteine: 500 mg daily
Lungs	Cordyceps: 1,000 mg daily	Vitamin C: 1,000 mg daily Fish oils: 750 mg tid Flaxseed oil: 1 tbsp daily
Pancreas	Bitter melon: 200 mg daily Fenugreek: 250 mg daily Green tea: 250 mg daily	Chromium: 200 mcg daily Zinc: 25 mg daily
	Astragalus: 250 mg daily Echinacea: 250 mg daily, 3 weeks on and 1 week off	Thymus extract: 250 mg daily Vitamin C: 1,000 mg daily Zinc: 25 mg daily

Source: *Natural Therapeutics Pocket Guide*, 2nd Edition, Lexicomp

Special Cooking Preparations of Herbs

Special Instruction	Herb
Add at the end of cooking (no more than 5 minutes)	Bai Dou Kou Bo He Sha Ren
Add at the end of cooking (no more than 10 minutes)	Chuang Xiong Da Huang Gou Teng Huo Xiang Qing Hao
Cook 30 minutes before other herbs	Bie Jia Ci Shi Dai Zhe Shi Fu Zhi Gui Ban Long Gu Mu Li Shi Gao Shi Jue Ming Zhen Zhu Mu

Special Instruction	Herb
Cook in a muslin bag	Che Qian Zi Huai Shi Pi Pa Ye Xuan Fu Hua
Best taken in pill or powder form	Bing Pian Di Long Ge Jie Hu Po Ji Nei Jin Lu Rong Quan Xie San Qi She Xiang Wu Bei Zi Wu Gong Zhu Sha Zi He Che
Dissolve or melt in strained decoction	E Jiao Mang Xiao Yi Tang

Herbs	Uses	Information	Daily Dose	Cautions
Agar	int: constipation, GI complaints	acts similar to cellulose, absorbing water in intestines	1 to 2 teaspoons of powder, always with liquid	none known
Agrimony leaf	int: mild diarrhea, pharyngeal inflammation; ext: mild inflammation of skin	contains tannins and flavonoids: acts as an astringent	3 g or equivalent	none known
Aletris	int: dysmenorrhea, amenorrhea, anorexia	may have estrogenic effect, no conclusive studies	1.5 g drug/100 ml water or equivalent	none known
Alfalfa	int: anorexia, diabetes, hypothyroidism	no conclusive studies of effectiveness	as directed	avoid with SLE or other autoimmune diseases
Almond - sweet and bitter	int: (bitter) cough, nausea; ext: (sweet) skin inflammation	contains fatty acids, especially oleic acid, and cyanide-type compounds	as directed	overdose with cyanide-type effects; bitter almond to be used only under strict supervision
Aloe	int: constipation; ext: wound healing, psoriasis	FDA-approved as laxative, increases colonic motility	int: titrate to soft stool; ext: as directed	int: avoid in obstruction, IBD, appendicitis, pregnancy/ lactation, or in children; may cause abdominal cramping, hypokalemia- especially with diuretics - as well as albuminuria or hematuria; may cause benign red coloration of urine
Alpha-Lipoic Acid	int: diabetic complications, especially neuropathy; liver disease, cataracts, glaucoma, ischemia-reperfusion injury, amanita mushroom poisoning	water- and fat-soluble antioxidant needed in pyruvate DH reaction; may improve glucose utilization in diabetes and prevent free radical damage: can pass through BBB	no information: capsules available 30 to 100 mg	allergic skin reactions and hypoglycemia known; no data on pregnancy; effects of long-term use unknown
Alpine Cranberry	int: UTIs and urinary stones, rheumatism	has antiviral and antibacterial properties	2 g single dose or equivalent	contraindicated in pregnancy, nursing, children less than 12 years old; drug effective only with alkaline urine; hepatotoxicity due to hydroquinones is possible
American Hellebore	int: HTN	very effective but no longer used due to severe toxicity	do not use!	avoid completely, may cause cardiac arrest
Angelica root/fruit/leaf	int: decreased appetite, early satiety	contains coumarin and essential oil; increases gastric juice/bile production	4.5 g of drug or equivalent	may increase photosensitivity or cause dermatitis; may be carcinogenic; no interactions known
Anise fruit/ seed	int: dyspepsia; ext: bronchitis	expectorant, mild antibacterial agent	3 g of drug or equivalent	occasional allergic reactions- avoid if allergic to anethole; no interactions known
Arnica	ext: traumatic injuries, such as bruises, dislocations	analgesic and antiseptic activity	infusion: 2 g of herb per 100 ml of water	may cause allergic reaction; long-term use may cause edema or dermatitis; no interactions known; has been used internally for throat inflammation, but this is not recommended due to toxicity
Artichoke	int: dyspepsia, biliary complaints, anorexia	may increase bile flow, may be protective against hepatotoxins, may have lipid-lowering effects	6 g drug or equivalent	may cause allergic reaction; avoid in cholestasis or cholithiasis
Asarum	int: bronchitis, cough, asthma	may be mucolytic, antibacterial, local anesthetic	as directed- use purified dry extract	extremely susceptible mouse strain developed hepatoma after administration; avoid in children less than 12 and in pregnancy
Ash leaf/bark	int: URIs, rheumatism, fever	bark and leaf contain coumarin-like compounds; no evidence of effectiveness	as directed	none known
Asparagus root	int: inflammation of urinary tract, prevention of nephrolithiasis	may have diuretic effects	45 to 60 g of rhizome or equivalent	avoid if known nephrolithiasis; rare allergic skin reactions
Astragalus	int: general immune stimulant, as in HIV and other infections; memory impairment; anorexia	may increase WBCs (especially T cells), inhibit coxsackievirus replication, increase Liver function, and increase fibrinolysis	capsule as directed	caution with immunosuppressive therapy or anticoagulants; no definitive studies about pregnancy or lactation
Autumn Crocus	int: acute gout, familial Mediterranean fever	contains colchicine, an antichemotactic, mitosis inhibitor	initial dose equal to 1 mg colchicine, then 0.5 to 1.5 mg 1 to 2 hrs until pain free	avoid in pregnancy, may cause diarrhea, leukopenia, or aplastic anemia
Balm	int: depression, anxiety, insomnia, GI distress, neuralgia	acts as mild sedative: may inhibit TSH	infusion as recommended	none known
Barberry fruit/root	int: (fruit) UTIs, immune stimulant; (root) indigestion, constipation	may increase bile flow and have pro-peristaltic, antipyretic effects; contains vitamin C	as directed	none known
Barley	int: indigestion, diarrhea	contains numerous vitamins; has soothing effect on GI tract	taken as malt extract	avoid during pregnancy
Basil herb	int: fever, URIs, indigestion	may have antimicrobial effects	not recommended	potential carcinogen; avoid oil and large amounts of herbs

BOTANICAL

WESTERN HERBS

BOTANICAL

Herbs	Uses	Information	Daily Dose	Cautions
Bayberry fruit/bark	int: diarrhea, colitis, bronchitis	may have mineralocorticoid activity; acts as astringent, circulatory stimulant	*not recommended*	potential carcinogen, cannot recommend
Bean pods (without seeds)	int: supportive therapy for inability to urinate, UTIs, urinary stones	may act as weak diuretic	*5 to 15 g of herb or equivalent*	none known
Belladonna	int: liver and gallbladder complaints, GI spasms	contains atropine and related compounds, with anti-ACh effects	*0.05 to 0.1 g herb or equivalent*	avoid with tachy arrhythmias, BPH, narrow-angle glaucoma, acute pulmonary edema, GI obstruction, megacolon; may cause dry mouth, dry skin, tachycardia, tremor, difficult urination
Bellflower	int: bronchitis, sore throat, tonsillitis	contains saponins, which may inhibit gastric acid and act as expectorant	*6 g powder or equivalent*	none known
Betaine	nutrient which lowers level of homocysteine; found in variety of plant and animal foods	works in tandem with B vitamins and folate, so usually taken together	*no RDA: 500 to 1000 mg for general cardiovascular health*	none known
Bilberry fruit/leaf	int: acute diarrhea, pharyngitis, night vision; may lower blood sugar (leaf used for DM)	contains tannins, anthocyanins, and flavonoids	*fruit: 20 to 60 g or equivalent*	may have some anti-platelet effect; caution with ASA, anticoagulants, hypoglycemics
Biotin	needed for nerves, sweat glands, skin; found in dairy products, nuts, seeds, meats, vegetables	produced by intestinal bacteria	*no RDA; adult estimated need: 30 mcg*	none known
Birch leaf	int: inflammation of urinary tract, adjunct to rheumatic complaints	contains flavonoids, acts as a diuretic	*2 to 3 g of herb several times daily*	no side effects known; avoid if edema due to CHF or renal disease
Bishop's Weed fruit	int: angina, paroxysmal tachycardia, asthma, nonspecific chest pain	may increase coronary circulation with positive inotropic effects; may have antispasmodic effect on smooth muscles	*no information*	reversible cholestatic jaundice and photosensitivity are infrequent; chronic use may lead to dizziness, GI complaints, sleep disorders; high doses may reversibly increase LFTs
Bistort	int: diarrhea, mild GI bleed; ext: throat infections	contains tannins and starch	*as directed*	none known
Bitter Orange peel/flower	int: loss of appetite, dyspepsia	contains essential oil, may have spasmolytic effect on GI tract, increase gastric juice production	*peel: 4 to 6 g or equivalent*	may cause photosensitivity and sensitization with erythema and swelling
Black Cohosh root	int: PMS, dysmenorrhea, promotes labor, menopausal symptoms	may have estrogenic and anti-LH effects	*40 mg drug or equivalent*	occasional GI upset; no interactions known; complications of long-term use unknown; avoid in breast cancer; some use instead of HRT
Black Mustard	ext: pneumonia, sinusitis, sciatica	contains glucosinolates which are released by grinding seeds	*as directed*	contraindicated in peptic ulcer diseases or nephrolithiasis; protect eyes and skin from long-term use; coughing and possible asthma attacks may occur from breathing vapors; avoid in children younger than 6
Black Walnut	int: hemorrhoids, liver/ gallbladder problems	may have antimicrobial effects	*capsules: 95 mg to 500 mg to 3.5 g*	none known; treat overdose with charcoal and shock provisions
Blackberry leaf/root	int: nonspecific diarrhea, inflammation of mouth/throat	contains tannins	*leaf: 4.5 mg or equivalent*	none known
Blackthorn berry	int: inflammation of oral mucosa	contains tannins	*2 to 4 g or equivalent*	none known
Bladderwrack	int: thyroid dysfunction, obesity; ext: sprains	contains high amounts of iodine; may have antimicrobial and hypoglycemic effects	*as directed*	may worsen hyperthyroidism with high doses, as iodine content is not regulated; caution with other hypoglycemics
Blessed Thistle	int: decreased appetite, dyspepsia	promotes saliva, gastric juice production	*4 to 6 g or equivalent*	possible allergic reactions; no interactions known
Blue Cohosh	int: amenorrhea, dysmenorrhea, threatened miscarriage, atonic uterus	may have weak estrogenic, spasmolytic effects	*or equivalent*	avoid during first three months of pregnancy due to possible teratogenicity
Bogbean leaf	int: decreased appetite, dyspepsia	promotes saliva, gastric juice production	*1.5 to 3 g or equivalent*	possible allergic reactions; no interactions known
Boldo leaf	int: mild GI spasm, dyspepsia	contains alkaloids, flavonoids; increases bile and gastric juice production	*3 g or equivalent*	avoid with liver disease or gallstones; no side effects known, but avoid distillates or essential oil
Boneset	int: diaphoretic, emetic, mucolytic	may increase sweating	*as directed*	caution advised due to possible toxic alkaloids
Borage seed	int: astringent, anti-inflammatory such as in arthritis	astringent properties: contains gamma-linolenic acid, which reduces inflammation	*as directed*	caution advised due to potentially hepatotoxic alkaloids

156

Herbs	Uses	Information	Daily Dose	Cautions
Bromelain	int: edema, especially post-traumatic, wounds, burns, Peyronie's disease, angina, HIV	may have anti-edema effects in high dosages	80 to 320 mg of bromelain	may prolong PT and bleeding time with possible increased bleeding; may raise level of tetracyclines in blood; hypersensitivity reactions known; occasional GI side effects; no pregnancy data
Buchu leaf	int: irritation of urinary tract/prostate, various GI complaints, gout	no studies of drugs available; popular in South Africa today	as directed	avoid during pregnancy
Buckthorn bark/berry	int: constipation	increases colonic motility, GI secretion	20 to 30 mg hydroxyanthracene derivatives daily	bark must be aged for one year, fresh bark will cause severe vomiting; avoid with intestinal obstruction or chronic inflammation; may cause hypokalemia; GI cramping; use only if fiber/diet ineffective
Bugleweed	int: mild hyperthyroidism with nervous system dysfunction, mastodynia, PMS	inhibits conversion of T4-> T3; may inhibit prolactin	water-ethanol extracts equivalent of 20 mg of drug	may rarely cause goiter; avoid with other thyroactive drugs
Burdock root	int: GI complaints; ext: ichthyosis, psoriasis, seborrhea	may have mild antimicrobial effects; no studies available	capsules 460 to 475 mg or as directed	small risk of sensitization
Butcher's Broom	int: chronic venous insufficiency, hemorrhoids, leg cramps, itching	may act as diuretic; may increase venous tone	raw extract-equivalent to 7 to 11 mg total ruscogenin	rarely nausea; no interactions known
Cabbage	int: gastritis, ulcers, bronchitis, cough	may protect mucous membrane of stomach from gastric HCl	tablet 500 mg or juice as directed	none known
Calamus	int: dyspepsia, related GI complaints; ext: rheumatism, gum disease, tonsillitis	may stimulate appetite and digestion	tea as directed	avoid long-term use; susceptible rats developed tumors
Calendula flower/herb	int: pharyngitis/mucositis; ext: wound healing	contains glycosides, aglycones, carotenoids; may have anti-s. aureus, anti-HIV activity; may simulate epithelialization	as directed	uncommon dermatitis
Californian Poppy	int: depression, anxiety, sleep disorders	may act as sedative, limited clinical data	as directed	avoid during pregnancy; often prescribed with other sedatives
Camphor	int: circulatory regulation disorders; ext: muscular rheumatism, bronchitis, cardiac symptoms	acts as bronchial secretagogue, respiratory antispasmodic	as directed	avoid on broken skin; may cause contact eczema; no interactions known
Canadian Goldenrod	int: UTIs, stones of urinary tract	may act as diuretic, weakly spasmolytic	6 to 12 g or equivalent	avoid if edema due to CHF, renal failure; take with fluids
Capsicum	ext: analgesia, zoster, diabetic neuropathy	FDA-approved as topical analgesic; contains capsaicinoids, which may have anti-inflammatory actions; blocks substance P in nerves	as directed	avoid eyes; use only for 2 days and then again after 2 weeks; rare hypersensitivity reactions; do not add heat; may irritate mucous membranes at low doses; long contact with skin may injure nerves; overdose may cause hypothermia
Caraway oil/seed	int: dyspepsia, early satiety, flatulence	acts as antispasmodic, antimicrobial	3 to 6 drops of standard preparation	no side effects or interactions known
Cardamom seed	int: dyspepsia, liver/gallbladder complaints, URIs, pharyngitis, tendency to infection	may be virustatic, may increase biliary motility	1.5 g of drug or equivalent	avoid with gallstones
Carrageen (Irish seaweed)	int: cough, URIs	may act as expectorant	as directed	none known
Cascara bark	int: laxative, gallstones, liver ailments	FDA-approved as laxative; may increase peristalsis	20 to 30 mg hydroxyanthracene derivatives daily	may cause hypokalemia with chronic use; avoid with chronic GI inflammation or obstruction; fresh bark may cause vomiting—use aged bark
Cashew	int: GI ailments; ext: ulcers, warts, corns	may have anti-Gram positive activity	as directed	seed cases contain alkyl phenols and may act as strong skin irritants; nuts do not contain them
Castor oil	int: constipation, intestinal inflammation/parasites	ricolinic acid acts as laxative; also may be antimicrobial	laxative: 5 g bid or 2 g 5x per day	contraindicated in obstruction, acute inflammation, abdominal pain of unknown origin, pregnancy/nursing; rare skin rashes; chronic use may cause hypokalemia; castor beans highly toxic
Catechu	int: sore throat; ext: skin diseases, oral ulcers, toothache	may act as astringent and antiseptic	0.3 to 2 g tid or equivalent	none known
Catnip	int: fever, cramps, anxiety	limited scientific data	tea as directed	avoid during pregnancy; smoking drug may cause mind-altering effects

WESTERN HERBS

Herbs	Uses	Information	Daily Dose	Cautions
Cat's Claw	int: immune stimulant	contains hirsutine and sterol components, may stimulate IL-1, IL-6; may inhibit platelets, affect serotonin/dopamine, have anti-HTN effects, induce apoptosis in certain cell lines	*as directed*	contraindicated in pregnancy, nursing; avoid if taking immunosuppressants or with autoimmune disease (one report of ARF in patient with SLE); may lower estradiol and progesterone levels
Cat's Foot flower	int: diuretic, diarrhea	may increase bile flow and decrease GI spasms; limited scientific info	*tea as directed*	no information
Celandine	int: biliary spasm, GI distress	mild antispasmodic, papverdine-like action	*2 - 5 g of herb or equivalent*	may cause mild hypotension; no interactions known
Celery	int: anxiety, GI complaints, edema	may have sedative, anticonvulsant, diuretic effects	*as directed*	avoid volatile oil with pyelonephritis
Centaury	int: decreased appetite, dyspepsia	may increase gastric juice production	*6 g of drug or equivalent*	none known
Chamomile flower	int: GI inflammation, spasms; ext: skin inflammation, pharyngitis	antispasmodic, antiflatulent, antibacterial, promotes wound healing	*as directed*	may cause hypersensitivity or anaphylactic reactions; caution if allergic to ragweed, chrysanthemums, or asters
Chaste Tree fruit	int: PMS, dysmenorrhea, menopausal symptoms, mastodynia	may decrease prolactin secretion via dopaminergic action	*30 to 40 mg or equivalent*	may cause itchy rash; no interactions known; avoid during pregnancy
Chestnut	int: URIs, poor circulation	limited scientific info	*infusion as directed*	none known
Chickweed	int: joint stiffness, gout, Tb; ext: eczema, wounds	limited scientific info	*tea or infusion as directed*	none known
Chicory	int: decreased appetite, dyspepsia	may increase bile production	*3 g of herb or equivalent*	avoid in gallstones; may cause allergic reaction
Chinese Cinnamon	int: anorexia, dyspepsia, bronchitis	may be antibacterial, fungistatic, increase GI motility, inhibit ulcers	*2 to 4 g drug or equivalent*	avoid with pregnancy, as is potential abortifacent
Chinese Foxglove root	int: fever, insomnia, restlessness, rheumatism, eczema, kidney/heart disease	may be antibacterial, immunosuppressive, and hepatoprotective	*as directed - decoction in Chinese fashion*	none known
Chinese thoroughwax	int: fever, pain, inflammatory conditions	contains saponins, which may show antihistaminic, antitumor, and immunoregulatory effects	*often mixed with other herbs; use as directed*	avoid during pregnancy; overdose may cause GI complaints
Choline	found in many foods, in lecithin	important for nervous system functioning (converted to ACh)	*no RDA; recommended (adults): approx. 500 mg*	toxicity can cause rare GI side effects; may need to take if on niacin for hypercholesterolemia
Chondroitin	int: osteoarthritis, other degenerative diseases	carbohydrate which draws fluid into tissues, making them spongier; affects collagen and matrix production	*usually combined with glucosamine - as directed*	may affect coagulability of blood; avoid if pregnant/nursing; will only work for some patients
Chromium	trace element: found in meat, seafood, dairy products, eggs, grain, Brewer's yeast	may have hypoglycemic effect in some patients; most Americans do not receive enough	*no RDA; recommended (adults): 50 to 200 mcg*	toxicity rare, but reported to cause skin problems, liver/kidney disease, and even lung cancer; picolinate form has caused chromosomal damage to animals and rare nephrotoxicity, so chloride form may be preferred
Cinchona bark (quinine)	int: decreased appetite, dyspepsia, bloating	related to quinine-like drugs; may increase saliva, gastric juice production	*1 to 3 g herb or equivalent*	avoid if pregnant, allergic to quinine; rare thrombocytopenia; may sensitize to quinine
Cinnamon bark	int: decreased appetite, dyspepsia, bloating, flatulence	antibacterial, fungistatic, increases GI motility	*2 to 4 g bark or equivalent*	avoid in pregnancy; allergic skin reactions relatively common
Clivers	int: urinary tract inflammation, skin ulcers, rashes	limited scientific data	*tea as directed*	none known
Cloves	ext: topical anesthesia, oral/pharyngeal inflammation	antibacterial, antiviral, antifungal	*mouth washes with essential oil*	none known
Cocoa	int: diarrhea, liver/gallbladder dysfunction, UTIs	contains short-chained fatty acids; no therapeutic effect documented	*as directed*	avoid with migraines
Coenzyme Q10	int: cardiac insufficiency, angina, post-cardiac surgery; immunostimulant	important in ATP production as part of electron transport chain; immunostimulant properties (unproven)	*usually bid or tid as directed as supplement to conventional treatment*	none known; take with some fat to improve absorption
Coffee Charcoal	int: nonspecific diarrhea, mild oral/pharyngeal inflammation	acts as absorbent	*9 g or equivalent*	none known, although may influence absorption of other drugs
Cola Nut	int: mental/physical fatigue	contains methylxanthine, caffeine, similar compounds	*2 to 6 g or equivalent*	may cause insomnia, excitability, tachycardia, diuresis; avoid in peptic ulcer disease
Coltsfoot leaf	int: inflammation of oral/pharyngeal mucosa		*4.5 to 6 g of drug or equivalent*	avoid chronic use and in pregnancy or nursing
Comfrey herb/leaf/root	ext: contusions, sprains, dislocations	fosters callus production	*as directed*	avoid in pregnancy; do not apply to open skin or use internally; do not use more than 4-6 weeks (hepatotoxicity)

Herbs	Uses	Information	Daily Dose	Cautions
Condurango bark	int: decreased appetite	increases saliva, gastric juice production	*as directed*	none known
Copper	trace mineral; found in shellfish, nuts, other foods	important for Hb, collagen synthesis	*no RDA; recommended (adults): 2 to 3 mg*	avoid large doses while breastfeeding; take with zinc if taking supplement; balance may be affected by other minerals or antacids; high doses may cause GI side effects; dietary intake preferred to supplements
Coriander seed	int: decreased appetite, dyspepsia	limited scientific data	*3 g herb or equivalent*	avoid in gallstones; may cause allergic reaction
Corn Poppy	int: cough, colds, bronchitis, disturbed sleep	contains small amounts of alkaloids	*tea as directed*	reports of children poisoned with fresh foliage
Cornflower	int: dyspepsia, fever, URI	little evidence of effectiveness	*tea as directed*	small risk of sensitization reaction
Couch Grass	int: inflammation of urinary tract, prevention of urinary stones	contains saponins, essential oil (antimicrobial)	*6 to 9 g or equivalent*	avoid if edema due to CHF, renal failure; take with fluids
Cranberry	int: UTIs, urinary tract stones	may prevent E. Coli from adhering to wall of bladder	*juice or capsules bid to qid*	will not help once bacteria have taken hold; use pure juice, not cocktail or tablets; no known side effects/interactions
Creatine	int: muscle exhaustion, promotes muscle strength, CHF	formed naturally in liver; tends to pull water into muscles; more effective in sprint vs. endurance exercise; effect may be increased with insulin	*as directed during loading cycle, then maintenance*	avoid in renal disease; may lead to dehydration; do not use in pregnancy or breastfeeding
Cumin	int: dyspepsia	may have antimicrobial effect, especially vs. aspergillus	*as directed*	may prolong effect of barbiturates; used as abortifacent, so avoid in pregnancy
Cysteine	nonessential amino acid; changed into N-acetylcysteine (NAC); used for respiratory disease/ARDS, hyperlipidemia, acetaminophen overdose, HIV, general health	NAC is changed to glutathione, a potent antioxidant (see glutathione)	*no RDA: both NAC and l-cysteine are available; doses depend on indication;: start with 500 mg for general health*	avoid high (> 7 mg) doses of NAC; oral NAC may cause GI side effects and may interact with ACE-inhibitors; IV NAC can cause hypotension with nitroglycerin
Daffodil	int: bronchitis, pertussis, asthma	limited scientific data	*as directed*	may rarely cause itchiness
Damiana leaf/herb	int: aphrodisiac, antidepressant	considered ineffective	*not recommended*	not recommended
Dandelion root/herb	int: digestive aid, diuretic, laxative	may increase bile production, acts as diuretic	*4 to 10 g of herb tid*	avoid in bile duct obstruction, ileus; may cause minor skin rash
Devil's Claw root	int: loss of appetite, dyspepsia	may increase bile production	*as directed*	avoid in peptic ulcer disease; use with caution with gallstones
DHEA	int: adrenal insufficiency, fatigue, sexual dysfunction	low DHEA levels associated with many diseases from Alzheimer's to SLE, but cause not determined; DHEA may be tested in blood or saliva	*as directed*	avoid if history of uterine, breast, cervical, or prostate cancer; avoid in pregnancy or if breastfeeding
Dill seed/herb	int: dyspepsia	may be antispasmodic, bacteriostatic; contains essential oil rich in carvone	*3 g or equivalent*	none known
Dong Quai root	int: PMS, amenorrhea, insomnia, anemia, HTN	may contain B-12, coumarin-like compounds	*as directed*	may cause photosensitization, bleeding, and rarely fever
Dyer's broom	int: emetic, bladder stones, gout, dyspepsia	limited scientific data	*1 to 2 cups infusion*	avoid during pregnancy/lactation
Echinacea Purpurea/pallida/augustofolia	int: supportive therapy for colds, flu-like illnesses; ext: wound healing	may act as immune stimulant by increasing phagocytosis; may induce TNF-alpha, IL-1, IL-6; may protect collagen	*as directed*	avoid with HIV, autoimmune diseases, Tb, MS; do not use for more than 8 weeks or during pregnancy; antibiotics may be given in addition; may cause GI symptoms if given IV
EDTA	used in chelation therapy for heavy metal toxicity and increasingly for heart disease, Parkinson's disease, arthritis	trials for CAD as alternative to surgery ongoing	*as directed*	must be given slowly (IV) in monitored setting; long-term effects unknown; overdose can cause organ failure
Elder flower	int: URIs	may increase bronchial secretion, cause sweating	*10 to 15 g drug or equivalent*	none known
Elecampane root	int: bronchitis, cough	may have antimicrobial, antihelminic effects	*1 g drug or equivalent*	severely irritating to mucous membranes; avoid during pregnancy; large amounts may cause vomiting, diarrhea, spasms, paralysis
English Chamomile	int: sluggishness of bowels, anxiety; ext: stomatitis, rhinitis, toothache	limited scientific data	*1.5 g drug tid or equivalent*	avoid during pregnancy; small risk of sensitization; used in manzanilla sherry (Spain) as flavoring agent

WESTERN HERBS

BOTANICAL

Herbs	Uses	Information	Daily Dose	Cautions
English Plantain	int: URIs, bronchitis, fevers, pharyngitis; ext: skin inflammation, wounds	has proven bactericidal effect - may increase blood clotting	*infusion with 2 to 4 g drug or equivalent; also syrups, lozenges, cough medications*	none known
Ephedra (Ma Huang)	int: mild bronchospasm, nasal decongestant	FDA issued warning in 1995	*equivalent of 15 to 30 mg total alkaloid (adults)*	contraindicated in glaucoma, HTN, thyroid dysfunction, BPH; may cause insomnia, motor restlessness, irritability, headaches, nausea/ vomiting, urinary dysfunction, tachycardia, arrhythmias; avoid with MAO-inhibitors, Parkinsonian agents, digoxin, antimigraine agents, antiarrythmics. Avoid in children. May be addictive.
Eryngo	int: UTIs, bronchitis, coughs	limited scientific data; no evidence of effectiveness	*tea as directed*	none known
Eucalyptus leaf	int: inflammation of respiratory tract	secretion, expectorant, weakly spasmolytic	*4 to 6 g of leaf or equivalent*	may rarely cause diarrhea, vomiting; may induce P450
Eucalyptus oil	int: inflammation of respiratory tract; ext: rheumatic complaints	secretomor, expectorant, weakly spasmolytic	*int: 0.3 to 0.6 g oil; ext: as directed*	avoid internally in liver disease, GI inflammation; avoid in young children; rare cause of vomiting and diarrhea; may induce P450
Evening Primrose oil	int: diverse complaints from GI sluggishness to PMS, mastalgia, dermatitis, chronic fatigue syndrome	gamma-linolenic acid (also found in fish) converted to PGE1 in vivo, has anti-inflammatory/ cell membrane stabilizing actions	*capsules 500 to 1,300 mg as directed*	may lower seizure threshold in patients with seizure disorders or on medications which do same; may require up to 3 months treatment
Eyebright	ext: eye inflammation, stye, coughs	limited scientific data	*tea or lotion as directed*	none known
Fennel seed/ oil/honey	int: mild dyspepsia, flatulence	stimulates GI motility	*0.1 to 0.6 g of herb or equivalent*	avoid in pregnancy; avoid fennel other than fennel honey in children; rare allergic reactions; avoid oil, as may cause vomiting or seizures
Fenugreek seed	int: anorexia, gout, diabetes, menstrual irregularity; ext: local inflammation	secretolytic, hyperemic	*int: 6 g drug or equivalent, ext: 50 g powder/l H2O*	avoid repeated external applications
Fever bark	int: fever, HTN	contains reserpine, echitamin	*infusion as directed*	alkaloid-type poisoning possible but rare
Feverfew	int: migraine, arthritis, rheumatism	contains parthenolide, which may inhibit thromboxane B2 and leukotriene B4; may inhibit platelet aggregation via serotonin	*200 to 250 mg qid (capsules) or equivalent*	may cause sensitization via skin contact; may cross-react with Tansy, Yarrow, Marguerite, Aster-Sunflower, Laurel, Liverwort; rebound headache, insomnia, muscle stiffness, and anxiety characterize post-feverfew syndrome in patients who stop taking drug abruptly; also reports of glossitis/stomatitis; may alter effects of anticoagulants or thrombolytics. Avoid during pregnancy.
Fish berry	int: scabies and similar infections, motion sickness/ dizziness	contains picotoxin, which acts as presynaptic inhibitor	*in combination preparations as directed with caution*	very toxic: may cause headache, dizziness, nausea, spasms, vomiting; two or three kernels may be fatal
Fish oils (Omega-3 Fatty Acids)	int: hypercholesterolemia	may decrease LDL while raising HDL	*no RDA: take as directed, but eating fish 3x/week preferred*	caution with anticoagulants; better to eat more fish, especially cod, mackerel, salmon; one serving usually gives 1-3 g omega-3's
Flaxseed	int: chronic constipation due to enteritis, IBS; heart disease; ext: local inflammation	contains albumin, alpha-linolenic acid, and other fatty acids; increases peristalsis and coats colonic mucosa	*as directed*	avoid with ileus; take with fluids; keep oil from heat and light; may affect coagulation studies in high doses
Folic Acid	vitamin found in leafy green vegetables, liver, other foods	essential for DNA replication and RBC production	*RDA (adults): 400 mg; 500 if breastfeeding; 800 mg if pregnant*	GI and CNS symptoms have been reported with very large doses
Frostwort	int: digestive disorders, especially peptic ulcer disease; ext: skin inflammation	limited scientific data	*liquid extract as directed*	none known
Fumitory	int: spastic discomfort of biliary and GI tracts	antispasmodic effect on GI tract	*6 g of herb or equivalent*	none known
Galangal	int: anorexia, dyspepsia	may inhibit prostaglandins, act as antispasmodic	*as directed*	none known
Gamboge	int: digestive disorders, especially constipation	contains mucilage, which confers strong laxative effect	*as directed, but use with caution*	abdominal pain and vomiting may occur with as little as 0.2 g drug; powdered resin may cause sneezing
Garlic	int: infections, hyperlipidemia, HTN, stroke prevention	contains allin, may enhance fibrinolysis, inhibit platelets, lower lipids; may have antiviral and antihelminic properties	*4 g fresh garlic or equivalent*	rare allergic reactions; may rarely cause changes to GI flora; avoid if on large amounts of ASA or anticoagulants

Herbs	Uses	Information	Daily Dose	Cautions
Gentian root	int: dyspepsia, anorexia, bloating, hepatitis, sexual infections	may increase saliva and gastric juice production; may have fungistatic and bacteriostatic effects	as directed	avoid in peptic ulcer disease, diarrhea, or obstruction; may rarely cause headaches
German Sarsaparilla root	int: gout, rheumatism, fever, UTIs	limited scientific data; no documented efficacy	as directed	none known
Ginger root	int: dyspepsia, prevention of motion sickness, antiemetic	may increase peristalsis, gastric juice/bile production	2 to 4 g rhizome or equivalent	caution with gallstones; no interactions known; do not use for morning sickness with pregnancy
Ginkgo Biloba leaf	int: vertigo/tinnitus, Alzheimer's disease, decreased cerebral blood flow, PVD, memory improvement	contains antioxidant flavones such as quercetin and kaempferol; may inhibit platelet-activating factor; may act as free-radical scavenger	120 to 240 mg extract (dementia); 120 to 160 mg extract (PVD/ vertigo/tinnitus), 8 weeks minimum	hypersensitivity- rare GI upset: may interfere with anticoagulants or alter PT/PTT
Ginseng root - American	int: diverse complaints, such as lethargy, atherosclerosis, DM, shock, sexual dysfunction	contains saponins, antioxidants, peptides, polysaccharides; may lower hyperglycemia in some diabetics	1 to 2 g of root or equivalent	may rarely cause insomnia, diarrhea, menopausal bleeding; note lack of standardized extracts; may slow heart and decrease oxygen needs
Siberian Ginseng root	int: general fatigue, lethargy	contains coumarin derivatives; may increase T-cells	2 to 3 g of root or equivalent	avoid with HTN; generally use for less than 3 months
Glucosamine	int: osteoarthritis, other degenerative diseases	sugar found in food and produced by body; stimulates production of proteoglycans	usually 1000 to 2000 mg or as directed; dose may be affected by patient weight	occasional mild GI side effects; often combined with chondroitin; does not affect NSAID efficacy
Glutamine	nonessential amino acid, found in many foods; used for many ailments including arthritis, autoimmune diseases, psychosis, GI inflammation, impotence, stress	any stress may deplete body's stores	no RDA; 500 to 1500 mg often used	contraindicated in kidney or liver disease or in hyperammonemia; take on empty stomach
Glutathione	primary intracellular antioxidant; used for liver disease, peptic ulcer disease, cataracts, cancer, Parkinson's disease, HIV, others	may be helpful in cystic fibrosis and post-chemotherapy, where oxidant stress is widespread; likely has immuno-stimulant, anti-carcinogenic effects	no RDA; 500 mg bid often used	little information; oral glutathione may not raise blood GSH levels; n-actetylcysteine (NAC) may be a better dietary source
Goat's Rue	int: UTIs, inflammation of urinary tract, hyperglycemia	contains galegin, which may lower blood sugar, although not documented in humans	not recommended	overdose in animals caused salivation, spasms, paralysis and death; theoretically could cause hypoglycemia; no demonstrated efficacy
Goldenrod	int: inflammation of urinary tract, prevention of nephrolithiasis	may act as diuretic	6 to 12 g herb or equivalent	avoid in edema from CHF or renal disease; drink large amounts of fluid
Goldenseal	int: URI, menorrhagia, mouth sores, diarrhea	increases saliva, gastric juice production	as directed, often combined with echinacea	may displace bilirubin from albumin; contraindicated in pregnancy or G-6-PD deficiency; may lower effectiveness of heparin; high doses have caused convulsions
Goldenthread	int: dyspepsia	contains berberine; limited scientific info	as directed	avoid during pregnancy
Gotu Kola	int: promote longevity, aphrodisiac, wound healing, hot flashes, rheumatism	Contains saponins that promote wound healing and decrease venous pressure insufficiency	as directed	none known
Grape seed/ leaf/fruit	int: hyperlipidemia, edema, venous insufficiency	contains proanthocyanidins (PCOs), antioxidants and LDL inhibitors, capillary wall stabilizers; may help poor vision due to retinal pathology	many dosages of extract available, usually 150 to 600 mg daily	none known
Greater Burnet	int: menopausal disorders, URIs, GI inflammation; ext: boils, wounds	limited scientific info	as directed	none known
Green Tea	int: diarrhea, indigestion, motion sickness	6x antioxidants as black tea; inhibit c. difficile, c. perfringens; may have cancer preventive effects; contains caffeine; may prevent dental caries	many forms, as directed	may cause GI symptoms; caution with renal disease, cardiovascular disease, anxiety, thyroid disease; avoid more than 5 cups daily if pregnant; avoid in nursing; reports of microcytic anemia in children
Guaiac wood	int: supportive therapy for rheumatic complaints		4.5 g of drug or equivalent	none known
Guarana	int: fatigue	contains caffeine, which has stimulatory and diuretic effects	7 to 11 g powder or equivalent	may lead to hypokalemia with chronic use; caution with thyroid disorders, anxiety, renal disease, cardiovascular disease; avoid in pregnancy/nursing

BOTANICAL

WESTERN HERBS

Herbs	Uses	Information	Daily Dose	Cautions
Gumweed herb	int: irritation of upper respiratory tract, cough	may have antibacterial properties	4 to 6 g of drug or equivalent	rare gastric irritation; no interactions known
Haronga bark/leaf	int: dyspepsia, mild exocrine pancreatic insufficiency	may increase bile production	25 to 50 mg drug or equivalent	avoid in gallstones, serious liver/biliary disease, ileus; may cause photosensitivity
Hawthorn leaf/flower	int: atherosclerosis, HTN	may act as positive inotrope, may increase coronary/myocardial perfusion	as directed - 6 months minimum	none known; avoid with MI or other serious heart disease; self-medication not recommended; leaf alone unproven
Hay flower	ext: anti-inflammatory, as in chronic arthritis	acts as topical hyperemic	use as compress qid to bid	avoid on open skin or with acute inflammation
Heart's Ease herb	ext: mild seborrheic skin ailments		1.5 g of drug/ cup of water as tea	none known
Heather herb/flower	int: prostate and urinary problems, liver/gallbladder disorders, gout, rheumatism	may have diuretic effect, although no proven efficacy	add to water as directed	none known
Hemp Nettle	int: mild respiratory inflammation	contains tannin and saponins	6 g of herb or equivalent	none known
Henbane leaf	int: spasms of GI tract, tremors	contains alkaloids such as hyoscyamine and scopolamine; inhibits ACh at muscarinic sites	as directed	avoid with tachyarrhythmias, BPH, narrow-angle glaucoma, acute pulmonary edema, GI obstruction, megacolon; may cause dry mouth, dry skin, tachycardia, tremor, difficult urination
Hibiscus	int: anorexia, URIs, constipation	may have laxative effect due to poorly absorbed fruit acids; may relax uterine muscle and vascular smooth muscle; no documented efficacy	prepare tea as directed	none known
Hollyhock flower	int: bronchitis, fever, cough; ext: wounds, ulcers	limited scientific info; no documented effects	prepare tea as directed	none known
Hops	int: restlessness, anxiety, anorexia	unknown efficacy or mechanism	single dose: 0.5 g	none known
Horehound	int: dyspepsia, bloating, flatulence	may increase bile production	4.5 g of drug or equivalent	none known
Horse Chestnut seed/leaf	int: chronic venous insufficiency, pruritus, edema	seeds contain aescin, which may have anti-exudative, vascular-tightening effect	seed: 250 to 312. 5 mg extract bid; leaf: prepare tea as directed	seed may cause occasional GI complaints, hepatotoxicity, urticaria; leaf contains coumarins and may interact with warfarin, ASA, other anticoagulants
Horseradish	ext: minor muscle aches, inflammation of respiratory tract	may have antimicrobial, hyperemic properties	20 g of fresh root or equivalent	avoid with peptic ulcer disease or in children under 4
Horsetail	ext: wound healing; int: edema, irrigation therapy for urinary tract stones	contains silicic acid and flavonoids; may act as diuretic	int: 6 g of herb or equivalent	avoid with edema from CHF or renal disease; drink copious amounts of water
Hound's Tongue	ext: wounds; int: diarrhea	contains alkaloids which may be toxic	avoid	avoid folk medicinal preparations at all costs! hepatotoxic and hepatocarcinogenic
Hyssop	int: URIs, circulatory stimulation, liver/gallbladder dysfunction	may have antimicrobial, antiviral effects, especially vs. herpes simplex; no documented efficacy	capsules 445 mg qid	avoid during pregnancy; high doses may slightly increase seizure risk
Iceland Moss	int: anorexia, pharyngitis with cough, antiemetic, anemia	may act as demulcent	4 to 6 g of herb or equivalent	none known; avoid large amounts or chronic use due to possible lead content
Ignatius beans	int: faintness, anxiety, cramping (homeopathic doses)	contains strychnine and brucine, acts as psychoanaleptic	avoid	very toxic due to strychnine; avoid at all costs in allopathic doses; overdose may occur after one bean
Immortelle	int: dyspepsia	has antibacterial properties; increases bile production	3 g of drug or equivalent	avoid in biliary obstruction or cholethiasis
Indian Hemp	int: cardiac insufficiency, diuretic; ext: condylomas, warts	contains digitalis-like glycosides	as directed, with caution	causes irritation of mucous membranes, vomiting; use only if expert with this drug; overdose similar to digitalis
Indian Snakeroot	int: mild HTN, especially with anxiety	contains reserpine and alkaloids, which have alpha- and ß-blocking properties	600 mg drug or equivalent	avoid with depression, ulcers, pheochromocytoma, pregnancy, lactation; side effects may include stuffy nose, depressive mood, fatigue, reduction in sexual potency; may decrease ability to drive or operate machines; avoid with alcohol, digitalis, barbiturates, L-dopa, sympathomimetics

Herbs	Uses	Information	Daily Dose	Cautions
Indian Squill	int: cardiac insufficiency, cardiogenic edema, cough	contains cardioactive glycosides; may function as expectorant	*60 to 200 mg single dose or equivalent*	limited therapeutic range; may cause GI complaints; contraindicated with 1st or 2nd degree AV block, hypercalcemia, hypokalemia, hypertrophic cardiomyopathy, carotid sinus syndrome, ventricular tachycardia, aortic aneurysm, WPW; caution with anti-arrhythmics
Inositol	part of vitamin B complex; found in beans, fruit, meat; used for neurologic disorders, depression, diabetic neuropathy, hyperlipidemia	component of lecithin- may be important in nerve conduction: little scientific info	*no RDA: usually no more than 500 to 1000 mg*	none known, no information about pregnancy/nursing; may have dairy base
Iodine	mineral used in treating thyroid disease, fibrocystic breast disease, breast cancer, vaginitis, wounds	iodine deficiency rare in U.S.	*RDA: (adults): 150 mcg, 175 mcg if pregnant, 200 mcg if nursing*	iodine toxicity may affect thyroid; may interact with lithium; some foods such as cabbage and soybeans may inhibit iodine uptake in GI tract
Ipecac	int: emetic, expectorant, amebic dysentery		*tincture or extract as directed*	frequent contact may cause allergic reaction of skin; acts as emetic at higher doses
Iron	mineral, used for Fe-deficiency anemia	will not cause guaiac + stools	*RDA (men): 10 mg, (women): 18 mg; usually dose is 65 mg tid*	vitamin C increases absorption, calcium decreases absorption; iron inhibits absorption of drugs such as L-dopa, penicillamine, quinolones, tetracycline; antacids may decrease oral Fe absorption; can cause constipation; caution in first trimester of pregnancy
Ivy leaf	int: chronic respiratory inflammation. cough, bronchitis	contains saponins; may act as expectorant or antispasmodic; may have antibacterial/ antiviral effects	*0.3 g of drug or equivalent*	none known
Jambolan bark	int: nonspecific diarrhea, pharyngitis; ext: mild inflammation of skin	contains tannins; may act as astringent	*3 to 6 g of drug or equivalent*	none known
Java Tea	int: irrigation therapy for inflammation of urinary tract	contains lipophilic flavones, large amounts of potassium salts; may act as diuretic	*6 to 12 g herb or equivalent*	avoid with edema from CHF or renal disease; give with copious amounts of water
Jimsonweed leaf/seed	int: cough, bronchitis, pertussis, nervous system disorders such as Parkinson's	contains variable amounts of alkaloids such as scopolamine with anti-ACh effects similar to belladonna	*not recommended*	contraindicated in glaucoma, tachyarrhythmias, BPH/urinary retention, acute pulmonary edema, GI obstruction, atherosclerosis, megacolon; overdose similar to atropine; use not recommended due to non-standardization
Juniper berry	int: dyspepsia, diuretic	may increase urine output and stimulate smooth muscle contraction	*as directed*	chronic use may be nephrotoxic; avoid in pregnancy or nephritis
Kava Kava	int: anxiety, restlessness	may act as anxiolytic, antispasmodic, anticonvulsant	*60 to 120 mg kava pyrones or equivalent*	avoid in pregnancy, lactation, depression; may cause yellow skin, hair, or nails; may affect oculomotor function; may potentiate effects of alcohol, barbiturates, psychoactive drugs; may affect ability to drive or operate machinery; avoid use longer than 3 months
Kelp	int: regulation of thyroid function	contains various amounts of iodine	*no information*	allergic reactions may occur; may worsen hyperthyroidism, depending on iodine content
Knotweed	int: cough, bronchitis	contains tannins, silicic acid; may inhibit acetyl cholinesterase	*4 to 6 g of drug or equivalent*	none known
Lactobacillus acidophilus	int/ext: yeast and other sexual/GI infections, lactose intolerance, irritable bowel syndrome; found in yogurt, milk, and as supplement	helpful bacteria which produce lactase and lactic acid	*vaginitis: 1-2 billion live organisms; otherwise as directed*	mild GI upset in large doses; penicillins may deplete l. acidophilus; may affect sulfasalazine metabolism
Lady's Mantle	int: nonspecific diarrhea, anorexia, menstrual dysfunction	may act as astringent	*5 to 10 g of herb or equivalent*	rare hepatotoxicity
LaPacho	int: fungal and other infections	has antifungal, antiviral, and antibacterial properties as uncoupler of ox-phos; may have some antineoplastic effects	*as directed*	caution in children; avoid in pregnancy or if nursing; unrefined bark may be safest preparation; overdose may cause bleeding or vomiting
Larch Turpentine	ext: rheumatism, neurologic complaints, inflammation of respiratory tract	member of the Balsam family	*as directed*	topical administration may cause allergic reaction
Lavender flower	int: mood disturbances, anxiety, insomnia, abdominal complaints	may act as sedative, antiflatulent	*as directed*	may be used as bath therapy

BOTANICAL

WESTERN HERBS

BOTANICAL

Herbs	Uses	Information	Daily Dose	Cautions
Lecithin	int: hyperlipidemia	used by body to handle cholesterol and other fats; may help prevent atherosclerosis	no RDA, as directed	nicotinic acid (niacin) treatment for hyperlipidemia may deplete lecithin
Lemongrass	int: antipyretic, indigestion	limited scientific info; no proven effects	prepare infusion as directed	avoid inhalation of oil vapors, as may cause lung problems
Lesser Celandine	ext: bleeding wounds, swollen joints	contains tannins and large amounts of vitamin C	as bath or extract	extended contact to fresh plant may cause blisters; internal consumption may irritate GI and urinary tracts
Licorice root	int: inflammation of respiratory tract, peptic ulcers	contains coumarins, calcium, and potassium salts; may act as antitussive, anti-inflammatory agent; may have mineralocorticoid effects in high doses	5 to 15 g of root or equivalent	avoid in hypokalemia, pregnancy, heart disease, renal insufficiency, cirrhosis; hypokalemia with digitalis and diuretics may occur; do not use longer than 4-6 weeks without advice
Life root	int: uterine dysfunction, abortifacent, diuretic, urinary tract dysfunction	may contain toxic alkaloids		hepatotoxicity may occur; some experts do not recommend use of this drug
Lily of the Valley	int: mild CHF, chronic cor pulmonale	contains cardioactive glycosides, acting similar to digitalis	as directed	avoid with digitalis, hypokalemia; may cause nausea, vomiting, arrhythmias; may potentiate effects of quinidine, calcium, saluretics, laxatives, and glucocorticoids
Linden flower/wood	int: URIs, cough (flower), liver/gallbladder disorders (wood)	little scientific data; contains tannins, glycosides, and flavonoids, which show anti-edema and antimicrobial effects in animals	2 to 4 g of drug or equivalent	none known
Lobelia	int: asthma, emetic, smoking addiction (homeopathic doses)	stimulates respiratory center but quickly metabolized	homeopathic preparations only	not used in allopathic doses; signs of overdose: dry mouth, vomiting, anxiety, sweating
Lovage root	int: irrigation therapy for urinary tract	contains essential oil and coumarin derivatives	4 to 8 g of drug or equivalent	avoid if edema due to CHF or renal disease
Lungwort	int: bronchitis, cough, diuretic; ext: wounds	contains polysaccharides and tannins with expectorant and soothing effects; limited efficacy documented	prepare tea as directed	none known
Lycium	int: fever, HTN, improving hepatic and renal circulation	may have immunoregulatory and hypoglycemic effects, especially L. barbarum; limited scientific data	as directed	avoid in chronic inflammatory states; avoid during pregnancy/nursing
Lysine	essential amino acids, found in meat, cheese, soybeans, other foods; used in osteoporosis, cardiovascular disease, asthma, migraines	used in collagen production and fatty acid metabolism	no RDA: recommended (adults): 12 mg/kg	may in some cases increase cholesterol or triglycerides; otherwise nontoxic
Madder root	int: nephrolithiasis	contains inhibitor of calcium oxalate crystals in kidney; rubiadins are possibly carcinogenic	not recommended	lucidin is mutagenic; avoid this drug
Magnesium	found in green vegetables, fish, dairy products, nuts; used in constipation, Crohn's disease, HTN, stroke, preeclampsia, others	Important to normal bone structure and it plays an essential role in 300 fundamental cellular reactions	RDA (men): 350 mg, (women): 300 mg	avoid large doses while breastfeeding; toxicity includes GI and cardiovascular effects; avoid in kidney or heart disease; salt, sugar, caffeine, alcohol, fiber, riboflavin in high doses, insulin, diuretics, and digitalis may cause Mg loss; other ions such as Ca may interfere with Mg metabolism
Maidenhair	int: cough, bronchitis, menstrual disorders	may act as demulcent and expectorant	prepare tea as directed	avoid during pregnancy; no side effects known
Maitake	int: immune stimulant, HTN, diabetes	contains polysaccharide beta-D-glucan which may have immunostimulant properties	may be eaten or taken as tea	no information
Male Fern root/frond	int (root): liver fluke, band worms, viral infections; ext (herb): muscle pains, neuralgia, toothache, earache, wounds	strongly antihelminic properties, but very toxic	homeopathic preparations only	highly toxic--avoid internal consumption!
Mallow flower/leaf	int: pharyngitis associated with cough	may act as demulcent	5 g of drug or equivalent	none known
Manganese	mineral found in grains, nuts, beans, vegetables	needed for blood sugar control and in many other functions	no RDA; recommended (adults): 2.5 to 5.0 mg	overdose may include mood disorders; avoid in pregnancy/nursing; may affect blood clotting
Manna	int: stool softener	contains mannitol	adults: 20 to 30 g of drug or equivalent	avoid in bowel obstruction; occasional nausea, flatulence; avoid chronic use

Herbs	Uses	Information	Daily Dose	Cautions
Marjoram	int: URIs, mild abdominal pain	may have antimicrobial, antiviral, and insecticidal effects	prepare tea as directed	none known
Marshmallow leaf/root	int: pharyngitis and cough	anti-inflammatory properties; root may stimulate phagocytosis and inhibit mucociliary activity	5 g of leaf, 6 g of root or equivalent	may decrease absorption of other drugs
Maté	int: mental and physical fatigue	contains caffeine; may have diuretic, lipolytic, glycogenolytic, positive chronotropic and inotropic effects	3 g of drug or equivalent	syrup may contain sugar, so diabetics should avoid
Mayapple root/resin	ext: removal of pointed condyloma	resin contains podophyllotoxin	1.5 to 3 g root or equivalent	avoid in pregnancy; treated area must be smaller than 25 cm2; protect adjacent area
Meadowsweet	int: supportive therapy for URIs	contains flavonoids, glycosides, and salicylates	2.5 to 3.5 g flower or 4 to 5 g herb	avoid if ASA-allergic
Melatonin	int: insomnia, jet lag, seasonal affective disorder	naturally produced by pineal gland from trytophan; low melatonin seen in many cancer patients; long-term effects unknown	1 to 3 mg about 20 min before bedtime	contraindicated in autoimmune diseases, HIV, heart disease, leukemia; avoid if you are trying to conceive; take only at bedtime; avoid driving; caution in patients on NSAIDs, steroids, ß-blockers, benzodiazepines; may test blood levels
Milk Thistle fruit	int: alone for dyspepsia, in formulations for hepatitis/cirrhosis	contains silymarin, which may be hepatoprotective by altering hepatocyte cell membranes or protein synthesis	12 to 15 g or equivalent	none known; may have mild laxative effect; milk thistle herb is of doubtful benefit
Mint oil	int: flatulence, GI distress, liver/gallbladder complaints, URIs, fevers, pharyngitis; ext: myalgia, neuralgia	contains menthol, which cools skin; may increase bile production and have antibacterial properties	as directed	avoid internal use in biliary obstruction, cholecystitis, liver disease; avoid external use with children and on face; oil may exacerbate asthma; occasional GI upset as side effect
Molybdenum	trace mineral; found in vegetables, meats, other foods	deficiency can lead to tooth decay and anemia	no RDA: recommended (adults): 15 to 50 mcg; supplement by prescription	high doses can cause swollen joints; may decrease copper levels with supplementation
Monk's Hood	int: neuralgia, especially trigeminal; rheumatism; migraine; ext: skin inflammation	contains aconitin, which affects Na permeability in nerve ends; topically, has burning then anesthetizing effect	not recommended	highly toxic; signs of toxicity occur even with therapeutic doses; tingling of extremities is often first sign; may cause arrhythmias with overdose; drug is not recommended due to toxicity
Morning Glory	int: constipation, worm infections	contains resins with drastic laxative effects	0.5 to 3.0 g drug or equivalent	possibly teratogenic, so avoid during pregnancy; cramp-like pain is occasional side effect
Motherwort	int: used for cardiac disorders associated with anxiety, adjunct in hyperthyroidism	limited scientific data	4.5 g herb or equivalent	avoid with pregnancy; have uterine stimulating properties
Mountain Ash berry	int: kidney disease, diabetes, rheumatism, gout, diarrhea	contains vitamin C; little documented efficacy	puree for diarrhea - otherwise no information	popular ingredient in juices, jellies; cooking berries nearly eliminates incidence of GI side effect
Mugwort	int: GI infections, dyspepsia	may have antimicrobial effects; little documented efficacy	not recommended for internal consumption	avoid during pregnancy; used in Chinese technique of moxibustion, which is related to acupuncture
Muira Puama	ext: sexual disorders such as impotence; int: diarrhea, anorexia, sexual disorders	limited scientific data, no documented effect	0.5 g drug or equivalent	none known
Mullein flower	int: irritation of respiratory tract	contains saponins and mucopolysaccharides; may act as expectorant	3 to 4 g of herb or equivalent	none known
Myrrh	int: inflammation of respiratory tract, gingivitis, stomatitis	may act as antiseptic, astringent	as directed as resin - tincture - gargle	none known; used in commercial mouthwash, soaps, flavorings, cosmetics
Myrtle leaf/oil	int: bronchitis and other respiratory infections, diarrhea, cystitis, prostatitis	leaves show antimicrobial activity	infusion as directed	leaves contraindicated in chronic inflammatory states, liver disease, biliary stasis; avoid oil on face of children, as may trigger bronchial spasm; overdoses may be life-threatening
Nasturtium	int: UTIs, bronchitis, cough	contains benzyl mustard oil, which has antibacterial, antiviral, and antifungal effects	tablets or infusion: add 30 g leaves to 1 L H2O	contraindicated with peptic ulcers or renal disease; avoid in children; high or chronic doses can lead to mucous membrane or skin irritation
Niacin	water-soluble vitamin, used for tinnitus, PMS headaches, and in high doses for hyperlipidemia; found in meat, fish, poultry, other foods	important for DNA synthesis, many other functions	RDA (men): 16 to 18 mg; (women): 14 mg, 18 mg if breastfeeding	toxicity may include ulcers, GI symptoms, jaundice (only nicotinic acid form)

BOTANICAL

BOTANICAL

Herbs	Uses	Information	Daily Dose	Cautions
Niauli oil	ext./int: inflammation of respiratory tract, neuralgia, wounds, burns	contains cajeput oil; may act as antibacterial, circulatory stimulant; contains cineol, which may induce P450	as directed	rare GI distress with internal use; cajeput oil alone may cause life-threatening poisonings and should not be applied to faces of children; cajeput oil contraindicated in inflammation of GI tract, biliary tract, liver
Night-blooming Cereus	int: UTIs, angina, hemoptysis, menorrhagia	may have similar effect to digitalis	fluid extract up to 0.6 ml to 10 times daily	fresh juice may cause itching, rash, and vomiting; otherwise none known
Notoginseng root	int/ext: external bleeding, angina; ext: fractures, swelling, wounds	may have procoagulant properties	no information	occasional dry mouth, anxiety, insomnia, nausea; avoid during pregnancy, as may cause miscarriage
Nutmeg	int: indigestion, diarrhea/GI inflammation, liver disease	may decrease GI motility via effect on prostaglandins	as directed	avoid during pregnancy; may occasionally cause dermatitis; ingestion of "nuts" may produce amphetamine-like compounds; overdose may be signaled by red face, thirst, nausea, and occasional hallucinations
Nux Vomica	int: various GI complaints, anxiety/depression, migraine	contains strychnine and brucine, glycine antagonists	not recommended in allopathic doses	very toxic--do not use! similar to Ignatius beans
Oak bark	int: nonspecific diarrhea, anal/genital inflammation; ext: inflammation of skin	contains tannins; may have virustatic effects	as directed	ext: may cause skin damage in some cases; avoid baths with eczema, heart disease; may inhibit alkaloid-type drugs; use not recommended for more than 2-3 weeks
Oat straw/ herb/fruit	ext: inflammatory and itchy skin disease, warts (straw), hyperlipidemia (fruit)	fruit may have anti-lipid polysaccharides; limited data about herb and straw	straw: bath as directed; others as directed	none known
Oleander leaf	int: heart failure	similar to digitalis, with positive inotropic, negatively chronotropic effects	no information - not recommended	consumption has led to fatal poisonings; no longer used for nausea, vomiting, diarrhea, arrhythmias; avoid in pregnancy; may increase effects of quinidine, calcium salts, laxatives, diuretics, steroids; poisoning similar to digitalis
Olive leaf/oil	ext: (oil): psoriasis, eczema, sunburns, burns; int (oil): cholangitis, cholecystitis, atherosclerosis; (leaf) constipation	leaf may possess antiarrhythmic, spasmolytic, hypotensive effects; oil contains polyunsaturated, monounsaturated fatty acids	various preparations	contraindicated in gallstones
Omega-6 Fatty Acids	eye disease, heart disease, cancer; found in vegetable oils, oils of evening primrose, black currant, borage	gamma-linoleic acid may be important anti-inflammatory agent	no RDA, often 1.4 g GLA for rheumatoid arthritis	none known
Onion	int: anorexia, prevention of atherosclerosis	contains allein and similar sulfur compounds, essential oil, peptides, and flavonoids; may show anti-platelet, antibacterial effects	50 g of fresh onions or equivalent	none known
Oregano	int: cough, bronchitis	essential oil has antimicrobial properties; contains thymol (in commercial anti-cold medications)	various preparations: infusions, gargles, powders	none known
Orris root	int: cough, bronchitis	mild expectorant, may have antiulcer properties	used primarily in homeopathic doses	none known; juice of fresh plant may irritate skin and, if ingested, GI tract; avoid during pregnancy
Pancreatic enzymes	int: digestive disorders, autoimmune diseases, inflammatory diseases; ext: trauma	may affect fibrinolysis, complement cascade	as directed	contraindicated in coagulopathies, liver disease; may cause GI side effects, pale stools, allergic reactions, skin irritation with external application; no pregnancy studies
Papaya leaf	int: pancreatic enzyme deficiency, inflammation/ infection of GI tract; ext: skin ulcers (papain)	contains papain, used for healing of severe wounds and ulcers, as it dissolves dead tissue; may also have fibrinolytic effect	ointments with papain by prescription	avoid during pregnancy (teratogenic); documented interactions with warfarin, prolonging PT; allergic reaction known
Parsley herb/ root/seed	int: inflammation of urinary tract, urinary tract stones	may act as diuretic; seed may increase uterine tone	herb/root: 6 g of prepared drug or equivalent	avoid in pregnancy, nephritis; may cause photodermatitis; take copious amounts of fluid; essential oil may be toxic
Parsnip herb/root	int (herb): kidney, GI complaints, (root): kidney stones, fever	limited scientific data	one handful/one liter H2O of tea as directed	can increase photosensitivity in fair-skinned patients
Pasque flower	int: fever, GI inflammation, genital disorders, skin inflammation	may have antimicrobial, antipyretic, and GI spasmolytic effects	use only with caution	contraindicated during pregnancy; fresh plant may cause ulcers if contacts skin or GI distress if ingested; animals have died after large ingestion of similar plants

Herbs	Uses	Information	Daily Dose	Cautions
Passion Flower	int: anxiety, headaches, epilepsy, neuralgia, GI complaints associated with anxiety	may have both sedative and stimulant effects	4 to 8 g of herb or equivalent	none known
Pennyroyal	int: dyspepsia, liver/gallbladder complaints; ext: skin inflammation	hepatotoxic effects preclude use	external use only	contraindicated during pregnancy; use oil externally only
Peony flower/root	int: hemorrhoids, rheumatism	flower isolates may promote uterine contraction, GI relaxation, and hypotension	infusion as directed	overdoses may cause vomiting, abdominal pain; no efficacy demonstrated
Peppermint leaf	int: spasms of GI tract and gallbladder	may have direct antispasmodic effects on GI smooth muscle; may increase bile production	3 to 6 g of leaf or equivalent	avoid with gallstones or in small children due to possible choking sensation from menthol
Peppermint oil	int: spasms of GI tract and gallbladder, oral mucositis; ext: myalgia, neuralgia	may have similar actions to peppermint leaf; may have antimicrobial actions	6 to 12 drops or equivalent	avoid use on face of children: avoid in biliary obstruction- liver disease- gallstones
Perilla	int: cough, URIs, constipation, oral inflammation	may have antimicrobial and sedative effects; may lower serum lipids; little scientific data	extract 3 to 10 g or equivalent	avoid in pregnancy due to potential mutagenicity; one study showed pulmonary edema in sheep
Periwinkle	int: circulatory dysfunction (especially cerebral), hemorrhage; ext: skin inflammation	contains vincamine, which lowers BP and HR, also spasmolytic and hypoglycemic effects	infusion or tea as directed	flushing and GI symptoms may occur; overdose may cause severe hypotension
Peruvian Balsam	ext: hemorrhoids, wound healing, ulcers, burns	may have antiparasitic actions, especially for scabies; may promote granulation process	as directed	allergic skin reactions well known; use for more than one week not recommended
Petasites root/leaf	int: supportive therapy for pain associated with urinary stones	may have antispasmodic actions; may inhibit leukotrienes; pyrrolizidine alkaloids may be carcinogenic, hepatotoxic, and teratogenic; must check alkaloid content	4.5 to 7 g drug or equivalent	avoid with pregnancy or nursing; use for more than 4-6 weeks not recommended; check pyrrolizidine alkaloid content before using
Pheasant's Eye herb	int: mild cardiac insufficiency, especially with anxiety	contains cardioactive glycosides and flavonoids; may be positively inotropic	0.6 g of standardized powder	avoid with digitalis, hypokalemia; may cause nausea, vomiting, arrhythmias; may potentiate effects of quinidine, calcium, laxatives, and glucocorticoids
Phenylalanine	essential amino acid, as body cannot make enough; found in cheese, meat, eggs, fish, yeast, aspartame	converted by body to tyrosine	no RDA: recommended (adults): 14 mg/kg	may cause anxiety, headaches, HTN; contraindicated in PKU, pregnancy, breastfeeding; may compete with L-dopa; little pregnancy data about aspartame
Phosphatidyl-serine	phospholipid in brain, used for Alzheimer's disease and depression in elderly	critical layer in neurotransmitter release; semisynthetic prepared from soy; limited scientific data	100 mg tid commonly used	none known; pregnancy data unknown
Phosphorus	mineral found throughout body; found in meat, fish, milk; used for kidney stones as K-phos	innumerable functions in body, especially as ATP, and in tissue repair	RDA (adults): 800 mg, 1200 mg if pregnant/nursing	hyperphosphatemia
Phyllanthus	int: diabetes, gonorrhea, menstrual dysfunction, hepatitis B	may block enzyme crucial for hep B replication	trials have used 900 to 2700 mg	no information; used extensively in Indian medicine
Pimpinella root/herb	int: cough, bronchitis	contains essential oil and saponins	6 to 12 g root or equivalent	none known
Pine oil/sprouts	int/ext: inflammation of respiratory tract; ext: rheumatic complaints	may decrease secretions	as directed, oil may be applied or inhaled	avoid in asthma, pertussis; skin and membrane irritation may occur
Plantain	int: inflammation of oral mucosa; ext: skin inflammation	may have astringent and antibacterial properties	3 to 6 g of herb or equivalent	none known; in 1997 FDA warned some products actually contained digitalis
Poke root/fruit	int: rheumatism, skin ulcers, pharyngitis, dyspepsia	fruit may have hepatoprotective, antiviral, and emetic effects; root may have anti-edema and immunostimulant effects; saponins and lectins are toxic	use with caution	symptoms of poisoning include diarrhea, hypotension, and vomiting; children particularly susceptible
Pollen	int: lethargy, anorexia	limited scientific data	30 to 40 g of drug or equivalent	avoid in pollen-allergic patients; rare GI side effects
Pomegranate	int: URIs, diarrhea, worm infections	contains alkaloids which are antihelminic	as directed	avoid in pregnancy; overdose may cause vomiting, dizziness, respiratory compromise
Poplar bud	ext: superficial skin inflammation, frostbite, sunburn	contains essential oil, flavonoids, and phenol glycosides; may promote wound healing with some antibacterial properties	as directed	occasional skin reactions

BOTANICAL

Herbs	Uses	Information	Daily Dose	Cautions
Poppyseed	int: cough, pain	contains morphine, codeine, papaverine	as directed	opium no longer used as medication; contraindicated in pregnancy, reduced respiratory function, elevated ICP, biliary colic; caution with Addison's disease and hypothyroidism; overdose may include respiratory failure, vomiting, edema, spasms
Potentilla	int: dysmenorrhea, nonspecific diarrhea	may increase uterine tone	4 to 6 g of herb or equivalent	may irritate GI tract
Primrose flower/root	int: bronchitis, cough	may act as secretolytic, expectorant	flower: 2 to 4 g of drug or equivalent; root: 0.5 to 1.5 g of drug	occasional GI upset; allergies to primrose documented
Psyllium seed/husk-black/blonde	int: chronic constipation, IBS, also secondarily for diarrhea associated with irritable bowel	FDA-approved as laxative; may promote peristalsis, may increase volume of stool	as directed	avoid in stenosis/obstruction of esophagus or GI tract; rare allergic reactions; blonde psyllium may create difficulty with diabetes management and may decrease absorption of other drugs; must take adequate amounts of fluids; may lower serum cholesterol
Pumpkin seed	int: irritated bladder, urinary dysfunction with mild BPH	contain scucurbitin, phytosterol in free and bound forms, s- and gamma-tocopherol, selenium	10 g of seed or equivalent	may relieve symptoms of BPH without treating BPH itself
Pygeum	int: BPH, male impotence	contains three types of compounds that may act against BPH by inhibition of prostaglandins, prolactin; less effective than saw palmetto when compared in one study	extract: 50 to 100 mg bid	may cause GI irritation; must allow 6-9 months for drug to work
Pyrethrum	ext: infections with scabies, lice, other insects	may have neurotoxic effects on lower insects	liquid extract as directed	none known; overdose may cause neurotoxicity; wash area after use
Pyruvate (with dihydroxy-acetone)	int: weight loss, endurance exercise-enhancer	product of glucose in glycolysis; may increase fat loss in addition to exercise in obese populations; limited data	no information	no information
Radish	int: dyspepsia, especially associated with biliary tract	contains mustard oil glycosides and essential oil; may act as secretagogue, promote GI motility	50 to 100 ml pressed juice or equivalent	avoid with gallstones
Raspberry leaf	int: menorrhagia, uterine stimulant, menstrual cramps, laxative	contains tannins that have astringent properties	use with caution, as directed	no information--use at own risk
Red Clover	ext: eczema, acne; int: bronchitis, cough	may have antispasmodic and expectorant effects; aids in skin healing	4 g drug or equivalent	none known; avoid fermented herb
Red Sandalwood	int: dyspepsia, diabetes, cough, toothache	extracts have hypoglycemic effects in animals; limited scientific info	primarily as tea	none known
Red Yeast Rice	int: high cholesterol	natural component, mevinolin, inhibits HMG-CoA reductase	1200 mg or equivalent	may be hepatotoxic in high doses; contraindicated in pregnancy or nursing; avoid during infections, post-surgery; rhabdomyolysis possible
Red-Rooted Sage	int: angina, menstrual dysfunction, furuncles, joint pain	increase in coronary blood flow noted; may also have antithrombotic, anti-inflammatory, and hepatoprotective effects; limited scientific info	9 to 15 mg drug or equivalent	none known
Reishi	int: asthma, cough, insomnia, HTN, hyperlipidemia, immunomodulator	may have sedative effect on CNS, may lower cholesterol; may enhance immune function via production of IL-2	dried mushroom: 1.5 to 9 g or equivalent;: syrup: 4 to 6 ml	caution with anticoagulants, as may heighten effects; avoid while pregnant or nursing
Rhatany root	int/ext: mild inflammation of pharyngeal/oral mucosa	may act as astringent; contains tannins	as directed	very rare allergic reactions; use greater than 2 weeks not recommended
Rhododendron-Rusty-leaved	int: rheumatism, gout, HTN, migraine, neuralgia	limited scientific data	not recommended	not recommended; overdose may cause arrhythmias, cold sweats, stupor, and death
Rhubarb root-	int: constipation	1-8-dihydroxy-anthracene derivatives have a laxative effect via increasing GI motility, increased Cl- secretion	as directed	may cause GI discomfort or hypokalemia, so caution with steroids, diuretics, glycosides; avoid during pregnancy and nursing; use only if diet/lifestyle not effective; avoid chronic use
Rose Flower	int: mild inflammation of oral, pharyngeal mucosa	contains tannins; may act as astringent	1 to 2 g drug/cup H2O for tea	none known

Herbs	Uses	Information	Daily Dose	Cautions
Rose Hip fruit/shell	Int: (fruit): immunostimulator; (shells): UTIs, kidney disease, gout	fruit contains pectin and acids which have diuretic and laxative effects; shells are source of vitamin C	*shell: prepared tea from powder as directed; fruit: found in vitamin supplements*	none known
Rosemary leaf	int: dyspepsia; ext: rheumatic complaints, circulatory dysfunction	may stimulate blood supply via irritation; may decrease spasms of biliary system; may be positively inotropic, may increase coronary perfusion	*as directed*	none known
Rue	int: PMS, menstrual disorders; ext: skin inflammation	may have fertility-inhibiting, spasmolytic effects	*tea or external application as directed*	generally avoid, due to toxicity which may include photosensitivity, abortion, GI complaints, renal failure, and death
Rupturewort	int: UTIs, respiratory inflammation, gout, rheumatism	limited data suggest possible diuretic and spasmolytic effects	*infusion or tea as directed*	none known
Sage leaf	int: dyspepsia, excessive sweating; ext: inflammations of membranes of nose-throat	contains thujone- cineol- and camphor: may inhibit viruses-fungi- and bacteria: may inhibit perspiration	*as directed*	essential oil and alcoholic extracts should not be used internally during pregnancy; some experts question if internal use is safe at all
Sandalwood	int: supportive therapy for UTI, URI, bronchitis	may be antibacterial and antispasmodic	*1 to 1.5 g essential oil or equivalent*	avoid in renal disease: may cause nausea or urticaria: use enteric-coated form: use for more than 6 weeks not recommended
Sanicle	int: inflammation of respiratory tract	contains saponins	*4 to 6 g of drug or equivalent*	none known
Sarsaparilla root	int: anabolic steroid, constipation, rheumatic complaints, URI, psoriasis	some evidence to support diuretic, expectorant, laxative effects: no evidence of steroid activity	*as directed*	none known
Savin Tops	ext: warts	very irritating to internal and external membranes; lignans and podophyllotoxins may have antiviral properties	*powder or ointment as directed*	avoid internal administration - may cause death; volatile oil may cause severe skin inflammation: avoid even external application during pregnancy
Saw Palmetto berry	int: urinary dysfunction in BPH stages I-II	may have antiandrogenic and anti-inflammatory effects: banned as drug in U.S. by FDA: first choice for mild BPH in some parts of Europe	*1 to 2 g berry or equivalent (tea ineffective)*	rare GI upset
Schisandra	int: liver disease, GI inflammation, insomnia, night sweats, fatigue	contains lignans which promote regeneration of hepatocytes: may also have antitumor and energy-boosting effects	*dried berries: 1 to 6 g or equivalent*	none known
Scopolia root	int: spasms of GI and urinary tracts	contains alkaloids similar in effect to scopolamine: acts as anti-ACh- with decreased spasms and tremors: caution in children	*as directed*	avoid with glaucoma, prostate adenoma, tachycardia, GI obstruction, megacolon: may cause dryness of mouth, decreased sweating, red skin, ocular dysfunction, hyperthermia-tachycardia, difficulties in urination, attacks of glaucoma: may potentiate tricycli
Scotch Broom herb	int: nonspecific cardiac and circulatory dysfunction	contains alkaloids; primarily sparteine	*1 to 1.5 g of drug or equivalent*	contains tryamine, so avoid with MAO-inhibitors
Scullcap	int: anxiety, insomnia	may have sedative effects: limited scientific data	*1 to 2 g dried herb or equivalent*	none known
Selenium	int: general health promoter; found in green vegetables, meat, eggs, milk	works with vitamin E as antioxidant: current trials as prostate cancer preventative	*no RDA: 70 mcg recommended for men; 55 mcg for women*	toxicity in very high doses can affect hair, nails, teeth
Seneca Snakeroot	int: respiratory tract irritation, decongestant	contain saponins: may act as expectorant, secretolytic	*1.5 to 3 g root or equivalent*	may cause GI upset
Senna leaf/pod	int: constipation	FDA-approved as laxative: 1-8-dihydroxy-anthracene derivatives have a laxative effect by stimulating GI motility	*titrate to soft stool*	avoid in chronic intestinal inflammation or obstruction: may cause cramping, hypokalemia with chronic use: avoid long-term use, no data on pregnancy or nursing
Shark/bovine cartilage	int: cancer, arthritis, SLE, others	Studies presently investigating utility in cancer: may have anti-angiogenic actions: turns out sharks really do get cancer!	*as directed*	long-term side effects or interactions unknown: certainly avoid in pregnant women or those with serious heart disease
Shepherd's Purse	int: mild menorrhagia and metrorrhagia, epistaxis; ext: superficial bleeding	may increase uterine tone: may have positive inotropic and chronotropic effects	*int: 10 to 15 g of drug or equivalents: ext: as directed*	none known
Shiitake	int: cancer, HIV and other infections	may stimulate T-cells; increase production of TNF	*soup, lentinan extract, or tincture as directed*	may cause GI complaints at high dosages

BOTANICAL

WESTERN HERBS

BOTANICAL

Herbs	Uses	Information	Daily Dose	Cautions
Slippery Elm	int: inflammation of respiratory tract	may act as anti-inflammatory: declared safe and effective demulcent by FDA	as directed	no information: found in some commercial throat lozenges
Soapwort root-red/white	int: upper respiratory tract inflammation	may act as expectorant by irritating gastric mucosa	red: 1.5 g root or equivalent white: 30 to 150 mg drug or equivalent	rare GI irritation
Solomon's seal	int: constipation, hyperlipidemia, atherosclerosis	may decrease absorption of dietary cholesterol: steroid saponins may have anti-inflammatory actions	tablets as directed	GI irritation in high doses; otherwise none known
Soy isoflavones	int: cancer prevention/treatment especially gynecologic, breast, prostate: osteoporosis, cardiovascular disease	have wide range of effects on cell regulation: may have estrogenic partial agonist activity: may be anti-platelet and angiogenesis inhibitors: genistein has been conjugated with antibodies in clinical trials	diet much preferred, no dosing information for supplements	little information: estrogenic effects possible but unlikely: may have thyrotoxic, mutagenic, and even carcinogenic effects if large amounts of supplements taken: no data on pregnancy/nursing
Soy Lecithin/phosphor-lipids	int: hyperlipidemia, chronic hepatitis or nutritional liver disease (e.g. TPN)	linolenic acid most predominant fatty acid: phospholipid may be hepatoprotective via membrane stabilization	equivalent of 3.5 g (3-sn-phosphatidyl choline)	occasional GI upset: use when dietary/lifestyle measures insufficient
Spearmint	int: dyspepsia, flatulence	may have antispasmodic, mild sedative effects	oil or concentrate as directed	rare allergic reactions: used as flavoring agent for commercial products
Speedwell	int: dyspepsia, UTIs, GI inflammation; ext: skin inflammation	may have protective effect against ulcers- both internal and external	prepare tea as directed	none known
Spinach leaf	int: indigestion, anorexia, anemia, sluggish growth in children	contains vitamin C, oxalic acid, nitrates, and Fe	no information	high nitrate content; so do not eat frequently or give to infants
Spiny Restharrow root	int: wash-out therapy for inflammation or urinary tract	may act as diuretic: contains isoflavonoids	6 to 12 g of drug or equivalent	avoid if edema due to CHF or renal disease: drink large amounts of fluids
Spirulina	type of blue-green algae: used for HIV, cancer, skin diseases, candida, hypoglycemia	contains protein and vitamin A: effectiveness unproven: may have antiviral effect	as directed - often 500 mg qid	no information
Spruce shoots/oil	int: inflammation of respiratory tract; ext: neuralgia, rheumatic pain	Secretolytic, hyperemic	as directed	may exacerbate asthma - pertussis: avoid if acute skin infections - cardiac disease
Squill	int: mild cardiac insufficiency, renal insufficiency	contains glycosides of the bufadienolide type	0.1 to 0.5 g of standardized sea onion or equivalent	may cause diarrhea, vomiting, hypokalemia: arrhythmias: caution with steroids, diuretics, digitalis, quinine-like drugs, antiarrhythmic
St. John's Wort	int: depression, anxiety; ext: mild burns, myalgias, bruises	may have some mild antidepressant effect, although MAO-inhibitor like activity seems doubtful: may have some antiviral activity	2 to 4 g of drug or equivalent	may cause photosensitization in light-skinned patients: dermatitis has been reported: avoid with anti-HIV medications, cyclosporin: must take 4-6 weeks for depression
Star Anise seed	int: respiratory tract inflammation with cough, dyspepsia	may act as expectorant-antispasmodic of GI tract	3 g of drug or equivalent	none known: japanese star anise, a different herb, is poisonous
Stinging Nettle herb/leaf/root	int/ext: BPH (root), irrigation for lower urinary tract and prevention of nephrolithiasis (herb/leaf); ext: rheumatic complaints	contains calcium, potassium salts, and silicic acid: may increase urinary flow	as directed	avoid in heart or renal disease: take copious amounts of water: root may help urinary symptoms with BPH but does not treat BPH itself
Strawberry leaf	int: indigestion, diarrhea, gout, rheumatoid arthritis, urinary stones; ext: rashes	may have astringent and diuretic actions	prepare infusion or extract as directed	allergic reactions possible
Sulfur	mineral, used for skin complaints, arthritis, digestive disorders	found in many amino acids	bath used for arthritis: tablets as directed	none known, with exception of sulfa allergies: no pregnancy info
Sundew	int: cough, bronchitis	may have antispasmodic-antitussive actions	3 g of herb or equivalent	none known
Sweet Clover	int: venous insufficiency, thrombophlebitis, swelling; ext: contusions	contains coumarin and glycosides may increase wound healing	3 to 30 mg coumarin or equivalent	headaches and mild increase in LFTs are rare: to be safe, avoid during pregnancy
Sweet Violet herb/flower	int: cough, bronchitis, asthma, migraine	contains saponins, which have expectorant and secretolytic effects	use leaf or flower for tea as directed	none known
Sweet Woodruff	int: UTIs, insomnia, anxiety, edema	contains tiny amounts of coumarin: limited scientific data	prepare tea as directed	chronic use may cause reversible liver toxicity
Tangerine Peel	int: dyspepsia, nausea, diarrhea	limited scientific data	no information	none known

Herbs	Uses	Information	Daily Dose	Cautions
Tansy flower/ oil	int: (flower): GI infections, migraine neuralgia; (oil): PMS, intestinal worms	oil is antimicrobial, antihelminic, and repels insects: contains varying amounts of thujone, which is toxic	not recommended	avoid in allopathic doses, as may lead to spasms, arrhythmias, bleeding, and renal failure
Taurine	nonessential amino acid, as supplement for seizures, OCD, anxiety, angina, primary pulmonary HTN	important for muscle and CNS function: may be necessary for heart function	no RDA: some use 500 mg bid	occasional GI side effects reported
Tea tree leaf/oil	int: pharyngitis, colitis, sinusitis; ext: disinfectant, skin infections, acne	contains terpenes which have antibacterial and possibly antiviral actions	primarily externally in skin ointments	none known: overdose may lead to confusion if taken internally
Thuja oil/ branches	int: respiratory infections, cold sores, rheumatism, neuralgia, UTIs, conjunctivitis, other complaints	some preparations contain thujone, which is toxic: antiviral effects due to proliferation of T-cells, especially CD-4 cells	follow doses carefully due to thujone content	drug is misused as abortifacent, so avoid if pregnant: avoid essential oil: allopathic preparations do not contain thujone
Thyme- wild/ domestic	int: bronchitis, cough, pertussis	may have antibacterial and expectorant activity: contains thymol	domestic: 1 to 2 g of herb /cup of tea or equivalent: wild: 6 g of herb or equivalent	none known: found in commercial vapor, rubs and mouthwashes
Tree of Heaven bark	int: malaria, dysmenorrhea, cramps, asthma	trial vs. malaria presently ongoing limited scientific info	6 to 9 g drug	large doses may cause GI upset, headache, tingling
Turmeric root (Javanese/ regular)	int: dyspepsia	contains curcumin, which may increase bile flow: may have anti-inflammatory actions	1.5 to 3 g of drug or equivalent	occasional GI upset: avoid with gallstones, biliary obstruction
Turpentne oil- purified	ext/int: chronic bronchitis, cough: ext: rheumatic complaints, myalgias	may act as mucolytic, antiseptic	several drops in hot water to be inhaled or rubbed on skin	topic application to large areas may cause nephrotoxicity or neurotoxicity
Usnea	int: sore throat	may have antimicrobial effect	take in lozenge form	none known
Uva Ursi leaf	int: inflammation of urinary tract	may have antibacterial effect, especially against E. coli, Proteus, enterococcus, strep, and staph: contains arbutin, which is converted to hydroquinone	as directed	avoid in pregnancy, lactation, children: nausea and vomiting may occur: avoid using for more than one week: may decrease effectiveness of L-dopa: requires alkaline urine to function: may turn urine green (harmless)
Uzara	int: nonspecific diarrhea	contains glycosides: may inhibit intestinal motility: may cause digitalis,like effects in high doses	as directed	avoid with digitalis or other glycosides
Valerian root	int: restlessness, anxiety, insomnia, GI complaints	may act as sedative: generally viewed as effective	as directed	none known
Vanadium	trace mineral: no documented uses: found in vegetable oils, vegetables, meat	may affect blood sugar and cholesterol in animals, but scientific info lacking: Needed for bones and teeth	no RDA: supplementation rarely necessary	toxicity may include depression, liver/kidney disease: avoid taking with chromium: vitamin C may decrease levels
Vervain	int: cough, bronchitis, sore throat; ext: edema, bruising, arthritis	contains iridoid glycosides, which act as astringent: limited scientific info	prepare extract or infusion as directed	none known
Walnut leaf/ hull	ext: mild skin inflammation, excessive sweating	has astringent and fungistatic properties	2 to 3 g herb per 100 ml water or equivalent	topical use of hulls has been linked to leukoplakia and cancer of oral region
Watercress	int: inflammation of respiratory tract	contains glycosides and mustard oil	4 to 6 g dried herb or equivalent	avoid in peptic ulcer disease, nephrolithiasis, in young children: rarely causes GI distress
Whey protein	int: protein source of choice for anaerobic exercise	contains albumin, lactoglobulin, and immunoglobulins: Substrate for glutathione, which is depleted in exercise	as directed, usually post-exercise	allergic reactions possible: contains lactose: contains bovine albumin (BSA) which may be linked to IDDM (link unclear)
White bryony	int: laxative, emetic, diuretic	contains cucurbitanes which have strong toxic and cytotoxic effects	not recommended	high toxicity, not recommended: toxicity decreases with storage: avoid skin contact
White Mustard seed	ext: URIs, bronchitis, rheumatism	contains mustard oil glycosides and mustard oils: may be bacteriostatic	poultice prepared as directed	chronic use may cause nerve and skin damage
White Nettle herb/flower	ext/int: inflammation of mucous membranes, respiratory tract	contains tannin, mucilage and saponins	3 g of drug or equivalent or sitz bath	none known
White Willow bark	int: fever, rheumatic complaints, headaches	contains salicylate-like compounds: may have antipyretic, analgesic properties	dose corresponding to 60 to 120 mg total salicin	may cause ASA-like effects, although few if any reported
Wild Cherry	int: bronchitis, cough, indigestion	acts as astringent, antitussive, sedative: contains small amounts of cyanogenic glycosides	syrup or tincture as directed	risk of cyanide-like poisoning small

BOTANICAL

WESTERN HERBS

Herbs	Uses	Information	Daily Dose	Cautions
Wild Yam root	int: hyperlipidemia, GI inflammation, dysmenorrhea, rheumatism	contains diosgenin, which may increase cholesterol excretion: may also have estrogenic effect on mammary cells, but no progesterone effects	*capsules: 200 to 400 mg; 505 to 535 mg usually 1 pill tid or as directed*	may decrease anti-inflammatory effect of NSAIDs such as indomethacin; caution with other estrogen-like drugs
Wintergreen	int: GI irritation, bloating; ext: rheumatism, myalgias, inflammation, neuralgia	limited scientific data	*as directed*	has been largely replaced by synthetic version, methyl salicylate, found in many commercial products; avoid oral intake of essential oil, which may be fatal
Witch Hazel leaf/bark	ext: minor wounds, skin inflammation, hemorrhoids, varicose veins	FDA-approved as astringent: contains tannins and other constituents: may have anti-inflammatory- hemostatic properties	*as directed*	none known
Woody Nightshade stem	internal/ext: as supportive therapy for chronic eczema, acne, warts, furuncles	contains tannins, steroid alkaloids and steroid saponins may have anti-Ach, antimicrobial, cortisone-like effects	*int: 1 to 3 g of drug or equivalent; ext: as directed*	contraindicated in pregnancy and nursing: avoid unripe berries with children
Wormwood	int: anorexia, biliary dysfunction	approved for food use with thujone-free products	*2 to 3 g of herb as water infusion or equivalent*	none known: avoid essential oil alone as may be poisonous
Yarrow	int: dyspepsia, GI discomfort; ext: female pelvic cramps	may have antibacterial, bile-producing properties	*4.5 g herb or equivalent or as sitz bath*	allergic reactions known
Yeast-Brewer's	int: anorexia, acne and skin infections: related type S. boulardii (Hansen CBS 5926) may be used for diarrhea	contains vitamins, particularly B complex, glucans and mannans: may be antibacterial via phagocytosis stimulation	*6 g or equivalent*	occasionally migraine-type headaches, flatulence, or itching: avoid with MAO-inhibitors
Yellow Dock root	int: constipation, liver/ gallbladder dysfunction	may have mild laxative effects	*capsules 500 mg as directed*	avoid eating large amounts of leaves: fresh root may cause GI upset
Yohimbe	int: sexual dysfunction, primarily non-organic: xerostomia	contains Yohimbe, which is a selective alpha-2-adrenergic antagonist: increases salivary flow, epinephrine/NE	*as directed (smaller doses for xerostomia)*	contraindicated in liver and kidney disease: may exacerbate anxiety or HTN: avoid with ethanol, naltrexone, morphine; generally less safe than sildenafil: overdoses have been fatal
Yucca root	ext: arthritis, sprains, inflammation	FDA-approved food additive: in-vitro studies showed hemolysis after addition of one of yucca's components, but never seen in vitro	*as directed*	may cause loose stools
Zedoary	int: anorexia, liver/gallbladder dysfunction	may increase bile flow and have a spasmolytic effect: Fungicial and antitumor effects also shown	*prepare tea as directed*	avoid chronic use
Zinc	mineral, needed for enzymes, insulin function, wound healing, found in meat, milk, soybeans: supplement may help with URIs (gluconate or acetate may be best)	data on URIs mixed	*RDA (adults): 15 mg to 25 mg if breast feeding*	GI toxicity or lack of coordination rare

Source: *Natural Medicines Comprehensive Database,* 4th Edition, Therapeutic Research Faculty, 2002. *The Complete Guide to Herbal Medicines,* Charles Fetrow, Juan Avila, Simon & Schuster, 2000.

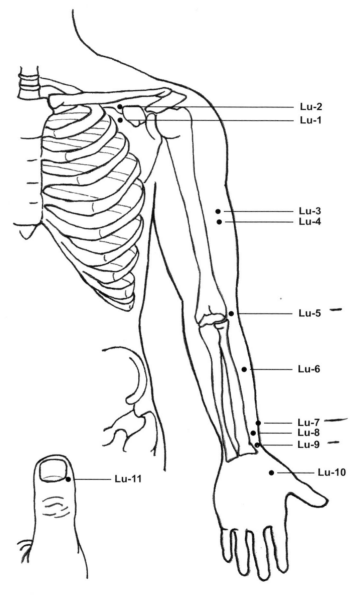

Lu-2
Lu-1

Lu-3
Lu-4

Lu-5

Lu-6

Lu-7
Lu-8
Lu-9

Lu-10

Lu-11

POINTS

Jing Well	Ying Spring	Shu Stream	Jing River	He Sea
11	10	9	8	5
Yuan	Luo-connect	Xi-Cleft	Front Mu	Back Shu
9	7	6	Lu-1	Ub-13

POINTS

Points	Location	Usage	Indications / Functions
Lu-1 **Zhongfu** *Central Residence* ↘ 0.5 – 0.8 cun towards lateral aspect of chest	6 cun lateral to the anterior midline, on the line lateral and superior to the sternum at the level of the 1st intercostal space.	Dry cough; cough with fullness in chest; asthma, lung heat; pulmonary TB (severe yin deficiency); coughing and wheezing with blood	• **Disperses fullness of the Lung**: used for late stage exterior patterns when the pathogen has penetrated into the interior such as retention of phlegm in the Lungs. • **Stops cough**: used for acute and chronic cough. • Treatment of chest pain due to stagnation of Heart blood or retention of phlegm in the chest. • Treats shoulder pain due to Lung channel dysfunction with lung-heat, damp-phlegm, or phlegm-heat obstructing the Lungs. • **Tonifies Lung and Spleen.**
Lu-2 **Yunmen** *Cloud Door* ↘ 0.5 – 0.8 towards lateral aspect of chest	In the depression below the acromial extremity of the clavicle, 6 cun lateral to the anterior midline.	Cough; asthma; pain in the chest; shoulder and arm; fullness in the chest	• **Clears Heat in the Lungs, Descends Lung Qi:** used to treat painful obstruction syndrome of the shoulder.
Lu-3 **Tianfu** *Heavenly Residence* ↓ 0.5 – 1.0	The point is on the medial aspect of the upper arm, 3 cun below the end of the axillary fold, on the radial side of the muscle biceps brachii.	Pain in the medial aspect of upper arm; asthma; epistaxis	• Clears Heat in the Lungs, Descends Lung Qi. • Cools the Blood, Stops bleeding.
Lu-4 **Xiabai** *Clasping the White* ↓ 0.5 – 1.0	On the medial aspect of the upper arm, 4 cun below the end of the axillary fold, on the radial side of the muscle biceps brachii.	Pain in the medial aspect of upper arm; cough; fullness in the chest	• Descends Lung Qi, Regulates Qi and Blood in the chest.
Lu-5 **Chize** *Foot Marsh* ↓ 0.5 – 1.0	On the cubital crease, on the radial side of tendon of m. biceps brachii. This point is located with the elbow slightly flexed.	Yellow phlegm maybe white and viscous; URI gone deeper; productive cough; asthma; bronchitis; pleurisy; pain in throat with cough; good for excess LU heat	• **Clears Heat in the Lungs**: for excess patterns characterized by heat in the Lungs with cough, fever, yellow sputum and thirst, and qi level patterns. It is also used in chronic conditions with phlegm and heat in the Lungs, bronchitis. • **Clears Lung and Nourishes Yin**: for injury to body fluids following febrile diseases. • **For excess-cold with retention of cold phlegm**: for Lung symptoms and cough with profuse white-sticky sputum and chilliness. • **Opens the water passages and facilitates urination**: for retention of urine caused by obstruction of the Lungs by descending and opening the water passages in the lower burner. • **Relaxes the tendons in the arm along the Lung channel**: used for painful obstruction syndrome.
Lu-6 **Kongzui** *Maximum Opening* ↓ 0.5 – 1.0 xi-cleft	The point is on the palmar aspect of the forearm, on the line joining Lu-9 and Lu-5, 7 cun above the transverse crease of the wrist.	Dry cough; dryness in lungs; good elbow and biceps point	• For acute, excess patterns of the lung including asthma. • Stops bleeding due to its action as an accumulation point.

Points	Location	Usage	Indications / Functions
Lu-7 **Lieque** *Broken Sequence* ↘ 0.3 – 0.5 luo-connect	Superior to the styloid process of the radius, 1.5 cun above the transverse crease of the wrist, between brachioradialis and abductor pollicis longus.	Wind cold; wind-heat; headache; coughing; asthma with little phlegm (allergic asthma); facial paralysis; stiff neck; taiyang s/sx; diseases of the wrist joint; sore throat; wind rash; empirical point for blood in urine	• **Releases the exterior in both Wind-heat and Wind-cold attacks.** For patterns including common cold and influenza, sneezing, stiff neck, headache, aversion to cold and a floating pulse, nasal obstruction, runny nose, headaches. • **Stimulates descending and dispersing of Lung Qi:** for all types of coughs and asthma. • Treats psychological and emotional disorders due to grief and sorrow, especially when there are repressed emotions. • Treats painful obstruction syndrome of the shoulder due to Large Intestine channel pathology. • **Opens the water passages:** for edema and water retention due to Kidney dysfunction (failing to grasp the qi).
Lu-8 **JingQu** *Channel canal* ↓ 0.3 – 0.5 jing-river	1 cun above the transverse crease of the wrist in the depression on the lateral side of the radial artery.	Wrist pain; cough; asthma	• Treats cough, asthma, fever, pain in the chest, sore throat, pain in the wrist.
Lu-9 **Taiyuan** *Greater Abyss* ↓ 0.2 – 0.3 shu-stream, yuan	At the radial end of the transverse crease of the wrist, in the depression on the lateral side of the radial artery.	Any LU problem due to deficiency; cold; weak deficient LU; cough; asthma; fever	• **Tonifies Lung Qi and yin.** • Resolves phlegm obstructing the Lungs with symptoms as chronic cough with yellow-sticky sputum. • **Tonifies Gathering Qi:** for deficiency with signs of weak voice and cold hands due to deficiency qi. • For weak and deep pulse.
Lu-10 **Yuji** *Fish Border* ↓ 0.5 – 0.8 ying-spring	On the radial aspect of the midpoint of the 1st metacarpal bone, on the junction of the red and white skin.	Sore throat; loss of voice; fever	• **Clears Heat and fire in the Lungs:** cough, hemoptysis, sore throat, loss of voice, fever, feverish sensation in the palms.
Lu-11 **Shaoshang** *Lesser Metal* ↓ 0.1 or bleed	On the radial side of the thumb, .1 cun posterior to the corner of the nail.	Fainting; loss of consciousness; nose bleeds; asthma; mania	• **Expels Exterior Wind-heat with sore throat.** • **For Interior Wind:** apoplexy and loss of consciousness from wind-stroke.

LU-3 ⎫ 3pts
LU-10 ⎬ that don't
LU-11 ⎭ have coughing.

POINTS

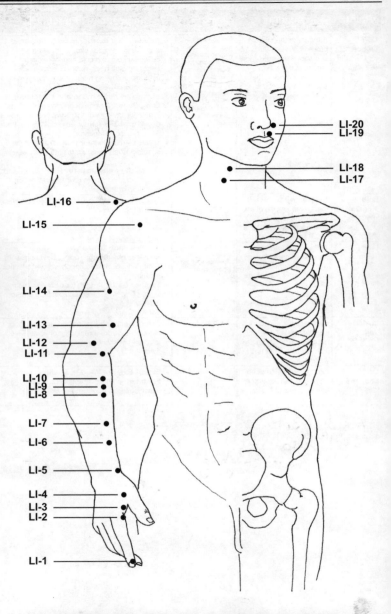

LI-20
LI-19
LI-18
LI-17
LI-16
LI-15
LI-14
LI-13
LI-12
LI-11
LI-10
LI-9
LI-8
LI-7
LI-6
LI-5
LI-4
LI-3
LI-2
LI-1

Jing Well	Ying Spring	Shu Stream	Jing River	He Sea
1	2	3	5	11
Yuan	Luo-connect	Xi-Cleft	Front Mu	Back Shu
4	6	7	St-25	Ub-25

Points	Location	Usage	Indications / Functions
LI-1 **Shangyang** *Metal Yang* ↓ 0.1 or bleed jing-well	On the radial side of the index finger, about .1 cun posterior to the corner of the nail	Apoplectic or any coma; high fever (yang ming meridian) and often used for high fevers instead of others; toothache if infected only; bleed with LI-11 needled for tonsillitis (fire toxin situation)	• **Removes obstruction:** for acute stage of wind-stroke. • **Clears both interior and exterior heat:** sore throat, interior heat affecting the large intestine. • **Expels Wind and Cold from the channel:** painful obstruction syndrome of the shoulder.
LI-2 **Erjian** *Second Interval* ↓ 0.2 – 0.3 ying-spring	In the depression of the radial side of the index finger, distal to the second metacarpal-phalangeal joint. The point is located with the finger slightly flexed.	Toothache; trigeminal neuralgia; febrile diseases; sore throat	• Clears heat from the Large Intestine: for constipation, dry stools, fever and abdominal pain.
LI-3 **Sanjian** *Third Interval* ↓ 0.5 – 0.8 shu-stream	When a loose fist is made, the point is on the radial side of the index finger, in the depression proximal to the head of the second metacarpal bone.	Toothache; sore throat; redness and swelling of fingers and dorsum of the hand	• Toothache, opthalmalgia, sore throat, redness and swelling of fingers and dorsum of the hand [arthritis].
LI-4 **Hegu** *Joining Valley* ↓ 0.5 –1.0 yuan	On the dorsum of the hand, between the 1st and 2nd metacarpal bones, approximately in the middle of the 2nd metacarpal bone on the radial side.	Common cold; febrile disease with or without sweat; headache (used for non-OP frontal and vertex; and only otherwise if URI related); disease of the sensory organs; facial paralysis; any face related problem; hemiplegia; major pain point; pain in the neck or any part of the body	• **Expels Wind-heat and Releases the Exterior:** exterior patterns including nasal congestion, sneezing, burning eyes, allergic rhinitis, hay fever. • **Stimulates Dispersing and Descending:** for nasal congestion, sneezing, cough, stiff neck, aversion to cold and a floating pulse, common cold, influenza or other infectious diseases. • **Unblocks the channels:** stops pain due to spasm and relieves painful obstruction syndrome of the arm or shoulder. • **Treats facial problems:** rhinitis, conjunctivitis, mouth ulcers, sties, sinusitis, epistaxis, toothache, trigeminal neuralgia. • **Tonifies Qi and Consolidates the Exterior:** for chronic wind attacks. • **Harmonizes the ascending of Yang and Descending of Yin:** subdues ascending rebellious qi of the Stomach, Lung or Liver with symptoms of epigastric pain, Liver-yang rising in migraine headaches, and asthma. • Empirical point for promoting delivery during labor.
LI-5 **Yangxi** *Yang Stream* ↓ 0.3 – 0.5 jing-river	On the radial side of the wrist. When the thumb is tilted upward, it is in the depression between the tendons of muscle extensor pollicis longus and brevis.	Diseases of the soft tissue of the wrist point; good for smoking withdrawal; pain and swelling of the eye; sore throat	• **Expels Wind and Releases the Exterior:** for headache, redness, pain and swelling of the eye, toothache, sore throat. • **Stops pain:** for painful obstruction syndrome of the wrist.
LI-6 **Pianli** *Slanting Passage* ↓ 0.3 or ↘ 0.3 – 0.5 luo-connect	When the elbow is flexed with the radial side of the arm upward, the point is on the line joining LI-5 and LI-11, 3 cun above LI-5.	Facial edema; hand edema; tinnitus; deafness	• **Opens the water passages:** for edema of the face and hands due to impaired circulation of defensive qi in the skin. • Treats manic depression.
LI-7 **Wenliu** *Warm Flow* ↓ 0.5 – 1.0 xi-cleft	When the elbow is flexed with radial side of the arm upward, the point is on the line joining LI-5 and LI-11, 5 cun above LI-5.	Headache; sore throat; swelling of the face; arm and shoulder pain	• **Stops pain and Removes obstructions from the channel:** painful obstruction syndrome of the channel and wind-heat causing painful and sore throat or swollen tonsils.

POINTS

Points	Location	Usage	Indications / Functions
LI-8 **Xialian** *Lower Angular Ridge* ↓ 0.5 – 1.0	On the line joining LI-5 and LI-11, 4 cun below LI-11.	Elbow and arm pain; motor impairment of the upper limbs; abdominal pain	• Harmonizes Small Intestine, Expels Wind, Clears Heat
LI-9 **Shanglian** *Upper Angular Ridge* ↓ 0.5 – 1.0	On the line joining LI-5 and LI-11, 3 cun below LI-11.	Shoulder and arm pain; motor impairment of the upper limbs; abdominal pain	• Harmonizes Large Intestine, Unblocks the channels, Stops pain.
LI-10 **Shousanli** *Arm Three Miles* ↓ 0.8 – 1.2	On the line joining LI-5 and LI-11, 2 cun below LI-11.	Pain in the arm; neck pain; good for overuse injuries of the arm and forearm (often quite sore and is the bulky area of the muscle)	• **Removes obstructions from the channel:** for painful obstruction syndrome, atrophy syndrome and sequelae of wind-stroke affecting the arm. A major point for the treatment of any muscular problem affecting the forearm and hands.
LI-11 **Quchi** *Pool at Bend* ↓ 1.0 – 1.5 he-sea	When the elbow is flexed, the point is in the depression at the lateral end of the transverse cubital crease, midway between Lu-5 and the lateral epicondyle of the humerus.	Paralysis; hemiplegia; arthritic pain in the upper limb; hypertension from excess yang (with St-36); high fever; any febrile disease; measles (heat toxin in TCM and showing up in the skin); main point for skin diseases involving redness; red eyes and pain	• **Expels exterior Wind-heat:** for exterior patterns with fever, chills, stiff neck, sweating, runny nose, body aches. • **Clears Internal Heat patterns:** including liver fire with hypertension. • **Cools the Blood:** for skin diseases due to heat in the blood such as urticaria, psoriasis and eczema. • **Resolves Dampness:** for patterns occurring in any part of the body including damp-heat causing skin eruptions or acne, damp-heat in the Spleen with digestive symptoms, or damp-heat in the urinary system causing cystitis or urethritis. Also for damp-heat causing fever, feeling of heaviness, loose stools, abdominal distention. • **Phlegm in the neck:** goiter. • **Benefits the sinews and joints:** for painful obstruction syndrome, atrophy syndrome and sequelae of wind-stroke paralysis, particularly of the arms and shoulders.
LI-12 **Zhouliao** *Elbow Seam* ↓ 0.5 – 1.0	When the elbow is flexed, the point is superior to the lateral epicondyle of the humerus, about 1 cun superolateral to LI-11, on the medial border of the humerus.	Numbness and contracture of the elbow and arm	• Unblocks the channels, Stops pain, Benefits elbow joint: for tennis elbow.
LI-13 **Shouwuli** *Arm Five Mile* ↓ 0.5 – 1.0	Superior to the lateral epicondyle of the humerus, on a line joining LI-11 and LI-15, 3 cun above LI-11.	Contracture and pain of the elbow and arm; scrofula	• Unblocks the channels, Stops pain, Stops coughing, Regulates Qi, Transforms Phlegm.
LI-14 **Binao** *Upper Arm* ↓ 0.8 – 1.5 or ↘ 0.8 – 1.5	On the line joining LI-11 and LI-15, 7 cun above LI-11, on the radial side of the humerus, superior to the lower end of the deltoid muscle, at the insertion.	Shoulder and arm pain; stiff neck; scrofula	• **Unblocks the channels:** for painful obstruction syndrome of the arm and shoulder. • Clears and enhances vision. • **Resolves Phlegm and disperses Phlegm masses:** for goiter.
LI-15 **Jianyu** *Shoulder Transporting Point* ↓ 0.8 – 1.5 or ↘ 0.8 – 1.5	In the depression, anterior and inferior to the acromion, on the upper portion of the deltoid muscle when the arm is in full abduction.	Hemiplegia; pain in shoulder; inflammation in shoulder; any shoulder problem	• **Benefits the sinews and joints, promotes Qi circulation, stops pain:** for painful obstruction syndrome of the shoulder.

Points	Location	Usage	Indications / Functions
LI-16 **Jugu** *Great Bone* ↓ 0.5 – 0.7	In the upper aspect of the shoulder, in the depression between the acromial extremity of the clavicle and scapular spine.	Disease of the shoulder and soft tissue of the shoulder; spitting blood	• Unblocks the channels: for painful obstruction syndrome of the shoulder. • Descends the Lung Qi: for breathlessness, cough or asthma caused by impairment of the Lung descending function.
LI-17 **Tianding** *Celestial Tripod* ↓ 0.3 – 0.5	On the lateral side of the neck, 1 cun below LI-18, on the posterior border of the SCM.	Sudden voice loss; sore throat; goiter; scrofula	• Benefits the throat and voice.
LI-18 **Futu** *Support the Prominence* ↓ 0.3 – 0.5	On the lateral side of the neck, level with the tip of the Adam's apple, between the sternal head and the clavicular head of the SCM muscle.	Cough; asthma; sore throat; goiter	• Benefits the throat, Stops coughing and wheezing: for tonsillitis, laryngitis, aphasia, hoarse voice and goiter.
LI-19 **Kouheliao** *Mouth Bone Hole*	Just below the lateral margin of the nostril, 0.5 cun lateral to Du-26.	Nasal obstruction; deviated mouth; epistaxis	• Expels Wind, Opens the nose.
LI-20 **Yingxiang** *Welcome Fragrance* ↘ 0.3 – 0.5 towards nose root	In the nasolabial groove, at the level of the midpoint of the lateral border of the ala nasi.	Rhinitis; sinusitis; can cause immediate clearing of the sinuses	• **Opens the nose:** for sneezing, loss of the sense of smell, epistaxis, sinusitis, runny nose, stuffed nose, allergic rhinitis and nasal polyps. • **Dispels Wind:** used for exterior patterns with nasal symptoms or trigeminal neuralgia and tics.

POINTS

POINTS

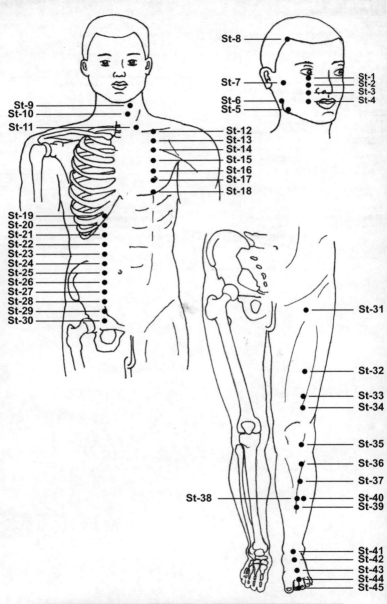

St-9
St-10
St-11

St-8

St-7
St-6
St-5

St-1
St-2
St-3
St-4

St-12
St-13
St-14
St-15
St-16
St-17
St-18

St-19
St-20
St-21
St-22
St-23
St-24
St-25
St-26
St-27
St-28
St-29
St-30

St-31

St-32

St-33
St-34

St-35

St-36

St-37

St-38

St-40
St-39

St-41
St-42
St-43
St-44
St-45

Jing Well	Ying Spring	Shu Stream	Jing River	He Sea
45	44	43	41	36
Yuan	Luo-connect	Xi-Cleft	Front Mu	Back Shu
42	40	34	Ren-12	Ub-21

Points	Location	Usage	Indications / Functions
St-1 **Chengqi** *Containing Tears* ↓ 0.5 – 1.0 slowly, w/o thrusting, lifting, or rotating	With the eyes looking straight forward, the point is directly below the pupil, between the eyeball and the infraorbital ridge.	Conjunctivitis; sties; eyelid twitching; redness and swelling of eye; lacrimation; night blindness	• Treats problems of the eye including acute and chronic conjunctivitis, myopia, astigmatism, squint, color blindness, night blindness, glaucoma, atrophy of the optic nerve, cataract, keratitis and retinitis. • **Expels Wind:** both for exterior and interior wind-heat or wind-cold with symptoms of swelling, pain and lacrimation and paralysis of the eyelid.
St-2 **Sibai** *Four Whites* ↓ 0.2 – 0.3	Below St-1, in the depression at the infraorbital foramen.	Facial paralysis; spasms; trigeminal neuralgia; sinusitis (especially maxillary or ethmoid sinusitis)	• **Expels Wind:** for either external or internal wind with swelling of the eyes, allergic rhinitis or facial paralysis, twitching of the eyelids, facial paralysis and trigeminal neuralgia. • Also used for biliary ascariasis.
St-3 **Juliao** *Great Crevice* ↓ 0.3 – 0.5	Directly below St-2, at the level of the lower border of the ala nasi, on the lateral side of the nasolabial groove.	Rhinitis; facial paralysis; trigeminal neuralgia in this area; upper toothache	• Expels Exterior and Interior Wind: for facial paralysis and trigeminal neuralgia. Also for treatment of epistaxis and nasal obstruction.
St-4 **Dicang** *Earth Granary* ↘ 0.5 – 1.5	Lateral to the corner of the mouth, directly below St-3.	Facial paralysis; trigeminal neuralgia; excessive salivation; difficulty closing eyes; herpes; gum ulcers	• **Eliminates Exterior Wind:** facial paralysis with deviation of the mouth, or aphasia.
St-5 **Daying** *Great Reception* ↓ 0.3 – 0.5 avoid artery	Anterior to the angle of the mandible, on the anterior border of the attached portion of the masseter muscle, in the groove-like depression appearing when the cheek is bulged.	Local problems; parotitis; lock jaw	• Expels Wind, Reduces swelling.
St-6 **Jiache** *Jaw Chariot* ↓ 0.3 – 0.5 towards ST 4	One finger breadth anterior and superior to the lower angle of the mandible where the masseter attaches, at the prominence of the muscle when the teeth are clenched.	Lower toothache; mumps; TMJ; grinding of teeth; facial paralysis	• Expels exterior wind affecting the face including mumps and spasm of the masseter muscle. • Toothache.
St-7 **Xiaguan** *Lower Gate* ↓ 0.3 – 0.5	At the lower border of the zygomatic arch, in the depression anterior to the condyloid process of the mandible, located with mouth closed.	Upper toothache; TMJ; TM arthritis; otitis media; tinnitus; earache; pus in ear	• **Removes obstruction:** for facial paralysis and trigeminal neuralgia, otitis, toothache, deafness and earache.
St-8 **Touwei** *Head Support*	.5 cun within the anterior hairline at the corner of the forehead, 4.5 cun lateral to Du-24.	Frontal and damp headache; psychosis if phlegm misting; facial paralysis; major headache point for frontal and vertex headache; other for dizziness especially with damp involvement; Meniere's disease (qi deficiency with damp)	• **Resolves Dampness and Phlegm:** for dizziness due to dampness and phlegm retained in the head and preventing the clear yang from rising to brighten the orifices, or causing frontal headaches.

POINTS

Points	Location	Usage	Indications / Functions
St-9 **Renying** *Person's Welcome* ↓ 0.3 – 0.5	Level with the tip of the Adam's apple, on the anterior border of the SCM.	Blood pressure; sore throat; asthma; goiter; flushed face	• **Removes obstructions from the head to send Qi downwards:** stops hiccup, belching and nausea or asthma due to stomach channel obstruction. • **Removes Masses and resolves swellings:** heat and swelling affecting the stomach channel with tonsillitis, swollen and sore throat, adenitis, pharyngitis and swelling of the thyroid. • **Tonifies and Regulates Qi:** to regulate excess above and deficiency below.
St-10 **Shuitu** *Water Prominence* ↓ 0.3 – 0.5	At the midpoint of the line joining St-9 and St-11, on the anterior border of the SCM.	Sore throat; asthma; cough	• Descends Lung Qi, Benefits throat and neck.
St-11 **Qishe** *Qi Abode* ↓ 0.3 – 0.5	At the superior border of the sternal extremity of the clavicle, between the sternal head and the clavicular head of the SCM.	Sore throat; asthma; neck stiffness; cough; hiccups	• Descends Qi, Benefits throat and neck.
St-12 **Quepen** *Empty Basin* ↓ 0.3 – 0.5	In the midpoint of the supraclavicular fossa, 4 cun lateral to the Ren meridian.	Supraclavicular fossa pain; cough; asthma	• Descends Lung qi, Clears heat from the chest: used for excess patterns characterized by rebellious Stomach Qi going upwards causing breathlessness and asthma. • Used for anxiety, nervousness and insomnia due to a Stomach disharmony.
St-13 **Qihu** *Qi Door* ↓ 0.3 – 0.5	At the lower border of the middle of the clavicle, 4 cun lateral to the Ren meridian.	Chest and hypochondrium pain; chest fullness; hiccups	• Descends rebellious Qi, Unbinds the chest.
St-14 **Kufang** *Storeroom* ↘ 0.3 – 0.5	In the 1st intercostal space, 4 cun lateral to the Ren meridian.	Chest fullness and pain; cough	• Descends rebellious Qi, Unbinds the chest.
St-15 **Wuyi** *Room Scream* ↘ 0.3 – 0.5	In the 2nd intercostal space, 4 cun lateral to Ren meridian.	Chest and costal region fullness and pain; mastitis; asthma	• Descends rebellious Qi, Unbinds the chest. • Benefits the breast, Stops pain.
St-16 **Yingchuang** *Breast Window* ↘ 0.3 – 0.5	In the 3rd intercostal space, 4 cun lateral to the Ren meridian.	Mastitis; insufficient lactation	• Stops coughing and wheezing, Benefits the breast.
St-17 **Ruzhong** *Breast Center*	In the 4th intercostal space, 4 cun lateral to the Ren meridian.	Landmark for locating points; no moxa or acupuncture	• Contraindicated for moxa or acupuncture.
St-18 **Rugen** *Breast Root* ↘ 0.3 – 0.5	In the 5th intercostal space, directly below the nipple.	Breast problems; mastitis; insufficient lactation	• Stops coughing and wheezing, Benefits the breast, Reduces swelling: used mostly as a local point for breast problems, especially in relation to stomach qi with symptoms as mastitis, PMS swellings and lumps in the breasts. • Regulates lactation and can either promote or reduce it.
St-19 **Burong** *Not Contained* ↓ 0.5 – 0.8	6 cun above the umbilicus, 2 cun lateral to Ren-14.	Stomachache; vomiting; gastritis (stuck food); upper abdominal distension	• Harmonizes the middle jiao, Descends Qi, Stops cough and wheezing.
St-20 **Chengman** *Assuming Fullness* ↓ 0.5 – 1.0	5 cun above the umbilicus, 2 cun lateral to Ren-13.	Abdominal distension; gastric pain; vomiting	• Harmonizes the middle jiao, Descends rebellious Lung and Stomach Qi.

Points	Location	Usage	Indications / Functions
St-21 **Liangmen** *Beam Door* ↓ 0.8 – 1.0	4 cun above the umbilicus, 2 cun lateral to Ren-12.	Stomachache; stomach ulcers; gastritis; nervous stomach; nausea; vomiting; secondary back up support point used with Ren-12	• **Regulates Stomach Qi:** for excess patterns including nausea or vomiting, burning sensation in the epigastrium, epigastric pain.
St-22 **Guanmen** *Pass Gate* ↓ 0.8 – 1.0	3 cun above the umbilicus, 2 cun lateral to Ren-11.	Abdominal distension; lack of appetite	• Regulates Qi, Stops pain, Regulates the intestines, Benefits urination.
St-23 **Taiyi** *Supreme Unity* ↓ 0.7 – 1.0	2 cun above the umbilicus, 2 cun lateral to Ren-10.	Gastric pain; indigestion; irritability	• Harmonizes the middle jiao, Transforms Phlegm, Calms the Mind.
St-24 **Huaroumen** *Slippery Flesh Gate* ↓ 0.7 – 1.0	1 cun above the umbilicus, 2 cun lateral to Ren-9.	Gastric pain; vomiting; mania	• Harmonizes the Stomach, Transforms Phlegm, Calms the Mind, Stops vomiting.
St-25 **Tianshu** *Heavenly Pillar* ↓ 0.7 – 1.2	2 cun lateral to the center of the umbilicus.	All intestinal problems; constipation; gastritis; abdominal distension and stagnation; diarrhea; constipation; low back pain as related to constipation; vomiting; colitis; blood in stools; irregular menstruation; edema	• **Regulates Intestines:** for excess patterns of the stomach manifesting in abdominal problems such as diarrhea, abdominal pain, bloating, abdominal distention. • **Clears heat from the Stomach and Intestines:** for burning sensations in the epigastrium, thirst, constipation, or foul-smelling loose stools and a yellow tongue coating. • **Treats acute stomach patterns:** for yangming or Qi level patterns with high fever, thirst, profuse sweating and a full pulse. • When used with direct moxibustion, it tonifies and warms the Spleen and the Intestines, and is a special point for chronic diarrhea due to Spleen-yang deficiency.
St-26 **Wailing** *Outer Mound* ↓ 0.7 – 1.2	1 cun below the umbilicus, 2 cun lateral to Ren-7.	Abdominal pain; hernia; dysmenorrhea	• Regulates Qi, Stops pain.
St-27 **Daju** *Big Great* ↓ 0.7 – 1.2	2 cun below the umbilicus, 2 cun lateral to Ren-5.	Spermatorrhea; premature ejaculation; inguinal hernia	• Regulates Stomach Qi: for excess patterns of the stomach with lateral abdominal pain and genital or hernia pain.
St-28 **Shuidao** *Water Passage* ↓ 0.7 – 1.2	3 cun below the umbilicus, 2 cun lateral to Ren-4.	Opens water passages; edema; urine retention; UTIs; menstrual and fertility problems related to dampness	• **Opens the water passages of the lower burner:** stimulates excretion of fluids, for edema, difficult urination and retention or urine when caused by an excess pattern. • **Regulates Qi in the lower abdomen:** regulates menses due to stasis of qi or blood.
St-29 **Guilai** *Return back* ↓ 0.7 – 1.2	4 cun below the umbilicus, 2 cun lateral to Ren-3.	Irregular menstruation; dysmenorrhea; amenorrhea; orchitis from blood or cold stagnation; endometriosis; inguinal hernia	• **Relieves Blood Stasis:** for blood stasis in the uterus and irregular menses, dysmenorrhea with dark clotted blood, amenorrhea due to blood stasis. • **Tonifies and raises Qi:** prolapse of the uterus.
St-30 **Qichong** *Rushing Qi* ↓ 0.5 – 1.0	5 cun below the umbilicus, 2 cun lateral to Ren-2.	Diseases of the reproductive organs; essence point; impotence; external genitalia pain female or male; retained placenta	• **Regulates Qi and Blood in the lower abdomen and genitals:** for excess patterns with abdominal pain, abdominal masses, hernia, swelling of the penis, retention of placenta and swelling of the prostate. • **Promotes Kidney Essence:** for impotence. • Improves Stomach and Spleen Function

POINTS

STOMACH

Points	Location	Usage	Indications / Functions
St-31 **Biguan** *Thigh Gate* ↓ 1.0 – 1.5	At the crossing point of the line drawn down from the ASIS and the line level with the lower border of the pubic symphisis, in the depression on the lateral side of sartorius, when the thigh is flexed.	Paralysis of the lower limb; atrophy and blockage of the muscles of the thigh and buttock if at least the thigh is involved	• **Removes obstruction from the channel:** for atrophy syndrome, painful obstruction syndrome, and sequelae of wind-stroke. • **Strengthens the Leg:** facilitates leg movement and raising of the leg.
St-32 **Futu** *Hidden Rabbit* ↓ 1.0 – 1.5	On the line connecting the anterior superior iliac spine (ASIS) and lateral border of the patella, 6 cun above the laterosuperior border of the patella, in muscle rectus femoris.	Lumbar and iliac region pain; knee coldness; beriberi; lower extremities motor impairment and pain	• Strengthens leg. • Expels Wind-heat: urticaria and heat in the blood.
St-33 **Yinshi** *Yin Market* ↓ 0.7 – 1.0	When the knee is flexed, the point is 3 cun above the latero superior border of the patella, on the line joining the laterosuperior border of the patella and ASIS.	Numbness; soreness; motor impairment of leg and knee	• Opens channels, Stops pain, Dispels Wind-Damp.
St-34 **Liangqiu** *Beam Mound* ↓ 0.5 – 1.0 xi-cleft	When the knee is flexed, point is 2 cun above the laterosuperior border of the patella.	Gastritis (stomach); mastitis (meridian); diseases of the knee (meridian); excess and hot ST problems; stuck food (needle against the flow of the qi)	• **Subdues Rebellious Qi:** for acute patterns of the Stomach with pain, hiccup, nausea, vomiting and belching. • **Open Channels:** for painful obstruction syndrome of the knee due to exterior dampness, wind and cold from the knee joint.
St-35 **Dubi** *Calf Nose* ↓ 0.7 – 1.0	When the knee is flexed, the point is at the lower border of the patella, in the depression lateral to the patellar ligament.	Numbness and motor impairment of the knee	• **Invigorate the Channels:** for painful obstruction syndrome of the knee. Used to expel dampness and cold.
St-36 **Zusanli** *Three Miles of the Leg* ↓ 0.5 – 1.2 he-sea	3 cun below St-35, one finger breadth from the anterior crest of the tibia, in tibialis anterior.	Gastritis; ulcers; enteritis; all digestive problems; shock; mania; hypertension (deficiency type); allergies; hay fever; asthma; cough (deficiency type); neurasthenia (nervous exhaustion); nausea; vomiting; abscess breasts (channel problem); insufficient lactation	• **Tonifies Qi and Blood:** for all cases of deficiency of Stomach and Spleen, and to strengthen the body in debilitated persons after chronic disease. • **Tonifies the Defensive Qi:** used for prevention of attacks from exterior factors when symptoms include sweating or edema. • **Brightens eyes:** blurred vision or declining vision in elderly. • **Regulates the Intestines:** for constipation due to deficiency. • **Raises the Yang:** for prolapse when used with direct moxibustion in combination with Ren-6 and Du-20. • **Expels Wind and Damp from the channels in painful obstruction syndrome.** Can be used either as a local point for the knee or a distal point for the wrist.
St-37 **Shangjuxu** *Upper Great Emptiness* ↓ 0.5 – 1.2	3 cun below St-36, one finger breadth from the anterior crest of the tibia, in the muscle tibialis anterior.	Colitis; and problem in the large intestine; abdominal pain or distension; diarrhea; appendicitis; dysentery like disorder (any damp-heat disorder); hemiplegia	• **Regulates the Stomach and Intestines:** for chronic diarrhea and damp-heat patterns of the Large Intestine with loose stools and mucus and blood. • Opens the chest to calm asthma and breathlessness.
St-38 **Tiaokou** *Narrow Opening* ↓ 0.5 – 1.0	2 cun below St-37, one finger breadth lateral to the crest of tibia, midway between St-35 and St-41.	Perifocal inflammation of the shoulder; frozen shoulder; limited ROM; good local point	• **Opens channels:** pain and stiffness of the shoulder joint.

Points	Location	Usage	Indications / Functions
St-39 **Xiajuxu** *Lower Great Emptiness* ↓ 0.5 – 1.0	3 cun below the St-37, one finger breadth from the anterior crest of the tibia, in muscle tibialis anterior.	Acute or chronic enteritis; paralysis of lower limb; mastitis in some books	• **Regulates Stomach and Intestines:** for all patterns of the Small Intestine including lower abdominal pain with borborygmi and flatulence, damp-heat in the Small Intestine with cloudy, dark urine.
St-40 **Fenglong** *Abundant Bulge* ↓ 0.5 – 1.0 luo-connect	8 cun superior to the external malleolus, two finger breadth lateral to St-38.	All phlegm situations; coughing; asthma (excess or deficient; but with phlegm); abundant mucous; phlegm nodules; damp headache with tight band around head; vertigo; swelling of the limbs; any significant swelling	• **Resolves Phlegm and Dampness:** for profuse expectoration from the chest, lumps under the skin, thyroid lumps and uterus lumps, phlegm misting the mind causing mental disturbances or dizziness and muzziness of the head. • Opens the chest and relieves asthma in phlegm patterns. • **Calms the Mind:** for phlegm misting the mind causing anxiety, fears and phobias. • **Relaxes the chest:** for bruising of the chest and rib-cage injuries.
St-41 **Jiexi** *Dispersing Stream* ↓ 0.5 – 0.7 jing-river	On the dorsum of the foot, at the midpoint of the transverse crease of the ankle, in the depression between the tendons of muscle extensor digitorum longus and hallucis longus, approximately at the level of the tip of the external malleolus.	Disease of foot and soft tissues; good distal point on the ST meridian; ankle joint pain; motor impairment; dizziness and vertigo	• **Opens channels:** for painful obstruction syndrome of the foot to remove cold-damp. Is frequently used for ankle problems. • **Clears Stomach-heat:** burning epigastric pain and thirst or headache or sore throats due to stomach heat.
St-42 **Chongyang** *Rushing Yang* ↓ 0.3 – 0.5 avoid artery yuan	Distal to St-41, at the highest point of the dorsum of the foot, in the depression between the 2nd and 3rd metatarsal bones and cuneiform bone.	Pain in upper teeth; facial paralysis; muscular atrophy and motor impairment of the foot	• **Tonifies the Stomach and Spleen.** • Powerfully tonifies the middle burner and dispels cold from the joints.
St-43 **Xiangu** *Sinking Valley* ↓ 0.3 – 0.5 shu-stream	In the depression distal to the junction of the 2nd and 3rd metatarsal bones.	Facial edema; conjunctivitis with heat	• Expels Wind and Heat from the joints in painful obstruction syndrome.
St-44 **Neiting** *Inner Courtyard* ↓ 0.3 – 0.5 ying-spring	Proximal to the web margin between the 2nd and 3rd toes, in the depression distal and lateral to the 2nd metatarsodigital joint.	Upper toothache; trigeminal neuralgia; gastric pain; stomach heat from overeating; acid reflux with heat involved; hot diarrhea and constipation; sore throat and tonsillitis combined with digestive symptoms; gum disorders	• **Clears heat from the Stomach:** for febrile diseases, epistaxis, gastric pain, acid regurgitation, abdominal distention. • **Expels Wind from the face:** toothache, pain in the face, trigeminal neuralgia, facial paralysis, deviation of the mouth, sore throat. • **Promotes Digestion:** diarrhea, dysentery.
St-45 **Lidui** *Strict Exchange* ↓ 0.1 or bleed jing-well	On the lateral side of the 2nd toe, .1 cun posterior to the corner of the nail.	Tonsillitis; febrile disease with heat; toothache (bleed); facial inflammation; distal point for any yangming face problems; dream-disturbed sleep; sore throat and hoarse voice; mania; coldness in the leg and foot	• **Calms the Mind:** for excess patterns such as Stomach-fire resulting in Heart-fire, with insomnia, irritability. • Clears Heat and brightens the eyes.

POINTS

POINTS

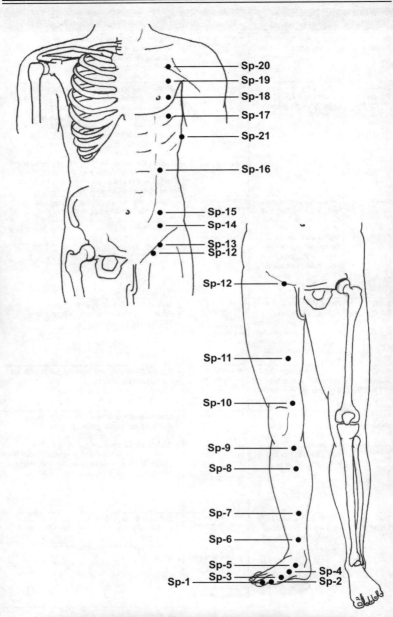

Jing Well	Ying Spring	Shu Stream	Jing River	He Sea
1	2	3	5	9
Yuan	Luo-connect	Xi-Cleft	Front Mu	Back Shu
3	4	8	Liv-13	Ub-20

Points	Location	Usage	Indications / Functions
Sp-1 **Yinbai** *Hidden White* ↓ 0.1 or bleed jing-well	On the medial side of the great toe, .1 cun posterior to the corner of the nail.	Any kind of bleeding; especially uterine (mostly from deficiency); watery, thin, scanty menorrhagia; bleeding of GI tract (most common places for SP related bleeding); mental diseases (SP overthinking); continuous nose bleeds; blood in stool; dream-disturbed sleep; convulsions	• **Regulates Blood in cases of excess in the Spleen or Stomach**, especially in blood stasis in the uterus. • Used with direct moxa to stop bleeding from any part of the body. • Mental restlessness and depression due in excess patterns due to blood stasis.
Sp-2 **Dadu** *Great Metropolis* ↓ 0.1 – 0.3 ying-spring	On the medial side of the great toe, distal and inferior to the first metatarso-digital joint, at the junction of the red and white skin.	Used for fever because the ying spring point; used locally for gout; foot pain; and cold feet	• Clears Heat in excess patterns to cause sweating in febrile diseases.
Sp-3 **Taibai** *Greater White* ↓ 0.3 – 0.5 shu-stream, yuan	Proximal and inferior to the head of the first metatarsal bone, at the junction of the red and white skin.	Headache from damp; stomach or gastric pain; abdominal distension; usually due to damp; sluggishness damp feeling; mental obsessions (can't let it go); cloying kind of thing; like emotional dampness; deficient type constipation or diarrhea	• **Tonifies the Spleen in cases of deficiency:** includes stimulating mental faculties associated with Spleen function that is weakened by excess mental work. • **Resolves dampness in 3 jiaos:** for symptoms of confused thinking, muzziness of the head, stuffiness. • Treats chronic retention of phlegm in the Lungs. • **Strengthens and straightens the spine.**
Sp-4 **Gongsun** *Grandfather Grandson* ↓ 0.5 – 0.8 luo-connect	In the depression distal and inferior to the base of the first metatarsal bone, at the junction of the red and white skin.	Fullness in chest and abdomen; great point for stomachache; acute and chronic enteritis; vomiting; endometriosis; amenorrhea (stuck type); intestines like a drum; abdominal pain and distension; Liv invading the SP; borborygmus; great point for gynecological problems	• **Tonifies Spleen and Stomach** • **For excess patterns of the Stomach and Spleen**: dampness in the epigastrium, stasis of blood in the Stomach, Stomach-heat and nausea or vomiting and stops abdominal pain. • **Opens the Chong:** regulates menstruation and stops excessive bleeding.
Sp-5 **Shangqiu** *Gold Mound* ↓ 0.2 – 0.3 jing-river	In the depression distal and inferior to the medial malleolus, midway between the tuberosity of the navicular bone and the tip of the medial malleolus.	Edema; diseases of ankle and surrounding soft tissue	• **Painful obstruction syndrome:** for dampness, especially of the knee or ankle.
Sp-6 **Sanyinjiao** *Three Yin Meeting* ↓ 0.5 – 1.0 contraindicated for pregnancy	3 cun directly above the tip of the medial malleolus, on the posterior border of the medial aspect of the tibia.	Diseases of reproductive system; distension or pain in abdomen; diarrhea; hemiplegia; neurasthenia; eczema; urticaria; deficient and weak conditions of SP and ST; borborygmus; poor digestion; irregular menstruation; almost any reproductive system problem	• **Tonifies Spleen and Stomach, Resolves Dampness:** for diarrhea, distension, and weak stomach conditions. • **Harmonizes the Liver, Regulates menses, and harmonizes the lower jiao:** for irregular menstruation, and any reproductive problems. • **Calms the Mind, Moves the Blood.** • **Unblocks the Channels, Stops pain.**

POINTS

Points	Location	Usage	Indications / Functions
Sp-7 **Lougu** *Leaking Valley* ↓ 0.5 – 1.0	3 cun above Sp-6, on the line joining the tip of the medial malleolus and Sp-9.	Abdominal distension; bloody stools; mental disorders; dream-disturbed sleep; convulsions	• Tonifies Spleen, Resolves Dampness. • Regulates menses, Harmonizes the Spleen, Moves the blood.
Sp-8 **Diji** *Earth Pivot* ↓ 0.5 – 1.0 xi-cleft	3 cun below Sp-9, on the line joining the tip of the medial malleolus and Sp-9.	Irregular menstruation; dysmenorrhea; irregular menstruation; edema of the legs or abdomen; nocturnal emissions; stuck food; emotional stagnation	• **Removes obstructions and stops pain:** acute excess patterns including dysmenorrhea of either acute or chronic nature. • Regulates the uterus, stops pain by moving blood and reducing blood stasis.
Sp-9 **Yinlingquan** *Yin Mound Spring* ↓ 0.5 – 1.0 he-sea	On the lower border of the medial condyle of the tibia, in the depression on the medial border of the tibia.	Distension and pain of the abdomen; ascites; edema; retention of urine; incontinence of urine; irregular menstruation due to damp; knee pain; diarrhea with undigested food; pain in the genitals; main diuretic point with Ren-9; main point for leukorrhea	• **Resolves Dampness in the lower burner:** damp-cold or damp-heat with symptoms of difficult urination, retention of urine, painful urination, cloudy urination, vaginal discharge, diarrhea, mucus in the stools and edema of the legs or abdomen. • Painful obstruction of the knee.
Sp-10 **Xuehai** *Sea of Blood* ↓ 0.5 – 1.2	When the knee is flexed, the point is 2 cun above the mediosuperior border of the patella, on the bulge of the medial portion of the muscle quadriceps femoris.	All skin diseases (especially redness and itchiness); irregular menstruation; dermatitis; menstrual and uterine bleeding disorders (from heat in blood)	• **Cools the Blood:** for blood heat patterns causing skin diseases such as eczema, urticaria and rashes. Also used for menorrhagia or metrorrhagia when due to heat in the blood. • **Removes Blood Stasis:** for stagnant blood especially in the uterus, including painful or irregular periods, chronic or acute dysmenorrhea.
Sp-11 **Jimen** *Winnower* ↓ 0.5 – 1.0	6 cun above Sp-10, on the line drawn from Sp-10 to Sp-12.	Dysuria; enuresis; lower extremities paralysis and pain; muscular atrophy	• Regulates urination, Drains Damp, Clears Heat.
Sp-12 **Chongmen** *Rushing Door* ↓ 0.5 – 1.0	Superior to the lateral end of the groove, on the lateral side of the femoral artery, at the level of the upper border of the symphisis pubis, 3.5 cun lateral to Ren-2.	Abdominal pain; hernia; dysuria	• Nourishes Yin: for Kidney deficiency. • Painful obstruction syndrome of the hip.
Sp-13 **Fushe** *Bowel Abode* ↓ 0.5 – 1.0	.7 cun laterosuperior to Sp-12, 4 cun lateral to the Ren meridian.	Lower abdominal pain; hernia	• Regulates Qi, Stops pain.
Sp-14 **Fujie** *Abdominal Bind* ↓ 0.5 – 1.0	1.3 cun below Sp-15, 4 cun lateral to the Ren meridian, on the lateral side of the muscle rectus abdominis.	Pain around umbilical region; hernia; diarrhea; constipation	• Regulates Qi, Subdues Rebellion, Warms and benefits lower jiao.
Sp-15 **Daheng** *Big Horizontal Stroke* ↓ 0.7 – 1.2	4 cun lateral to the center of the umbilicus, lateral to the muscle rectus abdominis.	Abdominal pain and distension; constipation; diarrhea; dysentery	• **Strengthens Spleen Function:** for chronic constipation due to deficiency. • **Strengthens Limbs:** for cold or weak limbs. • **Resolves Dampness:** for chronic diarrhea with mucus in the stools due to deficiency. • **Regulates Qi:** promotes the smooth flow of Liver qi manifesting in abdominal pain.
Sp-16 **Fuai** *Abdominal Lament* ↓ 0.5 – 1.0	3 cun above Sp-15, 4 cun lateral to Ren-11.	Abdominal pain; diarrhea; dysentery; constipation	• Regulates the Intestines.

POINTS

Points	Location	Usage	Indications / Functions
Sp-17 **Shidou** *Food Hole* ↘ 0.3 – 0.5	In the 5th intercostal space, 6 cun lateral to the Ren meridian.	Chest and hypochondriac fullness and pain	• Reduces food stagnation, Promotes digestion.
Sp-18 **Tianxi** *Heavens Ravine* ↘ 0.3 – 0.5	In the 4th intercostal space, 6 cun lateral to the Ren meridian.	Insufficient lactation; chest and hypochondriac fullness and pain; hiccups; mastitis	• Regulates and Descends Qi, Benefits the breast, Promotes lactation.
Sp-19 **Xiongxiang** *Chest Village* ↘ 0.3 – 0.5	In the 3rd intercostal space, 6 cun lateral to the Ren meridian.	Chest and hypochondriac fullness and pain	• Regulates Qi, Subdues rebellion.
Sp-20 **Zhourong** *All Round Flourishing* ↘ 0.3 – 0.5	In the 2nd intercostal space, 6 cun lateral to the Ren meridian.	Chest and hypochondriac fullness and pain; cough; hiccups	• Regulates Qi, Descends Qi.
Sp-21 **Dabao** *Great Wrapping* ↘ 0.3 – 0.5	On the mid-axillary line, 6 cun below the axilla, in the 6th intercostal space, midway between the axilla and the free end of the 11th rib.	General body soreness; excess in the luo vessels	• **Moves Blood in the connecting channels:** for muscular pain moving throughout the body.

POINTS

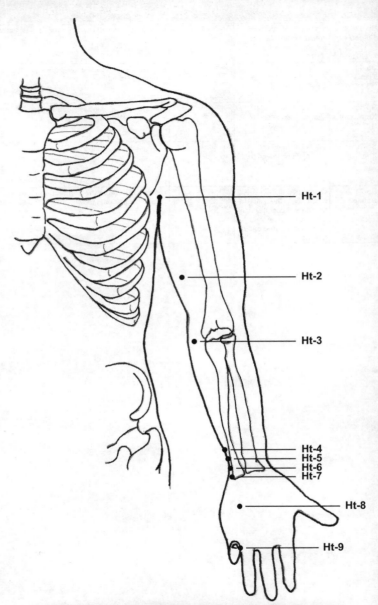

POINTS

Jing Well	Ying Spring	Shu Stream	Jing River	He Sea
9	8	7	4	3
Yuan	Luo-connect	Xi-Cleft	Front Mu	Back Shu
7	5	6	Ren-14	Ub-15

Points	Location	Usage	Indications / Functions
Ht-1 **Jiquan** *Summit Spring* ↓ 0.5 – 1.0 avoid artery	When the upper arm is abducted, the point is in the center of the axilla, on the medial side of the axillary artery.	Arthritis; local shoulder joint problems; generally for armpit problems; not very common	• **Nourishes Heart Yin and Clears deficiency heat:** for dry mouth, night sweating, mental restlessness, and insomnia. • Also used in sequelae of wind-stroke for paralysis of the arm.
Ht-2 **Qingling** *Green Spirit* ↓ 0.3 – 0.5	When the elbow is flexed, the point is 3 cun above the medial end of the transverse cubital crease (Ht-3), in the groove medial to muscle biceps brachii.	Cardiac and hypochondriac pain; shoulder and arm pain	• Unblocks the Channels, Stops pain.
Ht-3 **Shaohai** *Lesser Sea* ↓ 0.5 – 1.0 he-sea	When the elbow is flexed, the point is in the depression between the medial end of the transverse cubital crease of the elbow and the medial epicondyle of the humerus.	Neurasthenia; psychosis; intercostal neuralgia; ulnar neuralgia; important for hand tremors; good for trembling and shaking from Parkinson's; cardiac/chest pain; pain in axilla	• **Clears Heat:** for Heart-fire or Heart deficiency heat. • **Calms the Mind:** for epilepsy, depression, mental retardation or hypomania due to Heart fire.
Ht-4 **Lingdao** *Spirit Pathway* ↓ 0.3 – 0.5 jing-river	When the palm faces upward, the point is on the radial side of the tendon of muscle flexor carpi ulnaris, 1.5 cun above the transverse crease of the wrist.	Aphasia; main point for speaking difficulties; bradycardia; hysterical aphasia; stuttering due to emotional issues; nervous anxiety; uptight nervousness	• Unblocks obstructions from the Heart channel: for spasm and neuralgia of the forearm and arthritis of the elbow and wrist.
Ht-5 **Tongli** *Penetrating the Interior* ↓ 0.3 – 0.5 luo-connect	When the palm faces upward, the point is on the radial side of the tendon of m. flexor carpi ulnaris, 1 cun above the transverse crease of the wrist.	Palpitations; dizziness; blurry vision; sore throat; sudden voice loss; aphasia with stiff tongue; wrist and elbow pain	• **Main point to tonify Heart Qi:** for all symptoms of Heart-qi deficiency and especially aphasia due to its effect on the tongue. • **Benefits the Bladder:** for Heart fire causing heat in the Urinary Bladder via the Small Intestine channel with symptoms of thirst, bitter taste, insomnia, tongue ulcers, burning on urination and hematuria.
Ht-6 **Yinxi** *Yin's Crevice* ↓ 0.3 – 0.5 xi-cleft	When the palm faces upward, the point is on the radial side of the tendon of m. flexor carpi ulnaris, 0.5 cun above the transverse crease of the wrist.	Night sweats; nosebleed; cardiac pain; hysteria	• **Nourishes Heart yin:** for Heart yin deficiency with symptoms including night sweating, dry mouth, insomnia. • **Clears Heart-fire and Heart yin deficiency heat:** for mental restlessness and feelings of heat from deficiency.
Ht-7 **Shenmen** *Spirit Gate* ↓ 0.3 – 0.5 shu-stream, yuan	At the ulnar end of the transverse crease of the wrist, in the depression on the radial side of the tendon of muscle flexor carpi ulnaris.	Palpitations; absent mindedness; insomnia; excessive dreaming due to HT or Liv fire; angina and cardiac pain; mental illness of any kind; dementia; mania; irritability and insomnia; main point for insomnia; hysteria	• **Calms the Mind:** for any Heart pattern and nourishes Heart blood with symptoms of anxiety, insomnia, poor memory, palpitation, cardiac pain and hysteria and a pale tongue.
Ht-8 **Shaofu** *Lesser Palace* ↓ 0.3 – 0.5 ying-spring	When the palm faces upward, the point is between the 4th and 5th metacarpal bones. When a fist is made, the point is where the tip of the little finger rests.	Tachycardia; dysuria; enuresis; itching of the groin; sweaty palms	• **Clears Heat in the Heart:** for both excess and deficiency heat patterns of the Heart with symptoms of insomnia, thirst, bitter taste, mental restlessness or hypomania, dark urine, tongue ulcers, and a Red tongue with redder tip and yellow coating. • **Calms the Mind:** for more excess patterns including schizophrenia and psychosis.
Ht-9 **Shaochong** *Lesser Surge* ↓ 0.1 or bleed jing-well	On the radial side of the little finger, .1 cun posterior to the corner of the nail.	Coma; apoplectic hysteria	• **For excess patterns of the Heart with Heat:** including wind-stroke due to internal wind.

POINTS

POINTS

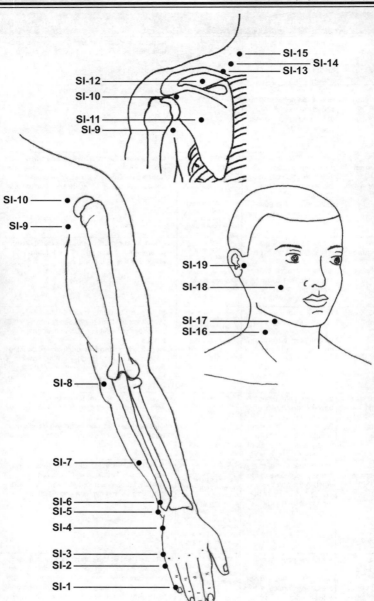

Jing Well	Ying Spring	Shu Stream	Jing River	He Sea
1	2	3	5	8
Yuan	Luo-connect	Xi-Cleft	Front Mu	Back Shu
4	7	6	Ren-4	Ub-27

Points	Location	Usage	Indications / Functions
SI-1 **Shaoze** *Lesser Marsh* ↓ 0.1 or bleed jing-well	On the ulnar side of the little finger, about .1 cun posterior to the corner of the nail.	Mastitis; insufficient lactations; sometimes for PMS breast tenderness; swollen breasts including breast lumps and fibrocystic lumps; as jing well point can be used for loss of consciousness	• Expels Wind-heat: for exterior attacks, especially when the symptoms affect the head and neck, causing stiff neck and headache. Also used to treat tonsillitis from invasion of exterior wind-heat. • Opens the orifices and promote resuscitation: for internal wind and phlegm blocking the orifices and causing sudden unconsciousness, as in wind-stroke. • Used as a distal point for channel problems of the neck including chronic stiff neck or acute torticollis. • Promotes lactation: when lactation is inhibited by the presence of some pathogenic factor or stagnation.
SI-2 **Qiangu** *Front Valley* ↓ 0.3 – 0.5 ying-spring	When a loose fist is made, the point is on the ulnar side, distal to the 5th MP joint, at the junction of the red and white skin.	Numb fingers; febrile diseases; tinnitus	• **Clears Heat:** for both interior and exterior heat patterns, especially when the neck and eyes are affected and also to clear interior heat from the Small Intestine, or acute febrile diseases. Also for clearing heat in the Urinary Bladder with burning on urination.
SI-3 **Houxi** *Back Stream* ↓ 0.5 – 0.7 shu-stream	When a loose fist is made, the point is on the ulnar side, proximal to the 5th MP joint, at the end of the transverse crease at the junction of the red and white and skin.	Seizures; psychosis; mania; all kinds of sweating; stiff neck; low back pain (acute and chronic); mania; malaria; night sweats; tinnitus; deafness (meridian related); the strongest distal point on the SI meridian	• **Opens the Governing Vessel:** for all symptoms of the Du channel including eliminating interior wind from the channel with convulsions, tremors, epilepsy, stiff neck, and giddiness and headache. In combination with Ub-62 it can be used to affect the whole spine and back in both acute and chronic cases. • **Eliminates Exterior Wind:** for both wind-heat and wind-cold when there are symptoms affecting the neck and head such as stiff neck, occipital headache, aches down the spine and back, and chills and fever. • **Benefits the sinews and tendons:** especially along the Du, Small Intestine and Bladder channels. In particular, for the upper more than the lower back area along the Small Intestine and Bladder channels. More for acute than chronic conditions. • **Clears the Mind:** helps strengthen the mind to face to choices and difficult decisions.
SI-4 **Wangu** *Wrist Bone* ↓ 0.3 – 0.5 yuan	On the ulnar side of the palm, in the depression between the base of the fifth metacarpal bone and the triquetral bone.	Wrist pain; neck rigidity; finger contracture	• **Unblocks the Channels:** mostly used for channel problems of the Small Intestine including painful obstruction syndrome of the wrist or elbow. • **Clears Damp-heat:** for jaundice from damp-heat obstructing the Gallbladder, hypochondriac pain or cholecystitis.
SI-5 **Yanggu** *Yang Valley* ↓ 0.3 – 0.5 jing-river	At the ulnar end of the transverse crease on the dorsal aspect of the wrist, in the depression between the styloid process of the ulna and the triquetral bone.	Hand and wrist pain; febrile diseases	• **Clears the Mind:** helpful in distinguishing correct action, direction, due to providing a sense of clarity. • Unblocks the channel. • **Expels Exterior Damp-heat:** eliminates dampness from the knees when they are swollen and hot.
SI-6 **Yanglao** *Nourishing the Old* ↓ 0.3 – 0.5 xi-cleft	Dorsal to the head of the ulna. When the palm faces the chest, the point is in the bony cleft on the radial side of the styloid process of the ulna.	Pain in shoulder and back; arthritis; main point for acute low back sprains; used a lot for whiplash	• **Benefits the sinews and unblocks the channels:** used for any channel problems of the Small Intestine, particularly when there is tightness of the tendons and ligaments causing stiff neck and shoulders. • **Brightens eyes:** benefits the eyesight in patterns related to Heart or Small Intestine.
SI-7 **Zhizheng** *Branch to Heart Channel* ↓ 0.5 – 0.8 luo-connect	On the line joining SI-5 and SI-8, 5 cun above SI-5.	Headache; spastic elbow and fingers	• **Unblocks the channel:** treats any channel problem, especially related to elbow problems. • **Calms the Mind:** for severe anxiety affecting the Heart. • Treats thyroid phlegm swellings.

POINTS

Points	Location	Usage	Indications / Functions
SI-8 **Xiaohai** *Small Intestine Sea* ↓ 0.3 – 0.5 he-sea	When the elbow is flexed, the point is located in the depression between the olecranon of the ulna and the medial epicondyle of the humerus.	Headache; nape pain; shoulder arm and neck pain; epilepsy	• **Clears Damp-heat:** effective in treating acute swelling of the glands of the neck and parotitis. • Removes obstruction from the channel: painful obstruction syndrome of the elbow and neck. • Calms the Mind: heart patterns with anxiety.
SI-9 **Jianzhen** *Upright Shoulder* ↓ 0.5 – 1.0	Posterior and inferior to the shoulder joint. When the arm is adducted, the point is 1 cun above the posterior end of the axillary fold.	Scapula pain	• Benefits the shoulder, Unblocks the channels, Stops pain: local point for painful obstruction syndrome of the shoulder.
SI-10 **Naoshu** *Upper Arm Hollow* ↓ 0.5 – 1.0	When the arm is adducted, the point is directly above SI-9, in the depression inferior to the scapular spine.	Swelling shoulders; shoulder and arm pain	• Benefits the shoulder, Unblocks the channels, Stops pain: local point for painful obstruction syndrome of the shoulder.
SI-11 **Tianzong** *Heavenly Attribution* ↓ 0.5 – 1.0	In the infrascapular fossa, at the junction of the upper and middle third of the distance between the lower border of the scapular spine and the inferior angle of the scapula.	Pain in the shoulder; insufficient lactations	• Benefits the shoulder, Unblocks the channels, Stops pain, Benefits the breast: local point for painful obstruction syndrome of the shoulder.
SI-12 **Bingfeng** *Grasping the Wind* ↓ 0.5 – 0.7	In the center of the suprascapular fossa, directly above SI-11. When the arm is lifted, the point is at the site of the depression.	Scapula pain; shoulder and arm motor impairment	• Benefits the shoulder, Unblocks the channels, Expels the Wind: local point for painful obstruction syndrome of the shoulder.
SI-13 **Quyuan** *Crooked Wall* ↓ 0.3 – 0.5 ↘ 0.3 – 0.5	On the medial extremity of the suprascapular fossa, about midway between SI-10 and the spinous process of the 2nd thoracic vertebra.	Scapula pain and stiffness	• Benefits the shoulder and scapula: local point for painful obstruction syndrome of the shoulder.
SI-14 **Jianwaishu** *Outer Shoulder Shu* ↓ 0.3 – 0.7	3 cun lateral to the lower border of the spinous process of the 1st thoracic vertebra where Du-13 is located.	Shoulder and back pain; neck stiffness and pain	• Benefits the shoulder and scapula, Stops pain, Expels Wind: local point for painful obstruction syndrome of the shoulder and trapezius.
SI-15 **Jianzhongzhu** *Middle Shoulder Shu* ↓ 0.3 – 0.6	2 cun lateral to the lower border of the spinous process of the 7th cervical vertebra.	Cough; asthma; pain in shoulder and arm; hemoptysis	• Unblocks the channels, Stops pain, Descends Lung Qi: local point for painful obstruction syndrome of the shoulder and neck.
SI-16 **Tianchuang** *Heaven Window* ↓ 0.3 – 0.7	In the lateral aspect of the neck, in the posterior border of the SCM, posterior and superior to LI-18.	Tinnitus; stiff neck; loss of voice	• Benefits the ear, throat, and voice, Unblocks the channels, Stops pain, Clears Heat.
SI-17 **Tianrong** *Heavenly Appearance* ↓ 0.5 – 0.7	Posterior to the angle of the mandible, in the depression on the anterior border of the SCM.	Difficulty hearing; difficulty swallowing; sometimes goiter; tonsillitis	• Resolves Damp-heat: for both interior and exterior damp-heat and is indicated in swelling of the cervical glands, parotitis and tonsillitis.
SI-18 **Quanliao** *Zygomatic Crevice* ↓ 0.5 – 0.8	Directly below the outer canthus, in the depression on the lower border of the zygomatic bone.	Trigeminal neuralgia; facial paralysis; toothache in upper jaw	• **Expels Wind, Relieves Pain:** local point for treating facial paralysis, tics or trigeminal neuralgia.
SI-19 **Tinggong** *Listening Palace* ↓ 0.5 – 1.0 when mouth is open	Anterior to the tragus and posterior to the condyloid process of the mandible, in the depression formed when the mouth is open.	Tinnitus; difficulty hearing; jaw problems like TMJ; otitis media	• **Benefits the ear:** local point for tinnitus and deafness.

POINTS

URINARY BLADDER

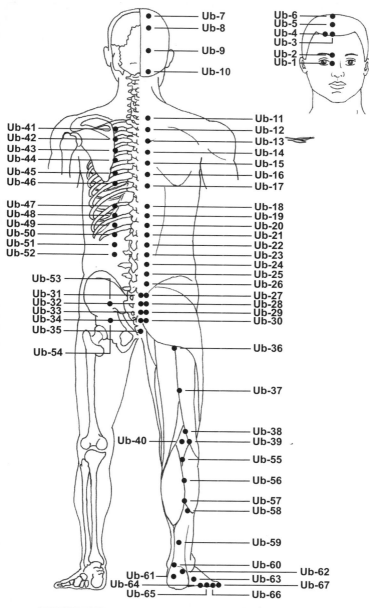

POINTS

Jing Well	Ying Spring	Shu Stream	Jing River	He Sea
67	66	65	60	40
Yuan	Luo-connect	Xi-Cleft	Front Mu	Back Shu
64	58	63	Ren-3	Ub-28

Points	Location	Usage	Indications / Functions
Ub-1 **Jingming** *Eye Brightness* ↓ 0.3 – 0.7 slowly, w/o thrusting, lifting, or rotating	0.1 cun superior to the inner canthus.	Any eye problems; blindness; blurring; itchy canthus	• **Expels Exterior Wind and Clears Heat:** for conjunctivitis and runny eyes due to exterior wind, red, painful, swollen and dry eyes due to Liver-fire, and stops pain and itching due to heat. • Treats insomnia and somnolence by opening the Yin and Yang Qiao vessels.
Ub-2 **Zanzhu** *Collecting Bamboo* sub- ↓ 0.3 – 0.5 or bleed	On the medial extremity of the eyebrow, or on the supraorbital notch.	Headache (local point); acute conjunctivitis; excessive tearing; excessive twitching; good point for sinus allergies; hay fever; sinus headaches	• Expels Wind from the face and removes obstructions from the channel: for facial paralysis, facial tics and trigeminal neuralgia. • Brightens the eyes and soothes the Liver: for any Liver pattern affecting the eyes such as floaters in the eyes, red eyes, blurred vision, and persistent headaches around or behind the eyes.
Ub-3 **Meichong** *Eyebrow Surging* sub- ↓ 0.3 – 0.5	Directly above the medial end of the eyebrow, 0.5 cun within the anterior hairline between Du-24 and Ub-4.	Headache; giddiness; nasal obstruction	• Expels Wind, Clears the head, Stops pain, Benefits the eyes and nose.
Ub-4 **Quchai** *Deviating Turn* sub- ↓ 0.3 – 0.5	1.5 cun lateral to Du-24 at the junction of the medial 1/3 and lateral 2/3 of the distance from Du-24 to St-8.	Headache; nasal obstruction; epistaxis; blurry and failed vision	• Expels Wind, Clears the head, Stops pain, Benefits the eyes and nose.
Ub-5 **Wuchu** *Five Places* sub- ↓ 0.3 – 0.5	10.5 cun lateral to Du-23, or 0.5 cun directly above Ub-4.	Headache; blurry vision; epilepsy; convulsion	• **Subdue Interior Wind:** a local point to treat epilepsy, convulsions or rigidity of the spine in children during a febrile disease. • **Restores Consciousness:** for acute attacks of interior wind with unconsciousness.
Ub-6 **Chengguang** *Receiving Light* sub- ↓ 0.3 – 0.5	1.5 cun posterior to Ub-5, 1.5 cun lateral to the DU meridian.	Rhinitis (nasal obstruction); any nose problem	• Expels Wind, Clears Heat, Benefits the eyes and nose.
Ub-7 **Tongtian** *Reaching Heaven* sub- ↓ 0.3 – 0.5	1.5 cun posterior to Ub-6, 1.5 cun lateral to the DU meridian.	Headache; nasal obstruction; rhinorrhea	• Dispels Wind: for both exterior and interior wind patterns of the head causing severe headache or facial paralysis, dizziness, vertigo. A local point for vertex headaches due to liver yang rising or liver-wind or Liver-blood deficiency. • Subdues interior wind: local point for convulsions and unconsciousness. • For the eyes and nose, rhinitis.
Ub-8 **Luoque** *Declining Connection* sub- ↓ 0.3 – 0.5	1.5 cun posterior to Ub-7, 1.5 cun lateral to the DU meridian.	Dizziness; blurry vision; mania; tinnitus	• Benefits sensory organs, Transforms Phlegm, Calms the Mind.
Ub-9 **Yuzhen** *Jade Pillow* sub- ↓ 0.3 – 0.5	1.3 cun lateral to Du-17, on the lateral side of the superior border of the EOP.	Occipital headache; stiffness and soreness in back of neck; pharyngitis; URIs; common cold; seizures (wind)	• Expels Wind and Cold, Stops pain, Benefits the nose and eyes.
Ub-10 **Tianzhu** *Heaven Pillar* ↓ 0.5 – 0.8	1.3 cun lateral to Du-15, in the depression on the lateral aspect of the trapezius muscle.	With common cold; bronchitis; with pleurisy can be needled if tender; neck and back pain	• **Expels Wind:** for both exterior and interior wind in the head, for occipital or vertex headache from any origin. Also for wind causing stiff neck and headache due to wind-cold invasion. • **Subdues Interior Wind:** for occipital headaches deriving from Liver wind rising. • **Clears the brain:** stimulates memory and concentration. • Increases vision, especially due to Kidney deficiency. • **Invigorates the lower back:** for bilateral acute lower backache.

POINTS

Points	Location	Usage	Indications / Functions
Ub-11 **Dazhu** *Great Shuttle* 0.5 – 0.7	1.5 cun lateral to Du-13, at the level of the lower border of the spinous process of T1.	Common cold; bronchitis; pleurisy; can use for taiyang stage disease (some say it is best used before the pathogen gets into the organ); URIs like wind-heat	• **Nourishes Blood:** for generalized muscular ache due to blood not nourishing the muscles. • **Releases the Exterior:** for wind-cold or wind-heat. • **Nourishes the Bones:** promotes bone formation and prevent bone degeneration in the elderly or in chronic arthritis. Also treats contractions of the tendons.
Ub-12 **Fengmen** *Wind Door* 0.5 – 0.7	1.5 cun lateral to the DU meridian, at the level of the lower border of the spinous process of T2.	Bronchitis; asthma; pleurisy; night sweats; pulmonary TB; steaming bone syndrome (severe kidney yin deficiency); spitting blood from lungs; any kind of cough; fullness in chest; throat blockage; anything that affects lungs	• For beginning stage of exterior invasion of wind-cold or wind-heat with symptoms of stuffy nose, sneezing, chills, aversion to cold and headache.
Ub-13 **Feishu** *Lung Back Shu* 0.5 – 0.7	1.5 cun lateral to Du-12, at the level of the lower border of the spinous process of T3.	Cough; asthma; chest pain; spitting blood	• For both exterior and interior patterns of the Lung, especially including cough, breathlessness or asthma. • **Clears Heat from the Lungs:** for acute bronchitis or pneumonia, high fever, thirst, a cough with sticky yellow sputum, breathlessness, restlessness, a rapid pulse and a red tongue body with a thick dry yellow coating. • **Tonifies Lung Qi:** for chronic deficiency of Lung qi or Lung yin.
Ub-14 **Jueyinshu** *Terminal Yin Shu* 0.5 – 0.7	1.5 cun lateral to the DU meridian, at level with the lower border of the spinous process of T4.	Neurasthenia (nervous system exhaustion); seizures; psychosis; hysteria; absent-mindedness; any mental problems; very good insomnia point; mania; memory loss; palpitations	• For Heart conditions, including arrhythmia, tachycardia, angina pectoris and coronary heart disease.
Ub-15 **Xinshu** *Heart Shu* 0.5 – 0.7	1.5 cun lateral to the Du-11, at the level of the lower border of the spinous process of T5.	Cardiac pain; loss of memory; palpitation; spitting blood; night sweat; epilepsy	• **Calms the Mind:** for nervous anxiety and insomnia due to excess conditions of the Heart such as Heart-fire, or Heart yin deficiency. Also for anxiety and insomnia due to deficiency conditions such as Heart blood deficiency or Heart yin deficiency. • Invigorates Blood: for pain in the chest due to blood stasis.
Ub-16 **Dushu** *DU - Governing Vessel Shu* 0.5 – 0.7	1.5 cun lateral to Du-10, at the level of the lower border of the spinous process of T6.	Cardiac pain; abdominal pain	• Regulates Qi in the chest and abdomen.

POINTS

URINARY BLADDER

Points	Location	Usage	Indications / Functions
Ub-17 **Geshu** *Diaphragm Shu* ↘ 0.5 – 0.7	1.5 cun lateral to Du-9, at the level of the lower border of the spinous process of T7.	Anemia; chronic hemorrhagic disorders; spasms of the diaphragm; nervous vomiting; constriction of the esophagus; abdominal distension or lumps; good for skin indications (heat in the blood); chronic and acute hepatitis; cholecystitis (Liv/GB damp-heat); stomach disease (Liv invading ST); eye diseases (ascendant Liv yang); intercostal neuralgia (pathway); irregular menstruation (due to Liv disharmony); emotional aspects of the Liv; measles; night sweats; hiccups	• **Nourishes Blood:** for deficiency of blood in any organ and is combined with other shu points to target blood of specific organs. • **Invigorates Blood and removes blood stagnation:** a general point to remove blood stasis in any organ and from any part of the body. • **Moves Qi in the diaphragm and chest:** for stuffiness and pain of the chest, fullness in the epigastrium, belching and hiccup. • **Pacifies Stomach Qi and Subdues rebellious Stomach Qi:** for hiccup, belching, nausea and vomiting. • **Tonifies Blood and Qi.**
Ub-18 **Ganshu** *Liver Shu* ↘ 0.5 – 0.7	1.5 cun lateral to Du-8, at the level of the lower border of the spinous process of T9. (Skips T8).	Hepatitis; cholecystitis; gastritis; bitter taste in mouth; dry or bilious vomiting; pain in the flanks; yellowish eyes/jaundice	• **Benefits the Liver and Gallbladder:** for stagnation of Liver qi or retention of damp-heat in the Liver and Gallbladder causing distension of the epigastrium and hypochondrium, sour regurgitation, nausea, jaundice and cholecystitis. Also for Liver deficiency patterns such as Liver blood deficiency. • **Benefits the eyes:** promotes vision in all eye disorders related to Liver disharmony such as poor night vision, blurred vision, floaters, red and painful and swollen eyes.
Ub-19 **Danshu** *Gall Bladder Shu* ↘ 0.5 – 0.7	1.5 cun lateral to Du-7, at the level of the lower border of the spinous process of T10.	Jaundice; bitter taste of the mouth; chest and hypochondriac pain; pulmonary TB	• **Resolves Damp-heat in the Liver and Gallbladder:** for jaundice and cholecystitis. • **Pacifies the Stomach and Stimulates the Descending of Stomach Qi:** for belching, nausea and vomiting. • **Relaxes the diaphragm:** moves qi in the diaphragm for feelings of stuffiness and pain of the chest, fullness in the epigastrium, belching and hiccup due to Liver qi stagnation.
Ub-20 **Pishu** *Spleen Shu* ↘ 0.5 – 0.7	1.5 cun lateral to Du-6, at the level of the lower border of the spinous process of T11.	Gastritis from deficiency; prolapsed stomach; nervous vomiting; indigestion; edema; weakness or heaviness of the limbs due to damp	• Tonifies Spleen Qi and Yang, Resolves Dampness, Raises Spleen Qi, Regulates and Harmonizes middle jiao.
Ub-21 **Weishu** *Stomach Shu* ↘ 0.5 – 0.8	1.5 cun lateral to the DU meridian, at the level of the lower border of the spinous process of T12.	Stomach ache; gastric distension; anorexia; regurged vomiting; abdominal pain from cold in ST; diarrhea; nausea	• **Regulates and Tonifies the Stomach:** for subduing ascending Stomach qi causing belching, hiccup, nausea and vomiting. • **Relieves food stagnation:** for food stagnation causing fullness of the epigastrium, sour regurgitation and belching.
Ub-22 **Sanjiaoshu** *Triple Burner Back Shu* ↓ 0.5 – 1.0	1.5 cun lateral to the Du-5, at the level of the lower border of the spinous process of L1.	Borborygmus; abdominal distention; indigestion; vomiting; diarrhea; dysentery; low back pain (local point); edema from urinary retention	• **Resolves Dampness and Opens the water passages:** for dampness, particularly in the lower burner causing urinary retention, painful urination, edema of the legs and any other manifestation of dampness in the lower burner.

Points	Location	Usage	Indications / Functions
Ub-23 Shenshu *Kidney Shu* ↓ 1.0 – 1.2	1.5 cun lateral to Du-4, at the level of the lower border of the spinous process of the L2.	Low back pain; nocturnal emission; impotence; irregular menstruation; weakness of the knee; dizziness; tinnitus; deafness; edema; diarrhea	• **Tonifies Kidney:** for any chronic Kidney deficiency. • **Nourishes Kidney Essence:** for impotence, nocturnal emissions, infertility, spermatorrhea and lack of sexual desire. Also used for chronic asthma due to Kidney not grasping the Lung Qi. Also used as a stimulus.
Ub-24 Qihaishu *Sea of Qi Shu* ↓ 0.8 – 1.2	1.5 cun lateral to the DU meridian, at the level of the lower border of the spinous process of L3.	Low back pain or sprain; irregular menstruation; dysmenorrhea; asthma	• Strengthen low back and unblocks the channels: a local point for low back weakness. • Regulates Qi and Blood: for blood stasis in the lower burner including uterine bleeding and irregular menstruation.
Ub-25 Dachangshu *Large Intestine Shu* ↓ 0.8 – 1.2	1.5 cun lateral to Du-3, at the level of the lower border of the spinous process of L4.	Low back pain; borborygmus; abdominal distention; diarrhea; constipation; numbness and motor impairment of lower extremities; sciatica	• **Promotes Large Intestine Function:** for both constipation and diarrhea and for chronic disease of the Large Intestine. • **Relieves fullness and swelling:** for excess patterns of the Large Intestine with abdominal fullness and distension. • **Strengthens low back:** a local point for acute lower backache.
Ub-26 Guanyuanshu *Origin Gate Shu* ↓ 0.8 – 1.2	1.5 cun lateral to the DU meridian, at the level of the lower border of the spinous process of L5.	Low back pain; abdominal distention; diarrhea; enuresis; urinary incontinence	• Strengthens back, Removes obstructions from the Channels: a local point for low backache.
Ub-27 Xiaochangshu *Small Intestine Shu* ↓ 0.8 – 1.2	1.5 cun lateral to the DU meridian, at the level of the lower border of the 1st posterior sacral foramen.	Lower abdominal pain and distention; dysentery; nocturnal emission; hematuria; sciatica; low back pain	• **Promotes Small Intestine Function:** for stimulating the receiving and separating functions of the Small Intestine, or any Small Intestine pattern causing borborygmus, abdominal pain and mucus in the stools. • **Resolves dampness, Clears Heat, benefits urination:** also to eliminate damp-heat from the lower burner and benefit urination to treat cloudy urination, difficult urination and burning, painful urination.
Ub-28 Pangguangshu *Bladder Shu* ↓ 0.8 – 1.2	1.5 cun lateral to the DU meridian, at the level of the 2nd posterior sacral foramen.	Incontinence; dark and rough flowing urine; swelling and pain in the genitals; sacral back pain; sciatica; good for UTIs; atonic bladder; prostate problems	• **Regulates the Bladder, Resolves Dampness:** for retention of urine, difficult urination and cloudy urine due to dampness. • **Clears Heat, stops pain:** for painful, burning urine, or pain due to renal stones. • **Opens the water passages:** improves transformation and excretion of dirty fluids in the lower burner and promotes dieresis. • **Strengthens lower back.**
Ub-29 Zhonglushu *Central Spine Shu* ↓ 0.8 – 1.2	1.5 cun lateral to the DU meridian, at the level of the 3rd posterior sacral foramen.	Anal disease; dysentery; stiffness and pain of lower back	• Benefits lumbar region, Dispels Cold, Stops diarrhea.
Ub-30 Baihuanshu *White Ring Shu* ↓ 0.8 – 1.2	1.5 cun lateral to the DU meridian, at the level of the 4th posterior sacral foramen.	Enuresis; pain due to hernia; leukorrhea; dysuria; cold sensation; rectum prolapse; constipation	• Strengthens lumbar region and legs, Regulates menses, Stops leakages: for hemorrhoids, prolapse of the anus, spasm of the anus, and incontinence of feces.
Ub-31 Shangliao *Upper Crevice* ↓ 0.8 – 1.2	In the 1st posterior sacral foramen.	Diseases of the lumbosacral joint; leukorrhea; peritonitis; orchitis; paralysis; paralysis of lower limb; sequelae of infantile paralysis; urinary problems; prolapsed uterus; constipation; infertility	• **Regulates the lower burner:** for genital disorders in men and women causing leukorrhea, prolapse of the uterus and sterility, impotence, orchitis and prostatitis. • **Strengthens the lumbar region and Nourishes the Kidneys:** for benefiting essence, and strengthening the low back and knees.

POINTS

Points	Location	Usage	Indications / Functions
Ub-32 **Ciliao** *Second Crevice* ↓ 0.8 – 1.2	In the 2nd posterior sacral foramen.	Low back pain; hernia; nocturnal emission; impotence; urinary problems; prolapsed uterus; constipation	• **Regulates the lower burner:** for genital disorders in men and women causing leukorrhea, prolapse of the uterus and sterility, impotence, orchitis and prostatitis. • **Strengthens the lumbar region and Nourishes the Kidneys:** for benefiting essence and strengthening the low back and knees. • Raises the Qi in prolapse of the anus or uterus.
Ub-33 **Zhongliao** *Central Crevice* ↓ 0.8 – 1.2	In the 3rd posterior sacral foramen.	Lower back pain; constipation; diarrhea; dysuria; irregular menstruation	• Regulates the lower burner: for genital disorders in men and women causing leukorrhea, prolapse of the uterus and sterility, impotence, orchitis and prostatitis. • Strengthen the lumbar region and Nourishes the Kidneys: for benefiting essence, and strengthening the low back and knees.
Ub-34 **Xialiao** *Lower Crevice* ↓ 0.8 – 1.2	In the 4th posterior sacral foramen.	Pain in lower back during menstruation; leukorrhea; impotence; diarrhea; hemorrhoids	• Regulates the lower burner: for genital disorders in men and women causing leukorrhea, prolapse of the uterus and sterility, impotence, orchitis and prostatitis. • Strengthens the lumbar region and Nourishes the Kidneys: for benefiting essence, and strengthening the low back and knees.
Ub-35 **Huiyang** *Meeting of Yang* ↓ 0.5 – 1.0	On either side of the tip of the coccyx, 0.5 cun lateral to the DU meridian.	Sciatica; paralysis of lower extremity	• Clears Damp-heat, Regulates lower jiao, Treats hemorrhoids.
Ub-36 **Chengfu** *Receiving Support* ↓ 1.0 – 1.5	In the middle of the transverse gluteal fold. Locate the point in the prone position.	Lower back and gluteal pain; constipation; muscular atrophy	• Opens the channels, Stops pain: used as a local point for sciatica with lower backache and pain radiating down the back of the leg.
Ub-37 **Yinmen** *Huge Gate* ↓ 1.0 – 2.0	6 cun below Ub-36 on the line joining Ub-36 and Ub-40.	Lower back and thigh pain; muscular atrophy; hemiplegia	• Opens the channels, Strengthens the lumbarspine, Stops pain: used as a local point for sciatica with pain radiating down the back of the leg.
Ub-38 **Fuxi** *Superficial Cleft* ↓ 0.5 – 1.0	1 cun above Ub-39 on the medial side of the tendon of muscle biceps femoris. The point is located with the knee slightly flexed.	Numbness of gluteal and femoral regions; contracture of popliteal fossa	• Relaxes the sinews, Strengthens the lumbarspine, Clears Heat.
Ub-39 **Weiyang** *Outside of the Crook* ↓ 0.5 – 1.0	Lateral to Ub-40, on the medial border of the tendon of muscle biceps femoris.	Low back pain; nephritis; cystitis; chyluria (white milky urine); spasms of gastrocnemius; any obstruction of urine flow (especially from dampness)	• Opens the water passages and stimulates the transformation and excretion of fluids in the lower burner: for all excess patterns of the lower burner with accumulation of fluids in the form of dampness or edema causing urinary retention, burning, painful urination, difficult urination, edema of the ankles. Also for lower burner deficiency causing incontinence of urine or enuresis.
Ub-40 **Weizhong** *Supporting Middle* ↓ 0.5 – 1.0 or bleed he-sea	Midpoint of the transverse crease of the popliteal fossa, between the tendons of muscle biceps femoris and muscle semitendinosus.	Heat exhaustion; low back pain; arthritis of the knee and other knee pain; paralysis of the knee; skin problems due to heat	• **Clears Heat and Resolves Dampness from the Bladder:** for burning urination. • **Relaxes the sinews and removes obstruction from the channel:** for both chronic and acute low backache, however, used primarily for acute pain. Ub-60 can be used in deficiency cases. Also, best used to treat unilateral or bilateral pain, but not for midline pain. • **Cools the Blood, eliminates blood stagnation:** for skin diseases caused by heat in the blood, and pain in the lower legs due to blood stasis. • **Clears Summer-heat:** for summer-heat attacks with fever, delirium and a red skin rash.

Points	Location	Usage	Indications / Functions
Ub-41 **Fufen** *Attached Branch* ↘ 0.3 – 0.5	3 cun lateral to the DU meridian, at the level of the lower border of the spinous process of T2, on the spinal border of the scapula.	Back pain; neck pain; shoulder stiffness and pain; elbow and arm numbness	• Opens the channels, Strengthens the lumbar and knees, Cools the blood, Clears Summer-heat, Stops pain.
Ub-42 **Pohu** *Door of the Corporeal Soul* ↘ 0.3 – 0.5	3 cun lateral to the DU meridian, at the level of the lower border of the spinous process of T3, on the spinal border of the scapula.	Pulmonary TB; cough; asthma; neck stiffness; hemoptysis	• **Regulates the descending of Lung Qi, Stops cough and asthma:** for coughing and wheezing due to rebellious Lung Qi. • For painful obstruction syndrome of the upper back and shoulders. • For emotional problems related to the Lungs causing sadness, grief and worry.
Ub-43 **Gaohuangshu** *Vital Region Shu* ↓ 0.3 – 0.5	3 cun lateral to the DU meridian, at the level of the lower border of the spinous process of T4, on the spinal border of the scapula.	For late stage chronic deficiency disorders; bronchitis; asthma; TB; neurasthenia (archaic - feeble; neurosis); general weakness caused by prolonged illness; consumptive diseases like HIV; pulmonary TB; poor memory indicating a weakened condition	• **Tonifies Qi, Strengthens Deficient Conditions:** for debilitating, chronic illness. • **Nourishes the Essence:** for Kidney deficiency causing nocturnal emissions, low sexual energy or poor memory. • **Nourishes Lung yin:** in the aftermath of chronic pulmonary disease where the Lung yin has been injured causing chronic dry cough and debility. • **Invigorates the Mind:** stimulates memory after a long-standing disease.
Ub-44 **Shentang** *Mind Hall* ↘ 0.3 – 0.5	3 cun lateral to the Du-11, at the level of the lower border of the spinous process of T5, on the spinal border of the scapula.	Cardiac palpitation and pain; stuffy chest; back stiffness and pain	• **Calms the Mind:** for emotional and psychological problems related to the Heart causing anxiety, insomnia and depression.
Ub-45 **Yixi** *Sighing Laughing Sound* ↘ 0.3 – 0.5	3 cun lateral to the Du-10, at the level of the lower border of the spinous process of T6, on the spinal border of the scapula.	Shoulder and back pain; cough; asthma	• Expels Wind, Clears Heat, Descends Lung Qi. • Moves Qi and Blood, Stops pain.
Ub-46 **Geguan** *Diaphragm Pass* ↘ 0.3 – 0.5	3 cun lateral to the Du-9, at the level of the lower border of the spinous process of T7, approximately level with inferior angle of the scapula.	Dysphagia; hiccups; belching	• Regulates diaphragm, Benefits the middle jiao. • Opens the Channels, Stops pain.
Ub-47 **Hunmen** *Door of the Ethereal Soul* ↘ 0.3 – 0.5	3 cun lateral to the Du-8, at the level of the lower border of the spinous process of T9.	Chest and hypochondriac pain; back pain; vomiting; diarrhea	• **Regulates Liver Qi:** combined with Ub-18 to eliminate Liver qi stagnation. • **Roots the Ethereal Soul:** for emotional problems related to the Liver manifesting as depression, frustration and resentment over a long period of time.
Ub-48 **Yanggang** *Yang's Key Link* ↘ 0.3 – 0.5	3 cun lateral to the Du-7, at the level of the lower border of the spinous process of T10.	Abdominal pain; diarrhea; jaundice; borborygmus	• Regulates Gallbladder, Clears damp-heat, Harmonizes the middle jiao.
Ub-49 **Yishe** *Thought Shelter* ↘ 0.3 – 0.5	3 cun lateral to the Du-6, at the level of the lower border of the spinous process of T11.	Abdominal distension; vomiting; diarrhea; difficult swallowing	• Tonifies Spleen, Stimulates memory and concentration: to tonify the mental aspect of the Spleen.
Ub-50 **Weicang** *Stomach Granary* ↘ 0.3 – 0.5	3 cun lateral to the DU meridian, at the level of the lower border of the spinous process of T12.	Infantile indigestion	• Harmonizes the middle jiao.
Ub-51 **Huangmen** *Vital Door* ↘ 0.3 – 0.5	3 cun lateral to the Du-5, at the level of the lower border of the spinous process of L1.	Abdominal pain; constipation; abdominal masses	• Regulates the Triple Burner: spreads the qi in the Heart region when there is a feeling of tightness below the heart.

POINTS

Points · Location		Usage	Indications / Functions
Ub-52 **Zhishi** Will Power Room ↓ 0.5 – 1.0	3 cun lateral to the Du-4, at the level of the lower border of the spinous process of L2.	Primary for sexual function; nephritis; low back pain; spermatorrhea; infertility (both sexes; but more for men); any sperm related problems; nocturnal emissions; prostatitis; secondary point for urinary dysfunction	• Tonifies Kidney, Strengthens low back: reinforces Ub-23. • Reinforces the will power: for depression that includes disorientation and lack of will power or mental strength to make efforts to get better.
Ub-53 **Baohuang** Bladder Vitals ↓ 0.8 – 1.2	3 cun lateral to the Du-5, at the level of the 2nd posterior sacral foramen.	Sciatica; lower back pain; borborygmus; urine retention; edema; abdominal distention	• Opens water passages: stimulates the transformation and excretion of dirty fluids in the lower jiao when there is retention of urine, difficult urination and burning urination. Spreads the qi in the lower jiao.
Ub-54 **Zhibian** Order's Limit ↓ 1.5 – 2.0	Lateral to the hiatus of the sacrum, at the level of the 4th posterior sacral foramen, 3 cun lateral to Du-2.	Lumbarosacral pain; muscular atrophy; dysuria; external genitalia swelling; hemorrhoids; constipation	• Local point for lower backache radiating to the buttocks and legs (along the bladder line).
Ub-55 **Heyang** Yang Union ↓ 0.7 – 1.0	2 cun directly below Ub-40, between the medial and lateral heads of the gastrocnemius muscle, on a line joining Ub-40 and Ub-57.	Low back pain; lower extremities paralysis and pain	• Opens the channels, Stops pain, Stops uterine bleeding, treats genital pain.
Ub-56 **Chengjin** Sinew Support ↓ 0.8 – 1.2	Midway between Ub-55 and Ub-57, on the line connecting Ub-40 and Ub-57, center of the gastrocnemius.	Pain in lower back and leg; sciatica with UB meridian pain in leg; hemorrhoids; spasms of gastrocnemius; charley horses	• Relaxes sinews, Opens the Channels, Stops pain, Benefits the foot and heel.
Ub-57 **Chengshan** Supporting Mountain ↓ 0.8 – 1.2	Directly below the belly of muscle gastrocnemius, on a line joining Ub-40 and Ub-60, about 8 cun below Ub-40.	Hemorrhoids; pain in lower back and leg with leg weakness; beriberi; rheumatoid arthritis (controversial)	• **Relaxes sinews:** for cramps of the gastrocnemius and muscles of the lower leg. • **Invigorates the Blood:** for menstrual pain or blood in the stools caused by blood stasis. • **Unblocks the Channels:** used as a distal point for lower backache and sciatica. Also frequently used as an empirical distal point for treatment of hemorrhoids.
Ub-58 **Feiyang** Flying Up ↓ 0.7 – 1.0 luo-connect	7 cun directly above Ub-60, on the posterior border of the fibula, about 1 cun inferior and lateral to Ub-57.	Headache; hemorrhoids; pain in lower back and leg with leg weakness; rheumatoid arthritis (controversial)	• **Removes obstructions from the channel:** a distal point for lower backache and sciatica. Also an empirical distal point for treatment of hemorrhoids.
Ub-59 **Fuyang** Instep Yang ↓ 0.5 – 1.0	3 cun directly above Ub-60.	Headache; low back pain; paralysis of lower limb; inflammation of ankle joint; heavy sensation in the head	• Unblocks the Channels: a distal point for lower backache, particularly in chronic cases with weakness of the leg and back. It is effective only in unilateral backache.
Ub-60 **Kunlun** Kunlun Mountains ↓ 0.5 – 1.0 jing-river	In the depression between the external malleolus and tendo calcaneus.	Pain in ankle and foot; plantar fasciitis (stretch; ice feet; needle other local points all way up to calf); paralysis of lower limb; headache; blurry vision; neck rigidity; difficult labor	• **Expels Wind, Unblocks the Channels:** for painful obstruction syndrome of the shoulder, neck and head due to externally contracted wind or internal wind attacking the upper part of the body. For chronic backache of the deficiency type. Also for headaches of the occiput and head from Kidney deficiency. • **Invigorates the Blood:** for menstrual problems due to blood stasis with painful periods and dark clotted blood.

Points	Location	Usage	Indications / Functions
Ub-61 **Pucan** *Servant's Partaking* ↓ 0.3 – 0.5	Posterior and inferior to the external malleolus, directly below Ub-60, in the depression lateral to calcaneus at the junction of the red and white skin.	Headache (lateral and midline); Meniere's disease; seizures; psychosis and mania; hemiplegia; arthritis; low back pain; epilepsy	• Relaxes sinews, Opens the Channels, Stops pain.
Ub-62 **Shenmai** *Extending Vessel* ↓ 0.3 – 0.5	In the depression directly below the external malleolus.	Epilepsy; mania; dizziness; insomnia; backache	• **Unblocks the Channels:** for chronic backache. • **Relaxes the tendons and muscles of the outer leg:** for muscle tension in the outer part of the leg. • **Benefits the eyes:** for dryness of the eyes. • **Clears the Mind and Expels Interior Wind:** for epilepsy with attacks occurring mostly in the daytime.
Ub-63 **Jinmen** *Golden Door* ↓ 0.3 – 0.5 xi-cleft	1 cun anterior and inferior to Ub-62, in the depression lateral to the lower border of the cuboid bone.	Mania; epilepsy; infantile convulsion; motor impairment and pain of lower extremities; sometimes used for bladder incontinence	• Clears Heat, Stops pain: for acute Bladder patterns with frequent and burning urination.
Ub-64 **Jinggu** *Capital Bone* ↓ 0.3 – 0.5 yuan	Below the tuberosity of the 5th metatarsal bone, at the junction of the red and white skin.	Headache; neck rigidity; blurring vision; pain in the lower back	• Clears heat from the Bladder: for burning painful urination. • Eliminates Interior Wind: for epilepsy. • Strengthens back: for chronic lower backache.
Ub-65 **Shugu** *Binding Bone* ↓ 0.3 – 0.5 shu-stream	Posterior to the head of the 5th metatarsophalangeal joint, at the junction of the red and white skin.	Mania; backache; headache; neck rigidity; blurry vision	• **Unblocks the Channels:** used as a distal point for any problem along the Bladder channel particularly if affecting the head. For painful obstruction syndrome of the neck. • **Clears Heat:** for heat in the Bladder, acute cystitis. • **Eliminates Interior Wind:** for epilepsy or the beginning stages of wind-cold attack with headache and stiff neck.
Ub-66 **Zutonggu** *Foot Connecting Valley* ↓ 0.2 – 0.3 ying-spring	In the depression anterior to the 5th metatarsophalangeal joint.	Headache; neck rigidity; blurring vision; mania	• Clears Heat: for Bladder heat in acute cases of cystitis. Also for beginning stages of wind-heat in the defensive qi level with fever, headache and stiff neck.
Ub-67 **Zhiyin** *Reaching Yin* ↘ 0.1 jing-well	On the lateral side of the small toe, 0.1 cun posterior to the corner of the nail	Headaches; malposition of fetus and difficult labor (needle and moxa); feverish sensation in the sole; nasal obstruction; epistaxis	• **Expels Wind:** for both interior and exterior wind, especially when there is headache. • **Unblocks the channel:** for channel disorders causing blurred vision or pain in the eye. • Used empirically for malposition of the fetus (breech). This is done in the 8th month of pregnancy by burning moxa cones on each side once a day for 10 days.

POINTS

POINTS

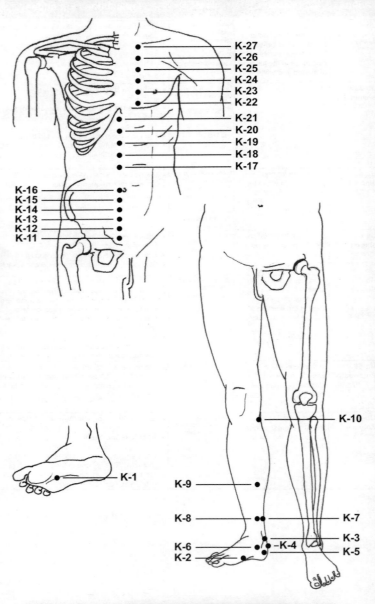

Jing Well	Ying Spring	Shu Stream	Jing River	He Sea
1	2	3	7	10
Yuan	Luo-connect	Xi-Cleft	Front Mu	Back Shu
3	4	5	Gb-25	Ub-23

Points	Location	Usage	Indications / Functions
K-1 **Yongquan** *Bubbling Spring* ↓ 0.3 – 0.5 jing-well	On the sole, between 2nd and 3rd toes, in the depression when the foot is in plantar flexion, approximately at the junction of the anterior third and posterior 2/3 of the sole.	Shock; heat exhaustion; stroke; open the orifices and help with loss of voice; hypertension from excess; seizures; infantile convulsions; vertex headache (Liv yang rising); hot soles of the feet; whole body muscle cramping	• **Tonifies Kidney yin, Clears deficiency heat:** for yin deficiency with heat signs. • **Subdue Interior Wind:** for epilepsy, descend liver yang or liver wind. • Restores consciousness.
K-2 **Rangu** *Blazing Valley* ↓ 0.3 – 0.5 ying-spring	Anterior and inferior to the medial malleolus, in the depression of the lower border of the tuberosity of the navicular bone.	Chronic excess and recurring pharyngitis; irregular menstruation due to heat or damp-heat; thirst from diabetes; diarrhea with damp-heat; itching in genital region; plantar fasciitis	• **Clears deficiency heat:** for Kidney yin deficiency heat causing malar flush, feelings of heat in the evening, mental restlessness, thirst without desire to drink and dry throat and mouth at night. Also used to clear excess heat and heat in the blood.
K-3 **Taixi** *Greater Stream* ↓ 0.3 – 0.5 shu-stream, yuan	In the depression between the medial malleolus and tendo calcaneus, at the level of the tip of the medial malleolus.	Nephritis; cystitis; irregular menstruation; spermatorrhea; enuresis; tinnitus; alopecia; impotence; constipation and diarrhea if Kid involved; yin type insomnia; low back pain; knee pain; asthma if Kid deficient	• **Tonifies Kidney, Benefits the Essence:** for any deficiency pattern of Kidney yin, yang, or essence. • **Regulates the uterus:** for irregular periods, amenorrhea and excessive uterine bleeding. • **Strengthens low back and knees.**
K-4 **Dazhong** *Big Bell* ↓ 0.3 – 0.5 luo-connect	Posterior and inferior to the medial malleolus, in the depression medial to the attachment of tendo calcaneus.	Plantar fasciitis; bone spurs	• **Strengthens the back:** for chronic backache from Kidney deficiency. • **Lifts the Spirit:** for exhaustion and depression from chronic Kidney deficiency.
K-5 **Shuiquan** *Water Spring* ↓ 0.3 – 0.5 xi-cleft	1 cun directly below K-3 in the depression anterior and superior to the medial side of the tuberosity of the calcaneus.	Amenorrhea; irregular menstruation; dysmenorrhea; uterus prolapse; dysuria; blurry vision	• **Benefits urination, Stops pain in the Abdomen:** for acute cystitis, urethritis, or pain around the umbilicus. • **Regulates the uterus:** for amenorrhea due to Kidney deficiency.
K-6 **Zhaohai** *Shining Sea* ↓ 0.3 – 0.5	In the depression of the lower border of the medial malleolus, or 1 cun below the medial malleolus.	Irregular menstruation; uterus prolapse; chronic pharyngitis; tonsillitis; epileptic seizures that occur more at night; deficient yin asthma; constipation; insomnia; dry throat; eye pain from dryness; vaginal discharge like chronic leukorrhea; vaginal dryness (menopause or other); major for yin deficiency	• **Nourishes the Yin:** for any yin deficiency patterns with dry throat and dry eyes. • **Benefits the eyes:** for chronic eye diseases, particularly in the elderly with yin deficiency. • **Calms the Mind:** for restlessness, insomnia, irritability due to yin deficiency. • **Cools the Blood:** for skin diseases caused by heat in the blood. • **Regulates the uterus:** for amenorrhea and prolapse of the uterus due to kidney deficiency. • Opens the chest: for chest pain, circulate qi in the chest when combined with Pc-6.
K-7 **Fuliu** *Returning Current* ↓ 0.5 – 0.7 jing-river	2 cun directly above K-3, on the anterior border of tendo calcaneus.	Leukorrhea; any urinary problems; night sweats; URI sweat or lack of sweat; low back pain; edema with Sp-9; good for ankle edema	• **Tonifies Kidney:** similar to K-3, but is better for Kidney yang. • **Resolves Dampness in the lower jiao:** for edema in the legs. • **Regulates Sweating:** to either promote (with LI-4) or stop sweating (with Ht-6) for night sweats or spontaneous sweats.

POINTS

Points	Location	Usage	Indications / Functions
K-8 **Jiaoxin** *Exchange Belief* ↓ 0.5 – 0.7	0.5 cun anterior to K-7, 2 cun posterior to the medial border of the tibia.	Irregular menstruation; uterus prolapse; uterine bleeding; diarrhea; constipation; pain and swelling of testis	• Unblocks the Channels, Stops pain, Removes Masses: to eliminate obstructions along the vessel and dissolve abdominal masses due to stagnation of qi or blood, and to stop abdominal pain. • Regulates menses: for menstrual problems due to blood stasis.
K-9 **Zhubin** *Guest Building* ↓ 0.5 – 0.7	5 cun directly above K-3 at the lower end of the belly of muscle gastrocnemius, on the line drawn from K-3 to K-10.	Mental disorders; hernia; lower leg and foot pain	• **Clears the Mind, Tonifies Kidney yin:** for deep anxiety and mental restlessness caused by Kidney yin deficiency. It also tonifies yin. • **Opens the chest:** for relaxing feeling of oppression in the chest, often with palpitations as with Heart and Kidneys not harmonized.
K-10 **Yingu** *Yin Valley* ↓ 0.8 – 1.0 he-sea	When the knee is flexed, the point is on the medial side of the popliteal fossa, between the tendons of muscle semitendinosus and semimembranosus, level with Ub-40.	Diseases of urogenital system; dysuria; arthritis of knee in medial area; important for water balance	• **Expels Dampness in the lower jiao:** for urinary symptoms such as urinary difficulty, painful urination, and frequency of urination. • Nourishes Kidney yin.
K-11 **Henggu** *Pubic Bone* ↓ 0.5 – 1.0	5 cun below the umbilicus, on the superior border of the symphysis pubis, 0.5 cun lateral to Ren-2.	Fullness and pain of the lower abdomen; dysuria; enuresis; nocturnal emission; impotence	• Benefits lower jiao.
K-12 **Dahe** *Great Manifestation* ↓ 0.5 – 1.0	4 cun below the umbilicus, 0.5 cun lateral to Ren-3.	Nocturnal emission; impotence; uterus prolapse; external genitalia pain	• Tonifies Kidney, Nourishes the Essence.
K-13 **Qixue** *Qi Hole* ↓ 0.5 – 1.0	3 cun below the umbilicus, 0.5 cun lateral to Ren-4.	Irregular menstruation; dysmenorrhea; dysuria; abdominal pain; diarrhea	• Tonifies Kidney, Nourishes the Essence. • Unblocks the Channel: for circulation of Qi and blood in the abdomen, removing masses and obstructions in the abdomen and chest. For excess patterns with abdominal fullness and masses.
K-14 **Siman** *Fourfold Fullness* ↓ 0.5 – 1.0	2 cun below the umbilicus, 0.5 cun lateral to Ren-5.	Abdominal distension pain; diarrhea; nocturnal emission; irregular menstruation; postpartum abdominal pain	• Strengthens lower jiao, Stops pain. • Regulates Qi, Moves blood stagnation. • Regulates water passages, Promotes urination.
K-15 **Zhongzhu** *Central Flow* ↓ 0.5 – 1.0	1 cun below the umbilicus, 0.5 cun lateral to Ren-7.	Irregular menstruation; abdominal pain; constipation	• Strengthens lower jiao and Intestines.
K-16 **Huangshu** *Vitals Transporting Point* ↓ 0.5 – 1.0	0.5 cun lateral to the umbilicus, level with Ren-8.	Habitual constipation with firm and difficult-to-pass stool (need to nourish yin); hiccups; vomiting; dry constipation point	• **Tonifies Kidneys, Benefits the Heart, Calms the Mind:** for Kidney yin deficiency failing to nourish the Heart.
K-17 **Shangqu** *Shang Bend* ↓ 0.5 – 1.0	2 cun above the umbilicus, 0.5 cun lateral to Ren-10.	Irregular menstruation; abdominal pain; constipation; diarrhea	• Dispels accumulation, Stops pain.
K-18 **Shiguan** *Stone Pass* ↓ 0.5 – 1.0	3 cun above the umbilicus, 0.5 cun lateral to Ren-11.	Vomiting; abdominal pain; constipation; sterility	• Strengthens lower jiao, Stops pain. • Regulates Qi, Moves blood stagnation, Harmonizes Stomach.
K-19 **Yindu** *Yin Metropolis* ↓ 0.5 – 1.0	4 cun above the umbilicus, 0.5 cun lateral to Ren-12.	Borborygmus; abdominal pain; constipation; vomiting	• Regulates Qi, Harmonizes Stomach, Stops coughing and wheezing.

POINTS

Points	Location	Usage	Indications / Functions
K-20 **Futonggu** *Abdomen Connecting Valley* ↓ 0.5 – 1.0	5 cun above the umbilicus, 0.5 cun lateral to Ren-13.	Abdominal distension and pain; indigestion; vomiting	• Harmonizes the middle, Unblocks the chest.
K-21 **Youmen** *Dark Gate* ↓ 0.3 – 0.7 avoid liver & deep puncture	6 cun above the umbilicus, 0.5 cun lateral to Ren-14.	Abdominal distension and pain; indigestion; vomiting; diarrhea; morning sickness	• Spreads Liver Qi, Benefits the chest, Tonifies Spleen, Harmonizes the Stomach.
K-22 **Bulang** *Walking Corridor* ↘ 0.3 – 0.5 avoid lung, liver & deep puncture	In the 5th intercostal space, 2 cun lateral to the Ren meridian.	Cough; asthma; fullness and distension of the chest; vomiting; anorexia	• Unblocks the chest, Subdues rebellious Qi.
K-23 **Shenfeng** *Mind Seal* ↘ 0.3 – 0.7 avoid lung, liver, heart, & deep puncture	In the 4th intercostal space, 2 cun lateral to the Ren meridian.	Cough; asthma; fullness and distension of the chest; mastitis	• Unbinds the chest, Subdues rebellious Qi, Benefits the breast.
K-24 **Lingxu** *Spirit Burial Ground* ↘ 0.3 – 0.7 avoid lung, liver, heart, & deep puncture	In the 3rd intercostal space, 2 cun lateral to the Ren meridian.	Cough; asthma; fullness and distension of the chest; mastitis	• Unbinds the chest, Subdues rebellious Qi, Benefits the breast.
K-25 **Shencang** *Mind Storage* ↘ 0.3 – 0.7 avoid lung, liver, heart, & deep puncture	In the 2nd intercostal space, 2 cun lateral to the Ren meridian.	Cough; asthma; chest pain	• Unbinds the chest, Subdues rebellious Qi, Benefits the breast.
K-26 **Yuzhong** *Comfortable Chest* ↘ 0.3 – 0.7 avoid lung, liver, heart, & deep puncture	In the 1st intercostal space, 2 cun lateral to the Ren meridian.	Cough; asthma; phlegm accumulation; fullness and distension of the chest	• Unbinds the chest, Benefits the breast, Transforms Phlegm.
K-27 **Shufu** *Transporting point Mansion* ↘ 0.3 – 0.7	In the depression on the lower border of the clavicle, 2 cun lateral to the Ren meridian.	Cough; asthma; chest pain	• **Stimulates Kidney Function of Reception of Qi** • **Subdues rebellious Qi:** used to stops cough and calm asthma. • **Resolves Phlegm:** a local point for treatment of asthma due to Kidney deficiency.

POINTS

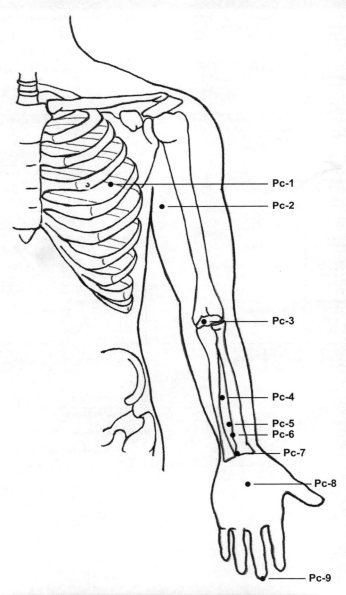

Pc-1
Pc-2
Pc-3
Pc-4
Pc-5
Pc-6
Pc-7
Pc-8
Pc-9

Jing Well	Ying Spring	Shu Stream	Jing River	He Sea
9	8	7	5	3
Yuan	Luo-connect	Xi-Cleft	Front Mu	Back Shu
7	6	4	Ren-17	Ub-14

Points	Location	Usage	Indications / Functions
Pc-1 **Tianchi** *Heavenly Pool* ↘ 02 – 0.4 avoid deep puncture	In the 4th intercostal space, 1 cun lateral to the nipple, 5 cun lateral to anterior midline.	Intercostal neuralgia; pain and swelling under the axilla; mastitis; insufficient lactation	• Local point for distension and pain of the breast caused by Liver qi stagnation.
Pc-2 **Tianquan** *Heavenly Spring* ↓ 0.5 – 0.7	2 cun below the level of the anterior axillary fold, between the two heads of the muscle biceps brachii.	Pain along the upper aspect of the arm; local for chest	• Unblocks the chest, Moves blood, Stops pain.
Pc-3 **Quze** *Marsh on Bend* ↓ 0.5 – 1.0 or bleed	On the transverse cubital crease, at the ulnar side of the tendon of muscle biceps brachii.	Acute gastritis and gastroenteritis; easily startled; pain along the arm; mostly for gastric problems; cardiac pain; palpitation; febrile diseases; tremor of the hand and arm	• **Pacifies the Stomach, Clears Heat, Cools the Blood:** for heat in the Qi level including acute sun stroke and heat in the intestines. Clears heat and cools blood in the blood level including late stages of febrile diseases with skin eruptions and convulsions. Also promotes descending of Stomach qi which is causing nausea and vomiting. • **Opens the Heart:** for loss of consciousness due to heat in the Pericardium obstructing the Heart orifice. • **Invigorates the Blood, Dispels Blood Stasis:** for excessive menstrual bleeding, stagnant blood giving rise to uterine fibroids. • **Calms the Mind:** for severe anxiety caused by Heart fire.
Pc-4 **Ximen** *Cleft Door* ↓ 0.5 – 1.0 xi-cleft	5 cun above the transverse crease of the wrist, on the line connecting Pc-3 and Pc-7, between the tendons of palmaris longus and flexor carpi radialis	Myocarditis; angina pectoris; palpitations (most are from deficiency); irritability and acute pain in the chest due to deficiency; angina; clears the heart channel and stops pain	• **Unblocks the Channels, Regulates Blood, Stop Pain:** for acute arrhythmias and palpitations, and chest pain due to stagnant qi and blood. • **Cools the Blood:** for skin diseases caused by blood heat. • **Strengthens the Mind:** for Heart deficiency causing fear and lack of mental strength.
Pc-5 **Jianshi** *Intermediate Messenger* ↓ 0.5 – 1.0	3 cun above the transverse crease of the wrist between the tendons of palmaris longus and flexor carpi radialis	Cardiac pain; palpitation; stomachache; malaria; mental disorders; contracture of the elbow and arm; seizures with drooling; hysteria; psychosis; clears insubstantial phlegm	• **Resolve Phlegm, Regulate the Heart, Open the Heart Orifice**: for non-substantial phlegm obstructing the Heart and misting the mental faculties resulting in delirium, aphasia and coma often associated with heat in the blood level, also causing mental illness, manic depression, and reckless behavior. Epilepsy with loss of consciousness due to phlegm misting the orifice. • **Regulates Heart Qi:** dispels stagnation of qi in the chest. • Subdues rebellious Stomach qi causing nausea and vomiting. • Clears Heart-fire causing insomnia, tongue ulcers, bitter taste, dry mouth and mental agitation. • **Empirical point for malaria.**
Pc-6 **Neiguan** *Inner Gate* ↓ 0.5 – 0.8 luo-connect	2 cun above the transverse crease of the wrist, between the tendons of palmaris longus and flexor carpi radialis	Angina pectoris; chest pain; stuffiness in chest; pain in hypochondrium; asthma; nausea or vomiting; opens the chest; stomachache; any kind of upper abdominal pain; spasms of the diaphragm; cough; seizures; hysteria; irritability; insomnia; nervousness; malaria; mental disorders	• **Opens the chest:** for any chest problems. Regulates Qi and blood in the chest to treat stasis of qi and blood causing pain in the chest. • **Calms the Mind:** for irritability due to Liver qi stagnation, especially when there is anxiety due to a Heart pattern. Treats pre-menstrual depression and irritability and promotes sleep. • **Harmonizes the Stomach:** subdues rebellious Stomach qi and stops nausea and vomiting. Also for epigastric pain, acid regurgitation, hiccup and belching. • **Regulates the Triple Burner:** for neck ache on the occiput. • **Regulates Blood:** regulate irregular or painful menses.

POINTS

Points	Location	Usage	Indications / Functions
Pc-7 **Daling** *Great Hill* ↓ 0.3 – 0.5 yuan	In the middle of the transverse crease of the wrist, between the tendons of muscle palmaris longus and flexor carpi radialis.	Palpitations; gastritis with heat and anxiety; intercostal neuralgia; mental illness	• **Calms the Mind:** for stabilizing emotions. • **Clears Heat:** for Heart-fire causing anxiety and mental restlessness or manic behavior.
Pc-8 **Laogong** *Palace of Toil* ↓ 0.3 – 0.5	On the transverse crease and center of the palm, between the 2nd and 3rd metacarpal bones. When the fist is clenched, the point is just below the tip of the middle finger.	Heat exhaustion; cardiac pain; yin exhaustion; stomatitis; foul breath; ulcerated oral cavity; hysteria and mental illness due to heat; excessive sweating of palms	• **Clears Heart-fire:** for all symptoms of Heart-fire including tongue ulcers, mental symptoms, or high fever and delirium.
Pc-9 **Zhongchong** *Center Rush* ↓ 0.1 or bleed	In the center of the tip of the middle finger.	Shock; apoplectic coma; main jing well point for returning consciousness	• Clears Heat: for chronic conditions with mental symptoms, or in acute cases of exterior heat at the qi or nutritive qi level. • Expels interior Wind and restores consciousness: for wind-stroke.

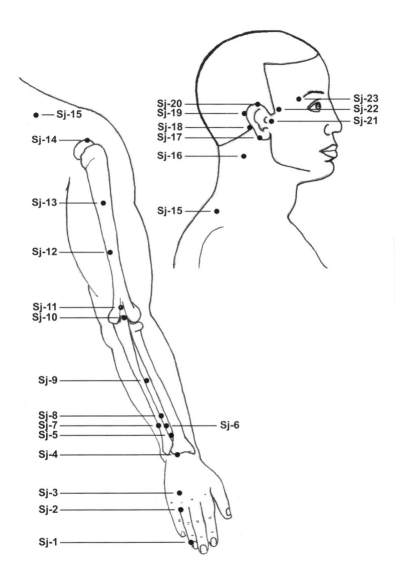

Sj-15

Sj-14

Sj-13

Sj-12

Sj-11
Sj-10

Sj-9

Sj-8
Sj-7
Sj-5

Sj-4

Sj-3

Sj-2

Sj-1

Sj-6

Sj-20
Sj-19
Sj-18
Sj-17
Sj-16
Sj-15

Sj-23
Sj-22
Sj-21

POINTS

Jing Well	Ying Spring	Shu Stream	Jing River	He Sea
1	2	3	6	10
Yuan	**Luo-connect**	**Xi-Cleft**	**Front Mu**	**Back Shu**
4	5	7	Ren-5	Ub-22

Points	Location	Usage	Indications / Functions
Sj-1 **Guanchong** *Gate Rush* ↓ 0.1 or bleed jing-well	On the lateral side of the ring finger, about .1 cun posterior to the corner of the nail.	Headache; red eyes; sore throat; febrile diseases; irritability; stiff tongue	• Clears Heat, Expels Wind: for invasion of exterior wind-heat causing fever, sore throat or earache. For both Taiyang and Shaoyang disorders. • Restores Consciousness: for acute stage of wind-stroke. • For painful and stiff shoulder joint.
Sj-2 **Yemen** *Fluid Door* ↘ 0.3 – 0.5 ying-spring	When the fist is clenched, the point is located in the depression proximal to the margin of the web between the ring and small fingers.	Pain and swelling of the fingers; sudden deafness; sore throat; malaria; headache; red eyes	• Clears Heat, Expels Wind, Benefits the ear: for invasion of exterior wind-heat causing earache due to infection of the middle ear, tinnitus, or deafness due to liver fire. • Unblocks the Channels: for painful obstruction syndrome of the fingers.
Sj-3 **Zhongzhu** *Middle Islet* ↓ 0.3 – 0.5 shu-stream	When the fist is clenched, the point is on the dorsum of the hand between the 4th and 5th metacarpal bones, in the depression proximal to the 4th metacarpophalangeal joint.	Tinnitus; deafness; headache; red eyes; elbow and arm pain	• **Clears Heat, Expels Wind, Benefits the ear:** for invasions of exterior wind-heat causing earache due to infection of the middle ear, tinnitus, or deafness due to liver fire. • **Unblocks the Channels:** for painful obstruction syndrome of the fingers. • **Regulates Qi:** for Liver qi stagnation causing hypochondriac pain and mood swings. Also lifts depression caused by Liver qi stagnation.
Sj-4 **Yangchi** *Yang Pool* ↓ 0.3 – 0.5 yuan	On the transverse crease of the dorsum of the wrist, in the depression lateral to the tendon of muscle extensor digitorum communis.	Pain and diseases of the soft tissues of wrist; carpal tunnel syndrome; malaria; deafness; thirst	• **Relaxes sinews, Unblocks the Channels:** for painful obstruction syndrome of the arm and shoulder. Also for headaches of the occiput due to exterior invasion of wind. • **Regulates the Stomach:** used in combination with St-42, tonifies the Stomach. • Transforms congested fluids. • Benefits Original Qi, Tonifies Penetrating and Directing Vessels: for all chronic diseases when the Kidneys have become deficient and energy is weakened. Also for irregular periods and amenorrhea.
Sj-5 **Waiguan** *Outer Gate* ↓ 0.5 – 1.0 luo-connect	2 cun above Sj-4, between the radius and the ulna.	Common colds; high fever (shao yang); tinnitus; temporal migraines; lateral stiff neck; hemiplegia; pain in joints; controlling point for the hand and opens up qi circulation to the hand; (master point of yang wei)	• **Release the Exterior, Expels Wind-heat:** for fever, sore throat, slight sweating, aversion to cold and a floating, rapid pulse. Used in taiyang wind-heat, Qi level heat, and shaoyang stage disorders with alternating fever and chills, irritability, hypochondriac pain, bitter taste, blurred vision and a wiry pulse. • **Unblocks the Channels:** for painful obstruction syndrome of the arm, shoulder and neck. • **Benefits the ear:** for ear infection from invasion of exterior wind-heat or tinnitus and deafness from liver fire or liver yang rising. • **Subdues Liver yang:** distal point to treat migraine headaches on the temples from liver yang rising.
Sj-6 **Zhigou** *Branching Ditch* ↓ 0.8 – 1.2 jing-river	3 cun above Sj-4, between the radius and the ulna, on the radial side of muscle extensor digitorum.	Intercostal neuralgia; constipation; shingles; herpes zoster; skin disorders	• **Regulates Qi:** used to regulate qi in the three burners and removes stagnation of Liver qi (combine with Gb-34). • Clears Heat: for qi level invasions of heat when there is constipation and abdominal pain. • **Expels Wind-heat:** for wind-heat in the blood affecting the skin and skin diseases from wind characterized by red rashes and hives that come and go or move quickly, including urticaria (combine with Gb-31). Used as a major point for herpes zoster, especially when the eruptions are on the flanks.

Points	Location	Usage	Indications / Functions
Sj-7 **Huizong** *Ancestral Meeting* ↓ 0.5 – 1.0 xi-cleft	At the level of Sj-6, about 1 finger breadth lateral to Sj-6, on the radial side of the ulna.	Ear pain; deafness; arm pain	• For excess patterns to stop pain. It acts on pain in the ears, temples and eyebrows.
Sj-8 **Sanyangluo** *Connecting Three Yang* ↓ 0.5 – 1.0	4 cun above Sj-4, between the radius and the ulna.	Pain in the arm involving all three arm meridians; pain in forearm inhibiting movement; toothache; deafness; sudden voice loss	• Clears Heat, Unblocks the Channels: for painful obstruction syndrome of the arm, neck, shoulders and occiput. Particularly useful when the pain involves more than one channel on the yang surface of the arm and shoulders. It relaxes sinews and relieves pain and stiffness.
Sj-9 **Sidu** *Four Rivers* ↓ 0.5 – 1.0	On the lateral side of the forearm, 5 cun below the olecranon, between the radius and the ulna.	Deafness; migraine; forearm pain	• Unblocks the Channels, Stops pain.
Sj-10 **Tianjing** *Heavenly Well* ↓ 0.3 – 0.5 he-sea	When the elbow is flexed, the point is in the depression about 1 cun superior to the olecranon.	Diseases of the soft tissue of the elbow	• **Relaxes tendons:** for painful obstruction syndrome along the channel, especially of the elbow. • **Resolves Phlegm and Dampness, Dispels Masses:** for external invasions of damp-heat causing swelling of glands and tonsils. • **Regulates Nutritive and Defensive Qi:** for invasions of exterior wind-cold to stop sweating and release the exterior.
Sj-11 **Qinglengyuan** *Clear Cold Abyss* ↓ 0.3 – 0.5	1 cun above Sj-10 when the elbow is flexed.	Shoulder and arm motor impairment and pain; migraine	• Unblocks the Channels, Dispels Wind-Damp, Clears damp-heat.
Sj-12 **Xiaoluo** *Dispersing Riverbed* ↓ 0.5 – 0.7	On the line joining the olecranon and Sj-14, midway between Sj-11 and Sj-13.	Headache; neck stiffness; arm pain and motor impairment	• Unblocks the Channels, Stops pain.
Sj-13 **Naohui** *Upper Arm Convergence* ↓ 0.5 – 0.8	On the line joining Sj-14 and the olecranon, on the posterior border of muscle deltoidus.	Goiter; shoulder and arm pain	• Unblocks the Channels, Stops pain, Regulates Qi, Transforms Phlegm.
Sj-14 **Jianliao** *Shoulder Crevice* ↓ 0.7 – 1.0	Posterior and inferior to the acromion, in the depression about 1 cun posterior to LI-15 when the arm is abducted.	Shoulder and upper arm pain and impairment	• **Dispels Wind-Damp, Stops pain, Benefits the shoulder joint:** for painful obstruction syndrome of the shoulder.
Sj-15 **Tianliao** *Heavens Bone Hole* ↓ 0.3 – 0.5	Midway between Gb-21 and SI-13, on the superior angle of the scapula.	Shoulder and elbow pain; stiff neck	• Dispels Wind-Damp, Unblocks the channels, Stops pain.
Sj-16 **Tianyou** *Window of Heaven* ↓ 0.3 – 0.5	Posterior and inferior to the mastoid process, level with mandibular angle, on the posterior border of SCM, almost level with SI-17 and Ub-10.	Tinnitus; deafness; lymphatic swellings around neck	• Benefits the head and sensory organs, Regulates Qi.
Sj-17 **Yifeng** *Wind Screen* ↓ 0.5 – 1.0	Posterior to the lobule of the ear, in the depression between the mandible and the mastoid process.	All ear problems; tinnitus; parotitis; locked jaw; facial paralysis; most important local point for ear; dizziness involving ear problems	• **Benefits the ears:** for all ear problems of exterior or interior origin. Used in ear infections caused by exterior wind-heat, or for deafness and tinnitus from rising of liver yang or liver fire. • **Expels Wind:** for exterior wind causing trigeminal neuralgia and facial paralysis.

POINTS

Points	Location	Usage	Indications / Functions
Sj-18 **Qimai** *Spasm Vessel* ↓ 0.3 – 0.5 or bleed	In the center of the mastoid process, at the junction of the middle and lower 1/3 of the curve formed by Sj-17 and Sj-20 posterior to the helix.	Tinnitus; headache; deafness; infantile convulsion	• Benefits the ears. • Expels Wind.
Sj-19 **Luxi** *Skull Rest* ↘ 0.3 – 0.5	Posterior to the ear, at the junction of the upper and middle 1/3 of the curve formed by Sj-17 and Sj-20 posterior to the helix.	Headache; tinnitus; deafness; infantile convulsion	• Benefits the ears, Clears Heat. • Expels Wind.
Sj-20 **Jiaosun** *Angle Vertex* sub-↓ 0.3 – 0.5	Directly above the ear apex, within the hair line.	Parotitis; toothache; tinnitus	• Benefits the ears, teeth, gums, and lip. • Clears Heat. • Expels Wind.
Sj-21 **Ermen** *Ear Door* ↓ 0.3 – 0.5	In the depression anterior to the supratragic notch and slightly superior to the condyloid process of the mandible. The point is located with the mouth open.	Tinnitus; otitis media; pus in ear; temporomandibular joint problems	• **Benefits the ears, Clears Heat:** local point for tinnitus caused by liver yang rising.
Sj-22 **Erheliao** *Ear Bone Hole* ↘ 0.1 – 0.3 avoid artery	Anterior and superior to Sj-21, level with the root of the auricle, on the posterior border of the hairline of the temple where the superficial temporal artery passes.	Tinnitus; locked jaw; migraine; check for TMJ	• Expels Wind, Stops pain.
Sj-23 **Sizhukong** *Silk Bamboo Hole* sub-↓ 0.3 – 0.5	In the depression at the lateral end of the eyebrow.	Redness and pain of the eye; blurry vision; headache; twitching eyelid; facial paralysis	• Expels Wind, Stops pain, Benefits the eye: local point for eye problems and headache around the outer corner of the eyebrow, especially when due to liver yang rising. Also for facial paralysis when there is inability to raise the outer corner of the eyebrow.

POINTS

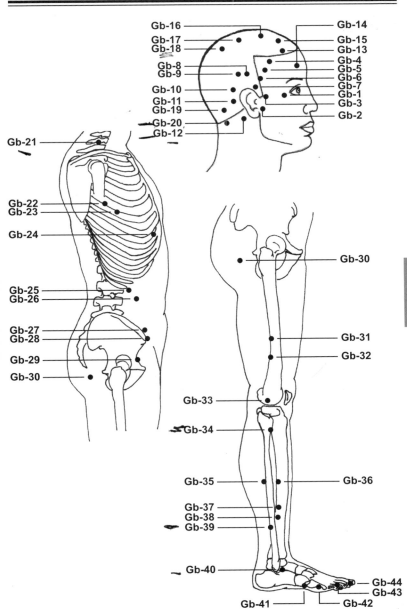

Jing Well	Ying Spring	Shu Stream	Jing River	He Sea
44	43	41	38	34
Yuan	**Luo-connect**	**Xi-Cleft**	**Front Mu**	**Back Shu**
40	37	36	Gb-24	Ub-19

POINTS

GALLBLADDER

Points	Location	Usage	Indications / Functions
Gb-1 **Tongziliao** *Pupil Crevice* sub- ↓ 0.3 – 0.5	0.5 cun lateral to the outer canthus, in the depression on the lateral side of the orbit.	Headache; anything with heat	• **Expels Wind-heat:** for conjunctivitis from wind-heat attack. • **Clears fire:** for liver fire causing red, dry and painful eyes. • Local point for migraine headaches due to liver fire or liver yang rising.
Gb-2 **Tinghui** *Hearing Convergence* ↓ 0.5 – 0.7	Anterior to the intertragic notch, at the posterior border of the condyloid process of the mandible. The point is located with the mouth open.	OM; ear pain; tinnitus; facial paralysis; mumps; dislocation or motor impairment of the jaw (TMJ)	• **Unblocks the Channels:** local point for tinnitus and deafness caused by liver-fire or liver yang rising blocking the channels. • **Expels exterior wind-heat:** used for otitis media due to exterior wind-heat.
Gb-3 **Shangguan** *Above the Joint* ↓ 0.3 – 0.5 no deep puncture	In the front of the ear, on the upper border of the zygomatic arch, in the depression directly above St-7.	Headache; deafness; tinnitus; mouth and eye deviation; toothache	• Expels Wind, Benefits the ears. • Activates the Channels, Stops pain.
Gb-4 **Hanyan** *Jaw Serenity* sub- ↓ 0.3 – 0.5	Within the hairline of the temporal region, at the junction of the upper 1/4 and lower 3/4 of the distance between St-8 and Gb-7.	Migraine; vertigo; tinnitus; outer canthus pain; convulsion; epilepsy	• Expels Wind, Clears Heat. • Activates the Channels, Stops pain.
Gb-5 **Xuanlu** *Skull Suspension* sub- ↓ 0.3 – 0.5	Within the hairline of the temporal region, at the midpoint of the line joining St-8 and Gb-7.	Migraine; outer canthus pain; convulsion; epilepsy	• Expels Wind, Clears Heat. • Activates the Channels, Stops pain.
Gb-6 **Xuanli** *Hair Suspension* sub- ↓ 0.3 – 0.5	Within the hairline, at the junction of the lower 1/4 and the upper 3/4 of the distance between St-8 and Gb-7.	Migraine; outer canthus pain; tinnitus; frequent sneezing	• Expels Wind, Clears Heat. • Activates the Channels, Stops pain: local point for migraine headaches on the side of the head due to liver yang rising, liver fire or liver wind.
Gb-7 **Qubin** *Turning On the Temple* sub- ↓ 0.3 – 0.5	Directly above the anterior border of the auricle, 2 cun within the hairline, about .5 cun posterior to Gb-8.	Headache; swelling of the cheek; temporal region pain; infantile convulsion	• Expels Wind, Benefits the mouth and jaw.
Gb-8 **Shuaigu** *Leading Valley* sub- ↓ 0.3 – 0.5	Superior to the apex of the auricle, 1.5 cun within the hairline.	Nausea and vomiting with headache; good for migraines	• **Unblocks the Channels, Benefits the ear:** local point for tinnitus and deafness or migraine headache from liver yang rising or liver fire.
Gb-9 **Tianchong** *Heavenly Rushing* sub- ↓ 0.3 – 0.5	Directly above the posterior border of the auricle, 2 cun within the hairline, about 0.5 cun posterior to Gb-8.	Headache; epilepsy; pain and swelling of the gums; convulsion	• **Unblocks the Channels, Subdues Rebellious Qi:** local point for migraine headaches due to liver yang rising, liver fire or liver wind. Descends upward rebellious qi. • **Subdues Interior Wind, Alleviates spasms:** for convulsions, epilepsy or contraction of muscles due to liver wind. Also for disturbance of movement such as ataxia and speech originating from disorders of the central nervous system. • **Calms the Mind:** for serious mental disorders such as hypomania.
Gb-10 **Fubai** *Floating White* sub- ↓ 0.3 – 0.5	Posterior and superior to the mastoid process, junction of middle 1/3 and upper 1/3 on the curved line drawn from Gb-9 to Gb-12.	Headache; tinnitus; deafness	• Clears the Head, Benefits the neck region. • Activates the Channels, Stops pain.
Gb-11 **Touqiaoyin** *Head-Yin-Orifice* sub- ↓ 0.3 – 0.5	Posterior and superior to the mastoid process, junction of middle 1/3 and lower 1/3 on the line drawn connecting Gb-9 and Gb-12.	Head and neck pain; tinnitus; deafness; ear pain	• Clears the Head, Benefits the sensory organs. • Activates the Channels, Stops pain.

Points	Location	Usage	Indications / Functions
Gb-12 **Wangu** *Mastoid Process* ↘ 0.3 – 0.5	In the depression posterior and inferior to the mastoid process.	Headache; insomnia; neck pain	• **Expels Exterior Wind:** used as a local point for otitis media and to subdue interior wind causing epilepsy. • **Subdues Rebellious Qi:** for migraine headaches along the Gall Bladder channel on the posterior side of the head caused by liver yang rising or liver wind. • **Calms the Mind:** for insomnia caused by liver yang rising or liver fire.
Gb-13 **Benshen** *Origin of the Spirit* sub- ↓ 0.3 – 0.5	0.5 cun within the hairline of the forehead, 3 cun lateral to Du-24.	Mental disorders; vertigo; seizures; hemiplegia; psychosis; schizophrenia; irrational suspicion and jealousy; rigid thinking; obsessive thought	• **Calms the Mind:** for severe emotional problems such as schizophrenia. Also for anxiety derived from constant worry and fixed thoughts. • **Gathers Essence to the Head:** for calming the mind and strengthening will power when combined with other essence strengthening points. • **Expels internal wind:** for wind stroke and epilepsy.
Gb-14 **Yangbai** *Yang White* sub- ↓ 0.3 – 0.5	On the forehead, directly above the pupil, 1 cun directly above the midpoint of the eyebrow.	Supraorbital neuralgia; headache; sinus headache; eye problems	• Benefits the head and eye, Expels Wind, Stops pain.
Gb-15 **Toulinqi** *Tear Controlling* sub- ↓ 0.3 – 0.5	Directly above Gb-14, 0.5 cun within the hairline, midway between Du-24 and St-8.	Headache; vertigo; lacrimation; outer canthus pain; nasal obstruction	• Regulates the Mind, Balances the Emotions: for balancing mood swings and manic depressive oscillations.
Gb-16 **Muchuang** *Eye Window* sub- ↓ 0.3 – 0.5	1.5 cun posterior to Gb-15, on the line connecting Gb-15 and Gb-20.	Headache; vertigo; red and painful eyes; nasal obstruction	• Benefits the eyes, Expels Wind, Stops pain.
Gb-17 **Zhengying** *Upright Nutrition* sub- ↓ 0.3 – 0.5	1.5 cun posterior to Gb-16, on the line connecting Gb-15 and Gb-20.	Migraine; vertigo	• Benefits the Head, Stops pain, Pacifies the Stomach.
Gb-18 **Chengling** *Spirit Support* sub- ↓ 0.3 – 0.5	1.5 cun posterior to Gb-17, on the line connecting Gb-15 and Gb-20.	Headache; vertigo; epistaxis; rhinorrhea	• Calms the Mind, Clears the brain: for deep mental problems such as obsessional thoughts and dementia.
Gb-19 **Naokong** *Brain Depression* sub- ↓ 0.3 – 0.5	Directly above Gb-20, at the level with Du-17, on the lateral side of the external occipital protuberance.	Headache; stiff neck; vertigo; painful eyes; tinnitus; epilepsy	• Benefits the Head, Stops pain, Clears Wind.
Gb-20 **Fengchi** *Wind Pool* ↓ 0.5 – 0.8 towards nose tip	In the depression between the upper portion of the muscle trapezius, on the same level with Du-16.	Common colds including wind-heat or wind-cold; anything with nasal obstruction; vertigo; occipital headache; stiff neck; hypertension; seizures; hemiplegia; very nice insomnia point; opens up whole head	• **Expels Wind:** for both interior and exterior wind including wind-cold, wind-heat, causing headache, stiff neck, dizziness and vertigo due to liver yang rising or liver fire. • **Subdues Liver yang:** for occipital headaches caused by liver yang rising. • **Benefits the eyes:** for eye problems due to Liver disharmony causing blurred vision, cataracts, iritis and optic nerve atrophy. Also can be used for eye problems caused by Liver blood deficiency. • **Benefits the ears:** for tinnitus and deafness due to liver yang rising. • **Clears the brain:** tonifies marrow and nourishes the brain when there are symptoms of poor memory, dizziness and vertigo.

POINTS

Points	Location	Usage	Indications / Functions
Gb-21 **Jianjing** *Shoulder Well* ↓ 0.3 – 0.5 contraindicated for pregnancy & pneumothorax	Midway between Du-14 and the acromion, at the highest point of the shoulder.	Hemiplegia due to stroke; any motor impairment of the arm; mastitis; breast abscess; difficult labor	• **Relaxes sinews:** for painful obstruction syndrome of the shoulders and neck. Also relieves stiffness of the neck. • **Promotes Lactation:** empirical point to promote lactation in nursing mothers. • **Promotes Delivery:** empirical point to promote delivery or expulsion of the fetus. For retention of the placenta, post-partum hemorrhage or threatened miscarriage.
Gb-22 **Yuanye** *Armpit depression* ↘ 0.3 – 0.5	On the mid axillary line when the arm is raised, in the 4th intercostal, 3 cun below the axilla.	Chest fullness; pain and motor impairment of the arm; hypochondriac pain; swelling of the axillary region	• **Regulates Qi:** unbinds the chest, benefits the axilla.
Gb-23 **Zhejin** *Flank Sinews* ↘ 0.3 – 0.5	1 cun anterior to Gb-22, on the 4th intercostal, approximately at the level with the nipple.	Chest fullness; hypochondriac pain; asthma	• Unbinds the chest, Regulates Qi in all three jiaos.
Gb-24 **Riyue** *Sun and Moon* ↘ 0.3 – 0.5	Directly below the nipple, in the 7th intercostal space, 4 cun to the anterior midline, one rib below Liv-14.	Intercostal neuralgia; cholecystitis; jaundice; peptic ulcer; hepatitis; heartburn; pain in the hypochondrium; check for herpes zoster; one of main points for gallstones; jaundice; hepatitis; mastitis; for wood attacking earth; good for nausea and vomiting	• **Resolves damp-heat:** for damp-heat in the Liver and Gallbladder causing jaundice, hypochondriac pain, felling of heaviness, nausea and a sticky yellow tongue coating. • **Promotes Qi circulation:** for stagnation of Liver qi causing hypochondriac pain and distension.
Gb-25 **Jingmen** *Capital Gate* ↓ 0.3 – 0.5	On the lateral side of the abdomen, on the lower border of the free end of the 12th rib.	Nephritis; serious and/or chronic UTI; intercostal neuralgia; lumbago; Kid stones; back pain from standing long-term	• Tonifies Kidney, Regulates water passages, Strengthens Spleen, Regulates Intestines. • Benefits the lumbar.
Gb-26 **Daimai** *Girdling Vessel* ↓ 0.5 – 0.8	Directly below the free end of the 11th rib, where the Liv-13 is located, at the level of the umbilicus.	Stops leukorrhea; main point for vaginal discharges; especially heat or excess type; endometriosis; cystitis; irregular menstruation from damp-heat; profuse uterine bleeding; inguinal hernia	• **Regulates the uterus and the menses:** for irregular periods and dysmenorrhea. • **Resolves damp-heat in the lower jiao:** for chronic vaginal discharges and vaginal prolapse.
Gb-27 **Wushu** *Pivot of the Five* ↓ 0.5 – 1.0	On the lateral side of the abdomen, anterior to the superior iliac spine, 3 cun below the umbilicus.	Leukorrhea; lower abdominal pain; lumbar pain; hernia; constipation	• Regulates the girdle vessel and the lower jiao. • Transforms stagnation.
Gb-28 **Weidao** *Linking Path* ↓ 0.5 – 1.0	Anterior and inferior to the ASIS, 0.5 cun anterior and inferior to Gb-27.	Prolapsed uterus; pain from intestinal hernia	• Regulates the girdle vessel and the lower jiao. • Transform stagnation.
Gb-29 **Juliao** *Stationary Crevice* ↓ 0.5 – 1.0	In the depression of the midpoint between the ASIS and the greater trochanter.	Numbness; paralysis; skin itching; paralysis of lower limb; pain in low back and leg; numbness and stiffness of lower leg; hemiplegia of lower limb	• **Unblocks the Channels:** a local point for painful obstruction syndrome of the hip.

POINTS

Points	Location	Usage	Indications / Functions
Gb-30 **Huantiao** *Circling Jump* ↓ 1.5 – 2.5	At the junction of the lateral 1/3 and medial 2/3 of the distance between the greater trochanter and the hiatus of the sacrum (Du-2). When locating this point, put patient in lateral recumbent position with thigh flexed.	Sciatica; Hip, lumbar, and thigh pain; diseases of the hip joint and surrounding tissue; look there for endometriosis as the constricted qi may exacerbate these problems	• **Unblocks the Channels:** local point for painful obstruction syndrome of the hip. Also, for atrophy syndrome and sequelae of wind-stroke. For sciatica with pain extending down the lateral side of the leg. • **Tonifies Qi and Blood:** almost as strong as St-36. • **Resolves damp-heat:** for damp-heat in the lower burner causing itchy anus or groin, vaginal discharge and urethritis.
Gb-31 **Fengshi** *Wind Market* ↓ 0.7 – 1.2	On the midline of the lateral aspect of the thigh, 7 cun above the transverse political crease. When the patient is standing erect with hands at sides, the point is where the tip of the middle finger touches.	Sciatica, especially with lateral leg pain; numbness and paralysis of lower leg; diseases of hip joint and surrounding soft tissue	• **Expels Wind:** for wind-heat moving in the blood causing sudden appearance of red rashes that move from place to place such as in urticaria. Also used to expel wind-heat in herpes zoster (combined with Sj-6). • **Strengthens Bones and sinews:** for atrophy syndrome and sequelae of wind-stroke to relax the sinews and invigorate the circulation of qi and blood to the legs.
Gb-32 **Zhongdu** *Middle Ditch* ↓ 0.7 – 1.0	On the lateral aspect of the thigh, 5 cun above the transverse popliteal crease, between vastus lateralis and biceps femoris.	Soreness and pain of the thigh and knee; numbness and weakness of the lower limbs; hemiplegia	• Relaxes sinews, Benefits joints, Expels Wind-Damp.
Gb-33 **Xiyangguan** *Knee Yang Gate* ↓ 0.5 – 1.0	3 cun above Gb-34, with flexed knee, between the tendon of biceps femoris and the femur, in the depression above the lateral epicondyle of the femur.	Diseases of knee and surrounding soft tissue	• Relaxes sinews, Benefits joints, Expels Wind-Damp: local point for painful obstruction syndrome of the knee, especially when there is involvement of the ligaments and tendons of the knee.
Gb-34 **Yanglingquan** *Outer Mound Spring* ↓ 0.8 – 1.2 he-sea	In the depression anterior and in inferior to the head of the fibula.	Major point for musculoskeletal problems; controversial main point for frozen shoulder; important sciatica point; hepatitis; cholecystitis; causes GB contractions and can expel gallstones; hypertension (Liv yang rising type); intercostal neuralgia; herpes	• **Promotes Smooth Flow of Qi:** for Liver qi stagnation causing hypochondriac pain and distention, or pain in the epigastrium. Also for Liver-Stomach disharmony causing vomiting and nausea. • **Resolves damp-heat:** for damp-heat in the Liver and Gallbladder channels. • **Relaxes sinews:** for relaxing tendons whenever there are contractions of muscles, cramps or spasms. • **Unblocks the channels:** for painful obstruction syndrome, atrophy syndrome and sequelae of wind-stroke.
Gb-35 **Yangjiao** *Yang Crossroads* ↓ 0.5 – 0.8	7 cun above the tip of the lateral malleolus, on the posterior border of the fibula.	Chest fullness; muscular atrophy; leg paralysis	• Unblocks the Channels, Stops pain: for acute pain along the channel with stiffness and cramping of the leg muscles.
Gb-36 **Waiqiu** *Outer Mound* ↓ 0.5 – 0.8 xi-cleft	7 cun above the tip of the lateral malleolus, on the anterior border of the fibula.	Rage; channel excess s/sx like high fever; excess sweating (thought to refer to rabies)	• **Unblocks the Channels, Stops pain, Clears Heat:** for all painful conditions of the Gallbladder channel or organ.
Gb-37 **Guangming** *Bright Light* ↓ 0.7 – 1.0 luo-connect	5 cun directly above the tip of the lateral malleolus, on the anterior border of the fibula.	Main distal point for vision; any eye problems; blurry vision; itching eyes; pain in the eyes	• **Brightens eyes:** improves eyesight and eliminates floaters. • **Conducts fire downwards:** for liver fire affecting the eyes.
Gb-38 **Yangfu** *Lateral Support* ↓ 0.5 – 0.7 jing-river	4 cun above and slightly anterior to the tip of the lateral malleolus, on the anterior border of the fibula, between m. extensor digitorum longus and m. peroneus brevis.	Migraines; hemiplegia; sedation point (but Gb-34 used more); whole body pain of excess type	• **For chronic migraine headaches** caused by liver yang or liver fire.

POINTS

POINTS

Points	Location	Usage	Indications / Functions
Gb-39 **Xuanzhong** *Suspended Bell* ↓ 0.3 – 0.5	3 cun above the lateral malleolus, in the depression between the posterior border of the fibula and the tendons of m. peroneus longus and brevis.	Stiff neck (with Gb-20 and 21 locally); distal for migraines; hemiplegia (flaccid type); sciatica; distal point for knee; any pain in lower leg GB area and pain in all three yang meridians of the leg (such as resulting from hemiplegia); leg qi syndrome; spastic leg; muscular atrophy of lower limbs	• **Benefits the Essence, Nourishes marrow, Expels Wind:** for chronic interior wind with Kidney yin deficiency. Used to prevent wind stroke.
Gb-40 **Qiuxu** *Mounds of Ruins* ↓ 0.5 – 0.8 yuan	Anterior and inferior to the lateral malleolus, in the depression on the lateral side of the tendon of m. extensor digitorum longus.	Pain in chest and ribs; tidal fevers; malaria; cholecystitis; acid reflux; vomiting; distal sciatica point; disease of ankle and surrounding tissues; timidity is often listed as well	• **Promotes Qi circulation:** for hypochondriac pain and distension due to Liver qi stagnation.
Gb-41 **Zulinqi** *Foot Tear-Control* ↓ 0.3 – 0.5 shu-stream	In the depression distal to the junction of the 4th and 5th metatarsal bones, on the lateral side of the tendon of m. extensor digiti minimi of the foot.	HA; migraines; menstrual HA from dai channel connection; vertigo; conjunctivitis (Gb-37 better); mastitis; breast distention; irregular menstruation; scrofula; outer canthus pain; good for pregnancy pain when the tendons and ligaments stretch too early	• **Resolves damp-heat:** for damp-heat in the genital region causing chronic vaginal discharge, cystitis and urethritis. • **Promotes the smooth flow of Liver Qi:** for headaches from Liver qi stagnation of liver fire. • Painful obstruction syndrome of the knee and hip.
Gb-42 **Diwuhui** *Earth Five Meetings* ↓ 0.3 – 0.5	Between the 4th and 5th metatarsal bones, on the medial side of the tendon of m. extensor digiti minimi of the foot.	Canthus pain; tinnitus; breast distension pain; swelling and pain of the dorsum of the foot	• Spreads Liver Qi, Clears Gallbladder heat.
Gb-43 **Xiaxi** *Narrow Stream* ↓ 0.3 – 0.5 ying-spring	On the dorsum of the foot, between the 4th and 5th toes, 0.5 cun proximal to the margin of the web.	Headache; dizziness and vertigo; outer canthus pain; deafness; tinnitus; breast distension pain; febrile diseases	• **Subdues Liver yang:** for temporal headaches from liver yang rising and migraine headaches affecting the Gallbladder channel on the temples. • **Benefits the ear:** for tinnitus from liver yang rising or otitis media from exterior damp-heat.
Gb-44 **Zuqiaoyin** *Foot Yin Orifice* ↓ 0.1 jing-well	On the lateral side of the 4th toe, about .1 cun posterior to the corner of the nail.	Migraines; headache; intercostal neuralgia; violent nightmares	• **Subdues Liver yang, Benefits the eyes:** for migraine headaches around the eyes caused by liver yang rising. Also for red and painful eyes from liver fire. • **Calms the Mind:** for insomnia and agitation caused by liver fire.

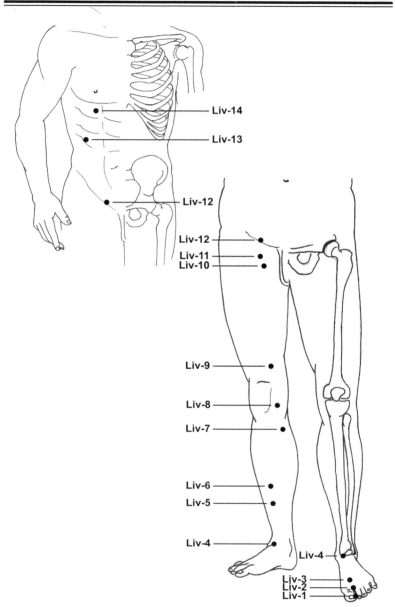

POINTS

Jing Well	Ying Spring	Shu Stream	Jing River	He Sea
1	2	3	4	8
Yuan	**Luo-connect**	**Xi-Cleft**	**Front Mu**	**Back Shu**
3	5	6	Liv-14	Ub-18

LIVER

Liver (Liv) - Foot Jueyin

Points	Location	Usage	Indications / Functions
Liv-1 **Dadun** *Big Mound* sub-↓ 0.1 – 0.2 jing-well	On the lateral side of the terminal phalanx of the great toes, 0.1 cun lateral to the corner of the big toenail.	Abnormal uterine bleeding from hot blood	• **Regulates menses:** stops uterine bleeding due to heat in the blood. • **Resolves damp-heat:** for damp-heat in the lower burner causing difficult urination, retention of scrotum, enlarged scrotum, itchy scrotum, vaginal discharge or pruritus valvae. • **Promotes the smooth flow of Liver Qi:** for pain on urination with distension of the hypogastrium due to Liver qi stagnation. • **Restores consciousness:** for acute wind-stroke.
Liv-2 **Xingjian** *Temporary In-Between* ↘ 0.3 – 0.5 ying-spring	On the dorsum of the foot, between the 1st and 2nd toes, 0.5 cun proximal to the margin of the web.	Vertex headache; vertigo; dizziness from upsurge of wind (not anything else); intercostal neuralgia from heat; abnormal menstrual bleeding due to heat; cloudy urine or urethra discharge; eyes red and swollen; seizures or convulsions of any type; abdominal distension	• **Clears Liver-fire, Subdues Liver yang:** for patterns including bitter taste, thirst, a red face, headaches, dream-disturbed sleep, scanty dark urine, constipation, red eyes, a red tongue with thick yellow coating, and a rapid-wiry pulse. Used to treat migraine headaches due to Liver-yang rising. Also for liver fire insulting the Lungs and causing coughing accompanied by pain below the ribs and breathlessness. This often is exacerbated by phlegm which combines with fire. • **Expels Interior Wind:** for epilepsy and children's convulsions.
Liv-3 **Taichong** *Bigger Rushing* ↓ 0.3 – 0.5 shu-stream, yuan	On the dorsum of the foot, in the depression distal to the junction of the 1st and 2nd metatarsal bones.	Improves vision; rising Liv yang; Liv wind; vertex and occular headache; dizziness of Liv yang rising and Liv wind type; hypertension (excess or deficient); insomnia; hepatitis; mastitis; major point for irregular menstruation due to stagnation; mouth deviation; uterine bleeding; epilepsy; hernia; urine retention	• **Subdues Liver-yang:** major point for sedating Liver excess patterns, although mostly for subduing liver yang with migraine headaches. • **Expels interior Wind:** calming spasms, contractions and cramps of the muscles, wind in the face (when combines with LI-4) causing facial paralysis and tics. • **Calms the Mind:** for calming tensions, for short temper, anger, irritability, deep frustration and repressed anger, and also for tension from stress. • **Promote Qi circulation:** used with moxibustion to treat genital swelling and orchitis or white vaginal discharge due to cold in the liver channel.
Liv-4 **Zhongfeng** *Middle Seal* ↓ 0.3 – 0.5 jing-river	1 cun anterior to the medial malleolus, midway between Sp-5 and St-41, in the depression on the medial side of m. tibialis anterior.	Genital pain and contraction; hypogastric pain; seminal emission problems; difficult urination; urine retention; lumbar pain; numbness of the body; pain of medial aspect of knee; all ankle problems; difficult defecation; pain and swelling of the lower abdomen; contracted sinews	• Promotes the smooth flow of Liver qi in the lower burner: for urinary symptoms with a feeling of distension in the hypogastrium due to Liver qi stagnation.
Liv-5 **Ligou** *Woodworm Canal* sub-↓ 0.3 – 0.5 luo-connect	5 cun above the tip of medial malleolus, on the medial aspect and along the medial border of the tibia.	Genital itching like herpes; leukorrhea; irregular menstruation and endometriosis if damp-heat in nature; weakness and atrophy of leg; hernia	• **Promotes Qi circulation:** for any urinary symptom deriving from Liver qi stagnation including distension of the hypogastrium, distension and pain before urination and retention of urine. Also for Liver qi stagnation causing the sensation of a lump in the throat "plum pit". • **Resolves damp-heat:** for vaginal discharge or cloudy urine.
Liv-6 **Zhongdu** *Middle Capital* sub-↓ 0.5 – 0.8 xi-cleft	7 cun above the tip of the medial malleolus, on the medial aspect and along the medial border of the tibia.	Abdominal pain; diarrhea; hernia; uterine bleeding; prolonged lochia	• Used primarily for acute excess patterns causing pain around the genitalia and deriving from either damp-heat or Liver qi stagnation including cystitis, painful urination, hernia.

POINTS

Points	Location	Usage	Indications / Functions
Liv-7 **Xiguan** *Knee Joint* ↓ 0.5 – 1.0	Posterior and inferior to the medial condyle of the tibia, in the upper portion of m. gastrocnemius, 1 cun posterior to Sp-9.	Knee pain	• Used as a local point for painful obstruction syndrome of the knee, particularly when caused by wind and with pain on the medial aspect of the knee.
Liv-8 **Ququan** *Spring and Bend* ↓ 0.5 – 0.8 he-sea	When the knee is flexed, the point is located in the depression above the medial end of the transverse popliteal crease, posterior to the medial epicondyle of the tibia, on the anterior part of the insertion of m. semimembranosus and m. semitendinosus.	Genital herpes; vaginitis; local for medial knee pain; nocturnal emissions	• **Benefits the Bladder, Resolves Dampness:** used to eliminate dampness obstructing the lower burner and causing urinary retention, cloudy urine, burning urination, vaginal discharge, pruritus vulvae. Can be used for either damp-heat or damp-cold. • **Nourishes Liver Blood**
Liv-9 **Yinbao** *Yin Wrapping* ↓ 0.5 – 0.7	4 cun above the medial epicondyle of the femur, between m. vastus medialis and sartorius.	Lumbosacral pain; lower abdominal pain; urine retention; irregular menstruation	• Regulates menses and lower jiao.
Liv-10 **Zuwuli** *Leg Five Miles* ↓ 0.5 – 1.0	3 cun directly below St-30, at the proximal end of the thigh, below the pubic tubercle and on the lateral border of m. abductor longus.	Lower abdominal fullness and distention; urine retention	• Clears damp-heat, Benefits lower jiao.
Liv-11 **Yinlian** *Yin Angular Ridge* ↓ 0.5 – 1.0	2 cun directly below St-30, at the proximal end of the thigh, below pubic tubercle and on the lateral border of m. abductor longus.	Irregular menstruation; leukorrhea; lower abdominal pain; thigh and leg pain	• Benefits the uterus.
Liv-12 **Jimai** *Urgent Pulse* ↓ 0.3 – 0.5	Inferior and lateral to the pubic bone, 2.5 cun lateral to the Ren line, at the inguinal groove, lateral and inferior to St-30.	Cold indications, especially genital area; hernia; lower abdominal pain	• Expels cold from Liver channel, Benefits lower jiao.
Liv-13 **Zhangmen** *Chapter Gate* ↓ 0.5 – 0.8	On the lateral side of the abdomen, below the free end of the 11th rib.	Liv invading SP is the classic presentation for this point; enlargement of liver and spleen; hepatitis; enteritis; abdominal distension from Liv invading SP; constipation from stagnant Liv qi; pain in hypochondrium; diarrhea due to cold; borborygmus	• **Promotes the smooth flow of Liver Qi, Relieves retention of food.** • **Benefits the Spleen and Stomach:** for Liver qi stagnation patterns when Liver invades Stomach and Spleen, preventing Spleen qi from ascending and causing loose stools and abdominal distension, or preventing Stomach qi from descending causing retention of food, belching and fullness in the epigastrium. Since this is both for strengthening Spleen function as well as for eliminating stagnation, it is the main point for Liver-Spleen disharmony. With moxa it can be used to tonify and warm the Spleen for Spleen yang deficiency.
Liv-14 **Qimen** *Cyclic Gate* ↘ 0.3 – 0.5	Directly below the nipple, in the 6th intercostal space, 4 cun lateral to the midline.	Main point for intercostal neuralgia; hepatitis; tight chest from anger and frustration; nervous dysfunction of ST (Liv invading the ST); vomiting; hiccups; stuck food; hypochondrium pain and distension; shingles; insufficient lactation	• **Promotes Qi Circulation, Benefits the Stomach:** for Liver qi stagnation patterns when Liver invades Stomach and prevents Stomach qi from descending causing nausea, vomiting, hypochondriac distension and pain, retention of food, belching and fullness in the epigastrium. • **Cools the Blood.**

POINTS

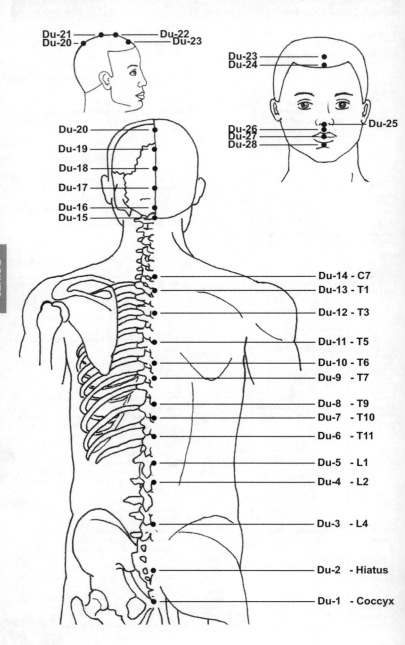

Du-21 — Du-22
Du-20 — Du-23

Du-23
Du-24

Du-26 — Du-25
Du-27
Du-28

Du-20
Du-19
Du-18
Du-17
Du-16
Du-15

Du-14 - C7
Du-13 - T1
Du-12 - T3
Du-11 - T5
Du-10 - T6
Du-9 - T7
Du-8 - T9
Du-7 - T10
Du-6 - T11
Du-5 - L1
Du-4 - L2
Du-3 - L4
Du-2 - Hiatus
Du-1 - Coccyx

POINTS

Points	Location	Usage	Indications / Functions
Du-1 **Changqiang** *Long Strength* luo-connect	Midway between the tip of the coccyx and the anus, locating the point in prone position.	Diarrhea; constipation; coccyx pain; hemorrhoids; rectal prolapse; rectal bleeding	• **Regulates the Du and Ren:** eliminates obstructions from the channels. It is also a local point for prolapse of the anus. • **Resolves damp-heat:** for hemorrhoids. • **Calms the Mind:** for agitation and hypomania.
Du-2 **Yaoshu** *Lumbar Shu* ↘ 0.5 – 1.0	On the hiatus of the sacrum.	Hemorrhoids (after DU1); low back pain (local pain; stiffness; and from cold)	• **Eliminates Interior Wind:** for spasms and convulsions, epilepsy.
Du-3 **Yaoyangguan** *Lumbar Yang Gate* ↘ 0.5 – 1.0	Below the spinous process of the 4th lumbar vertebrae, level with the iliac crest.	Low back pain; paralysis of lower limbs; muscular atrophy of the legs; impotence; nocturnal emission; epilepsy	• **Strengthens back, Tonifies Yang, Strengthens the legs:** for lower backache, atrophy syndrome.
Du-4 **Mingmen** *Gate of Life* ↓ 0.5 – 1.0	Below the spinous process of the 2nd lumbar vertebrae.	Low back pain or sprain; 5am diarrhea; enuresis; spermatorrhea; impotence; leukorrhea; irregular menstruation; endometriosis; peritonitis; spinal myelitis; sciatica; sequelae of infantile paralysis; asthma due to deficient kidney not grasping lung qi	• **Tonifies Kidney yang:** tonifies and warms the gate of vitality. For Kidney yang deficiency causing chilliness, abundant-clear urination, tiredness, lack of vitality, depression, weak knees and legs, a pale tongue and a deep-weak pulse. • **Benefits Original Qi:** for chronic weakness and both physical and mental. • **Benefits the Essence:** for impotence, premature ejaculation or nocturnal emissions. • **Strengthens lower back and knees:** for chronic backache due to Kidney yang deficiency. • **Expels Cold:** for interior cold due to either Kidney or Spleen yang deficiency causing chronic diarrhea, profuse clear urination, incontinence or enuresis, abdominal pain or dysmenorrhea or infertility.
Du-5 **Xuanshu** *Suspended Pivot* ↓ 0.5 – 1.0	Below the spinous process of the 1st lumbar vertebrae.	Diarrhea; indigestion	• Strengthens lumbar spine, Benefits lower jiao.
Du-6 **Jizhong** *Spinal Center* ↓ 0.5 – 1.0	Below the spinous process of the 11th thoracic vertebrae.	Diarrhea; jaundice; epilepsy; stiffness and back pain	• Drains damp, Tonifies Spleen, Benefits lower jiao.
Du-7 **Zhongshu** *Central Pivot* ↓ 0.5 – 1.0	Below the spinous process of the 10th thoracic vertebrae.	Low back pain; back stiffness; epigastric region pain	• Strengthens lumbar spine, Benefits middle jiao.
Du-8 **Jinsuo** *Tendon Spasm* ↓ 0.5 – 1.0	Below the spinous process of the 9th thoracic vertebrae.	Epilepsy; gastric pain; back stiffness	• **Expels Interior Wind, Relaxes sinews:** for convulsions, muscle spasms, tremors or epilepsy.
Du-9 **Zhiyang** *Reaching yang* ↘ upward 0.5 – 1.0	Below the spinous process of the 7th thoracic vertebrae, approximately at level with the inferior angle of the scapula.	Jaundice; cough; asthma; back stiffness	• **Regulates the Liver and Gallbladder:** promotes the smooth flow of Liver qi when there is hypochondriac pain and distension. • **Opens the chest and diaphragm:** for distension or oppression, hiccup and sighing. • **Resolves damp-heat:** for damp-heat in the Liver and Gallbladder channel causing jaundice.
Du-10 **Lingtai** *Spirits Tower* ↘ upward 0.5 – 1.0	Below the spinous process of the 6th thoracic vertebrae.	Back pain; neck rigidity; cough; asthma	• Stops coughing and wheezing, Clears heat and detoxifies poison.
Du-11 **Shendao** *Spirit Pathway* ↘ upward 0.5 – 1.0	Below the spinous process of the 5th thoracic vertebrae.	Poor memory; anxiety; palpitation; pain and stiffness of the back	• **Regulates the Heart, Calms the Mind:** clears Heart fire and for other excess Heart patterns.

POINTS

DU

Du Channels (Du) - Governing Vessel

POINTS

Points	Location	Usage	Indications / Functions
Du-12 **Shenzhu** *Body Pillar* ↘ upward 0.5 – 1.0	Below the spinous process of the 3rd thoracic vertebrae.	Cough; asthma; pain and stiffness of the back	• **Expels Interior Wind, Relieves spasms:** for spasms, convulsions and tremors or epilepsy. • Tonifies Lung Qi following debilitating illness.
Du-13 **Taodao** *Way of Happiness* ↘ upward 0.5 – 1.0	Below the spinous process of the 1st thoracic vertebrae.	Malaria; headache; febrile diseases; stiffness of the back	• **Clears Heat, Release the Exterior, Regulates the Shaoyang:** for beginning stage wind-heat attack. Also for alternating fever and chills and Shaoyang patterns.
Du-14 **Dazhui** *Big Vertebra* ↘ upward 0.5 – 1.0	Below the spinous process of the 7th cervical vertebrae, approximately level with the shoulders.	URI; cold; seizures; asthma used with Ding chuan; pain in shoulder; neck pain and rigidity (flexion and extension); any febrile disease; taiyang stage (URI wind-cold) use Du-14 to disperse and cause a sweat; yang ming stage (lung heat) use Du-14 to tonify	• **Clears Heat, Release the Exterior, Expels Wind, Regulates Nutritive and Defensive Qi:** for wind-heat patterns or any heat pattern. • **Tonifies Yang:** with reinforcing method it tonifies the yang and can be used for any yang deficiency pattern. • **Clears the Mind and stimulates the brain.**
Du-15 **Yamen** *Gate of Muteness* ↓ 0.5 – 0.8	0.5 cun directly above the midpoint of the posterior hairline, in the depression below the spinous process of the 1st cervical vertebrae.	Mental disorders; epilepsy; deafness and muteness; apoplexy after stroke; may not help voice box injury but worth a try	• Clears the Mind, Stimulates speech: for speech impairment.
Du-16 **Fengfu** *Wind Palace* ↓ 0.5 – 0.8 no deep puncture	1 cun directly above the midpoint of the posterior hairline, directly below the external occipital protuberance, in the depression between m. trapezius.	Headache; sore throat; can be used for any of the common wind symptoms; stiff neck; numbness; stroke	• **Expels Wind, Clears the Mind and the Brain:** eliminates both exterior and interior wind causing wind stroke, epilepsy and severe giddiness.
Du-17 **Naohu** *Brain's Door* sub- ↓ 0.3 – 0.5	On the midline of the head, 1.5 cun directly above Du-16, in the depression on upper border of EOP.	Epilepsy; neck stiffness	• Expels Wind, Clears the brain, Clears the Mind: subdues wind affecting the brain causing epilepsy, wind stroke.
Du-18 **Qiangjian** *Unyielding Space* sub- ↓ 0.3 – 0.5	On the midline of the head, 1.5 cun directly above Du-17, midway between Du-16 and Du-20.	Headache; neck rigidity; blurry vision; mania	• Expels Wind, Stops pain. • Calms the Mind, Soothes the Liver.
Du-19 **Houding** *Behind the Crown* sub- ↓ 0.3 – 0.5	On the midline of the head, 1.5 cun directly above Du-18.	Headache; vertigo; epilepsy; mania	• Calms the Mind: for severe anxiety.
Du-20 **Baihui** *Hundred Meetings* sub- ↓ 0.3 – 0.5	On the midline of the head, 7 cun directly above the posterior hairline, approximately on the midpoint of the line connecting the apexes of the two auricles.	Vertex headache; frontal headache from sinus congestion; dizziness; hypertension; insomnia; seizures (wind); prolapse (lifts energy up); hemorrhoids; diarrhea; vaginal bleeding; tinnitus; nasal obstruction and congestion; stroke; locked jaw; hemiplegia	• **Ascends Yang, Clears the Mind:** for prolapse of the internal organs including stomach, uterus, bladder, anus or vagina. • Eliminates Interior Wind. • Promotes resuscitation and restores consciousness.
Du-21 **Qianding** *In Front of the Crown* sub- ↓ 0.3 – 0.5	On the midline of the head, 1.5 cun anterior to Du-20.	Epilepsy; dizziness; blurry vision; rhinorrhea; vertical headache	• Expels Wind, Treats convulsions, Benefits the Mind.

Points	Location	Usage	Indications / Functions
Du-22 **Xinhui** *Fontanel Meeting* sub-↓ 0.3 – 0.5 no infants with metopism	2 cun posterior to the midpoint of the anterior hairline, 3 cun anterior to Du-20.	Headache; blurry vision; mental disorders; epistaxis; opthalmalgia	• Benefits the nose, Expels Wind, Benefits the Mind.
Du-23 **Shangxing** *Upper Star* sub-↓ 0.3 – 0.5 no infants with metopism	1 cun directly above the midpoint of the anterior hairline.	Headache; rhinitis; any nose problems involving obstruction	• Opens the nose: for chronic allergic rhinitis or sinusitis.
Du-24 **Shenting** *Mind Courtyard* sub-↓ 0.3 – 0.5 or bleed	0.5 cun directly above the midpoint of the anterior hairline.	Local headache (frontal and sinus); seizures	• **Calms the Mind:** for severe anxiety and fears. Treats schizophrenia.
Du-25 **Suliao** *White Crevice* ↓ 0.2 – 0.3 or bleed	On the tip of the nose.	Nasal obstruction; loss of consciousness; epistaxis; rhinorrhea; rosacea	• Benefits the nose.
Du-26 **Renzhong** *Middle of Person* ↘ upward 0.3 – 0.5	At the junction of upper 1/3 and lower 2/3 of the philtrum near the nostrils, or upper lip midline.	Loss of consciousness; acute low back sprain; drowning; coma; heat exhaustion; seizures	• **Restores consciousness, Calms the Mind.** • **Benefits the face and nose, Expels Wind.** • **Strengthens lumbar spine.**
Du-27 **Duiduan** *Mouth Extremity* ↘ upward 0.2 – 0.3	On the median tubercle of the upper lip, at the junction of the skin and upper lip.	Mental disorders; lip stiffness; lip twitching; pain and swelling of the gums	• Clears Heat, Generates fluid, Benefits the mouth. • Calms the Mind.
Du-28 **Yinjiao** *Gum Intersection* ↘ upward 0.1 – 0.2 or bleed	At the junction of the gum and frenulum of the upper lip.	Mental disorders; pain and swelling of the gums; rhinorrhea	• Clears Heat, Benefits the gums, nose, and eyes.

POINTS

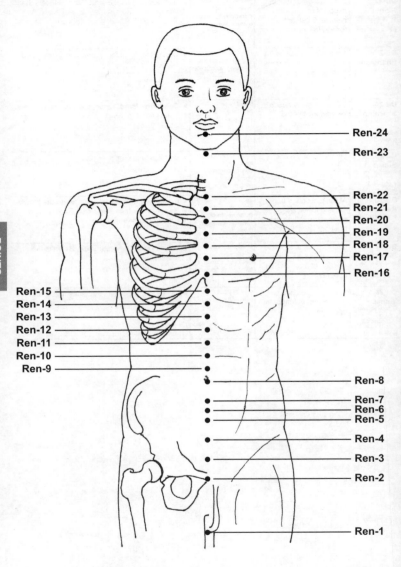

Ren-24
Ren-23
Ren-22
Ren-21
Ren-20
Ren-19
Ren-18
Ren-17
Ren-16
Ren-15
Ren-14
Ren-13
Ren-12
Ren-11
Ren-10
Ren-9
Ren-8
Ren-7
Ren-6
Ren-5
Ren-4
Ren-3
Ren-2
Ren-1

Points	Location	Usage	Indications / Functions
Ren-1 **Huiyin** *Meeting of Yin* ↓ 0.5 – 1.0	Between the anus and the root of the scrotum in males, and between the anus and the posterior labial commissure in females.	Vaginitis; urine retention; hemorrhoids; nocturnal emission; enuresis; mental disorders	• Nourishes the Yin, Benefits the Essence: for incontinence, enuresis and nocturnal emissions deriving from yin deficiency. • Resolves damp-heat: for damp-heat in the genital area causing vaginal discharge, pruritus vulvae or itching of the scrotum. • Empirical point to promote resuscitation after drowning.
Ren-2 **Qugu** *Curved Bone* ↓ 0.5 – 1.0 caution in pregnancy	On the midpoint of the upper border of the pubis symphysis.	Urine dribbling and retention; enuresis; nocturnal emission; irregular menstruation; hernia; dysmenorrhea	• Warms and invigorates Kidney, Benefits urination, Regulates lower jiao.
Ren-3 **Zhongji** *Middle Extremity* ↓ 0.5 – 1.0 caution in pregnancy	On the midline of the abdomen, 4 cun below the umbilicus.	Spermatorrhea; enuresis; retention of urine; leukorrhea; (all due to damp-heat); any urinary tract disorder (90% of the time they are damp-heat related); excessive uterine bleeding; dysmenorrhea (but these are not usually related to damp-heat)	• **Regulates Bladder Function:** for any urinary problem, especially acute. For either excess or deficiency patterns. • **Resolves damp-heat:** for pain and burning on urination and interrupted flow of urine.
Ren-4 **Guanyuan** *Gate to the Original Qi* ↓ 0.8 – 1.2 caution in pregnancy	On the midline of the abdomen, 3 cun below the umbilicus.	For all Kid problems; abdominal pain; pain from deficiency; cold diarrhea (Kid related); UTI (Ren-3 might be better); urination from cold (clear and copious); deficient types of "rrheas"; can use it to regulate almost any GYN problems	• **Nourishes Yin and Blood:** for any pattern of deficiency of blood or yin. • **Strengthens Yang:** rescue the yang in acute stages of wind-stroke due to collapse of yang. Also for deficiency of Kidney yang. • **Regulates the uterus and menses:** for amenorrhea or scanty periods. • **Tonifies the Kidney and Benefits the Original Qi:** for chronic diseases or for patients with poor constitution or emaciation. • **Calms the Mind:** for anxiety from yin deficiency. • **Roots the Ethereal Soul:** for vague feelings of fear at night due to floating of the ethereal soul.
Ren-5 **Shimen** *Stone Door* ↓ 0.5 – 1.0 caution in pregnancy	On the midline of the abdomen, 2 cun below the umbilicus.	Abdominal pain; diarrhea; hernia; edema; uterine bleeding; postpartum hermmorhage	• **Benefits the Original Qi:** for Kidney deficiency and a poor constitution. • **Regulates the transformation and excretion of fluids in the lower burner and Opens the water passages:** for edema of the abdomen, urinary retention, difficult urination, diarrhea or vaginal discharge.
Ren-6 **Qihai** *Sea of Qi* ↓ 0.8 – 1.2 caution in pregnancy	On the midline of the abdomen, 1.5 cun below the umbilicus.	Neurasthenia; abdominal pain and distension related to digestion; impotence; irregular menstruation; intestinal paralysis; all urinary problems like incontinence; infertility spermatorrhea; prolapse rectum; postpartum hemorrhage; diarrhea; (Ren-4 better as it more deeply tonifies the Kid)	• **Tonifies Qi, Yang and Original Qi:** for extreme physical and mental exhaustion and depression. • **Regulates Qi:** for lower abdominal pain and distention due to qi stagnation. • **Benefits Original Qi:** for chilliness, loose stools, profuse pale urination, physical weakness, mental depression, lack of will power. • **Resolves Dampness:** for urinary difficulty, vaginal discharge or loose stool with mucus.
Ren-7 **Yinjiao** *Yin Crossing* ↓ 0.8 – 1.2 caution in pregnancy	On the midline of the abdomen, 1 cun below the umbilicus.	Abdominal distension; edema; hernia; irregular menstruation	• **Nourishes Yin, Regulates the uterus:** for menstrual problems including amenorrhea, scanty periods or infertility. Also used during menopause to nourish blood and yin.

POINTS

POINTS

Points	Location	Usage	Indications / Functions
Ren-8 Shenque *Spirit Gateway* No puncture caution in pregnancy	In the center of the umbilicus.	Diarrhea from SP yang deficiency; 5 am diarrhea; apoplexy (flaccid stroke) from yang collapse; any kind of prolapse due to SP yang deficiency	• **Rescues Yang:** for acute stage wind-stroke or the flaccid type characterized by collapse of yang. • **Strengthens Spleen:** for internal cold and extreme weakness, and chronic diarrhea from Spleen deficiency.
Ren-9 Shuifen *Water Separation* ↓ 0.5 – 1.0 caution in pregnancy	On the midline of the abdomen, 1 cun above the umbilicus.	Ascites (retention of fluid in abdomen); edema; retention of urine; diarrhea; general dampness in the body (fluid retention in the body; actual fluid retention in the body as opposed to less material dampness like foggy head)	• **Controls the water passages:** promotes the transportation, transformation and excretion of fluids in all parts of the body. For dampness, phlegm, edema or ascites.
Ren-10 Xiawan *Lower Epigastrium* ↓ 0.5 – 1.2 caution in pregnancy	On the midline of the abdomen, 2 cun above the umbilicus.	Indigestion; food retention after eating; prolapsed stomach	• **Descends Rebellious Qi, Relieves food stagnation:** for stimulating the downward movement of Stomach qi, retention of food in the stomach, abdominal distension, feeling of fullness after eating and sour regurgitation. For treating the pylorus and duodenum.
Ren-11 Jianli *Strengthen the Interior* ↓ 0.5 – 1.2 caution in pregnancy	On the midline of the abdomen, 3 cun above the umbilicus.	Stomachache; vomiting; abdominal distention; borborygmus; edema; anorexia	• Regulates Stomach function, Descend Qi: for feeling of fullness and distension in the epigastrium, nausea, vomiting and epigastric pain.
Ren-12 Zhongwan *Middle of Epigastrium* ↓ 0.5 – 1.2 caution in pregnancy	On the midline of the abdomen, 4 cun above the umbilicus.	Acute or chronic gastritis; gastric ulcers; prolapsed ST; vomiting; nausea; one of the main nausea points and good for any kind; can be used for constipation if chronic or deficient; indigestion; madness from phlegm type of blockage; builds middle energy	• **Tonifies Stomach and Spleen:** for deficiency patterns of the Stomach and Spleen causing lack of appetite, fatigue, and dull epigastric pain relieved by eating. • **Regulates Stomach:** for deficiency cold patterns of the Stomach and Spleen. • **Resolves Dampness.**
Ren-13 Shangwan *Upper Epigastrium* ↓ 0.5 – 1.2 caution in pregnancy	On the midline of the abdomen, 5 cun above the umbilicus.	Stomach pain; nausea; vomiting; abdominal distention	• **Subdues rebellious Stomach Qi:** for hiccup, belching, nausea, vomiting and a feeling of fullness in the upper epigastrium.
Ren-14 Juque *Great Palace* ↓ 0.3 – 0.8	On the midline of the abdomen, 6 cun above the umbilicus.	Mental diseases; seizures; angina pectoris; vomiting; nausea (if more tender than Ren-12); palpitations due to anything; hiatal hernia; strong spirit and mental associations	• **Descends Rebellious Stomach Qi:** for digestive problems with rebellious Stomach qi of emotional origin. • **Clears Heart-fire and Calms the Mind:** for phlegm-heat misting the heart causing mental symptoms.
Ren-15 Jiuwei *Dove Tail* ↘ 0.4 – 0.6	1 cun below the xyphoid process, 7 cun above the umbilicus; locate the point in the supine position with the arms uplifted.	Mental illness; good for fatigue; yang madness; epilepsy	• **Benefits the Original Qi:** nourishes all yin organs and calms the mind when there is anxiety, worry, emotional upsets, fears or obsessions caused by yin deficiency.
Ren-16 Zhongting *Center Courtyard* sub- ↓ 0.3 – 0.5	On the midline of the sternum, at the level of the 5th intercostal space.	Fullness and distension in the chest and intercostal region; hiccups; nausea; anorexia	• Unblocks the chest, Regulates the Stomach, Descends rebellion.

Points	Location	Usage	Indications / Functions
Ren-17 **Shanzhong** *Middle of Chest* sub- ↓ 0.3 – 0.5	On the anterior midline, at level with the 4th intercostal space.	Asthma; bronchitis; intercostal neuralgia; wheezing; panting; spitting blood; difficulty or inability to swallow food; dilates bronchioles; insufficient lactation; hiccups	• **Tonifies the Qi of the chest, Regulates Qi:** aids the dispersing and descending of qi, dispels stagnation of qi in the chest causing tightness in the chest, breathlessness and pain in the chest. • **Opens the chest:** dispels fullness from the chest and helps breathing. For Lung and Heart qi patterns or obstruction of the chest by phlegm. For chronic bronchitis. • **Benefits the diaphragm:** for hiatal hernia or insufficient lactation from qi and blood deficiency.
Ren-18 **Yutang** *Jade Hall* sub- ↓ 0.3 – 0.5	On the anterior midline, at the level of the 3rd intercostal space.	Fullness and distension in the chest and intercostal region; hiccups; nausea; anorexia	• Unblocks the chest, Regulates and Subdues rebellion.
Ren-19 **Zigong** *Purple Palace* sub- ↓ 0.3 – 0.5	On the anterior midline, at the level of the 2nd intercostal space.	Chest pain; cough; asthma	• Unblocks the chest, Regulates and Subdues rebellion.
Ren-20 **Huagai** *Florid Canopy* sub- ↓ 0.3 – 0.5	On the anterior midline, at the midpoint of the sternal angle, at the level of the 1st intercostal space.	Fullness and distension in the chest and intercostal region; asthma; cough	• Unblocks the chest, Regulates and Subdues rebellion.
Ren-21 **Xuanji** *Jade Pivot* sub- ↓ 0.3 – 0.5	On the anterior midline, in the center of the sternal manubrium, 1 cun below Ren-22.	Chest pain; cough; asthma	• Descends Stomach Qi, Dispels food stagnation. Unblocks the chest, Descends Lung Qi. • Benefits the throat.
Ren-22 **Tiantu** *Heaven Projection* First, ↓ 0.2, then insert downward along posterior aspect of sternum ↓ 0.5 – 1.0	In the center of the suprasternal fossa.	Pharyngitis; goiter; hiccups; spasms of the esophagus; diseases of the vocal cords; heavy wheezing; nodules that are phlegm based	• **Stimulates the descending of Lung qi:** for cough and asthma. • **Resolves Phlegm:** for phlegm in the throat and lungs causing acute bronchitis with profuse sputum, or chronic retention of phlegm in the throat. • **Clears Heat:** for Lung heat or wind-heat in the Lungs.
Ren-23 **Lianquan** *Angular Ridge Spring* ↘ 0.5 – 1.0 toward tongue root	Above the Adam's apple, in the depression of the upper border of the hyoid bone.	Loss of voice; paralysis of hypoglossus; excessive salvation; tongue problems	• Descends Qi, Stops cough.
Ren-24 **Chengjiang** *Saliva Receiver* ↘ upward 0.2 – 0.3	In the depression in the center of the mentolabial groove.	Facial paralysis; facial edema involving REN meridian; deviated eyes and mouth	• Local point for exterior wind invading the face causing facial paralysis.

POINTS

Points	Location	Usage	Indications / Functions
E-Anmian *Peaceful Sleep* ↓ 0.5 – 0.8	Midpoint between Sj-17 and Gb-20	Insomnia; vertigo; headache; palpitation; mental disorders; calms the spirit and clears the brain	• Calms the Mind, Pacifies the Liver.
E-Bafeng *Eight Winds* ↓ 0.5 – 0.8	On the dorsum of the foot, in the depressions on the webs between toes, 0.5 cun proximal to the margins of the webs, eight points in all.	Beriberi; toe pain; redness and swelling of the dorsum of the foot	• Clears Heat, Reduces swelling.
E-Baichongwo *Shelter of Hundred Insects* ↓ 1.0 – 1.2 cun.	1 cun above Sp-10.	Rubella; eczema; gastrointestinal parasitic diseases	• Clears Heat from the blood, Expels Wind, Drains Dampness.
E-Bailao *100 Labors* ↓ 0.3 – 0.5	2 cun above Du-14, 1 cun lateral to the midline.	Scrofula; cough; asthma; whooping cough; neck rigidity.	• Transforms Phlegm, Reduce nodules, Stops coughing and wheezing.
E-Baxie *Eight Pathogenic Factors* ↘ 0.3 – 0.5 or prick to bleed	On the dorsum of the hand, at the junction of the white and red skin of the hand webs, eight in all, making a loose fist to locate the points.	Excess heat; pain; numbness and swelling of the hands	• Clears Heat, Reduce swelling.
E-Bitong *Nose Passage* sub-↓ upward 0.3 – 0.5	At the highest point of the nasolabial groove.	Rhinitis; nasal obstruction; nasal boils	• Benefits the nose.
E-Bizhong *Middle Of Arm* ↓ 1.0 – 1.2	On the forearm, midway between the transverse wrist crease and elbow crease, between the radius and the ulna.	Spasm or contracture of the upper extremities; paralysis; pain of the forearm	• Spasm or contracture of the upper extremities; paralysis; pain of the forearm.
E-Dannangxue *Gall Bladder Point* ↓ 0.8 – 1.2	The tender spot 1-2 cun below Gb-34.	Acute and chronic cholecystitis; cholelithiasis; biliary ascariasis; Giovanni: resolves damp-heat in the GB	• Clears Heat, Drains Damp.
E-Erbai *Two Whites* ↓ 0.5 – 1.0	On the palmar aspect of the forearm, 4 cun above the transverse wriste crease, on both sides of the tendon of m. flexor carpi radialis.	Hemorrhoids; prolapse of the rectum	• Treats prolapse of rectum and hemorrhoids.
E-Dingchuan *Stop Wheezing* ↓ 0.5 – 0.8	0.5 to 1.0 cun lateral to Du-14.	Asthma; cough; neck rigid; urticaria; rubella; Giovanni: Expels exterior wind; calms asthma-used to calm an acute attack of asthma	• Stops coughing and wheezing.
E-Erjian *Ear Apex* ↓ 0.1 – 0.2 or bleed	Fold of the oracle, the point is at the apex of the auricle (on the helix).	Redness; swelling and pain of the eyes; febrile disease; nebula	• Clears Heat, Reduce swelling, Benefits the eyes.
E-Heding *Crane's Summit* ↓ 0.3 – 0.5	In the depression of the midpoint of the superior patellar border.	Knee pain; weakness of the foot and leg; paralysis	• Moves Qi and Blood, Strengthens the knees.
E-Huanzhong *Central Round* ↓ 1.5 – 2.0	Midway between Gb-30 and Du-2.	Lumbar pain; thigh pain	• Moves Qi and Blood: used for lumbar pain and thigh pain.
E-Huatuojiaji *Lining The Spine* ↓ 0.5 – 1.0 cervical: 1.0 – 1.5 lumbar	A group of 34 points on both sides of the spinal column, 0.5 - 1.0 cun lateral to the lower border of each spinous process from T1 to L5.	T1-T3 diseases in the upper limbs; T2-T8 diseases in the chest region; T6-L5 diseases in the abdominal region; L1-L5 diseases in the lower limbs	• Regulates and harmonizes zang fu organs.

Points	Location	Usage	Indications / Functions
E-Jiacheng-jiang *Adjacent Container Fluids* ↘ 0.5 – 1.0	1 cun lateral to Ren-24.	Pain in the face; deviation of the eyes and mouth; spasm of facial muscle	• Expels Wind, Opens the Channels, Stops pain.
E-Jianqian *Front of the Shoulder* ↓ 0.8 – 1.2	Midway between the top of the anterior axillary crease and LI-15.	Used for shoulder pain or frozen shoulder if pain radiates towards the anterior aspect of the shoulder	• Moves Qi and Blood, Benefits the Shoulder.
E-Jinjin, Yuye *Golden Fluid & Jade Humor* Prick to bleed	On the veins on both sides of the frenulum of the tongue, Jinjin is on the left, Yuye is on the right.	Swelling of the tongue; vomiting; aphasia with stiffness of tongue	• Clears Heat, Reduce swelling, Generate fluids, Benefits the tongue.
E-Lanweixue *Appendix Point* ↓ 1.0-1.2	2 cun below St-36. Locate by finding the tender spot between St-36 and St-37.	Acute and chronic appendicitis	• Moves Qi and Blood, Clears excess heat from Large Intestine.
E-Luozhen *Stiff Neck* ↓ 0.5-0.8	On the dorsum of the hand between the 2nd and 3rd metacarpal bones, 0.5 cun posterior to the metacarpophalangeal joint.	Neck pain	• Moves Qi and Blood in the neck region.
E-Naoqing *Clear the Brain Point*	2 cun proximal to St-41 on the St-36-41 line.	Improve memory; clears the brain	• Improve memory; clears the brain.
E-Pigen *Root of Glomus* ↓ 0.5 – 0.8	3.5 cun lateral to the lower border of L1.	Hepatosplenomegaly; lumbar pain	• Hepatosplenomegaly; lumbar pain.
E-Qianzheng *Pull Aright* ↘ 0.5 – 1.0	0.5-1 cun anterior to the auricular lobe.	Deviation of the eyes and mouth; ulceration on tongue and mouth	• Deviation of the eyes and mouth; ulceration on tongue and mouth.
E-Qiuhou *Behind the Ball* Push eyeball upward ↓ 0.5 – 1.2	At the junction of the lateral 1/4 and 3/4 of the infra orbital margin.	Eye diseases	• Benefits the eyes.
E-Shang-lianquan *Upper Ridge Spring* 0.8 – 1.2	1 cun below the midpoint of the lower jaw, in the depression between the hyoid bone and the lower border of the jaw.	Alalia; salivation with stiff tongue; sore throat; difficulty in swallowing; loss of voice	• Alalia; salivation with stiff tongue; sore throat; difficulty in swallowing; loss of voice
E-Shiqizhuixia *Below The 17th Vertebrae* ↓ 0.8 – 1.2	Below the spinous process of L5.	Lumbar and thigh pain; paralysis of the lower extremities; irregular or painful menses; benefits the lower back and regulates the lower burner	• Tonifies Kidney, Promotes urination, Opens the channels, Stops pain.
E-Shixuan *Ten Diffusions* sub- ↓ 0.1 – 0.2 Prick to bleed	On the tips of the ten fingers, about 0.1 cun distal to the nail.	Apoplexy; coma; epilepsy; high fever; acute tonsillitis; infantile convulsion; clear heat; subdue interior wind; open the orifices	• Revives consciousness, Drains Heat, Pacifies Wind.
E-Sifeng *Four Seams* Prick to bleed	On the palmar surface, in the midpoint of the transverse creases of the proximal interphalangeal joints of the index, middle, ring and little fingers.	Malnutrition and indigestion syndrome in children; whooping cough	• Tonifies Spleen, Reduce accumulation.

POINTS

Points	Location	Usage	Indications / Functions
E-Sishencong *Four Alert Spirit* sub- ↓ 0.5 – 1.0	A group of points, at the vertex, 1 cun respectively posterior, anterior and lateral to Du-20.	Headache; vertigo; insomnia; poor memory; epilepsy; subdue interior wind-used as local point for the treatment of epilepsy	• Calms the Mind, Expels Wind, Benefits the eyes and ears.
E-Taiyang *Greater Yang* ↓ 0.3 – 0.5	In the depression about 1 cun posterior to the midpoint between the lateral end of the eyebrow and the outer canthus.	Headache; eye diseases; deviation of eye & mouth	• Clears Heat, Expels Wind, Reduce swelling. • Opens channels, Stops pain.
E-Weiguan-xiashu ↘ 0.5 – 0.7	1.5 cun lateral to the lower border of the spinous process of T8.	Diabetes; vomiting; pain in the chest or abdomen; Note: Considered to be the back shu point of the pancreas	• Clears Heat, Generates fluid.
E-Xiyan/ Xiyuan *Eyes Of the Knee* ↓ 0.5 – 1.0	A pair of points in the two depressions, medial and lateral to the patellar ligament, locating the point with the knee flexed. Lateral xiyan overlaps with St-35.	Knee pain; weakness of the lower extremities; used for painful obstruction of the knee; needle obliquely upwards or medially with moxa for best results	• Dispels Wind-Damp, Reduce Swelling, Stops pain.
E-Yaoqi *Lumbar Extra* sub- ↓ upwards 1.0 – 2.0	2 cun directly above the tip of the coccyx	Epilepsy; headache; insomnia; constipation	• Moves Qi and Blood.
E-Yaotongxue *Lumbar Pain Point* ↘ 0.5 – 1.0 towards center	On the dorsum of the hand midway between the transverse wrist crease and metacarpophalangeal joint, between the 2nd and 3rd metacarpal bones, and between the 4th and 5th metacarpal bones, four points in all on both hands.	Acute lumbar sprain	• Moves Qi and Blood in the lumbar region.
E-Yaoyan *Lumbar Eyes* ↓ 0.8 – 1.2	3.5 cun lateral to the lower border of L4, located in the prone position.	Lumbar pain; frequent urination; irregular menses	• Tonifies Kidney, Strengthens the lumbar region.
E-Yiming *Shielding Brightness* ↓ 0.5 – 0.8	1 cun posterior to Sj-17.	Eye diseases; tinnitus; insomnia; calms the spirit and brightens the eyes; benefits the ears	• Calms the spirit and brightens the eyes; Benefits the ears.
E-Yintang *Seal Hall* sub- ↓ 0.3 – 0.5	Midway between the medial ends of the two eyebrows.	Headache; epistaxis; insomnia; head heaviness; frontal headache	• Calms the Mind, Expels Wind, Benefits the nose. • Opens the Channels, Stops pain.
E-Yuyao *Waist Spine* sub- ↓ 0.3 – 0.4	At the midpoint of the eyebrow, direcly above the pupil (in the hair).	Twitching of the eyes; redness; swelling; pain of the eyes; ptosis; cloudiness of the cornea; Giovanni: Used mostly for eye disorders; such as blurred vision or floaters; derived from liver blood deficiency	• Benefits the eyes, Relaxes sinews, Stops pain.
E-Zhongkui *Central Boss* Moxibustion is applied	On the midpoint of the proximal interphalangeal joint of the middle finger at the dorsum aspect.	Nausea; vomiting; hiccups	

POINTS

Points	Location	Usage	Indications / Functions
E-Zhongquan *Central Spring* ↓ 0.3 – 0.5	In the depression between LI-5 and Sj-4, on the radial side of the extensor digitorum communis.	Stuffy chest; gastric pain; spitting of blood	• Nausea; vomiting; hiccups.
E-Zhoujian *Tip of the Elbow* Moxibustion is applied	On the tip of the ulnar olecranon when the elbow is flexed.	Scrofula	• Stuffy chest; gastric pain; spitting of blood.
E-Zigongxue *Womb Or Palace Of Child; Uterus Point* ↓ 0.8 – 1.2	3 cun lateral to Ren-3.	Prolapse of uterus; irregular menses; ovarian cysts; regulates menses; clears heat and transforms damp-heat; raises the middle qi; Giovanni: Used to tonify the kidneys; regulate menses; and for infertility in women	• Raises and regulates Qi, Regulates menses, Stops pain.

Special Needling Cautions & Contraindications

Caution during pregnancy
Ren-4	no needle and moxa
Ren-11	no moxa
Sp-2	no moxa - & 3 months after birth
Sp-6	no needle
Gb-21	no needle
Ub-60	no needle
Ub-67	no needle
LI-4	no needle
St-25	no needle

Contraindicated - No needling or use with caution with direction
Ren-5	may cause infertility in females
Ren-8	may be fatal
Ren-15	may shorten life
Du-11	may damage heart
Du-24	
Pc-1	may cause pneumothorax
St-17	
Ht-2	
Lu-2	may cause inability to raise arm
Liv-12	
Gb-3	may cause deafness
Gb-18	
Gb-21	deep needle forbidden in heart cases
K-11	
Ub-56	
Sj-7	
Sj-8	
E-Zhongkui	

No head points on infants
No points on lower abdomen and lower back 3 months after pregnancy

No Moxa
Pc-1	forbidden moxa on females
Pc-9	

Caution - over pulses and major vessels
Pc-3
Lu-7
Lu-8
Lu-9
St-30
St-42
St-11
Liv-3
Liv-12
Ub-1
Ub-2
LI-4
LI-5
LI-13
Sj-23

POINTS

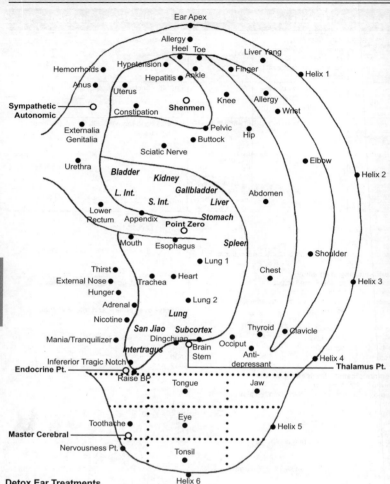

POINTS

Detox Ear Treatments

The National Acupuncture Detoxification Association (**NADA**) and American College of Addictionology and Compulsive Disorders (**ACACD**) auricular acupuncture protocol are used around the world to help people deal with and recover from substance abuse. The **NADA** and **ACACD** protocol has been shown in a variety of clinical settings to be beneficial in the process of detoxification from substance abuse as well as to help with the emotional, physical and psychological attributes involved in addictions.

NADA Protocol

Lung 2	Addiction-related lung issues
Shen Men	Stress, anxiety, excessive sensitivity
Autonomic	Balance sympathetic and parasympathetic nervous systems, blood circulation
Liver	Hepatitis, cirrhosis
C. Kidney	Kidney disorders, urination issues

ACACD Protocol

Point Zero	General homeostatic balance
Shen Men	Stress, anxiety, excessive sensitivity
Autonomic	Balance sympathetic and parasympathetic nervous systems, blood circulation
C. Kidney	Kidney disorders, urination issues
Brain	Pituitary gland, endocrine glands, addictions, sleep
Limbic System or *Master Cerebral*	Aggressiveness, compulsive behavior

Condition	Protocols
Acne	Face, Skin, Lung 1 & 2, Point Zero, Shenmen
Alcoholism	Alcoholic Point, Liver, Lung 1, Lung 2, Brain, Occiput, Forehead, Kidney, Point Zero, Shenmen, Lesser Occipital Nerve
Allergy	Apex of the Ear, Allergy Point, Omega 2, Inner Nose, Asthma, Point Zero, Shenmen, Sympathetic, Endocrine
Anxiety	Nervousness, Master Cerebral, Tranquilizer Point, Heart, Point Zero, Shenmen, Sympathetic
Back Pain	Thoracic Spine, Lumbosacral Spine, Buttock, Sciatic Nerve, Lumbago, Lumbar Spin, Pint Zero, Shenmen, Thalamus Point
Cancer	Corresponding body area, Thymus Gland, Vitality Point, Heart, Point Zero, Shenmen, Thyroid Gland
Carpal Tunnel	Wrist I-III Forearm, Hand, Thoracic Spin, Point Zero, Shenmen, Thalamus
Chronic fatigue	Vitality Point, Antidepressant, Brain, ACTH, Adrenal Gland, Point Zero, Shenmen, Master Oscillation
Common Cold	Inner Nose, Throat, Forehead, Lung 1 & 2, Asthma, Prostaglandin 1 & 2, Ear Apex
Constipation	Constipation, Large Intestines, Rectum, Omega 1, Abdomen
Cough	Asthma, Antihistamine, Point Zero, Adrenal Gland, Throat 1 & 2, Lung 1 & 2
Depression	Antidepressant, Brain, Excitement Pint, Pineal Gland, Master Cerebral, Shenmen, Sympathetic
Diarrhea	Small Intestines, Large Intestines, Point Zero, Shenmen, Sympathetic
Dizziness	Dizziness, Inner Ear, Cerebellum, Occiput, Lesser Occipital Nerve, Point Zero,
Drug Addiction	Lung 1, Lung 2, Shenmen, Sympathetic, Endocrine, Liver, Kidney, Brain
Fibromyalgia	Thoracic Spine, Lumbosacral Spine, Muscle Relaxation, Antidepressant, Point Zero, Shenmen, Thalamus
Headaches	Temples, Lesser Occipital Nerve, Vagus Nerve, Shenmen, Kidney, Thalamus Point, Cervical Spine
Hypertension	Hypertension 1 & 2, Heart, Sympathetic, Point Zero, Shenmen
Hyperthyroidism	Thyroid Gland, Point Zero, Shenmen, Endocrine, Brain, Master Oscillation, Apex of the Ear
Infertility	Uterus, Ovary, Shenmen, Point Zero, External Genitalia, Endocrine, Adrenal, Kidney, Abdomen, Brain
Insomnia	Insomnia 1 & 2, Pineal Gland, Heart, Master Cerebral, Point Zero, Shenmen, Thalamus Point, Forehead, Occiput, Brain, Kidney
Memory Loss	Frontal Cortex, Hippocampus, Memory 1 & 2, Master Cerebral, Heart, Point Zero, Shenmen
Multiple Sclerosis	Corresponding body area, Brainstem, Medulla Oblongata, Master Oscillation, Point Zero, Thalamus Point, Thymus Gland, Vitality
Muscle Sprain	Corresponding body area, Heat Point, Point Zero, Shenmen, Thalamus Point, Adrenal Gland, Liver, Spleen, Kidney
PMS	Uterus, Ovary, Endocrine, Shenmen
Rheumatoid Arthritis	Corresponding body area, Omega 2, Prostaglandin 1 & 2, Allergy Point, Adrenal Gland, Point Zero, Shenmen, Thalamus Point, Endocrine Point
Sciatica	Sciatic Nerve, Buttocks, Lumbago, Lumbar Spin, Hip, Thigh, Calf , Point Zero, Shenmen, Thalamus Point, Adrenal, Kidney, Bladder
Shoulder Pain	Shoulder, Shoulder Phase II, Master Shoulder, Clavicle, Cervical Spine, Thoracic Spine
Sinusitis	Inner Nose, Frontal Sinus, Forehead, Occiput, Point Zero, Shenmen, Adrenal
Smoking	Nicotine, Lung 1, Lung 2, Mouth, Point Zero, Shenmen, Sympathetic, Brain
Sore throat	Throat, Mouth, Trachea, Tonsil 1-4
Stress	Adrenal Gland, Tranquilizer Point, Point Zero, Shenmen, Master Cerebral, Muscle Relaxation
Stroke	Corresponding body area, Brain, Adrenal Gland, ACTH, Shenmen, Sympathetic, Master Cerebral, Endocrine
Tennis Elbow	Elbow Phase I-III, Forearm, Thoracic Spine, Point Zero, Shenmen, Thalamus Point, Muscle Relaxation Point, Adrenal, Kidney, Occiput
Tinnitus	Inner Ear, External Ear, Auditory Nerve, Kidney, Point Zero, Shenmen, San Jiao
TMJ	TMJ, Upper Jaw, Lower Jaw, Cervical Spine, Trigeminal Nerve, Occiput
Toothache	Toothache 1-3, Upper Jaw, Lower Jaw, Trigeminal Nerve, Shenmen
Weight Control	Appetite, Stomach, Mouth, Esophagus, Small Intestines, Shenmen, Point Zero

Source: Oleson, Terry, *Auriculotherapy Manual 3rd Edition*, 2003, Churchill Livingston, London, England.

POINTS

HEAD POINTS

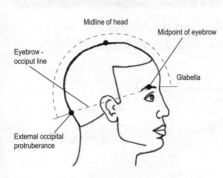

Lines of Measurement

Midline of head
Midpoint of eyebrow
Eyebrow - occiput line
Glabella
External occipital protruberance

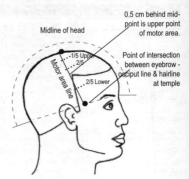

Motor Area Measurements

Midline of head
0.5 cm behind mid-point is upper point of motor area.
1/5 Upper
2/5
2/5 Lower
Motor area line
Point of intersection between eyebrow - occiput line & hairline at temple

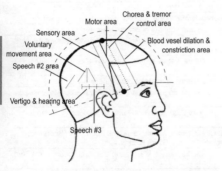

Stimulation Areas - Side View

Motor area
Sensory area
Voluntary movement area
Speech #2 area
Chorea & tremor control area
Blood vesel dilation & constriction area
Vertigo & hearing area
Speech #3

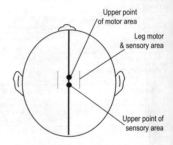

Stimulation Areas - Top View

Upper point of motor area
Leg motor & sensory area
Upper point of sensory area

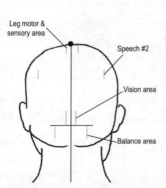

Stimulation Areas - Posterior View

Leg motor & sensory area
Speech #2
Vision area
Balance area

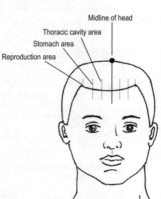

Stimulation Areas - Anterior View

Midline of head
Thoracic cavity area
Stomach area
Reproduction area

POINTS

238

Area	Location	Indications
Motor area	A line starting from a point. 0.5 cm (not cun), posterior to the midpoint of anterior to posterior plane that goes diagonally across the head to a point at the intersection of the zygomatic arch (superior margin) and the hairline at the temple.	
Lower limb & trunk area	Upper 1/5 of motor area line	Paralysis of the lower limbs on the opposite side.
Upper limb area	Middle 2/5 of motor area line	Paralysis of the upper limbs on the opposite side.
Facial area (includes Speech #1)	Lower 2/5 of motor area line	Upper motor neuron paralysis of the face (opposite), motor aphasia, impaired speech, dribbling.
Sensory area	A line parallel and 1.5 cm. posterior to motor area line.	
Lower limb, head, & trunk area	Upper 1/5 of sensory area line	Pain, numbness, abdominal sensation in the lower extremities on opposite side, neck pain, occiput headache, vertigo, tinnitus.
Lower limb, head, & trunk area	Middle 2/5 of sensory area line	Pain, numbness, tingling in the upper extremities on opposite side.
Upper limb area	Lower 2/5 of sensory area line	Migraine headache, facial paralysis, trigeminal neuralgia, toothache (opposite side), TMJ.
Vertigo & hearing	Horizontal line 1.5 cm. superior and centered on the apex of the ear, 4 cm. in length.	Meniere's syndrome, vertigo, tinnitus, diminished hearing.
Blood vessel dilation & constriction area	Parallel with and 1.5 cm. anterior to motor area line	Hypertension, superficial edema.
Chorea & tremor control area	Parallel with and 1.5 cm. anterior to motor area line	Chorea, tremors, bells palsy, Parkinson's.
Leg motor & sensory area	Parallel with midline of head, 1 cm. lateral to midpoint, approximately 3 cm. in length (bilateral)	Paralysis, pain or numbness o flower limbs, acute low back pain and strain, uterine prolapse, nocturnal emission.
Stomach area	Beginning at the hairline directly above the pupil of the eyes, parallel with the midline of the head, extending posteriorly 2 cm. (bilateral)	Upper abdominal pain or discomfort.
Liver & gallbladder area	Beginning at the hairline it extends anteriorly from the stomach area line 2 cm. in length (bilateral)	Pain in the upper right abdomen and/or right rib cage, chronic hepatitis.
Thoracic area	Beginning at the hairline midway between and parallel with the stomach area line and midline of the head, extending posteriorly and anteriorly 2 cm. in each direction.	Asthma, chest pain and discomfort, tachycardia.
Reproductive area	Beginning at the hairline parallel and lateral to the stomach area line at a distance equal to that between the stomach area and thoracic area line, extending posteriorly 2 cm. in length. (bilarea0	Menstrual disorders, combined with leg motor area line for uterine prolapse.
Balance area	3 cm. lateral to the EOP, parallel to the midline of the head, 4 cm. in length extend inferiorly.	Loss of balance due to cerebellar disturbances.
Vision area	1 cm. lateral to the EOP, parallel to the midline of the head, 4 cm. in length extending superiorly.	Visual disturbances.
Voluntary movement area	Tuber parietal origin. 3 needles inserted inferiorly, anteriorly and posteriorly 3 cm. in length. The 3 lines will form a 40 degree angle.	Apraxia, (nerve injury in which unable to carry out purposeful movement despite normal muscle power & coordination).
Speech #1	Lower 1/5 of motor area line	Motor aphasia, impaired speech, dribbling saliva.
Speech #2	Vertical line 2 cm. besides tuber parietale on the back of the head, 3 cm. in length.	Nominal aphasia.
Speech #3	Overlaps vertigo & hearing area line at midpoint & continues 4 cm. posteriorly.	Receptive aphasia.

POINTS

POINTS

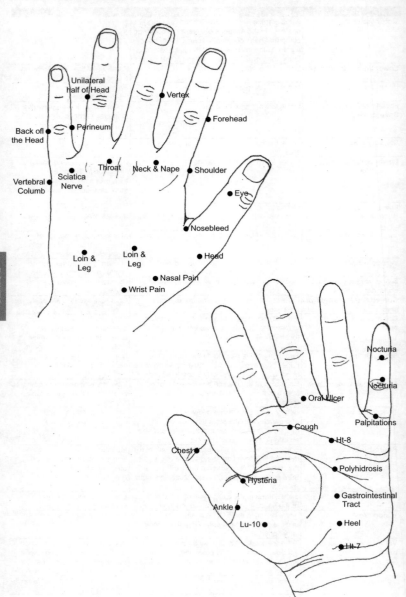

Esoteric Acupuncture was developed to address the complex imbalances of the people today and addresses imbalances on the physical, etheric, astral, mental, causal, buddhic, atmic and monadic planes.

Esoteric Acupuncture encompasses a much broader spectrum of healing and emphasizes the wellness stage versus the disease stages of the older systems. The general thinking of people in the West is to consider becoming healthy only after they have a physical or emotional imbalance. The real power of Esoteric Acupuncture is to harmonize and strengthen the body systems before a disease stage. Dr. Mikio Sankey is a renowned author and lecturer on Esoteric Acupuncture with books that include: *Climbing Jacob's Ladder, Esoteric Acupuncture, Vol. III Workbook, Discern the Whisper, Esoteric Acupuncture, Vol. II, Acupuncture, Gateway to Expanded Healing. Vol I., Sea of Fire-Cosmic Fire, Esoteric Acupuncture, Vol IV.* The following information is composed of excerpts from his books with the needling sequences.

Discern the Whisper Pattern

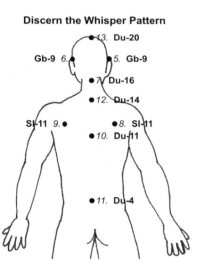

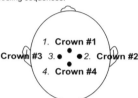

Discern the Whisper Pattern

1. Crown #1 (Sishencong)
2. Crown #2
3. Crown #3
4. Crown #4
5. Gb-9 (Right)
6. Gb-9 (Left)
7. Du-16
8. SI-11 (Right)
9. SI-11 (Left)
10. Du-11
11. Du-4
12. Du-14
13. Du-20

POINTS

Integration Synthesis Pattern

Integration Synthesis Pattern

1. Du-20
2. Pc-8 (Right)
3. Pc-8 (Left)
4. Ren-17

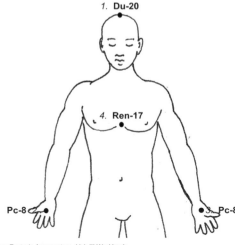

Source: Dr. Mikio Sankey. *Climbing Jacob's Ladder, Esoteric Acupuncture, Vol. III Workbook, Discern the Whisper, Esoteric Acupuncture, Vol. II, Acupuncture, Gateway to Expanded Healing. Vol I.* Information on books and upcoming lectures can be found at http://www.esotericacupuncture.com

Celestial Tuning Fork Yin Pattern

Celestial Tuning Fork Yang Pattern

1.   Du-20
2.   Du-16
3.   Du-14
4.   Du-11
5.   Du-4
6.   Gb-30 (Left)
7.   Gb-30 (Right)
8.   Ub-40 (Left)
9.   Ub-40 (Right)
10.   K-1 (Left)
11.   K-1 (Right)

Celestial Tuning Fork Yang Pattern

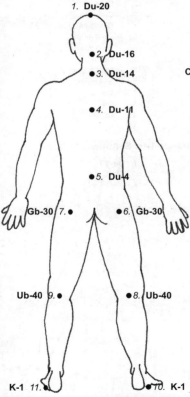

POINTS

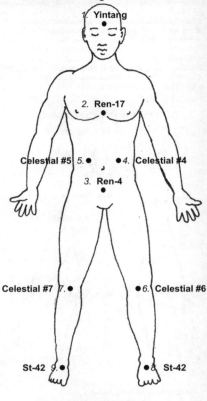

Celestial Tuning Fork Yin Pattern

1.   E-yintang
2.   Ren-17
3.   Ren-4
4.   Celestial #4 (Left)
5.   Celestial #5 (Right)
6.   Celestial #6 (Left)
7.   Celestial #7 (Right)
8.   St-42 (Left)
9.   St-42 (Right)

Source: Dr. Mikio Sankey. *Climbing Jacob's Ladder, Esoteric Acupuncture, Vol. III Workbook,
Discern the Whisper, Esoteric Acupuncture, Vol. II, Acupuncture, Gateway to Expanded Healing. Vol I.*
Information on books and upcoming lectures can be found at http://www.esotericacupuncture.com

Zang – Yin Channels		Wood Jing Well	Fire Ying Spring	Earth Shu Stream	Metal Jing River	Water He Sea	Fu – Yang Channels		Metal Jing Well	Water Ying Spring	Wood Shu Stream	Fire Jing River	Earth He Sea
Tai Yin	Lu	11	10	9	8	5	Yang Ming	LI	1	2	3	5	11
	Sp	1	2	3	5	9		St	45	44	43	41	36
Shao Yin	Ht	9	8	7	4	3	Tai Yang	SI	1	2	3	5	8
	K	1	2	3	7	10		Ub	67	66	65	60	40
Jue Yin	Pc	9	8	7	5	3	Shao Yang	Sj	1	2	3	6	10
	Liv	1	2	3	4	8		Gb	44	43	41	38	34

	Yuan	Luo-connect	Xi-Cleft	Front Mu	Back Shu
Lu	9	7	6	Lu-1	Ub-13
LI	4	6	7	St-25	Ub-25
St	42	40	34	Ren-12	Ub-21
Sp	3	4	8	Liv-13	Ub-20
Ht	7	5	6	Ren-14	Ub-15
SI	4	7	6	Ren-4	Ub-27
Ub	64	58	63	Ren-3	Ub-28
K	3	4	5	Gb-25	Ub-23
Pc	7	6	4	Ren-17	Ub-14
Sj	4	5	7	Ren-5	Ub-22
Gb	40	37	36	Gb-24	Ub-19
Liv	3	5	6	Liv-14	Ub-18
Ren		Ren-15			
Du		Du-1			

8 Influential Points	
Zang	Liv-13
Fu	Ren-12
Qi	Ren-17
Blood	Ub-17
Sinews	Gb-34
Marrow	Gb-39
Bones	Ub-11
Vessels	Lu-9

4 Command Points	
Abdomen	St-36
Head & Neck	Lu-7
Back	Ub-40
Face & Mouth	LI-4

Lower He Sea Points		
3 Leg Yang	LI	St-37
	SI	St-39
	Sj	Ub-39
3 Leg Yin	St	St-36
	Ub	Ub-40
	Gb	Gb-34

Group Luo Points	
3 Arm Yang	Sj-8
3 Arm Yin	Pc-5
3 Leg Yang	Gb-39/35
3 Leg Yin	Sp-6

4 Sea Points	
Blood	Ub-11, St-37, St-39
Qi	Ren-17, Ub-10, St-9
Bone	Du-15, Du-16, Du-19, Du-20
Nourishment	St-30, St-36

Window of Sky	
Ub-10	Pc-1
St-9	Ren-22
Sj-16	Du-16
LI-18	SI-16
Lu-3	SI-18

Muscle Meridian Points	
3 Arm yang	Gb-13
3 Arm yin	Gb-22
3 Leg yang	SI-18 or St-3
3 Leg yin	Ren-3

8 Extra Meridian Points				
	Master	Xi-Cleft	Luo	Indications
Ren	Lu-7		Ren-15	Abdomen, chest, lungs, throat, face
Yin Qiao	K-6	K-8		
Du	SI-3		Du-1	Back of legs, back, spine, neck, head, eyes, brain
Yang Qiao	Ub-62	Ub-59		
Dai	Gb-41			Outer aspect of leg, sides of body, shoulders, side of neck
Yang Wei	SJ-5	Gb-35		
Chong	Sp-4			Inner aspect of leg, abdomen, chest, heart, stomach
Ying Wei	Pc-6	K-9		

Jing Well	Ying Spring	Shu Stream	Jing River	He Sea
Mental illness, stifling chest, fullness under the heart	Febrile complexion, hot sensations	Bi, wind, damp, heaviness, joint pain	Asthma, cough, hot/cold sensations, change of voice	Fu organs, stomach, intestines, rebellious Qi, diarrhea

Twelve Officials of the Court		
Ht	King	Source of Shen and clear insight
Lu	Minister to the King	Receives the pure Qi from Heaven
Liv	General	Sets strategy
Gb	Judge	Decisions of courage & wise judgment
Pc	Messenger to the King	Protects the King
Sp	Official	Grainery, transform & transport
St	Official	Grainery, rotting & ripening
LI	Official	Drainage
SI	Receiving Official	Separates pure from the impure
Kid	Minister of Health	Strength of body, controls water
Sj	Irrigation Official	Water channels, balance & harmony
Ub	Minor district Official	Controls storage of water & excretes fluids

POINTS

FOUR NEEDLE TECHNIQUE

Step One: Determine which organ system is out of balance
Step Two: Determine whether the imbalance is excess or deficiency
Step Three: See Below

Deficiency Conditions

• Tonify the horary point on the mother organ's channel.
• Tonify the mother organ's element point on the affected channel.
• Sedate the horary point on the "controlling" organ's channel.
• Sedate the controlling organ's element point on the affected organ.

Tonification prescriptions for conditions of deficiency

Meridian	Tonify		Sedate	
	Horary Pt	Mother Pt.	Horary Pt.	Control Pt.
Lung	Sp-3	Lu-9	Ht-8	Lu-10
Large Intestine	St-36	LI-11	SI-5	LI-5
Stomach	SI-5	St-41	Gb-41	St-43
Spleen	Ht-8	Sp-2	Liv-1	Sp-1
Heart	Liv-1	Ht-9	K-10	Ht-3
Small Intestine	Gb-41	SI-3	Ub-66	SI-2
Urinary Bladder	LI-1	Ub-67	St-36	Ub-40
Kidney	Lu-8	K-7	Sp-3	K-3
Pericardium	Liv-1	Pc-9	K-10	Pc-3
San Jiao	Gb-41	Sj-3	Ub-66	Sj-2
Gallbladder	Ub-66	Gb-43	LI-1	Gb-44
Liver	K-10	Liv-8	Lu-8	Liv-4

Excess Conditions

• Tonify the horary point on the controlling organ's channel.
• Tonify the controlling point on the affected channel.
• Sedate the horary point on the "son" channel.
• Sedate the son point on the affected channel.

Sedation prescriptions for conditions of excess

Meridian	Tonify		Sedate	
	Horary Pt	Control Pt.	Horary Pt.	Son Pt.
Lung	Ht-8	Lu-10	K-10	Lu-5
Large Intestine	SI-5	LI-5	Ub-66	LI-2
Stomach	Gb-41	St-43	LI-1	St-45
Spleen	Liv-1	Sp-1	Lu-8	Sp-5
Heart	K-10	Ht-3	Sp-3	Ht-7
Small Intestine	Ub-66	SI-2	St-36	SI-8
Urinary Bladder	St-36	Ub-40	Gb-41	Ub-65
Kidney	Sp-3	K-3	Liv-1	K-1
Pericardium	K-10	Pc-3	Sp-3	Pc-7
San Jiao	Ub-66	Sj-2	St-36	Sj-10
Gallbladder	LI-1	Gb-44	SI-5	Gb-38
Liver	Lu-8	Liv-4	Ht-8	Liv-2

Control Cycle – Interacts or Overacts

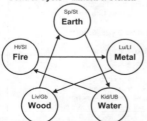

Mother-Son Cycle

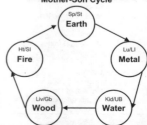

Elements	Wood	Fire	Earth	Metal	Water
Yin	Liver	Heart	Spleen	Lung	Kidney
Yang	Gallbladder	Small intestine	Stomach	Large intestine	Bladder
Color	Green/blue	Red	Yellow	White	Black, deep blue
Flourishes/ manifests	Nails	Complexion	Lips	Body hair, skin	Head hair
Sense organ	Eyes	Tongue	Mouth	Nose	Ears
Tissue dominated/ rules over	Ligaments, tendons, tissues, sinews	Blood & vessels	Muscles	Skin, mucous membranes	Bones, teeth, marrow, nerves
Orifice/ opens into	Eyes	Tongue	Mouth	Nose	Ears
Physiognomy	Eyes	Nose, tongue	Tongue, mouth	Cheeks & nostrils	Ears
Eye	Iris	Canthus	Lids	Sclera	Pupil
Tongue	Sides	Tip	Center	Posterior of tip	Root
Secretion	Tears	Sweat	Saliva	Mucous	Urine
Pulse	Stringy, wiry	Large, rapid	Slippery	Floating, slow	Sunken, deep
Emotion	Anger, jealousy	Joy	Anxiety, pensiveness, sympathy, desire	Sorrow, worry, grief	Fear & depression
Odor/smell	Rancid (cheese), goatish, fetid	Scorched (burnt)	Fragrant	Rotten (fish), rank	Putrid (urine), rotten
Flavor	Sour & acid	Bitter & sharp	Sweet	Pungent & spicy	Salty
Strained by	Reading	Walking	Sitting	Lying	Standing
Sound emitted to emotion	Shouting	Laughter & talkative	Singing	Weep, wail, cry	Groan & complain
Sound emitted in illness	Talking	Belching	Swallowing	Coughing	Yawning
Direction	East	South	Center	West	North
Climate	Windy	Hot	Moisture & thunder	Dryness & cold	Cold & wet
Season	Spring	Summer	Late summer, Indian summer	Autumn	Winter
Development	Birth	Growth	Change	Decline	Death
Granted power	Control	Sadness, grief	Belching	Cough	Trembling
Sense	Vision	Speech	Taste	Smell	Hearing
Instinct	Emotion	Spirit	Conscience	Health	Will
Thought	Relaxed	Enlightened	Careful	Energetic	Quiet
Motion	Clench	Anxiety	Hiccup	Cough	Tremble
Heavens	Stars	Sun	Earth	Zodiac	Moon
Planet	Jupiter	Mars	Saturn	Venus	Mercury
Number	8 & 3	7 & 2	10 & 5	9 & 4	6 & 1
Tendency	Up	Periphery	Balance	Down	Center
Ministries	Agriculture	War	Capital	Justice	Works
Classes	Fish	Birds	Man	Mammals	Invertebrate
Instruments	Compasses	Weights & measures	Plumb lines	T-square	Balances
Covering	Scales	Feathered	Naked	Hairy	Shelled
Wild animal	Tiger	Stag	Bear	Bird	Monkey
Grain	Wheat, rye, barley	Corn, beans	Rice, millet	Rice, oats	Peas, millet, buckwheat
Vegetable	Short green	Round	Leafy green	Tall green	Bushy
Fruit	Plum	Apricot	Date	Peach	Chestnut
Animal food	Sheep	Fowl	Beef, ox	Horse, dog	Wild pig
Cooking	Steam	Raw	Stew	Bake	Sautéed

POINTS

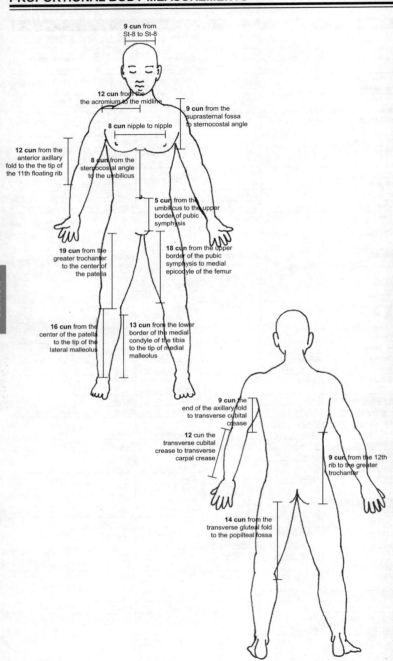

9 cun from St-8 to St-8

12 cun from the acromium to the midline

9 cun from the suprasternal fossa to sternocostal angle

8 cun nipple to nipple

12 cun from the anterior axillary fold to the the tip of the 11th floating rib

8 cun from the sternocostal angle to the umbilicus

5 cun from the umbilicus to the upper border of pubic symphysis

19 cun from the greater trochanter to the center of the patella

18 cun from the upper border of the pubic symphysis to medial epicodyle of the femur

16 cun from the center of the patella to the tip of the lateral malleolus

13 cun from the lower border of the medial condyle of the tibia to the tip of medial malleolus

9 cun the end of the axillary fold to transverse cubital crease

12 cun the transverse cubital crease to transverse carpal crease

9 cun from the 12th rib to the greater trochanter

14 cun from the transverse gluteal fold to the popilteal fossa

Condition	Formulas & Diagnoses	Points	Extra Points (BM)
Acid Reflux	Xiang Lian Wan - Stomach heat; Wei Te Ling; hyperacidity; Xiang Sha Yang Wei Wan - qi stag.; Chai Hu Shu Gan Tang - Liver qi stag.; Shu Gan Tang - Liver qi stag.; Yi Guan Jian Wan - yin def., qi stag.; Wei Tong Ding cold, yang def.; Bao He Wan - food stag.; Ping Wei San - phlegm damp; Jian Pi Wan - pregnancy; Bo Ying Compound - Infants; Qi Xing Tea - infants	Common pts: St-34, Gb-23, Gb-24, Gb-40, Liv-14, Ren-9, Ren-14, Ren-17; Stomach heat: Liv-2, LI-11, Gb-34, St-36, St-44, Ren-12, Ren-13, Ren-17, Ub-18; Liver qi stag.: Liv-3, LI-10, Pc-6, St-36, Ren-12, Ren-13, Ren-17, Ub-18, Ub-19; Damp phlegm: St-40, Pc-6, Pc-5, St-36, Sp-3, Ren-12, Ren-17; food stag.: Pc-6, Ren-12, St-21, St-36, St-40, St-44, LI-10	
Acne	Qing Re An Chuang Pian - toxic heat & hot blood.; Zhen Zhu An Chuang Tablet - toxic & damp heat; Huang Lian Jie Du Tang - damp heat; Wu Wei Xiao Du Yin - toxic heat; Lien Chiao Pai Tu Pien - wind heat, toxic heat; Chuan Xin Lian Cream topical	All points: Lu-11, Ht-9, Sp-2, Ub-54/40, Liv-11, K-12, Lu-4, LI-11; Blood Heat: Sp-10, LI-11, Ub-17, Sp-6, LI-4, Du-14	BM: (L) Liv-1, Liv-4, LI-1, LI-4; (R) Gb-44, Gb-40, Lu-11, Lu-8
Allergy	Yu Ping Feng San - wei qi def.; Reishi Mushroom immune regulator; Bi Ye Ning Capsule - phlegm heat; Pe Min Kan Wan - wind; Xiang Sha Liu Jun Tang - Spleen def. with phlegm damp; Ba Ji Yin Yang Wan - Lung & Kid. yang def.	LI-20, Ub-2	BM Cold type: (L) LI-3, LI-11, Sp-3, Sp-4, Sp-9; (R) Lu-5, Lu-9, St-36, St-41 BM Heat type: (L) LI-1, LI-3, Sp-3, Sp-4, Sp-9; (R) St-36, St-37, St-43
Alopecia	Yang Xue Sheng Fa Capsules - blood & yin def., postpartum; Qi Bao Mei Ran Dan blood & yin def., postpartum; Tangkwei Essence of Chicken - blood def., postpartum Deer Velvet - jing def.; Shou Wu Chih - blood & yin def.; Shou Wu Pian - blood def. You Gui Wan - yang def.; Zuo Gui Wan - yin def.; Tong Qiao Huo Xue Wan - blood stag.	Ub-17, Ub-18, Ub-19, Ub-23, St-36, Sp-9, K-3	7 star needles in balding area.
Alzheimer's	Huan Shao Dan - Heart & Kid. def.	Sea of Marrow: Du-1, Du-15, Du-16, Du-17 and Du-28. Du-16 and Du-20 treat brain disorders. Sj-19, K-16 and Liv-7 neutralize the effect of biochemical toxicities and balance the pineal gland.	BM: (L) K-1, K-4, LI-1, LI-4; (R) Lu-11, Lu-8, Ub-67, Ub-64
Amenorrhea	Ba Zhen Wan - qi & blood def.; Si Wu Tang - blood def.; Ba Zhen Yi Mu Wan - qi & blood def. with mild blood stag.; Gui Pi Tang - Heart & Spleen def.; Shi Quan Da Bu Tang - qi & blood def. with cold; Woo Garm Yuen Medical Pills - cold & blood stag.; Wen Jing Tang - cold, def. and blood stag.; Tong Jing Wan - blood stag.; Yunnan Paiyao blood stag.; Shao Fu Zhu Yu Tang - blood stag, with cold, severe; Tao Hong Si Wu Tang - blood stag. with blood def.; Liu Wei Di Huang Wan - Kid. yin def.; Zuo Gui Wan - Kid. yin def.; Fu Gui Ba Wei Wan - Kid. yang def.; Tiao Jing Cu Yun Wan - Kid. yang def.	All points: LI-4, LI-11, St-26, St-29, Sp-6, Sp-10, K-5, K-6, K-8, K-13, Gb-26, Gb-43, Liv-3, Liv-8, Du-7, Ren-1, Ren-3, Ren-4, Ren-7; Qi & blood stag.: Ren-3, Sp-6, Sp-8, Sp-10, Liv-3, LI-4; Yin & blood def.: K-6, Sp-6, Ub-17, Ub-18, Ub-23; Phlegm-damp: Ren-3, Sp-8, St-40, Sp-6 LI-4, St-36; Yang def.: Ub-23, Ren-3, Ren-4, Sp-6, St-36; Liver & Kidney def.: Ub-18, Ub-23, Ren-4, Sp-6, Ub-17; Qi & blood def.: Ub-20, Ren-4, St-36, Sp-6, Sp-10	BM: (L) Sp-9, Sp-8, Sp-6, LI-4, E-linkgu; (R) St-36, Lu-5, Lu-6 or ashi, Gb-42

METHODS

METHODS

Condition	Formulas & Diagnoses	Points	Extra Points (BM)
Angina	Xue Fu Zhu Yu Tang - qi & blood stag.; Dan Shen Pill - blood & phlegm stag.; Dan Shen Yin - qi & blood stag.; Xin Mai Ling - blood stag.; Raw Tienchi Tablets - blood stag.; Tao Hong Si Wu Tang - blood stag. with blood def., mild; Guan Xin An Kou Fu Ye - blood stag.; Huo Luo Xiao Ling Tang - blood stag.; Sunho Multi Ginseng Tablets - blood stag. & qi def.	Pc-6, Ub-14, St-40, Ub-13, Lu-9	BM: (L) Pc-6, St-22 or ashi; (R) LI-3, Sp-6, Liv-5 or ashi, Ear-shenmen. BM for severe blood stagnation or unknown cause: (L) Lu-11, Pc-9, Ht-9, St-36, Gb-34, Ub-40; (R) LI-4, SI-3, Sp-3, Sp-6, Liv-4, K-3
Ankle Pain	Jian Bu Qiang Shen Tang - Kid. def.	Common pts: Ub-60, Ub-62, K-6, Gb-40, St-41, Sp-5	BM: LI-11, Lu-5, Ht-3 and ashi
Anxiety	Tian Wang Bu Xin Dan - Heart & Kid. yin def.; Gui Pi Tang - Heart & Spleen qi def.; Bai Zi Yang Xin Tang - blood & yin def.; An Shen Ding Zhi Tang - blood & yin def. with phlegm; An Shen Bu Xin Tang - yin def., yang rising; Wen Dan Tang - phlegm heat; Chai Hu Long Gu Mu Li Tang - qi stag., phlegm heat, yang rising; Ban Xia Hou Po Tang - qi & phlegm stag.; Po Lung Yuen Medical Pills - phlegm heat	Common pts: Du-24, Gb-13, Ht-7, Pc-6, Pc-7, Sp-6, E-shishencong, E-anmian, Ear-shenmen; Heart def.: Ub-15, Pc-5, Pc-6, Ht-7, St-36, Ren-14, E-yintang	BM shu-stream/he-sea combo: (L) Gb-41, Gb-34, Ht-3, Ht-7; (R) Liv-3, Liv-8, SJ-3, SJ-10
Appendicitis (Acute)	Acute, uncomplicated: Huang Lian Jie Du Tang - damp & toxic heat; Wu Wei Xiao Du Yin - toxic heat; Ching Fei Yi Huo Pien - yang ming organ syndrome; Niu Huang Qing Huo Wan - yang ming organ syndrome; Liang Ge San - yang ming organ syndrome	All points: E-lanweixue, St-37, St-25, LI-11, St-36, Sp-10, Ub-54/40, Sp-9, Sp-8, Sp-6, Liv-2, SJ-10, LI-4	
Arthritis	Juan Bi Tang - wind cold damp; Qu Feng Zhen Tong Capsule - wind cold damp; Xuan Bi Tang - damp heat; Guan Jie Yan Wan - damp heat; Shu Jin Huo Xue Wan - blood & phlegm stag.; Shen Tong Zhu Yu Wan - blood stag.; Xiao Huo Luo Dan - severe cold; Du Huo Ji Sheng Tang - wind damp with Kid. def.; Jian Bu Qiang Shen Wan - Kid. def.; Fu Gui Ba Wei Wan - Kid. yang def.; Trans Wood Lock Liniment topical; Porous Capsicum Plaster topical; Gou Pi Gao topical	Wind Bi: Du-14, SJ-6, Gb-39 Cold Bi: SI-6, Ren-6, LI-11; Damp Bi: Sp-9, Sp-11, Gb-39, St-40; Heat Bi: St-43, LI-4; For local pts: Shoulder: LI-15, LI-14, SJ-14, E-jaineiling, SI-9, SI-10; Elbow: same as shoulder plus LI-11, SI-8, SJ-10; Wrist: SJ-5, LI-5, SI-4; Neck: Du-14, Ub-10, Gb-20,SI-3,Gb-39, Ub-60, E- huatoijaji; Hip: Gb-30, Gb-29, Ub-51, St-31, Gb-34, Gb-39, Gb-40; Knee: St-34, Sp-10, Gb-34, Sp-9, St-36, Ub-40; Ankle: St-41, Sp-5, St-36, Ub-60, K-3; Toes: Sp-4, Ub-65, E-Bafeng	
Asthma	Ma Huang Tang - wind cold; Su Zi Jiang Zi Tang - cold phlegm; Xiao Qing Long Wan - wind cold with congested fluids; Ding Chuan Wan - phlegm heat; Zing Zi Hua Tan Wan - phlegm heat; Mai Wei Di Huang Wan - Lung & Kid. yin def.; Sheng Mai San - qi & yin def.; Bu Fei Tang - Lung qi def.; Yulin Bu Shen Wan - Kid not grasping qi, yang def.; Cordyceps Essence of Chicken - Lung & Kid. def.	E-dingchuan, Ren-22, Lu-6. All points: Lu-1, Lu-2, Lu-3, Lu-4, Lu-5, Lu-6, Lu-7, Lu-8, Lu-9, LI-18, St-9, St-13, St-40, SI-17, Ub-13, Ub-23, Ub-42, Ub-43, Ub-44, K-2, K-3, K-4, K-22, K-23, K-24, K-25, K-26, Pc-6, Gb-25, Du-10, Ren-17, Ren-20, Ren-22, E-Dingchuan; Wind cold: Lu-5, Lu-7, Du-14, LI-20, Ub-12, Ub-13, LI-4, SJ-5, St-3; Phlegm heat: Ub-13, Lu-5, St-40, LI-4, E-dingchuan, Ren-22; Lung def.: E-dingchuan, Ub-13/43, Lu-9, Ub20, St-36; Kidney def.: K-3, Ub-13, Ub-23, Ren-7, E-dingchuan	

Condition	Formulas & Diagnoses	Points	Extra Points (BM)
Atherosclerosis	Dan Shen Pill - blood & phlegm stag;. Keep Fit Capsule - phlegm & blood stag;. Raw Tienqi Tablets - blood stag;. Dan Shen Yin - qi & blood stag;. Guan Xin An Kou Fu Ye - blood stag;. Sunho Multi Ginseng Tablets - blood stag;. Xue Fu Zhu Yu Tang - blood stag.	All points: Pc-6, Pc-4, Ub-15, Ren-17, LI-11, St-36, Ub-16, Ub-14	
Back pain	Back pain: Zhuang Yao Jian Shen - Kid. def;. Liu Wei Di Huang Wan - yin def;. Zuo Gui Wan - yin def;. Fu Gui Ba Wei Wan - Kid. yang def;. You Gui Wan - yang def;. Jian Bu Qing Shen Wan - Kid. def;. San Bi Wan - wind damp with Kid. def;. Kang Gu Zeng Sheng Pian - spondylosis; Shu Jin Huo Xue Wan - wind damp with blood stag;. Shi Lin Tong renal calculi; Bi Xie Sheng Shi Wan - damp heat; Die Da Zhi Tong Capsules - acute blood stag;. Plaster for Bruise and Analgesic topical; Porous Capsicum Plaster topical; Gou Pi Gao topical. Back weakness: Jian Bu Qiang Shen Wan - Kid. def;. Hua Tuo Zai Zao Wan - qi & yin def;. wind damp; Ba Ji Yin Yang Wan - Kid. yang def;. Zhuang Yao Jian Shen Tablets - Kid. yang def;. Si Jun Zi Wan - Spleen qi def	All points: E-yaotongxue, E-lingku, E-dabi, E-zhongbai; Gb-30, E-yaoyan, Ub-17, Ub-23, Ub-40; Cold-damp: Ub-23, Ub-25, Ub-40, Ub-54, Ub-32, Du-3, Ren-4; Damp-heat: Ub-23, Gb-34, Ub-32, Du-3, Sp-6 Ub-40; Blood stag;: Ub-23, Ub-25, Ub-40, Ub-54, Ub-32, Du-3, Du-26, E-yaotongxue, E-ashi; Kidney yang def.: Ub-23, Ub-40, Ub-54, Du-3, Du-4, E-yaoyan; Kidney yin def.: K-3, Ub-32, Ub-52, Ub-23, Du-3	BM opposite of pain: LI-4, SI-3, SI-4, E-lingku-dabi, E-zhongbai; K-4 or ashi; K-7 or ashi; BM same side pain: Lu-5, Lu-6, Ub-65, or ashi
Bronchitis	Acute: Ching Fei Yi Huo Pien - Lung fire; Qing Qi Hua Tan Wan - phlegm heat; Niu Huang Qing Huo Wan - toxic heat; Huang Lian Jie Du Tang - toxic & damp heat; Xiao Chai Hu Tang - post acute	Common pts: E-dingchuan, Ub-12, Ub-13, LI-4; Supp pts.: LI-11, Du-14, Lu-5, Lu-7, St-40, E-jiaji C7 to T6	BM with heat: Lu-10, Lu-9, LI-4, LI-5, Liv-3, St-44; BM with Phlegm: (L) Liv-5, K-9, Sp-6, LI-4, LI-11; (R) Lu-10, Lu-9, St-40, Ub-57
Bursitis	Juan Bi Tang - wind cold damp; Jian Bu Qiang Shen Wan - with Kid. def.; Zheng Gu Shui topical; Trans Wood Lock Liniment topical	LI-15, SJ-14, LI-4, LI-11, SI-6, Sj-3, Ub-10, LI-11, Gb-34, E-jianneiling for bursitis of the shoulder - consider St-38, Ub-57 with movement for acute pain in shoulder	BM: (L) St-36, Pc-6; (R) Sp-6 SI-5, LI-4
Cancer Pain	Reishi Mushroom immune regulator; American Ginseng Essence of Chicken; Cordyceps Essence of Chicken; Bu Zhong Yi Qi Tang	Pc-6, Pc-7, Sj-5, Sj-10, LI-11, Lu-8, Sj-6, LI-5, SI-4, LI-9 and LI-4 (hand and forearm); SI-3, LI-3 and E-baxie (fingers)	BM: (L) St-36, Pc-6; (R) Sp-6 SI-5, LI-4
Carpal Tunnel Syndrome (CTS)	Qu Feng Zhen Tong Tang - wind, cold, damp; Shen Tong Zhu Yu Wan - blood stag.		BM opposite side of pain: Sp-5, Liv-4, K-2, K-3, LI-5, SI-5, Sj-4; BM same side of pain: Ub-60, Gb-40, St-41
Cholesterol / Triglycerides High	Keep Fit Capsule - phlegm & blood stag;. Bojenmi Chinese Tea; Dan Shen Pill - blood stag;. Raw Tienchi Tablets - blood stag;. Sunho Multi Ginseng Tablets - blood stag;. Reishi Mushroom immune regulator		BM for high cholesterol: (L) Sp-9, Sp-10, Sj-5; (R) St-36, St-40, Pc-7, Pc-8; BM for fatty liver: (L) Sj-10, LI-9, LI-10, Liv-7, Sp-9; (R) Gb-34, ashi around Pc-3/Pc-4
Chronic Fatigue Syndrome	Xiao Chai Hu Tang - shao yang; Bu Zhong Yi Qi Tang - Spleen qi def.; Gui Pi Tang - Heart & Spleen def.; Xiang Sha Liu Jun Tang - Spleen qi def. with phlegm damp	St-36, Pc-6, Sp-4, Ren-4, Ren-6, Ren-12, Du-4, Ub-17, Ub-23	BM: (L) LI-4, St-36, K-3, Sp-9; (R) Lu-7, Ht-5, St-36

Condition	Formulas & Diagnoses	Points	Extra Points (BM)
Common Cold	Gan Mao Ling - general; Ma Huang Tang - wind cold, wheezing; Gui Zhi Tang - wind, postpartum; Ge Gen Tang - wind cold, neck pain; Chuan Xiong Cha Tiao Wan - wind cold, headache; Jing Fang Bai Du Wan - wind cold/heat; Yin Chiao Chieh Tu Pien - wind heat; Gan Mao Zhi Ke Chong Ji - tai yang/shao yang; Gan Mao Qing Re Chong Ji - wind heat; Shih San Tai Pao Wan - during pregnancy; Ren Shen Bai Du San - wind cold with qi def.; Xiao Chai Hu Tang - lingering	Wind cold: Gb-20, Lu-7, LI-20, Ub-12, LI-4, Sj-5; Wind-heat: Gb-20, Du-14, Lu-5, LI-4, LI-11, Sj-5; Cold def.: St-36, Ub-13 Yin def.: Ub-43, K-7; Supp pts: LI-20, E-bitong, E-yintang, E-taiyang, Ren-22, St-40, Ub-12, Ub-13, E-jiaji	BM: (L) Sj-10, LI-11, Ht-6/7 or ashi in btw, K-10, Liv-8, Sp-9; (R) Pc-3, Ht-8, Lu-9/10 or ashi in btw, Gb-34, St-36, Ub-40; BM with Phlegm: (L) Liv-5, K-9, Sp-6, LI-4, LI-11; (R) Lu-10, Lu-9, St-40, Ub-57
Constipation	Run Chang Wan - blood & fluid def.; Wu Ren Wan - blood & fluid def.; Cong Rong Bu Shen Wan - yang def., atonic; Mu Xiang Shun Qi Tang - qi stag., habitual; Chen Xiang Hua Zi Wan - qi stag., qi def.; Da Huang Jiang Zhi Wan - excess; Ching Fei Yi Huo Pien - yang ming syndrome, Lung fire; Da Chai Hu Tang - shao yang/yang ming syndrome; Yang Yin Qing Fei Wan - yin def., dry post febrile	Common pts: Ren-12, Ren-6, St-25, K-6, Sj-6, Ub-25; Heat: St-25, LI-4, LI-11, Sj-6, K-6, Ub-25; Qi stag.: St-25, Ub-25, Ren-6, Ren-12, Liv-3, Sj-6; Qi def.: St-25, Ub-20, Ub-25, Sp-6, St-36, Ren-4; Blood def.: St-25, Ub-25, St-36, Sp-14, Ren4, Sp-6; Cold: St-25, Ub-25, Ren-4, Ren-6, K-6, Ub-23, moxa Ren-8	BM for deficiency type: (L) Sj-5, Sj-6, K-6, LI-4; (R) St-36, St-37 Lu-6 or ashi; BM for excess type: (L) Sj-5, Sj-6, LI-11; (R) St-37, St-38 Lu-6 or ashi, Pc-3
Cough	Acute: Ma Huang Tang - wind cold; Xiao Qing Long Wan - wind cold with congested fluids; Gan Mao Zhi Ke Chong Ji - wind heat; Sang Ju Yin - wind heat; Ching Fei Yi Huo Pien - Lung heat/fire; Qing Qi Hua Tan Wan - phlegm heat; Pi Pa Cough Tea - phlegm heat; Su Zi Jiang Qi Wan - cold phlegm	Wind cold: Lu-7, LI-4, Ub-13, Sj-5; Wind-heat: Ub-13, Lu-5, Lu-11, K-7, LI-11, Du-14; Dryness: Ub-13, LI-11, Lu-5, Lu-10, Lu-7, LI-4; Liver fire: Ub-13, Ub-18, Liv-3, K-6, Lu-6; Yin def.: Ub-13, Lu-5, Lu-6, Lu-7, K-6, Ub-17	BM: (L) Lu-8, Lu-9, Pc-6, St-39/40/41; (R) LI-4, LI-5, Sp-6, K-8
Depression	Chai Hu Shu Gan Tang - Liver qi stag.; Xiao Yao San - qi stag. & blood def.; Tao Hong Si Wu Tang - blood stag., blood def.; Xue Fu Zhu Yu Tang - chronic, blood stag.; Wen Dan Tang - phlegm heat; Xiang Sha Yang Wei Wan - qi & damp stag.	Liver qi stag.: LI-4, Liv-3, St-36, Ren-17, Ht-7, Du-20; Phlegm: Liv-3, St-40, St-36, Ren-12, Ren-17, Pc-6; Heart & Spleen def.: Ht-7, Sp-6, St-36, Liv-3, Ub-15, Ub-17, Ub-20; Spleen & Kid def.: Ren-4, K-3, St-36, Sp-6, Du-4, Ub-20, Ub-23	BM: Shu Stream/He Sea Combo: (L) Ht-3, Ht-5, Ht-7, Gb-34, Gb-40, Gb-41; (R) Sj-3, Sj-10, Liv-3, Liv-8, E-yintang, E-anmian, Ear-shen men + 12 magic pts; Also consider BM with low energy: (L) Gb-40, Gb-34, Ht-7, Ht-5, Ht-3; (R) Liv-3, Liv-5, Sj-3, Si-5, Si-10
Diabetes	D. Insipidus: Sang Piao Xiao Wan - Heart & Kid. yang qi def. D. Mellitus: Yu Quan Wan; Sugardil; Liu Wei Di Huang Wan; Shen Ling Bai Zhu Wan; Gu Ben Wan; Fu Gui Ba Wei Wan. D. Mellitus: Yu Quan Wan - qi & yin def.; Sugardil; Liu Wei Di Huang Wan - Kid. yin def.; Shen Ling Bai Zhu Wan - Spleen qi def.; Gu Ben Wan - Stomach & Kid. yin def.; Fu Gui Ba Wei Wan - Kid. yang def.	Common pts: E-yishu, St-36, K-3, Ub-13, Ub-20, Ub-23; Supp pts.: LI-11, Lu-10, Ub-17, Ub-21, Ren-12, E-pire, Ren-4, K-5; Lung-heat: Ub-13, St-36, Lu-5, Ub-13; Stomach dryness: K-3, Sp-6, St-36, St-44, K-3, Ub-20, Lu-5; Kidney essence def.: K-3, K-3, Ren-4, Sp-6, Gv-20, Ub-23; Liver qi stag.: Liv-3, LI-4, Liv-14, Pc-6, Ub-18, Liv-2; Spleen qi def.: Sp-3, Sp-6, St-36, Ren-12, Ub-20	BM: (L) Sp-6, Sp-9 or ashi, K-7, LI-4, Sj-5; (R) St-36, Ub-40, Ub-41

Condition	Formulas & Diagnoses	Points	Extra Points (BM)
Diarrhea	Acute: Po Chai Pills - damp heat; Xing Jun San - summer damp; Huo Hsiang Cheng Chi Pien - wind cold with damp; Ge Gen Tang - wind cold; Huang Lian Jie Du Tang - damp or toxic heat; Bo Ying Compound - infantile. Chronic: Shen Ling Bai Zhu Wan - Spleen qi def.; Tong Xie Yao Fang Wan - Liver invading Spleen; Li Zhong Wan - Spleen yang def.; Zi Sheng Wan - Spleen def. with food stag.; Ba Ji Yin Yang Wan - Spleen & Kid. yang def.; cockcrow; Yulin Da Bu Wan - yang def.; cockcrow; Healthy Child Tea - infantile	Common pts: St-25, St-36, St-37, Sp-9, Ren-8 - moxa; Chronic diarrhea: (E-sanjiaojiu pts - triangle smile to Ren-8); Damp: St-25, Ren-12, St-36, LI-4, Sp-9; Damp-heat: St-25, St-36, St-44, Sp-9, LI-11; Food stag.: St-25, Ren-12, St-36, E-lineiting; Liver & Spleen disharmony: St-25, St-36, Ren-12, Gb-34, Liv-3, Ub-18; Spleen & Stomach def.: St-25, St-36, Sp-3, Ub-20, Ub-26, Ren-12; Spleen & Kidney yang def.: K-3, Du-4, Ren-4, St-36, Ub-20, Ub-23	BM for excess type: (L) St-34, St-36, St-37, St-38, Pc-4, Pc-6 or ashi; (R) Sp-3, Sp-4, Sp-10, LI-4, LI-11, LI-10 or ashi
Dysmenorrhea	Gui Zhi Fu Ling Tang - mild blood stag., masses; Tao Hong Si Wu Tang - mild blood stag. with blood def.; Tong Jing Wan - severe blood stag.; Shao Fu Zhu Yu Tang - cold & blood stag., severe; Woo Garm Yuen Medical Pills - blood stag. with cold; Dang Gui Si Ni Wan - cold; Tong Luo Zhi Tong Tablet - blood stag.; Xiao Yao San - Liver qi stag.; Tian Tai Wu Yao Wan - cold in Liver channel; Ba Zhen Yi Mu Wan - mild blood def.; Yi Mu Tiao Jing Tablet - blood def. with blood stag.; Shi Xiao Wan - blood stag.; Shi Quan Da Bu Tang - qi & blood def. with cold; Ba Zhen Tang - qi & blood def.	All points: St-25, St-26, St-28, Sp-6, Sp-8, Sp-10, Ub-24, Ub-25, Ub-30, Ub-31, Ub-32, Ub-34, K-5, K-6, K-8, Pc-5, Liv-5, Ren-2, Ren-6, E-Tituo; Cold-damp: Ren-3, St-28, Sp-8; Liver stag.: Ren-6, Liv-3, Sp-6; Damp-heat: Ren-3, Sp-8, St-29, Liv-3, LI-4, Ub-32; Yang def.: Ub-23, Ren-3, Ren-4, Sp-8, Sp-6, St-36; Liver & Kidney def.: Ub-18, Ub-23, Ren-4, St-36, K-6; Qi & blood def.: Ub-23, Ren-4, St-36, Sp-6	BM Tx1: (L) St-36, Lu-7; (R) LI-4, Sp-9, Sp-7 or ashi, Sp-6; BM Tx2: (L) Sp-6, Sp-8, Sp-9, LI-4, E-Lingku; (R) St-36, Lu-5, Lu-6, Lu-7 or ashi, Gb-42, Gb-41
Edema	Ma Huang Tang - wind cold, acute/facial; Wu Ling San - Spleen def. with congested fluids; Wu Pi Yin generalized, pregnancy, menopause; Fang Ji Huang Qi Wan - wind; Zhen Wu Tang - Heart & Kid. yang def.; Fu Gui Ba Wei Wan - Kid. yang def.; Bojenmi Chinese Tea - Spleen def.	All points: LI-6, St-12, St-22, St-25, St-28, St-36, St-43, St-36, Sp-6, Sp-7, Sp-8, Sp-9, Ub-20, Ub-22, Ub-23, Ub-50, Ub-52, Ub-53, K-6, K-7, K-14, Gb-8, Gb-29, Du-21, Ren-3, Ren-5, Ren-7, Ren-9	BM: (L) LI-4, Sp-9; (R) Lu-5, St-40
Elbow Pain		Common pts: St-11, LI-10, Lu-5, Sj-10, Sj-5, LI-4, SI-3, SI-7, Gb-34	BM opposite knee to pain: Sp-9/10, Liv-8, K-10, Ub-39/40, Gb-33/34, St-35/36
Endometriosis	Woo Garm Yuen Medical Pills - blood stag., cold; Wen Jing Tang - cold; def., blood stag.; Tong Jing Wan - blood stag., severe; Tao Hong Si Wu Tang - blood stag., with blood def.; Gui Zhi Fu Ling Tang - mild blood stag.; Shao Fu Zhu Yu Tang - blood stag. & cold; Nei Xiao Luo Li Wan - phlegm & blood stag.; Ru Jie Xiao Tablet - qi, blood & phlegm; Xue Fu Zhu Yu Tang - qi & blood stag.; Huo Luo Xiao Ling Tang - blood stag.; Cu Yun Yu Tai Capsules - Kid. yang def.; Ba Zhen Yi Mu Wan - qi & blood def.; Shi Quan Da Bu Tang - qi & blood def. with cold	Gb-26, Sp-8, Sp-6, Ren-3, Ren-2, St-28, St-29, St-30	BM: (L) Sp-6, Sp-8, Sp-9, LI-4, E-Lingku; St-36, Lu-5, Lu-6, Lu-7 or ashi, Gb-42, Gb-41
Energy (Tiredness, Fatigue)	Bu Zhong Yi Qi Tang - Spleen & Lung qi def.; Bu Fei Tang - Lung qi def.; Shi Quan Da Bu Tang - qi & blood def.; Fu Gui Ba Wei Wan - yang def.; Liu Wei Di Huang Wan - yin def.; Panax Ginseng Extractum - qi def.; Sheng Mai San - qi & yin def.; American Ginseng Essence of Chicken - qi & yin def.; Xiao Chai Hu Tang - shao yang syndrome; Ping Wei San - phlegm damp; Wen Dan Tang - phlegm heat	Common pts: St-36, Ren-4, Ren-6, Du-4, Ub-23	BM: (L) LI-4, Sp-9, Sj-5, K-7; (R) Ht-4, St-36, Lu-7

METHODS

252

Condition	Formulas & Diagnoses	Points	Extra Points (BM)
Eye Pain	Ming Mu Di Huang Wan - Liver yin def.; Si Wu Wan - blood stag.; Shi Quan Da Bu Tang - qi & blood stag.; Huang Lien Shang Ching Pien, wind heat, toxic heat; Long Dan Xie Gan Tang - Liver fire; Jie Wei Xiao Yao San - qi stag. with heat	All points: LI-8, St-44, Ht-5, SI-6, Ub-4, Ub-9, SI-6, Ub-45, Ub-67, K-19, SJ-5, SJ-6, SJ-10, SJ-11, Gb-1, Gb-11, Gb-14, Gb-18, Gb-37, Du-17, Du-23, E-Taiyang	
Fever	Acute excess, high: Ma Huang Tang - wind cold; Yin Chiao Chieh Tu Pien - wind heat; Lien Chiao Pai Tu Pien - wind heat, Warm disease; Huang Lian Jie Du Tang - damp heat, toxic heat; Long Dan Xie Gan Tang - Liver fire; Ching Fei Yi Huo Pien - Lung fire; Bai Hu Tang - yang ming channel syndrome; Niu Huang Qing Huo Wan - yang ming organ syndrome; Pu Ji Xiao Du Wan - Warm disease; King Fung Powder - phlegm heat, infants	Common pts: Du-14, LI-4, LI-11, E-shixuan, E-Erjian, jingwell	
Fibroids	Woo Garm Yuen Medical Pills - blood & cold stag.; Gui Zhi Fu Ling Tang - mild blood stag.; Tao Hong Si Wu Tang - blood stag. & blood def.; Tong Jing Wan - blood stag.; Shao Fu Zhu Yu Tang - cold & blood stag.; Xue Fu Zhu Yu Tang - qi & blood stag.; Nei Xiao Luo Li Wan - hard phlegm stag.; Hai Zao Jing Wan - phlegm stag.; Ru Jie Xiao Tablets - qi, phlegm & blood stag.; Ji Sheng Ju He Wan - qi & phlegm stag.; Shi Quan Da Bu Tang - qi & blood def. with cold	Upper body: Gb-21, St-18, Liv-14, SI-3, Pc-6, Ub-18, Lu-5, St-36, Ren-17, St-16; Lower body: Pc-6, K-6, Liv-14, Liv-3, Liv-2, Sp-10, Ub-17, Ub-18	
Fibromyalgia	Shu Gan Tang - qi stag.; Chai Hu Shu Gan Tang - qi stag.; Xiao Yao San - qi stag.; Shen Tong Zhu Yu Wan - blood stag; Xue Fu Zhu Yu Tang - qi & blood stag.; Hua Tuo Zai Zao Wan - qi & yin def.; Juan Bi Tang - wind damp; Qu Feng Zhen Tong Capsules - wind cold damp	Liv-3, LI-4, Pc-6, SJ-5, LI-15, Gb-21, St-36, Sp-6, Ub-20, Ren-4	
Flu	Gan Mao Ling - general; Ma Huang Tang - wind cold, wheezing; Gui Zhi Tang - wind, postpartum; Ge Gen Tang - wind cold, neck pain; Chuan Xiong Cha Tiao Wan - wind cold, headache; Jing Fang Bai Du Wan - wind cold/heat; Yin Chiao Chieh Tu Pien - wind heat; Gan Mao Zhi Ke Chong Ji - tai yang/shao yang; Gan Mao Qing Re Chong Ji - wind heat; Shih San Tai Pao Wan - during pregnancy; Ren Shen Bai Du San - wind cold with qi def.; Xiao Chai Hu Tang - lingering	Wind cold: Gb-20, Lu-7, Sj-5; Wind-heat: Gb-20, Du-14, LI-4, LI-11; Supp pts.: LI-20, E-bitong, E-yintang, E-taiyang, Ren-22, St-40, Ub-12, Ub-13, E-jiaji	BM: (L) SJ-10, LI-11, Ht-6/7 or ashii in btw, K-10, Liv-8, Sp-9; (R) Pc-3, Ht-8, Lu-9/10 or ashii in btw, Gb-34, St-36, Ub-40; BM with Phlegm: (L) Liv-5, K-9, Sp-6, LI-4, LI-11; (R) Lu-10, Lu-9, St-40, Ub-57
Focus	Concentration: Jian Nao Yi Zhi Capsule - qi def. with blood stag.; Xiang Sha Liu Jun Tang - Spleen def. with phlegm damp; Gui Pi Tang - Heart blood & Spleen qi def.; Ping Wei San - phlegm damp; Wen Dan Tang - phlegm heat; Tian Wang Bu Xin Dan - Heart & Kid. yin def.; Cerebral Tonic Pills - phlegm & Kid. def. Poor memory: Jian Nao Yi Zhi Capsules - qi def., blood stag.; Cerebral Tonic Pills - blood def. & phlegm heat; Gui Pi Tang - qi & blood def.; Tian Wang Bu Xin Dan - Heart & Kid. yin def.; Huan Shao Dan - Heart & Kid. def.; Zhi Gan Cao Tang - Heart qi & blood def.; Bai Zi Yang Xin Wan - general; Wen Dan Tang - phlegm heat	All points: Lu-7, LI-11, Ht-3, Ht-7, Ub-15, Ub-43, K-1, K-3, K-6, K-21, St-36, Pc-5, Pc-6, Gb-20, Du-11, Du-20, Ren-14, E-Sishencong	BM: (L) Ht-7, Ht-4, Gb-40, Gb-34; (R) Liv-3, Liv-6, Sj-3, SI-7, Ear-shenmen

Condition	Formulas & Diagnoses	Points	Extra Points (BM)
Fungal Infection	Skin: Bi Xie Sheng Shi Wan - damp heat; Xiao Feng San - wind, damp; Xiao Yan Tang Shang Cream topical; Fu Yin Tai Liniment topical; Hua Tuo Gao topical; Tujin Liniment topical. Intestines: Da Huang Jiang Zhi Wan - damp heat; Huang Lian Jie Du Tang - damp heat. Toes: Hua Tuo Gao topical; Tujin Liniment topical; Xiao Yan Tang Shang Cream topical		
Gastro-esophageal Reflux Disease (GERD)	Xiang Lian Wan - Stomach heat; Wei Te Ling hyperacidity; Xiang Sha Yang Wei Wan - qi stag.; Chai Hu Shu Gan Tang - Liver qi stag.; Shu Gan Tang - Liver qi stag.; Yi Guan Jian Wan - yin def., qi stag.; Wei Tong Ding cold, yang def.; Bao He Wan - food stag.; Ping Wei San - phlegm damp; Bo Ying Compound - infants; Qi Xing Tea - infants	Common pts: St-34, Gb-23, Gb-24, Gb-40, Liv-14, Ren-9, Ren-14, Ren-17; Stomach heat: Liv-2, LI-11, Gb-34, Pc-8, St-36, St-44, Ren-12, Ren-13, Ren-17, Ub-18; Liver qi stag.: Liv-3, LI-10, Pc-6, St-36, Ren-12, Ren-13, Ren-17, Ub-19; Damp phlegm: St-40, Pc-6, Pc-5, St-36, Sp-3, Ren-12, Ren-17; food stag.: Pc-6, Ren-12, St-21, St-36, St-40, St-44, LI-10	BM: (L) Sj-5, LI-4, Sp-9, St-34; (R) St-34, Sp-10, Pc-6 Lu-7
Goiter	Hai Zao Jing Wan - phlegm; Nei Xiao Luo Li Wan - hard phlegm	Qi and blood stagnation: St-9 joined to SI-17, LI-4, St-36, E-zeqian, Pc-6, Sp-6, K-3; Influence thyroid: Ren-13, Ren-23, St-9, Ren-19, Du-15, Ub-15, Ht-7, St-10, Ren-6, Sj-3, K-7 and LI-4	Seven groups of five points each, each group needled one day in succession over the course of a week with three days between each course of seven treatments, for goiter: Tx 1. K-3, Pc-5, St-10, Ub-10 and Ub-2; Tx 2. K-7, St-36, Ren-22, Pc-6 and Du-1; Tx 3. K-6, Sp-6, LI-4, LI-11 and St-10; Tx 4. K-3, Liv-3, St-40, St-10 and Ub-10; Tx 5. K-7, St-36, Pc-5 and Ren-22; Tx 6. K-6, Pc-6, Liv-3, St-10 and Ub-10; Tx 7. K-3, Sp-6, LI-4, St-40 and Ren-22
Gout	Huang Lian Jie Du Tang - damp heat; Xuan Bi Tang - damp heat; Fang Feng Tong Sheng Wan - internal & external excess heat; Tiger Balm topical	Ub-17, Ub-18, Ub-19, Ub-23, St-36, Sp-9, K-3	
Hair Loss	Yang Xue Sheng Fa Capsules - blood & yin def., postpartum; Qi Bao Mei Ran Dan blood & yin def., postpartum; Tangkwei Essence of Chicken - blood def., postpartum Deer Velvet - jing def.; Shou Wu Chih - blood & yin def.; Shou Wu Pian - blood def. You Gui Wan - yang def.; Zuo Gui Wan - yin def.; Tong Qiao Huo Xue Wan - blood stag.	Frontal: St-8, St-44, LI-4, Du-23, E-yintang, E-yuyao; Vertex: Du-20, SI-3, Liv-3, Ub-67; Occipital: Du-20, SI-3, Ub-60; Temporal: Gb-8, Gb-41, Sj-5 E-taiyang; Wind-cold: Gb-20, Ub-12, LI-4, Lu-7; Wind-heat: LI-4, LI-11, Gb-14, Gb-20; Wind-damp: Lu-7, Gb-20, Si-8, LI-4; Yang rising: Gb-4, Gb-5, Liv-3, K-3, Gb-20, Gb-43; Kidney yin def.: Du-20, Du-23, Sp-6, K-3, Ub-18, Ub-23; Kidney yang def.: Du-4, Du-20, Du-23, Ren-4; Qi def.: Du-20, Du-6, Du-23, Ub-20 LI-4, St-36; Blood stag.: Liv-3, LI-4, St-36, Sp-6, Sp-10, E-ashi; Blood def.: Ub-17, Ub-18, Ub-20, St-36, Sp-6, Du-23	
Headache	Acute: Tian Ma Tou Tong Capsules - cold wind, yang rising; Chuan Xiong Cha Tiao Wan - wind cold; Zhen Gan Xi Feng Wan - Liver yang rising, Liver wind; Tian Ma Gou Teng Yin - Liver yang rising; Qu Feng Zhen Tong Capsules - wind cold damp; Tong Luo Zhi Tong Tablets - blood def., blood stag.; Long Dan Xie Gan Tang - Liver fire; Jia Wei Xiao Yao San - Liver qi stag. with heat; Yan Hu Suo Zhi Tong Wan - analgesic		BM Tx 1: (L) Lu-11, Pc-9, Ht-9, St-36, Gb-34, Ub-40; (R) LI-4, SI-3, Sj-3, Sp-6 Liv-4, K-3. BM Tx 2: Opposite of side of pain location: Liv-3, Liv-7, Sj-5, Sj-10; Same side of pain location: Gb-31, Gb-42, Ht-8

METHODS

METHODS

Condition	Formulas & Diagnoses	Points	Extra Points (BM)
Hearing Loss	Er Long Zuo Ci Wan - Kid. yin def.; Zuo Gui Wan - Kid. yin def.; Fu Gui Ba Wei Wan - Kid. yang def.; You Gui Wan - Kid. yang def.; Deer Velvet - jing def.; Huan Shao Dan - Heart & Kid. yin def.; Tong Qiao Huo Xue Wan - blood stag.	Common pts: Sj-3, Sj-5, Li-1, Sj-17, Si-19, Gb-2, Sj-19. All points: Li-1, Li-4, Li-5, Li-6, St-7, Si-1, Si-3, Si-8, Si-16, Si-19, Ub-62, Ub-65, K-3, Sj-1, Sj-2, Sj-3, Sj-4, Sj-5, Sj-7, Si-10, Sj-16, Sj-17, Sj-18, Sj-19, Si-20, Sj-21, Gb-2, Gb-3, Gb-10, Gb-11, Gb-20, Gb-42, Gb-43, E-Sishencong	
Hemorrhoids	Hua Zhi Ling Tablets - damp heat, blood stag.; Fargelin for Piles damp heat; Huai Jiao Wan - Intestinal wind; Bu Zhong Yi Qi Tang - sinking Spleen qi; Gui Pi Tang - Spleen qi def.; Hemorrhoids Ointment topical; Ching Wan Hung topical; Xiao Yan Tang Shang Cream topical	Ub-30, Du-1, Ub-57, Ub-50/36, Ub-54/40, Ub-56, Ub-58 and Si-5 for pain and inflammation; Du-1, Du-3, Gb-32, E-erbai, Sp-6 strong stimulation; Si-3 and Ub-62 open the Du Mai for blood deficiency hemorrhoids; Ear-shenmen, brain, spleen, rectum and large intestine.	BM: Ren-24, bleed Ub-40, Ren-20, K-5, Gb-40
Herpes (Genital)	Acute: Bi Xie Sheng Shi Wan - damp heat; Long Dan Xie Gan Tang - Liver damp heat; Chuan Xin Lian Antiphlogistic Tablets - toxic heat; Chuan Xin Lian - toxic heat; Fu Yan Qing Tablets - toxic & damp heat. Recurrent: Bi Xie Sheng Shi Wan - damp heat; Bi Xie Fen Qing Wan - damp; Chuan Xin Lian Antiphlogistic Tablets - toxic heat; Chuan Xin Lian - toxic heat	Liver-fire: Liv-2, Liv-3, Liv-5, Ren-3, Sj-6, Ub-28	BM: (L) bleed Liv-1, Liv-3, Li-4; (R) Pc-6, Gb-41, bleed Pc-9
Herpes (Oral)	Lien Chiao Pai Tu Pien - wind heat, toxic heat; Peking Niu Huang Jie Du Pian - toxic heat; Huang Lien Shang Ching Pien - wind heat, toxic heat; Ban Lan Gen Chong Ji - toxic heat; Chuan Xin Lian Antiphlogistic Tablets - toxic heat; Chuan Xin Lian - toxic heat	Li-4, Li-11	BM: Lu-10, Lu-9, Li-4, Li-5, Liv-3, St-44
Herpes Zoster	Lien Chiao Pai Tu Pien - wind heat, toxic heat; Long Dan Xie Gan Tang - damp heat, Liver fire; Chuan Xin Lian Antiphlogistic Tablets - toxic heat; Chuan Xin Lian - toxic heat; Bi Xie Sheng Shi Wan - damp heat; Ban Lan Gen Chong Ji - toxic heat; Superior Sore Throat Powder topical	Li-11, Sp-10, Gb-40, Gb-20, Gb-34, Gb-41, Ub-54/40, Pc-7	
Hiccup	Wei Tong Ding cold, yang def.; Bao He Wan - food stag.; Xiang Sha Yang Wei Wan - qi & damp stag.	Common pts: St-36, Pc-6, Pc-8, Ren-12, Ub-2, Ub-17	
High Blood Pressure	General: Zhen Gan Xi Feng Wan - Liver yang rising, Liver wind; Tian Ma Gou Teng Yin - Liver yang rising; Tian Ma Wan - yin def., yang rising; Yang Yin Jiang Ya Wan - yang rising; Fu Fang Jiang Ya Capsules - yang rising; Qi Ju Di Huang Wan - Liver yin def.; Chai Hu Long Gu Mu Li Tang - Liver fire, phlegm heat; Ban Xia Bai Zhu Tian Ma Wan - wind phlegm; Huang Lian Jie Du Tang - damp heat; Xue Fu Zhu Yu Tang - qi & blood stag.; Da Chai Hu Tang - shao yang/yang ming syndrome	Common pts: Gb-20, Gb-34 Du-20, Li-4, Li-11, Sp-6, St-36; Supp pts: Liv-2, E-taiyang, Sj-17, E-anmian, Sp-6, K-3, Pc-6, St-40, Ren-4, Ren-6	BM for high cholesterol: (L) Sp-9, Sp-10, Sj-5; (R) St-36, St-40, Pc-7, Pc-8; BM for fatty liver: (L) Sj-10, Li-9, Li-10, Liv-7, Sp-9; (R) Gb-34, ashi around Pc-3/Pc-4
Hip pain	Qing Gan Li Dan Tablets - Gallbladder channel dysfunction; Zhuang Yao Jian Shen - yang def.; Juan Bi Tang - wind cold damp; Shen Tong Zhu Yu Wan - blood stag.; Xuan Bi Tang - damp heat	Common pts: St-31, Gb-25, Gb-30, Gb-34, Gb-39, Gb-40, Gb-41	

Condition	Formulas & Diagnoses	Points	Extra Points (BM)
Hot Flushes/ Flashes	Er Xian Tang - Kid. yin & yang def.; Da Bu Yin Wan - Kid. yin def.; Zhi Bai Ba Wei Wan - Kid. yin def.; Geng Nian Ling yin & yang def.; Jia Wei Xiao Yao San - qi stag. with heat; Kun Bao Wan - yin def. with yang rising; Tong Ren Wu Ji Bai Feng Wan - blood def., postpartum		BM: (L) LI-4, Ht-5; (R) St-36, K-3, Ren-4/5/6
Hypertension	General: Zhen Gan Xi Feng Wan - Liver yang rising. Liver wind; Tian Ma Gou Teng Yin - Liver yang rising; Tian Ma Wan - yin def., yang rising; Yang Yin Jiang Ya Wan - yang rising; Fu Fang Jiang Ya Capsules - yang rising; Qi Ju Di Huang Wan - Liver yin def.; Chai Hu Long Gu Mu Li Tang - Liver fire, phlegm heat; Ban Xia Bai Zhu Tian Ma Wan - wind phlegm; Huang Lian Jie Du Tang - damp heat; Xue Fu Zhu Yu Tang - qi & blood stag.; Da Chai Hu Tang - shao yang/yang ming syndrome	Common pts: Gb-20, Gb-34 Du-20, LI-4, LI-11, Sp-6, St-36: Supp pts.: Liv-2, E-taiyang, Sj-17, Anmian, Sp-6, K-3, St-40, Ren-4, Ren-6; primary hypertension: Liv-3, LI-18, St-9, St-36, LI-11	BM for excess type: (L) Sp-9, Sp-10, Sj-5; (R) St-36, St-40, Pc-7, Pc-8; BM for deficient type: (L) Gb-39, St-40, Ub-57, Lu-7, Ht-5; (R) LI-4, Liv-3, K-2, Sp-4, Sj-5
Hyper-thyroidism	Tian Wan Bu Xin Dan - Heart yin def.; Zhi Bai Ba Wei Wan - Kid. yin def.; Er Xian Tang - yin & yang def.; Da Bu Yin Wan - yin def. with heat; Zhi Gan Cao Tang - Heart qi & yin def.; Chai Hu Long Gu Mu Li Tang - Liver fire, phlegm heat; Long Dan Xie Gan Tang - Liver fire; Nei Xiao Luo Li Wan - phlegm heat	Pc-5, Sp-6, E-qiying, E-jiaji C-3 to C-5: Supp pts.: Ht-6, K-7, Pc-6, LI-4, Liv-3, Ht-7, Ub-2, St-2, Gb-20, E-anmian, E-shantianzhu; Influence thyroid: Ren-13, Du-23, St-9, Ren-19, Du-15, Ub-15, Ht-7, St-10, Ren-6, Sj-3, K-7, LI-4: Influence parathyroid: Ub-11, Ub-58, Gb-30, St-36, Du-2, Liv-3, Ub-15, Ub-3, Pc-7, Influence adrenals: K-7, Ub-47/52, Ren-10, Sp-6, Du-6, Ren-16, Pc-7; Influence pituitary: Ren-15, Ren-16, Ren-19, K-13, Sp-6, K-11, Ub-47/52, Gb-37, Gb-5, Ub-60, Ren-10; Influence pancreas: Sp-3, K-3, Ub-20, Sj-3, Liv-2, Ren-3	BM: (L) Gb-39, Gb-38, Gb-37, Pc-7, Ear-thyroid; (R) Liv-2, Liv-3, K-7, LI-5
Hypo-chondriac Pain	Shu Gan Tang - qi & blood stag.; Xiao Chai Hu Tang - shao yang; Chai Hu Shu Gan Tang - Liver qi stag.; Xue Fu Zhu Yu Tang - blood stag.; Long Dan Xie Gan Tang - damp heat; Li Dan Tablets - damp heat; Jigucao Wan - chronic hepatitis	Common pts: Gb-34, Gb-41, Sj-6	
Hypo-thyroidism	Fu Gui Ba Wei Wan - Kid. yang def.; You Gui Wan - Kid. yang def.; Zhen Wu Tang - Heart & Kid. yang def.	Common pts: Du-4, Ren-4, Ren-6, St-36, Sp-6, Pc-6, LI-4, Ub-17; Influence thyroid insufficiency: Pc-6, Pc-8, Ren-22, LI-4, Du-15, Ub-38/43, Ub-15, Ub-17; Influence thyroid: Ren-13, Du-23, St-9, Ren-19, Du-15, Ub-15, Ht-7, St-10, Ren-6, Sj-3, K-7, LI-4	BM: (L) LI-4, LI-5, K-7 Sp-6, Ear-thyroid; (R) Lu-9, Gb-39, Gb-38, Gb-37, St-36
Immuno-deficiency	Bu Zhong Yi Qi Tang - Spleen & Lung qi def.; Reishi Mushroom immune regulator; Tong Luo Zhi Tong Tablets - blood def.; Deer Antler and Ginseng qi & jing def.; Yu Ping Feng San - wei qi def.; Sheng Mai San - qi & yin def.; Cordyceps Essence of Chicken - qi & yang def.; American Ginseng Essence of Chicken - qi & yin def.; Panax Ginseng Extractum - qi def.	St-36, Sp-6, Gb-20, LI-4, Ren-6, Ren-12, Ub-12, Ub-20, Ub-21	BM: (L) LI-4, Sp-10; (R) Lu-5, Lu-7, St-36

METHODS

Condition	Formulas & Diagnoses	Points	Extra Points (BM)
Impotence	Gu Ben Fu Zheng Capsules - Kid. yang def.; Kang Wei Ling Wan - blood stag.; Zi Shen Da Bu Capsules - Kid. yang def.; Nan Bao Capsules - yang def.; Fu Gui Ba Wei Wan - Kid. yang def.; Gui Pi Tang - Heart & Spleen def.; Chai Hu Shu Gan Tang - Liver qi stag.; Wu Zi Yan Zong Wan - jing def.; Deer Velvet - jing def.; Deer Antler and Ginseng qi & jing def.	Common pts: Ren-4, Sp-6, Liv-5, Ht-7, Du-4; Liver qi stag.: Liv-3, LI-4, Liv-5, Liv-8, Liv-14, Pc-6, Sp-6, Ren-6; Damp-heat: Ren-3, Sp-9, Liv-5, Ub-32, SJ-6, K-10, Gb-26, Gb-41; Kid. yin def.: Ren-4, Ren-7, K-6, Ht-6, Sp-6, Ub-23; Kid. yang def.: Du-4, Ren-4, Ub-23, K-7, Lu-7, Sp-6, Du-20	BM: K-2, K-4, K-7 or BM 2: (L) E-lingku, Sp-10, K-3, Liv-4, LI-5; (R) Lu-7, Pc-7, St-36, Ub-62, Gb-34
Incontinence	Excessive/frequent/nocturnal/incontinence of: Ba Ji Yin Yang Wan - yang def.; Zi Shen Da Bu Capsules - Kid. yang def.; Fu Gui Ba Wei Wan - yang def.; Yulin Da Bu Wan - Kid. yang def.; Zhuang Yao Jian Shen - yang def.; Chin So Ku Ching Wan - astringent; San - Yuen Medical Pills - Kid. def. & astringent; Bu Zhong Yi Qi Tang - sinking qi, bladder prolapse, postpartum; Bu Yang Huan Wu Wan - qi def., blood stag., post stroke. Scanty (anuria): Wu Ling San - tai yang fu syndrome; Fu Gui Ba Wei Wan - Kid. yang def.; Zhen Wu Tang - Heart & Kid. yang def. Difficult: Fu Gui Ba Wei Wan - yang def.; Ba Zheng San - damp heat; Xue Fu Zhu Yu Tang - blood stag.; Prostate Gland Pills - damp heat; Qian Lie Xian Capsules - damp heat		
Indigestion	Bao He Wan - food stag.; Jian Pi Wan - food stag. during pregnancy; Ping Wei San - cold damp; Zi Sheng Wan - food stag. with Spleen def.; Mu Xiang Shun Qi Tang - qi & damp stag.; Li Zhong Wan - Spleen yang def.; Wei Tong Ding cold; Xiang Lian Wan - Stomach heat; Xiang Sha Yang Wei Wan - qi & damp stag.; Shu Gan Tang - Liver Spleen disharmony; Wei Te Ling antacid	Common pts: St-36, Sp-4; Spleen qi def.: Ren-12, St-36, Sp-3, Sp-6, Ub-20, Ub-21; Food stag.: Ren-12, Ren-6, St-25, St-36, St-40, St-44, LI-10; Liver qi stag.: Ren-12, Ren-6, St-25, St-36, Liv-3, Liv-13, Gb-34, Pc-6	
Infertility - All	Female: Tiao Jing Cu Yun Wan - yang def., weak progesterone phase; Cu Yun Yu Tai Capsules - yang def., weak progesterone phase; Ji Bai Feng Wan - blood & yang def.; Ba Zhen Tang - qi & blood def.; Shi Quan Da Bu Tang - qi & blood def. with cold; Gui Pi Tang - Heart & Spleen def.; Wen Jing Tang - cold & def., blood stag.; You Gui Wan - Kid. yang def.; Zuo Gui Wan - Kid. yin def.; Deer Velvet - jing def.; Lu Rong Jiao - jing def.; Gui Zhi Fu Ling Tang - blood stag., masses; Tao Hong Si Wu Tang - blood def., blood stag., masses; Hai Zao Jing Wan - polycystic ovaries; Shao Yao Gan Cao Wan - polycystic ovaries	E-zigong, Ren-3, Ren-4, Ren-5, Ren-7; Kid. yang def.: Ub-23, Du-4, Ren-4, St-36, Sp-6, E-zigong; Kid. yin def.: Ub-23, K-2, K-3, K-13, Sp-6, E-zigong; Liver qi stag.: LI-4, Liv-3, Sp-6, Sp-8, Ren-6, E-zigong; Phelgm-damp: Ren-3, Sp-6, St-40, Ub-20, E-zigong; Blood stag.: Ren-3, Sp-6, Sp-8, Sp-10, St-30, E-zigong	BM: (L) LI-4, Sp-9, Sp-7, Sp-6; (R) Pc-6, Lu-7, Ht-5, St-36, St-40
Infertility - Male	Male: Wu Zi Yan Zong Wan - jing def.; Gu Ben Fu Zheng Capsules - yang def.; Zi Shen Da Bu Capsules - yang def.; Gui Zhi Fu Ling Tang - blood stag.	Ren-2, Ren-3, Ren-4, Sp-6, K-2, K-7, K-12, Ub-23, Ub-32	BM for male: E-Lingku (L) Lu-7, K-5, Sp-6; (R) LI-5, St-36

256

Condition	Formulas & Diagnoses	Points	Extra Points (BM)
Insomnia	Gui Pi Tang - Heart & Spleen def.; Tian Wang Bu Xin Dan - Heart yin def.; Wen Dan Tang - phlegm heat; An Shen Bu Xin Wan - yang rising; Tao Chih Pien - Heart fire; Xue Fu Zhu Yu Tang - qi & blood stag., chronic refractory; An Shen Jie Yu Capsules - qi stag., premenstrual; Bao He Wan - food stag.; Qi Xing Tea - children	E-shishencong, E-yintang, Ear-shenmen, Ht-7, Sp-6, Ub-15, Pc-6; Liver fire: Ht-7, Sp-6,Liv-3, Ub-18, Pc-5, E-anmian; Phlegm fire: Ren-12, St-40, Sp-6, Ht-7, Ub-21, St-36, LI-4, E-yintang; Yin def.: Ht-7, Sp-6, K-3, Pc-6, Ub-15, Ub-23; Heart & Spleen def.: Ht-7, Sp-6, St-36, Ub-15, Ub-20	BM shu-stream/he-sea combo: (L) Gb-41, Gb-34, Ht-3, Ht-7; (R) Liv-3, Liv-8, Sj-3, Sj-10; BM Tx 2. (L) Sp-6, Sp-9, Sp-10, K-2, K-4, K-7, SI-7, Sj-3, LI-4; (R) St-36, St-41, Ht-3, Ht-5, Ht-8 + Ear-shenmen
Irritability	Chai Hu Shu Gan Tang - qi stag.; Chai Hu Long Gu Mu Li Tang - Liver fire, phlegm heat; Jia Wei Xiao Yao San - qi stag. with heat; Long Dan Xie Gan Tang - Liver fire; Fu Gui Ba Wei Wan - Kid. yang def.; Kun Bao Wan - Kid. yin def.		
Irritable Bowel Syndrome (IBS)	Diarrhea predominant: Tong Xie Yao Fang Wan - Liver invading Spleen; Chai Hu Shu Gan Tang - Liver invading Spleen; Xiao Yao San - Liver qi stag.; Zi Sheng Wan - qi def. & food stag. Constipation predominant: Mu Xiang Shun Qi Tang - qi & food stag.	All points: K-4, Ub-23, Liv-11, Liv-2, Liv-8, St-25, St-27, St-36, Ren-12, Ren-4, Sp-9, K-2, Ub-65, Lu-9, Ub-54/40, LI-11, Sp-1, Sp-3, St-44, Sp-4, Sp-14, K-14, K-7, Ren-9, Ub-35	BM: (L) LI-4, Liv-4, Sp-4, Sp-9, E-Lingku; (R) Lu-7, Lu-6, Pc-6, St-36, St-38 or ashi
Itching		Common pts: Sp-10, LI-11, Sp-6, E-baichongwo	BM: (L) Liv-1, Liv-4, LI-1, LI-4; (R) Gb-44, Gb-40, Lu-11, Lu-8
Jaundice	Long Dan Xie Gan Tang - damp heat; Qing Gan Li Dan Tablets - damp heat; Da Chai Hu Tang - damp heat; Li Dan Tablets - damp heat, blood stag.; Jigucao Wan - damp heat, blood stag.; Ge Xia Zhu Yu Wan - blood stag.	All points: St-31, St-36, St-45, Sp-4, Sp-5, Sp-9, Sp-17, Ht-9, SI-3, SI-4, Ub-13, Ub-15, Ub-17, Ub-18, Ub-19, Ub-20, Ub-21, Ub-22, K-1, K-2, Pc-6, Pc-7, Pc-8, Sj-11, Gb-24, Gb-34, Liv-3, Liv-4, Liv-14, Du-6, Du-7, Du-8, Du-9, Du-16, Du-17, Du-26, Du-28, Ren-13, Ren-14, Ren-22, E-Jiachengjiang	
Knee pain	Fang Ji Huang Qi Wan - wind damp, qi def.; Jian Bu Qing Shen Wan - Kid. def.; Zhuang Yao Jian Shen Tablets - Kid. yang def.; Du Huo Ji Sheng Tang - wind damp with Kid. def.; Xiao Huo Luo Dan - severe cold; Fu Gui Ba Wei Wan - Kid. yang def.; Zuo Gui Wan - Kid. yin def.; Xuan Bi Tang - damp heat; Tiger Balm topical; Plaster for Bruise and Analgesic topical; Porous Capsicum Plaster topical; Gou Pi Gao	E-heding, E-yixan, Sp-10, St-34, Ub-63, Gb-37, Liv-8	BM: LI-11, Lu-5, Ht-3 and ashi
Leg Pain		Common pts: Gb-34, Gb-40, Gb-41, Ub-57, Ub-58, Sp-6, Liv-3	
Leukorrhea	White mucoid watery: Shen Ling Bai Zhu Wan - Spleen damp; Xiang Sha Liu Jun Tang - Spleen def. with phlegm damp; Cu Yun Yu Tai Capsules - yang def., cold; Bi Xie Fen Qing Wan - Kid. def., damp; Ba Ji Yin Yang Wan - Kid. yang def.; Bai Feng Wan - qi & blood def. Yellow malodorous: Yu Dai Wan - damp heat; Bi Xie Sheng Shi Wan - damp heat; Long Dan Xie Gan Tang - Liver damp heat; Fu Yan Qing Tablets - toxic heat; Chien Chin Chih Tai Wan - damp heat with def.	All points: St-29, Ub-33, Ub-35, Ub-55, K-10, K-12, K-13, K-14, Pc-5, Ub-27, Ub-31, Sp-12, Ub-23, Ub-24, Gb-28, Du-3, Ren-2, Ren-3, Ren-4, Ren-5, Ren-7	

METHODS

Condition	Formulas & Diagnoses	Points	Extra Points (BM)
Libido	Cu Yun Yu Tai Capsules - yang def., cold; Tiao Jing Cu Yun Wan - yang def., cold; You Gui Wan - Kid., yang def.; Gu Ben Fu Zheng Capsules - yang def.; Qian Lie Xian Capsules - damp heat	Liver qi stag.: Liv-3, LI-4, Liv-5, Liv-8, Liv-14, Pc-6, Sp-6, Ren-6; Damp-heat: Ren-3, Sp-9, Liv-5, Ub-32, Sj-6, K-10, Gb-26, Gb-41; Kid. yin def.: Ren-4, Ren-7, K-6, Ht-6, Sp-6, Ub-23; Kid. yang def.: Du-4, Ren-4, Ub-23, K-7, Lu-7, Sp-6, Du-20	BM: E-lingku, (L) Sp-10, K-3, Liv-4, LI-5; (R) Lu-7, Pc-7, St-36, Ub-62, Gb-34
Malaria	Xiao Chai Hu Tang - shao yang; Da Chai Hu Tang - shao yang/yang ming; Ping Wei San - phlegm damp; Ge Xia Zhu Yu Wan - blood stag.	Pc-6, Sj-2, SI-3, Du-13, Du-14, Gb-41 w/ high fever LI-11; w/delirium bleed jing well pts, w/ splenomegaly Liv-13, E-pigen moxa	
Mastitis	Acute: Xiao Chai Hu Tang + Chuan Xin Lian Antiphlogistic Tablets; Xiao Chai Hu Tang + Wu Wei Xiao Du Yin; Lien Chiao Pai Tu Pien - toxic heat. Chronic or recurrent after antibiotics: Xiang Sha Liu Jun Tang - Spleen def. with phlegm; Li Zhong Wan - Spleen yang def.		BM same side of fibroid: Pc-5, Pc-6, Pc-4, Lu-7, Ht-5, St-39, St-40: BM opposite side of fibroid: LI-3, Sp-6, Sp-7, Sp-8 or ashi
Memory	Concentration: Jian Nao Yi Zhi Capsule - qi def. with blood stag.; Xiang Sha Liu Jun Tang - Spleen def. with phlegm damp; Gui Pi Tang - Heart blood & Spleen qi def.; Ping Wei San - phlegm damp; Wen Dan Tang - phlegm heat; Tian Wang Bu Xin Dan - Heart & Kid. yin def.; Cerebral Tonic Pills - phlegm & Kid. def. Poor memory: Jian Nao Yi Zhi Capsules - qi def., blood stag.; Cerebral Tonic Pills - blood def. & phlegm heat; Gui Pi Tang - qi & blood def.; Tian Wang Bu Xin Dan - Heart & Kid. yin def.; Huan Shao Dan - Heart & Kid. def.; Zhi Gan Cao Tang - Heart qi & blood def.; Bai Zi Yang Xin Wan - general; Wen Dan Tang - phlegm heat; Tong Qiao Huo Xue Wan - blood stag., post traumatic	All points: Lu-7, LI-11, Ht-3, Ht-7, Ub-15, Ub-43, K-1, K-3, K-6, K-21, St-36, Pc-5, Pc-6, Gb-20, Du-11, Du-20, Ren-14, E-Sishencong; Heart & Spleen def.: Du-20, Ub-52, Ht-3, Ht-7, Ub-15, Ht-7, Ub-20, St-36, Sp-6, Ren-4, E-yintang; Kid. essence def.: K-1, K-3, K-6, Ub-23, Du-20, Ren-4, Ub-62, SI-1, Ht-7; Blood & phlegm stag.: Ub-15, Ub-23, Ub-17, Pc-4, Sp-6, Du-20, St-40, Sp-3	BM: (L) Ht-7, Ht-4, Gb-40, Gb-34; (R) Liv-3, Liv-6, SI-3, SI-7, Ear-shenmen
Menopausal Syndrome	Kun Bao Wan - Kid. yin def.; Er Xian Tang - yin & yang def.; Geng Nian Ling yin & yang def.; Zhi Bai Ba Wei Wan - Kid. yin def.; Tian Wang Bu Xin Dan - Heart & Kid. yin def.; Da Bu Yin Wan - yin def., severe heat; Gan Mai Da Zao Tang	Kid. yin def.: Ren-4, K-3, K-7, K-10, LI-4, Sp-6, Ht-7; Heart & Kid. yin def.: Ren-4, Ren-15, K-3, L-10, Lu-7 K-6, K-13, Ht-8, Pc-7, Du-24; Phlegm & qi stag.: Ren-6, Ren-10, Ren-17, Sj-6, Sp-6, Sp-9, St-28, St-40, Pc-6, Lu-7; Kid yin & yang def.: Ren-4, Ren-7, K-3, K-6, Ht-6, Lu-7, Sp-6, Ub-23, Ub-52	BM: (L) St-36, Lu-7: (R) LI-4, Sp-9, Sp-7 or ashi, Sp-6
Menorrhagia	Yunnan Paiyao hemostatic; Raw Tienchi Tablets - hemostatic; Gui Pi Tang - Spleen qi def.; Tao Hong Si Wu Tang - blood stag., blood def.; Si Wu Tang + Huang Lian Jie Du Tang - hot blood with blood def.; Jia Wei Xiao Yao San - Liver qi stag. with heat; Li Zhong Wan - Spleen yang def.	Common pts: Liv-1, K-10, Ren-4, K-2, Sp-6, Ren-3, Ren-6, Sp-1, Sp-2, St-12, St-10, Ht-1, Pc-3, Ub-54/40	
Menstrual Amount	Scanty: Ba Zhen Tang - qi & blood def.; Shi Quan Da Bu Tang - qi & blood def.; Bai Feng Wan - qi & blood def.; Tao Hong Si Wu Tang - blood stag. with blood def.; Shao Fu Zhu Yu Tang - blood stag., cold. Prolonged: Cu Yun Yu Tai Capsules - yang def.; Tiao Jing Cu Yun Wan - yang def.; Woo Garm Yuen Medical Pills - blood stag. with cold & def.; Tao Hong Si Wu Tang - blood stag. with blood def.; Ba Zhen Tang - qi & blood def.; Shi Quan Da Bu Tang - qi & blood def., with cold	Scanty: Qi & blood def.: Liv-8, Ren-4, Sp-6, St-36, Ub-18, Ub-20, Ub-23; Blood stag.: Ren-4, Ren-6, St-29, Sp-6, Sp-10, K-14, (Sp-4/R and Pc-6/L), Ub-17; Kidney yang def.: K-3, K-13, Du-4, Ren-4, St-36, Sp-6, Liv-8, Ub-23; Phlegm obstruction: Ren-4, Ren-6, Ren-9, Ren-12, Sp-6, Sp-9, St-28 (Lu-7/R and K-6/L), Ub-20, Ub-23, Ub-32; Prolonged: Qi def.: Ren-6, Ren-12, Du-20, St-36, Ub-20, Ub-23; Blood-heat: Liv-2, Sp-6, Sp-8, Sp-10, LI-11, (Sp-4/R and Pc-6/L), Ub-17; Blood stag.: Liv-3, St-29, Sp-6, Sp-8, Sp-10, K-14, (Sp-4/R and Pc-6/L), Ub-17	BM: (L) Sp-9, Sp-8, Sp-6, LI-4, E-linkgu: (R) St-36, Lu-5, Lu-6 or ashi, Gb-42

Condition	Formulas & Diagnoses	Points	Extra Points (BM)
Menstrual Irregularity	Irregular: Si Wu Tang - blood def.; Xiao Yao San - Liver qi stag.; Jia Wei Xiao Yao San - Liver qi stag. with heat; Ba Zhen Tang - qi & blood def.; Bai Feng Wan - qi & blood def.; Wu Ji Bai Feng Wan - qi, blood & yang def.	Early: Hot-blood: Ren-3, Sp-10, LI-11, Sp-6, Liv-3, Liv-2, K-2, Ub-17; Qi def.: St-36, Sp-6, Ren-12, Ub-20, Du-20, Ren-4, Ren-6, Sp-1; Blood stag.: Ren-3, Sp-6, Sp-10, Sp-8, St-29; Late: Blood def.: Ren-4, Ren-6, Sp-6, Sp-10, Sp-20, Du-20, Ht-7, Ub-17; Cold def.: Ren-6, Ren-6, Sp-6, Sp-8, Sp-10, St-36, Du-4, Ub-32, St-25, St-29; Late: Liver qi stag.: Pc-6, Ren-12, Ren-6, Liv-2, Liv-3, Sp-4, Sp-6, Sp-8, Sp-10, Liv-3, Liv-14, Pc-6, Ub-23, Sj-5	BM: (L) Sp-9, Sp-8, Sp-6, LI-4, E-linkgu; (R) St-36, Lu-5, Lu-6 or ashi, Gb-42
Multiple Sclerosis	Bu Zhong Yi Qi Tang - Spleen qi def.; Hua Tuo Zai Zao Wan - qi & yin def.; Bu Yang Huan Wu Wan - qi def., blood stag.; You Gui Wan - Kid. yang def.; Niu Huang Qing Xin Wan - phlegm heat	St-36, Sp-3, Sp-6, Sp-9, St-40, Ub-20, Ub-21, Ren-12, LI-10, Sj-5, St-31; (Lu-7/L and K-6/R)	BM: (L) K-1, K-4, LI-1, LI-4; (R) Lu-11, Lu-8, Ub-67, Ub-64
Muscle Tension	Strain: Die Da Zhi Tong Capsules - blood stag. acute; Zheng Gu Shui topical; Trans Wood Lock Liniment topical. Muscular pain: Shao Yao Gan Cao Wan - antispasmodic; Jing Fang Bai Du Wan - wind cold; Xiao Yao San - Liver qi stag., blood def.; Shu Gan Tang - Liver qi stag.; Xing Jun San - summer damp, acute; Huo Hsiang Cheng Chi Pien - wind cold with damp, acute; Trans Wood Lock Liniment topical; Po Sum On Medicated Oil		BM for moving and muscle pain: (Both) Gb-20, Gb-34, Ear-shenmen; (L) Ht-9, Pc-9, St-36, Ub-40, Lu-11; (R) LI-4, Liv-4, SI-3, Sj-3, K-3, Sp-6, E-yintang
Neck Pain	Neck & upper back: Ge Gen Tang - wind cold; Headache and Dizziness Reliever; Chuan Xiong Cha Tiao Wan - wind cold; Xiao Yao San - Liver qi stag.; Ba Zhen Tang - qi & blood def.; Hua Tuo Zai Zao Wan - qi & yin def., wind damp	Common pts: E-luozhen, SI-3, Ub-10, Gb-20, Gb-39, E-bailao, LI-4, E-ashi; local (SI-8, SI-16, Ub-66, Ub-67, Si-2, Sj-5, Sj-21, Gb-4, Gb-40); Qi & Blood stag.: E-luozhen, LI-4, E-ashi, Ub-10, SI-3, Gb-39; Wind-cold attack: LI-4, Sj-5, Ub-10, SI-3, Gb-39, E-ashi	BM: (L) Ht-4, Ht-5, Ht-7, Ub-65; (R) SI-3, Sj-3, Sp-6 or ashi pts; also consider straight line along dorsum of hand from LI-3 to SI-3
Nosebleed	Yunnan Paiyao hemostatic; Niu Huang Qing Huo Wan - toxic heat; Huang Lian Jie Du Tang - Stomach heat	All points: Lu-5, Lu-11, LI-2, LI-3, LI-4, LI-5, LI-6, LI-20, St-3, St-44, St-45, Sp-1, Ht-6, SI-1, SI-2, SI-3, Ub-2, Ub-4, Ub-7, Ub-12, Ub-15, Ub-18, Ub-31, Ub-40, Ub-45, Ub-56, Ub-57, Ub-58, Ub-62, Ub-66, Ub-67, K-1, K-3, K-7, Pc-4, Sj-5, Gb-5, Gb-19, Gb-20, Gb-39, Liv-2, Liv-8, Du-16, Du-20, Du-22, Du-24, Du-25, Ren-7, Ren-9, Ren-22, Ren-24, E-Bitong, E-Yintang	
Obesity	Fang Feng Tong Sheng Wan - excess constitutions; Bojenmi Chinese Tea; Keep Fit Capsule - qi & blood stag., phlegm; Ping Wei San - phlegm damp	Common pts: Pc-6, Ren-12, Ren-6, St-25, Ren-4, St-36, St-40, Sp-6, Lu-7; Phlegm & damp: Ren-12, St-21, Sp-3, Sp-5, St-36, St-40, Pc-5	BM: (L) Sj-5, LI-4 Sp-9; (R) Pc-6, St-36
Overweight	Fang Feng Tong Sheng Wan - excess constitutions; Bojenmi Chinese Tea; Keep Fit Capsule - qi & blood stag., phlegm; Ping Wei San - phlegm damp	Common pts: Ren-12, Ren-6, St-25, Ht-7, St-34, Sp-4, Pc-7, Ren-4; Phlegm-damp: Ren-12, St-21, Sp-3, Sp-5, St-40, St-36, Pc-5	

METHODS

Condition	Formulas & Diagnoses	Points	Extra Points (BM)
Pain	Generalized: Yan Hu Suo Zhi Tong Wan - analgesic; Shao Yao Gan Cao Wan - antispasmodic; Du Huo Ji Sheng Tang - wind damp with Kid. def.; Xiao Huo Luo Dan - severe cold; Xing Jun San - summer damp, acute; Huo Hsiang Cheng Chi Pien - wind cold with damp, acute; Xiao Yao San - Liver qi stag.; Po Sum On Medicated Oil muscle tension, qi stag.; Shu Jin Huo Xue Wan - chronic blood stag.; Zhuang Yao Jian Shen.- Kid. def.		
Palpitation	Tian Wang Bu Xin Dan - Heart yin def.; Gui Pi Tang - Heart blood def.; Zhi Gan Cao Tang - Heart qi, yin, blood def.; Chai Hu Long Gu Mu Li Tang - Liver fire, phlegm heat; Wen Dan Tang - phlegm heat; Dan Shen Pill - blood & phlegm stag.; Sheng Mai San - qi & yin def.; Zhen Wu Tang - Heart yang def.	Common pts: Pc-4, Pc-6	
Parkinson's Disease	Hua Tuo Zai Zao Wan - qi & yin def.; San Bi Wan - Kid. def., wind damp; Niu Huang Qing Xin Wan - phlegm heat	St-36, Sp-6, Ren-4, Liv-8	BM: (L) K-1, K-4, LI-1, LI-4; (R) Lu-11, Lu-8, Ub-67, Ub-64
Pelvic Inflammatory Disease (PID)	Acute: Fu Yan Qing Tablets - toxic & damp heat; Bi Xie Sheng Shi Wan - damp heat; Long Dan Xie Gan Tang - Liver damp heat; Wu Wei Xiao Du Yin - toxic heat; Huang Lian Jie Du Tang - toxic heat; Huang Lian Su Tablets - toxic heat; Chuan Xin Lian Antiphlogistic Tablets - toxic heat. Chronic: Woo Garm Yuen Medical Pills - cold & blood stag.; Wen Jing Tang - blood def., cold stag.; Yu Dai Wan - damp heat, blood def.; Chien Chin Chih Tai Wan - smoldering damp heat with qi, blood & Kid. yang def.; Gui Zhi Fu Ling Tang - blood stag.; Zhi Bai Ba Wei Wan - Kid. yin def.	E-zigongxue, Ren-4, Sp-10, Sp-9, Du-14, Ren-4, Ren-6, Ren-12, Ub-23, LI-4, St-28, St-36	BM: (L) St-36, Lu-7; (R) LI-4, Sp-9, Sp-7 or ashi, Sp-6; BM Tx 2: (L) Sp-2, Sp-3, K-3, K-4, Liv-3, LI-4, LI-5; (R) Ub-67, Gb-44, Pc-7, Lu-7
PMS (Premenstrual Syndrome)	Syndrome, general: Xiao Yao San - Liver qi stag., blood def.; Gui Pi Tang - Heart & Spleen def.; Chai Hu Shu Gan Tang - Liver qi stag.; Tong Luo Zhi Tong Tablets - blood def. Dizziness: Xiao Yao San - Liver qi stag., blood def.; Jia Wei Xiao Yao San - Liver qi stag. with heat. Edema: Ba Zhen Yi Mu Wan - qi & blood def., blood stag.; Si Wu Tang + Xiao Yao San. Fever: Jia Wei Xiao Yao San - Liver qi stag. with heat. Edema: Ba Zhen Yi Mu Wan - qi & blood def., blood stag.; Si Wu Tang + Xiao Yao San. Lower backache: Wen Jing Tang - cold, def. blood stag.; Shao Fu Zhu Yu Tang - cold, blood def.; Yang Rong Wan - blood and Kid. def.; You Gui Wan - yang def. Fever: Jia Wei Xiao Yao San - Liver qi stag. with heat	Liv qi stag.: Liv-3, LI-4, Ub-17, Ub-18, Liv-14, Sp-6, Gb-25, Gb-34, Sj-6; Spleen & Kid yang def.: Ren-4, K-3, St-36, Sp-6, Ub-20, Ub-23, Lu-7, K-6; Heart & Spleen def.: Ub-15, Ub-20, Ht-7, Ren-6, St-36, Sp-6, E-yintang; Phlegm rising: Pc-7, St-8, St-40, Du-24, LI-11, Sp-9, Pc-6, Ren-12, Ub-20; Liver blood def.: Ren-4, Lu-7, K-6, Sp-6, LI-4, Ub-18, Ub-20, Gb-34; Liver & Kid. yin def.: Liv-3, Liv-8, Ren-4, Sp-6, K-3, K-6, Ub-18, Ub-23	BM to regulate menses: (L) St-36, Lu-7; (R) LI-4, Sp-9, Sp-7 or ashi, Sp-6; Stress related - BM shu-stream/ he-sea combo: (L) Gb-41, Gb-34, Ht-3, Ht-7; (R) Liv-3, Liv-8, Sj-3, Sj-10
Polycystic Ovarian Syndrome	Shao Yao Gan Cao Wan; Woo Garm Yuen Medical Pills - cold & blood stag.; Liu Wei Di Huang Wan - Kid. yin def.; Zuo Gui Wan - Kid. yin def.; Hai Zao Jing Wan - phlegm; Ji Sheng Ju He Wan - phlegm qi stag.	Influence the ovaries: K-13, Ub-67, K-7, Gb-37, Sp-6, K-2, Du-4, Liv-3; Consider indirect moxa to resolve blood stag.	

Rheumatoid Arthritis	Arthritis: Juan Bi Tang - wind cold damp; Qu Feng Zhen Tong Capsule - wind cold damp; Xuan Bi Tang - damp heat; Guan Jie Yan Wan - damp heat; Shu Jin Huo Xue Wan - blood & phlegm stag.; Shen Tong Zhu Yu Wan - blood stag.; Xiao Huo Luo Dan - severe cold; Du Huo Ji Sheng Tang - wind damp with Kid. def.; Jian Bu Qiang Shen Wan - Kid. def.; Fu Gui Ba Wei Wan - Kid. yang def.; Trans Wood Lock Liniment topical; Porous Capsicum Plaster topical; Gou Pi Gao topical. RA: Reishi Mushroom immune regulator; Xue Fu Zhu Yu Tang - qi & blood stag.	Wind Bi: Du-14, Sj-6, Gb-39 Cold Bi: St-6, Ren-6, Ll-11; Damp Bi: Sp-6, Sp-9, Ub-11, Gb-39, St-40; Heat Bi: St-43, Ll-4; For local pts: Shoulder: Ll-15, Ll-14, Sj-14, E-jianeiling, Sl-9, Sl-10; Elbow: same as shoulder plus Ll-11, Sl-8, Sj-10; Wrist: Sj-5, Ll-5, Sl-4; Neck: Du-14, Ub-10, Gb-20,Sl-3, Gb-39, Ub-60, E- huatojiaji; Hip: Gb-30, Gb-29, Ub-51, St-31, Gb-34, Gb-39, Gb-40; Knee: St-34, Sp-10, Gb-34, Sp-9, St-36, Ub-40; Ankle: St-41, Sp-5, St-36, Ub-60, K-3; Toes: Sp-4, Ub-65, E-Bafeng	
Rhinitis	Allergic: Xin Yi San - wind cold; Cang Er Zi Wan - wind heat; Xiao Qing Long Wan - wind cold with congested fluids; Hayfever Relieving Tea - phlegm heat; Qian Bai Bi Yan Pian - heat & Pain; Gui Zhi Tang - ying wei disharmony. Chronic: Qian Bai Bi Yan Pian - heat & pain; Bi Yen Ning Capsules - phlegm heat; Pe Min Kan Wan - Nasal Clear; Cang Er Zi Wan - wind & phlegm heat; Yu Ping Feng San - wei qi def.; Xu Han Ting - wei qi def.; Ba Ji Yin Yang Wan - Kid. yang def.	E-bitong, Ll-4, Du-23, Ub-7, E-yintang. All points: Ll-2, Ll-3, Ll-4, Ll-5, Ll-6, Ll-20, Ub-2, Ub-4, Ub-7, Ub-12, Ub-56, Ub-58, Gb-5, Gb-20, Du-23, Du-25, Bitong, E-Yintang	BM for heat: (L) Sj-10, Ll-11, Ht-6/7 or ashi in btw, K-10, Liv-8, Sp-9; (R) Pc-3, Ht-8, Lu-9/10 or ashi in btw, Gb-34, St-36, Ub-40; BM for allergies: (L) St-36, Sp-4, Sp-9, Ll-3, Ll-11, Ll-20; (R) St-41, Lu-5, Lu-9, Ll-20, Ub-2
Sciatica	Dang Gui Si Ni Wan - cold in the channels; Xiao Huo Luo Dan - severe cold in the channels; Huo Luo Xiao Ling Tang - blood stag.; Juan Bi Tang - wind cold damp; Qu Feng Zhen Tong Capsules - wind cold damp; Shu Jin Huo Xue Wan - blood stag. wind damp; Du Huo Ji Sheng Tang - Kid. def. with wind damp; Tong Luo Zhi Tong Tablet - blood def., blood stag.; Kang Wei Ling Wan - neuralgic pain; Yan Hu Suo Zhi Tong Wan - analgesic; Shao Yao Gan Cao Wan - antispasmodic	Common pts: Gb-30, Gb-31, Gb-34, Gb-40, Gb-41, K-4, Ub-36, Ub-37, Ub-40, Ub-57, Ub-58, Ub-62, E-tunzhong	(also consider Ub-50/36, Ub-57, Du-2, E-baliao, Ub-31, Ub-32, Ub-33 and Ub-34, Gb-43, St-36, St-32, St-34, St-31, E- yaotongxue, E-tunzhong, St-41, Ub-58 for sciatica). E-lingku, E-dabi, E-zhongbai
Shoulder Pain	Xiao Yao San - qi stag.; Ba Zhen Tang - blood def.; Huo Luo Xiao Ling Tang - blood stag.; Die Da Zhi Tong Capsules - blood stag., traumatic; Zheng Gu Shui topical; Po Sum On Medicated Oil topical	Common pts: E-jianqian, Ll-15, Ll-16, Sj-14, Sl-10, Ll-4, Sj-5, Sl-3	BM opposite wrist: Ll-5, Sj-4, Sl-4/5, Lu-8/9, Ht-7, Pc-7; BM opposite ankle: Liv-4, Sp-5, K-3, Ub-60 Gb-40, St-41; BM 2: (L) Ht-4, Ht-5, Ht-7, Ub-65; (R) Sl-3, Sj-3, Sp-6 or Ashi pts: also consider straight line along dorsum of hand from Ll-3 to Sl-3

METHODS

METHODS

Condition	Formulas & Diagnoses	Points	Extra Points (BM)
Sinusitis	Acute: Ching Fei Yi Huo Pien - Lung heat; Chuan Xin Lian Antiphlogistic Tablets - toxic heat; Peking Niu Huang Jie Du Pien - toxic heat; Qian Bai Bi Yan Pian - heat; Cang Er Zi Wan - wind heat; Xin Yi San - wind cold. Chronic: Bi Yen Ning Capsules - heat; Qing Qi Hua Tan Wan - phlegm heat; Jia Wei Xiao Yao San - Liver qi stag. with heat	Wind-heat: LI-4, LI-11, Lu-7, Du-23, Ub-12, Ub-2, Gb-14, St-2 E-yintang E-bitong; Liver & Gallbladder heat: Liv-2, Gb-43, LI-4, E-yintang, Gb-14, Gb-20; Lung heat: LI-4, LI-11, Lu-7, Du-14, Lu-10, LI-20, E-yintang, E-bitong; Spleen def. & damp heat: Ren-12, Ub-20, LI-4, LI-11, Sp-9, Ub-22, LI-20, E-yintang, E-bitong	BM sinusitis: (L) St-36, Sp-4, Sp-9, LI-3, LI-11; (R) St-41, Lu-5, Lu-9; BM general: (L) Sj-10, LI-11, Ht-6/7 or ashi in btw, K-10, Liv-8, Sp-9; (R) Pc-3, Ht-8, Lu-9/10 or ashi in btw, Gb-34, St-36, Ub-40; BM for allergies: (L) St-36, Sp-4, Sp-9, LI-3, LI-11, LI-20; (R) St-41, Lu-5, Lu-9, LI-20, Ub-2
Sore Throat	Acute: Yin Chiao Chieh Tu Pien - wind heat; Peking Niu Huang Jie Du Pien - toxic heat; Chuan Xin Lian Antiphlogistic Tablets - toxic heat; Ban Lan Gen Chong Ji - toxic heat; Ching Fei Yi Huo Pien - Lung fire; Superior Sore Throat Powder topical; Gan Mao Tea - children. Chronic: Tung Hsuan Li Fei Pien - heat & dryness; Yang Yin Qing Fei Wan - Lung yin def.; Zhi Bai Ba Wei Wan - yin def.; Mai Wei Di Huang Wan - yin def.; Qing Yin Wan - Lung dryness	Common pts: LI-4, Lu-11, LI-1, LI-18; Wind-heat & toxin: LI-4, LI-11, St-44, Lu-10, Lu-11, Lu-7, Ren-22, LI-18; Lung & Kid. def.: LI-4, LI-11, St-36, Lu-7, K-6, K-3, Lu-9, Lu-10, Ub-13, Ub-23; Spleen def.: St-36, LI-11, Ub-20, Ub-13, Lu-9, Ren-12	BM: Lu-10, Lu-9, LI-4, LI-5, Liv-3, St-44
Stress	Chai Hu Shu Gan Tang - qi stag.; Xiao Yao San - qi stag.; American Ginseng Essence of Chicken - general; Panax Ginseng Extractum - general	Common pts: St-36, Ren-4, Ren-6, Du-4, Ub-23, E-yintang, E-anmian, Ear-shenmen	BM shu-stream/he-sea combo: (L) Gb-41, Gb-34, Ht-3, Ht-7; (R) Liv-3, Liv-8, Sj-3, Sj-10 + E-yintang, Ear-shenmen
Stroke	Prevention of: Raw Tienchi Tablets - blood stag.; Zhen Gan Xi Feng Wan - yin def., yang rising & wind. Recovery from: Bu Yang Huan Wu Wan - qi def., blood stag.; Xiao Shuan Zai Zao Wan; Hua Tuo Zai Zao Wan - qi & yin def.	Pre-stroke closed pattern: Pc-8, Pc-9, Du-20, Du-26, Liv-3, Ren-22, St-40, Ren-12; Pre-stroke open pattern: Ren-4, Ren-6, Ren-8, Pc-6, Du-25, moxa Du-20	
Tendonitis	Qu Feng Zhen Tong Wan - wind cold damp; Shen Tong Zhu Yu Wan - blood stag.	Common pts: Gb-34, LI-4 plus local points of affected area	
Tinnitus	Er Long Zuo Ci Wan - Kid. yin def.; Tian Ma Gou Teng Yin - Liver yang rising; Long Dan Xie Gan Tang - Liver fire; Fang Feng Tong Sheng Wan - wind heat; Tong Qiao Huo Xue Wan - blood stag.; Ban Xia Bai Zhu Tian Ma Wan - wind phlegm; Xiang Sha Liu Jun Tang - Spleen def. with phlegm Dam pin the ear; Wen Dan Tang - phlegm heat; Tinnitus Herbal Treatment Kid. yin def.; Zuo Gui Wan - Kid. yin def.; Shi Quan Da Bu Tang - qi & blood def.	SI-17, Sj-3, Gb-20; Supp pts.: Liv-2, St-40, K-3, Ub-23	BM: (L) LI-4, Ht-5; (R) St-36, K-3, Ren-4/5/6

Condition	Formulas & Diagnoses	Points	Extra Points (BM)
TMJ	TMJ pain: Qing Gan Li Dan Tablets - Gallbladder channel dysfunction; Xiao Yao San - Liver qi stag., blood def.	LI-4, Liv-3, E-taiyang, Ub-2, St-2, St-7, E- jiachengjiang (also consider St-44, St-36, Sj-5, K-3 and Gb-20)	(Sj-5 & Gb-41 yang wei mai); BM: (L) LI-3, Sj-3, Liv-8; (R) ashi Lu-5 to Lu-6, Pc-3 to Pc-4, Ht-3 to Ht-4, Gb-41, St-43
Toothache	Qing Wei San - Stomach heat; Huan Lian Jie Du Tang - damp or toxic heat; Peking Niu Huang Jie Du Pian - toxic heat; Chuan Xiong Cha Tiao Wan - wind cold; Sanjin Watermelon Frost topical	Common pts: LI-4, St-44, K-3, St-6, St-7; upper jaw: Sj-21, Du-26; lower jaw: Du-24	
Toxins		Du-14, Du-9, LI-11, LI-4, Liv-3, SI-17, Pc-3	
Ulcerative Colitis (UC)	Shu Gan Tang - Liver qi stag.; Chai Hu Shu Gan Tang - Liver invading the Spleen; Jia Wei Xiao Yao San - qi stag. with heat; Xiang Lian Wan - damp heat; Hua Zhi Ling Tablet - damp heat; Zi Sheng Wan - qi def. with food stag.; Mu Xiang Shun Qi Tang - qi & damp stag.	All points: K-4, K-5, Ub-23, Liv-11, Liv-2, Liv-8, St-25, St-27, Ren-12, Ren-4, Sp-9, K-2, Ub-65, Lu-9, Ub-54/40, LI-11, St-36, Sp-1, Sp-3, St-44, Sp-4, Gb-41, Sp-14, K-14, K-7, Ren-9, Ub-35	BM: (L) LI-4, Liv-4, Sp-4, Sp-9, E-Lingku; (R) Lu-7, Lu-6, Pc-6, St-36, St-38 or ashi
Upper respiratory infection	Acute: Ching Fei Yi Huo Pien - Lung fire; Qing Qi Hua Tan Wan - phlegm heat; Niu Huang Qing Huo Wan - toxic heat; Huang Lian Jie Du Tang - toxic & damp heat; Xiao Chai Hu Tang - post acute	Du-14, Lu-10, Sj-5, Lu-11, Gb-20, Du-16, LI-4, LI-11, Ub-12, Ub-13	BM: (L) Liv-5, K-9, Sp-6, LI-4, LI-11; (R) Lu-10, Lu-9, St-40, Ub-57
Urinary Tract Infection (UTI)	Ba Zheng San - damp heat; Long Dan Xie Gan Tang - Liver fire, damp heat; Bi Xie Sheng Shi Wan - damp heat; Qing Re Qu Shi Tea - damp heat; Ming Mu Shang Ching Pien - damp heat; Huang Lian Su Tablets - toxic heat, damp heat; Fu Yan Qing Tablets - damp heat; Tao Chih Pien - Heart fire; DBD Capsules - severe toxic heat; Ke Yin Wan - damp; Chuan Xin Lian Antiphlogistic Tablets - toxic heat; Qi Xing Tea - children	Acute: Ren-3, Sp-9, Ub-28, Ub-39; Chronic: Liv-3, Ub-28, Ub-23	BM: (L) Sp-2, Sp-3, K-3, K-4 Liv-3, LI-4, LI-5; (R) Ub-67, Gb-44, Pc-7, Lu-7
Varicose Veins	Tao Hong Si Wu Tang - mild blood stag.; Xue Fu Zhu Yu Tang - qi & blood stag.; Sunho Multi Ginseng Tablets - blood stag.; Bu Zhong Yi Qi Tang - qi def.	Du-14, Du-12, Gb-21, Du-4, plus local points on the legs	
Venereal Diseases	Bi Xie Sheng Shi Wan - damp heat; Long Dan Xie Gan Tang - Liver damp heat; Chuan Xin Lian Antiphlogistic Tablets - toxic heat; Chuan Xin Lian - toxic heat; Fu Yan Qing Tablets - toxic & damp heat.	Sp-6, Sp-9, Sp-10, Ub-23, Ren-3, Ren-4, Ren-6, Ub-47/52 plus direct moxa to Ub-23 for chronic condition or indirect moxa with ginger to Ren-3 and Ren-4 for acute condition	
Vertigo	Ban Xia Bai Zhu Tian Ma Wan - wind phlegm; Zhen Gan Xi Feng Wan - Liver yin def., yang rising & wind; Tian Ma Gou Teng Yin - Liver wind; Yang Yin Jiang Ya Wan - hypertension, yang rising; Wen Dan Tang - phlegm heat; Xue Fu Zhu Yu Tang - qi & blood stag.; Tong Qiao Huo Xue Wan - blood stag.	Liver Yang & Fire: Liv-2, Gb-20, Gb-34, Sp-6, Du-20; Phlegm-damp: Ren-12, St-40, St-8, Ub-20, Ub-21, Du-20; Qi & blood def.: St-36, Sp-6, Ren-6, Ub-17, Du-20; Kidney essence: K-3, Ren-4, Ub-23, Gb-39, Du-20	
Warts Common	General: Chuan Xin Lian Antiphlogistic Tablets; Ban Lan Gen Chong Ji	1. Pierce mother wart horizontally. 2. Channel affected. 3. Insertions perpendicular through tip of wart to its base	

METHODS

METHODS

Condition	Formulas & Diagnoses	Points	Extra Points (BM)
Weakness, weakened immune system	Generalized: Bu Zhong Yi Qi Tang - Spleen qi def.; Shi Quan Da Bu Tang - qi & blood def.; Tangkwei Essence of Chicken - qi & blood def.; American Ginseng Essence of Chicken - qi & yin def.; Cordyceps Essence of Chicken - yin & yang def. Immune: Bu Zhong Yi Qi Tang - Spleen & Lung qi def.: Reishi Mushroom immune regulator; Tong Luo Zhi Tong Tablet - blood def.; Deer Antler and Ginseng qi & jing def.; Yu Ping Feng San - wei qi def.; Sheng Mai San - qi & yin def.; Cordyceps Essence of Chicken - qi & yang def.; American Ginseng Essence of Chicken - qi & yin def.; Panax Ginseng Extractum - qi def.	Common pts: St-36, Ren-4, Ren-6, Du-4, Ub-23	
Weight Control	Fang Feng Tong Sheng Wan - excess constitutions; Bojenmi Chinese Tea; Keep Fit Capsule - qi & blood stag., phlegm; Ping Wei San - phlegm damp	Ren-12, Ren-6, St-25, Ht-7, St-34, Sp-4, Pc-7, Ren-4	BM: (L) Sj-5, LI-4 Sp-9; (R) Pc-6, St-36
Yeast Infection	Bi Xie Sheng Shi Wan - damp heat; Yu Dai Wan - damp heat, blood def.; Chien Chin Chih Tai Wan - damp heat, def.; Bi Xie Fen Zing Wan - damp; Ping Wei San - phlegm damp	Damp-heat: Liv-4, Liv-5, Ren-2, Ren-3, Sp-6, Sp-9, Ub-33; Spleen qi & damp: Ren-2, Ren-3, Ren-12, St-36, Sp-6, Sp-9, Ub-20, Ub-22, Ub-32, Ub-33; Liver & Kidney yin def.: Ren-3, Ren-4, Liv-5, Liv-8, K-3, (Lu-7/R and K-6/L)	

Source for Formulas & Diagnoses sections comes from *The Clinical Manual of Chinese Herbal Patent Medicines, 2nd Edition*
Reproduced with the permission of Will Maclean and Kathryn Taylor; Pangolin Press (2003)

The Balance Method (BM) is a minimal needle, distal point-only system of acupuncture that obtains clinical results very rapidly and is easy to use in the clinic. It is amazingly effective in the treatment of a wide range of both internal and external channel blockages and imbalances. The Balance method has the same philosophical roots as TCM acupuncture, but clinically it is quite different and usually yields a positive effect during the first treatment, and continues to generate progress in successive treatments, often requiring fewer treatments.

Source for Balance Method Acupuncture provided by Dr. Richard Tan

The Balance Method is a specialized system developed and presented by Dr. Richard Tan. Additional information can be found by attending his seminars hosted throughout the country, visit www.drtanshow.com or by reading his books (*Twelve and Twelve in Acupuncture, Twenty-Four More in Acupuncture, Dr. Tan's Strategy of Twelve Magical Points, Acupuncture 1, 2, 3*).

Zang Fu	Description	Tongue / Pulse	Points	Formulas
Lung Invasion By Wind-Cold	Cough, fever, itchy throat, stuffed nose or runny nose with clear watery mucus, sneezing, aversion to cold, aversion to wind, headache, body aches	Thin, white coat	(Lu-7 & LI-4), Ub-12, Du-16, Gb-20, Ub-13	Ma Huang Tang, Gui Zhi Tang, Jing Fang Bai Du San, Chuang Xiong Cha Tiao San, Tong Xuan Li Fei Wan, Hua Gai San, Xing Shu San
Lung Invasion By Wind-Heat	Cough, fever, aversion to cold, aversion to wind, sore throat, stuffed or runny nose with yellow mucus, headache, body aches, slight sweating, thirst, swollen tonsils	Red body with thin white or yellow coat	LI-4, LI-11, Lu-11, Sj-7, Ub-12, Du-14, Du-16, Gb-20, Ub-13	Yin Qiao San, Sang Ju Yin, San Ao Tang, Ma Xing Gan Shi Tang
Lung Invasion By Wind-Water	Sudden swelling of the eyes and face, gradually spreading to the whole body, bright, shiny complexion, scanty and pale urination, aversion to Wind, fever, cough, breathlessness	White, slippery coat	Lu-7, Sp-9, LI-4, LI-6, LI-7, Ren-9, Ub-12, Ub-13	N/A
Lung Qi Deficiency	Shortness of breath, feeble cough, watery sputum, weak voice, spontaneous sweating, bright white complexion, propensity to catching colds, tiredness	Pale or normal colored	Lu-9, Lu-7, Ren-6, Ren-17, St-36, Ub-43, Ub-13	Bu Fei Tang, Bu Zhong Yi Qi Tang, Ping Chuan Wan
Lung Yin Deficiency	Dry unproductive cough with little sputum, blood-tinged sputum, low-grade fever in the afternoon or evening, malar flush, night sweating, 5 palm heat, insomnia, dry mouth, dry throat, hoarse voice	Red, peeled, cracks in the Lung area, dry	Lu-9, Lu-10, K-6, Du-12, Ren-4, Ren-6, Ren-12, Ren-17, Ub-43, Ub-13 (Sedate): Lu-10, Lu-1	Sheng Mai San, Li Fei Wan, Sha Shen Mai Dong Tang, Yang Ying Qing Fei Tang, Pa Xian Chang Shou Wan, Bai He Gu Jin Tang
Lung Dryness	Dry cough, dry skin, dry throat, dry mouth, thirst, hoarse voice	Dry	K-3, K-6, Lu-9, Lu-10, Ren-4, Ren-22, Ub-13	Xie Bai San, Sang Xing Tang, Qing Zao Jiu Fei Tang
Lung Obstruction By Damp-Phlegm	Chronic cough, profuse white sputum that is easy to expectorate, white, pasty complexion, stuffiness of the chest, shortness of breath, dislikes lying down (orthopnia)	Thick, sticky white coat	Lu-1, Lu-5, Lu-7, Pc-6, Ren-6, Ren-12, Ren-17, Ren-22, Ub-20, St-36, St-40, Ub-13	Er Chen Tang, San Zi Yang Qin Tang, Su Zi Jiang Qi Tang
Lung Obstruction By Phlegm-Fluids	Cough, breathlessness, vomiting of white, watery, frothy sputum, chilliness	Pale body, thick, sticky white coat	Lu-5, Lu-9, Ren-9, Ren-12, Ren-17, St-36, St-40, Ub-13, Ub-43	N/A
Lung Obstruction By Phlegm-Heat	Barking cough, flaring of the ala nasi, profuse yellow or green sputum that is foul smelling, blood-tinged sputum, shortness of breath, asthma, stuffiness in the chest, dryness of the mouth, constipation	Red body, thick, sticky yellow coat	Lu-1, Lu-5, Lu-7, Lu-10, LI-11, Ren-12, Ren-17, St-40, Ub-13	Qing Jin Hua Tan Tang, Chuan Be Pi Pa Gao, Qi Guan Yan Ke Sou Tan Chaun Wan

ZANG FU

Zang Fu	Description	Tongue / Pulse		Points	Formulas
Large Intestine Heat	Constipation with dry stools, burning sensation in the mouth, dry tongue, burning and swelling around the anus, scanty-dark urine	Thick, yellow, dry coat	Full, rapid	LI-2, LI-4, LI-11, Sj-6, St-25, St-37, St-44, Ub-25, Sp-6, K-6, Ren-4, Ren-6, Ren-12	Ma Zi Ren Wan, Run Chang Wan
Large Intestine Cold Invading	Sudden abdominal pain, diarrhea with pain, feeling cold, cold sensation in abdomen	Red, little or no coat	Deep, wiry	St-25, St-37, Ub-25	Da Huang Fu Zi Tang, Ji Chuan Jian, Wen Pi Tang
Large Intestine Damp-Heat	Abdominal pain, tenesmus, diarrhea, mucus and blood in the stools, foul odor of stools, burning sensation around the anus, scanty-dark urine, fever, sweating, thirst without the desire to drink, sensation of heaviness, stuffiness of the chest and epigastrium	Red, sticky, yellow coat	Slippery, rapid	LI-11, Sp-6, Sp-9, St-25, St-37, Ub-25 (Sedate) Ren-3, LI-4, Ub-20, Ub-22, Ub-17, Ren-12	Ge Gen Qin Lian Tang, Shen Chu Cha, Bao Ji Wan, Bao Tou Weng, Sang Yao Tang, Bai Tou Weng Tang
Large Intestine Deficiency Fluid	Dry stools, obstructed constipation, difficult passing stools, dizziness, bad breath, dry mouth and throat		Fine, rapid	K-6, Ren-4, Sj-6, Sp-6, St-36, St-25, St-37, Ub-25	Run Chang Wan, Ba Zhen Wan, Wu Ren Wan
Stomach Qi Deficiency	Uncomfortable feeling in the epigastrium, no appetite, lack of taste, loose stools, tiredness in the morning, weak limbs	Pale	Empty, especially in the right middle position	Ren-12, Ren-6, Sp-6, St-21, St-36, Ub-20, Ub-21	Liu Jun Zi Tang, Huang Qi Jian Zhong Tang, Xiang Sha Liu Jun Zi Tang
Stomach Yin Deficiency	No appetite, empty and uncomfortable feeling in the stomach, hunger with no desire to eat, afternoon fever, constipation, dry stools, burning epigastric pain, dry mouth and throat, thirst with no desire to drink, feelings of fullness after eating, constipation	Red and peeled in the center, or coat without root	Thready, rapid	K-3, Ren-12, Sp-3, Sp-6, St-25, St-36, Ub-21 (Sedate); St-44, St-41	Mai Men Dong Tang, Yi Wei Tang, Yang Wei Tang, Shen Ling Bai Zhu Wan, Yi Guan Jian + Bai Shao Gan Cao Tang
Stomach Blood Stagnation	Stabbing pain in the epigastrium that is worse with heat or pressure, pain after eating, vomiting of dark blood, blood in the stools	Purple with purple spots	Wiry or choppy	Ren-10, Sp-10, St-21, St-34, St-36, Ub-17, Ub-18	Shi Xiao San, Dan Shen Yin, Huo Luo Xiao Ling Dan, Bao He Wan, Yan Hu Suo Zhi Tong Pian
Stomach Cold Invading	Sudden severe pain in the epigastrium, feeling of cold, preference for warmth, vomiting of clear fluids,	Thick, white coat	Deep, slow, tight	Sp-6, St-21, St-25, St-27, St-34, St-36, St-37, Ren-6, Ren-13, Ub-20, Ub-21 or Ren-8 ginger or moxa, Ren-12, or thread Sj-5 to Pc-6	Liang Fu Wan, Fu Zi Li Zhong Wan, Huo Xiang Zheng Qi Wan, Kang Nang Wan
Stomach Damp-Heat	Stuffiness, fullness and distention of the epigastrium and lower abdomen, no appetite, bitter taste, jaundice, feeling of heaviness, thirst without desire to drink, nausea, vomiting, abdominal pain, loose stools with offensive odor, burning sensation of the anus, scanty and dark-yellow urine, low-grade fever, headache	Red, yellow coat	Rapid, slippery	LI-4, LI-11, Pc-6, Sp-6, Sp-9, St-36, St-40, St-43, Ren-12, Ub-20	Lian Po Yin

Zang Fu	Description	Tongue / Pulse	Points	Formulas
Stomach Fire	Burning sensation in the epigastrium, pain in the epigastrium, thirst with desire to drink cold liquids, empty and uncomfortable feeling in the stomach, polyphagia (constant hunger), swelling and painful gums, bleeding gums, sour regurgitation, constipation, nausea, vomiting, bad breath	Red, thick yellow coat	Full, deep, rapid	St-21, St-34, St-4, St-44, St-45 or bleed, Ren-12, Ren-13, Pc-6	Qing Wei San, Bai Hu Tang, Yu Nu Jian, Xie Xie Tang, Huang Lian Su Pian
Stomach Food Retention	No appetite, fullness and distention of the epigastrium which is relieved by vomiting, nausea, vomiting, foul breath, sour-regurgitation, belching, insomnia	Thick coat	Full, slippery	Ren-10, Ren-11, Ren-12, Ren-13, St-21, (Pc-6 & Sp-4) Liv-13, Liv-14, Ub-20	Bao He Wan, Zhi Shi Dao Zhi Wan, Kan Ning Wan, Xiao Cheng Qi Tang
Stomach Qi Rebels	Sudden swelling of the eyes and face, gradually spreading to the whole body, bright, shiny complexion, scanty and pale urination, aversion to Wind, fever, cough, breathlessness	White, slippery coat	Floating, slippery	(Pc-6 & Sp-4), Ren-10, Ren-13	N/A
Stomach Deficiency Cold	Discomfort in the epigastrium which is worse after bowel movements and better after eating or with pressure or massage, no appetite, preference for warm drinks and foods, vomiting of clear fluids, loose stools, no thirst, cold limbs, fatigue	Pale, swollen	Deep, weak especially on the right middle position	St-21, St-36, Ren-6, Ren-12, Ub-20, Ub-21	Fu Zi Li Zhong Tang, Huang Qi Jian Zhong Tang, Li Zhong Wan, Liang Fu Wan, Xiang Sha Liu Jun Tang, Xiao Jian Zhong Tang, Shen Ling Bai Zhu Wan
Spleen Qi Deficiency	Poor appetite, emaciation, abdominal distention after eating, fatigue, lassitude, sallow complexion, weakness of the limbs, loose stools, nausea, stuffiness of the chest and epigastrium and feelings of heaviness	Pale or normal colored, swollen sides with transverse cracks	Weak, soft, thready	Sp-3, Sp-6, St-36, Ren-12, Ub-21, Ub-20, Liv-13; BM (L) St-36, St-37, Pc-6, Sp-10 with (R) LI-4, SJ-5, Sp-9, St-34	Jia Wei Si Jun Zi Tang, Liu Jun Zi Tang, Xiang Sha Lui Jun Tang, Shen Ling Bai Zhu Wan, Bu Zhong Yi Qi Tang
Spleen Yang Deficiency	Poor appetite, abdominal distention that is worse after eating, dull pain in the abdomen that improves with warmth or pressure, fatigue, sallow or bright-white complexion, weakness of the limbs, loose stools, edema, chilliness, cold limbs, diarrhea, vomiting, nausea, stuffiness of the chest and epigastrium and feeling of heaviness	Pale, swollen, wet	Weak, deep, slow	Ren-6, Ren-9, Ren-12, Sp-6, Sp-9, St-28, St-36, Ub-22, Ub-20	Li Zhong Tang, Shen Ling Bai Zhu San, Fu Zi Zhong Tang, Si Ling San, Wu Pi Yin, Fang Ji Huang Qi Tang
Spleen Cold-Damp Invading	No appetite, stiffness of the chest and epigastrium, feeling of cold in the epigastrium that is improved by warmth, feeling of heaviness in the head, sweetish taste in the mouth or absence of taste, no thirst, loose stools, white vaginal discharge, lassitude and feeling of heaviness	Sticky, thick white coat	Slippery, slow	Ub-20, Liv-13, Ren-12, Sp-3, Sp-6, Sp-9, St-8	Huang Qi Jian Zhong Tang, Liu Jun Zi Tang, Ren Shen Jian Pi Wan, Xiang Sha Liu Jun Zi Tang, Sheng Ling Bai Zhu Wan, Wei Ling Tang

Zang Fu	Description	Tongue / Pulse	Points	Formulas
Spleen Damp-Heat Invading	Stuffiness, fullness and distention of the epigastrium and lower abdomen, no appetite, bitter taste, jaundice, feeling of heaviness, thirst without desire to drink, nausea, vomiting, abdominal pain, loose stools with offensive odor, burning sensation of the anus, scanty and dark-yellow urine, low-grade fever, headache	Sticky, yellow coat; Slippery, rapid or soft	Du-9, Gb-34, Li-11, Sp-6, Sp-9, St-25, St-36, St-44, Ren-12, Ub-20, Liv-13	Shao Yao Tang, Da Cheng Qi Tang, Bai Tou Weng Tang, Ge Gen Qi Lian Tang, Shen Chu Cha
Spleen Not Controlling Blood	Purpura, blood spots under the skin, hematuria, blood in the stools, menorrhagia or metrorrhagia, poor appetite, abdominal distention after eating, fatigue, sallow or bright-white complexion, weakness of the limbs, loose stools, edema, diarrhea, vomiting, nausea, stuffiness of the chest and epigastrium and feeling of heaviness	Pale; Thready, weak	Sp-1, Sp-3, Sp-6, Sp-10, St-36, Ren-6, Ren-12, Ren-17, Ub-17, Ub-21, Du-20, Sj-4, Ub-20, Liv-13	Gui Pi Tang, Huang Tu Tang
Spleen Qi Sinking	Bearing down sensations, prolapse of stomach, uterus, anus or vagina, frequent urination, urgency of urination, poor appetite, abdominal distention after eating, fatigue, sallow or bright-white complexion, weakness of the limbs, loose stools, edema, diarrhea, vomiting, nausea, stuffiness of the chest and epigastrium and feeling of heaviness	Pale; Empty or weak	Du-1, Du-20, Sp-3, Sp-6, St-21, St-36, Ren-12, Ub-20, Ren-6	Bu Zhong Yi Qi Tang
Heart Qi Deficiency	Palpitations, shortness of breath on exertion, spontaneous sweating, pallor, tiredness, listlessness	Pale or normal color. Possibly a mid-line crack reaching the tip with swelling on the sides; Thready, weak, or missed beat	Ht-5, Pc-6, Ren-6, Ren-14, Ren-17, St-36, Ub-15	Zhi Gan Cao Tang, Yang Xin Tang, Si Jun Zi Tang, Ling Zhi Feng Tang Jiang
Heart Blood Deficiency	Palpitations, insomnia, dream-disturbed sleep, poor memory, dizziness, vertigo, anxiety, startles easily, dull-pale complexion, pale lips	Pale, thin, slightly dry; Choppy or thready	Ht-7, (Pc-6 & Sp-4) Pc-6, Ren-4, Ren-14, Ren-15, Sp-6, St-36, Ub-15, Ub-17, Ub-20	Si Wu Tang, Suan Zao Ren Tang, Gui Pi Tang, Dang Yang Xin Tang, Bai Zi Yang Xin Wan, Bu Qi Cong Ming Tang
Heart Yang Deficiency	Palpitations, cyanosis of the lips, shortness of breath on exertion, tiredness, listlessness, spontaneous sweating, feeling of stuffiness or discomfort in the heart region, feeling of cold, bright-pale face, cold limbs	Pale, wet, swollen; Deep, weak or knotted	Ht-5, Pc-6, Ren-6, Ren-17, Du-14, St-36, Sp-6, Ub-15	Shen Fu Tang, Gui Zhi Gan Cao Tang, Zhen Wu Tang, Du Shen Tang, Ren Shen Lu Rong Wan, Bao Yuan Jian

Zang Fu	Description	Tongue / Pulse	Points	Formulas
Heart Yin Deficiency	Palpitations, insomnia, dream-disturbed sleep, startles easily, poor memory, anxiety, mental restlessness, malar flush, low-grade fever, night sweating, dry mouth, dry throat, 5 palm heat	Red, little or no coat, tip redder and swollen, deep midline crack reaching the tip	Floating, empty and rapid or fine-rapid	Ht-7, Ht-7, Pc-6, Ren-4, Ren15, Sp-6, Ren-14, Ub-15, K-6, K-7	Tian Wang Bu Xin Dan, Bu Xin Tang, An Shen Bu Nao Pian, Bai Zi Yang Xin Xan, Bu Nao Wan
Heart - Fire Phlegm	Mental restlessness, palpitations, bitter taste, insomnia, dream-disturbed sleep, startles easily, incoherent speech, mental confusion, rash behavior, uncontrollable laughter or crying, agitation, shouting, muttering to oneself, mental depression and dullness, aphasia or coma	Red, yellow, sticky coat, midline crack with yellow prickles on it. Possibly redder on the tip and swollen with red points	Full, rapid, slippery or rapid, overflowing, wiry	Ht-7, Ht-8, Liv-3, Liv-3, Pc-5, Pc-6, Pc-7, Pc-8, St-40, Sp-6, Gb-13, Ub-20, Ren-12, Ren-14, Ren-15, Ub-15, Du-16, Du-20, Du-24 or bleed jingwell points	Ban Xia Bai Zhu Tian Ma Tang, Huang Lian Wen Dan Tang, Shi Wei Wen Dan Tang, Su He Xiang Wan, An Shen Bu Xin Wan, Meng Shi Gan Tang
Heart - Phlegm Misting	Mental confusion, incoherent speech, unconsciousness, lethargic stupor, vomiting, rattling sound in the throat, aphasia	White, thick, sticky, slippery coat, midline crack reaching the tip with prickles. Tongue body swollen	Wiry, slippery	K-1, Ht-5, Ht-8, Ht-9, Pc-5, Pc-6, Liv-3, CLHT, St-40, Du-20, Du-26, Ub-20, Ren-12	Ban Xia Bai Zhu Tian Ma Tang, Dao Tan Tang, Di Tan Tang, Su He Xiang Wan
Heart Blood Stasis	Palpitations, pain in the heart region, stabbing or stuffy in the anterior region or behind the sternum that may radiate to the inner aspect of the left arm or to the shoulder, stuffiness of the chest, discomfort or feeling of oppression or constriction of the chest, cyanosis of the lips and nails, cold hands	Purple or purplish spots	Thready, hesitant or missed beat	Ht-6, Ht-7, Pc-4, Pc-6, Sp-6, Sp-10, Ren-17, Ren-14, Ub-14, Ub-15, K-25, Ub-17	Xue Fu Zhu Tang, Tao Hong Si Wu Tang, Gua Lou Xie Bai Bai Jiu Tang, Fu Fang Dan Shen Pian, Su He Xiang Wan
Heart Channel Obstruction	Palpitations, oppression or stuffiness in chest, pain can radiate to shoulders or down arms			(Pc-6 & Sp-6) Sp-6, Sp-6, Sp-15, Ub-15, Ub-16, Ub-17	Gua Lou Xie Bai Gui Zhi Tang
Heart Fire	Palpitations, thirst, ulcers in mouth and tongue, mental restlessness, insomnia, red face, dark urine, hematuria, bitter taste	Red, tip redder and swollen with red points, yellow coat, midline crack reaching to the tip	Full, rapid, overflowing	Ht-7, Ht-8, Ht-9, Ren-15, Ren-14, Sp-6, K-6, Ub-15	Huang Lian E Jiao Tang, Dao Chi San, Zhu Sha An Shen Wan, Xie Xin Tang
Heart Yang Collapse	Palpitations, shortness of breath on exertion, profuse sweating, cold limbs, cyanosis of the lips, severe cases of coma	Pale or bluish purple, short	Hidden, knotted, muted	Ren-4, Ren-6, Ren-8, Du-4, Pc-6, St-36, Du-14, Du-20, Ub-15, Ub-20, Ub-23	Si Ni Tang, Tong Mai Si Ni Tang, Shen Fu Tang

ZANG FU

Zang Fu	Description	Tongue / Pulse	Points	Formulas
Heart and Kidney Not Harmonized - Yin Deficiency	Palpitations, mental restlessness, insomnia, poor memory, dizziness, tinnitus, deafness, soreness of the lower back, nocturnal emissions with dreams, afternoon fever-tidal fever, night sweating, scanty, dark urine, dry throat	Red, peeled, tip redder, crack in the midline reaching the tip	Floating, empty, thready, or rapid	K-3, K-9, K-10, Sp-6, Ren-4, Ren-15, Ht-5, Ht-6, Ht-7, Pc-6, Du-24, Gb-13, Ub-15, Ub-23, E-yintang	Tian Wang Bu Xin Dan, Liu We Di Huang Wan, Dao Chi San, Jiao Tai Wan
Heart and Liver Blood Deficiency	Palpitations, insomnia, dream-disturbed sleep, poor memory, dry eyes, twitching eyes, dizziness, painful ribs and flanks, numbness of limbs, stiffness and spasms of tendons, low-grade fever, night sweats, irregular scanty menses	Pale, thin, little coat	Thready, choppy, forceless	Ht-7, Ren-4, Liv-3, St-36, Sp-6, Ub-15, Ub-17, Ub-18, Ub-20	Suan Zao Ren Tang, Dang Gui Bu Xue Dan
Heart and Lung Qi Deficiency	Palpitations, white complexion, shortness of breath, spontaneous sweating, stifling oppression in chest and heart, dizziness, asthma, cough, panting	Pale	Weak	Du-4, Ren-9, K-7, Sp-6, Sp-9, St-28, Ub-22, Ub-23	Bao Yuan Dan, Si Jun Zi Tang, Sheng Mai San
Small Intestine Cold	Slight lower abdomen pain, feelings of cold and heaviness, desire for warmth and pressure, abdominal fullness, borborygmi, frequent urination, diarrhea	Pale, thin white coat	Deep, slow, weak	Ren-6, Ren-12, St-25, St-36, St-37, St-39, Sp-3, Ub-20, Ub-27	Li Zhong Tang
Small Intestine Heat	Fullness and distension in lower abdomen, ulceration and erosion of mouth and tongue, irritability, sore throat, dry mouth, desire for drinks, scanty urination, painful urination or pain in urethra, palpitations, flushed face	Red, yellow coat	Slippery, rapid	Liv-2, Ht-5, Ht-8, Sp-6, (Sedate): SI-2, SI-5	Dao Chi San
Urinary Bladder Damp-Cold	Frequent urination, urgency of urination, difficult urination, felling of heaviness in the hypogastrium and urethra, pale and turbid urine	White, sticky coat on root	Slippery, slow, slightly wiry on rear position	Ren-3, Ren-9, Sp-6, Sp-9, Ub-22, Ub-23, Ub-28, St-28	Bei Xie Fen Xing Yin
Urinary Bladder Damp-Heat	Frequent urination, urgency of urination, burning of urination, difficult urination, dark-yellow and/or turbid urination, hematuria, sand in urine, stones, fever, thirst, lumbago-low back pain	Red, thick, sticky, yellow coat	Rapid, slippery, slightly wiry on left rear position	Ren-3, Sp-6, Sp-9, K-7, Liv-2, Ub-22, Ub-23, Ub-28, Ub-63, Ub-66	Ba Zhen Tang, Long Dan Xie Gan Tang, Dao Chi San, Si Wei San-Stones, Bleeding
Urinary Bladder Turbid Damp-Heat	Frequent urination that contains cloudy or murky substances, urgency of urination, burning of urination, difficult urination, dark-yellow and/or turbid urination, hematuria, sand in urine, stones, fever, thirst, lumbago-low back pain	Red, yellow greasy coat	Slippery, soggy, rapid	N/A	N/A

Zang Fu	Description	Tongue / Pulse	Points	Formulas
Kidney Qi Deficiency	Soreness of lower back, weakness of lower back, weakness of knees, clear urination, frequent urination, weak-stream urination, incontinence of urine, dribbling after urination, enuresis, nocturia, nocturnal emissions without dreams, premature ejaculation, spermatorrhea, prolapse uterus, leukorrhea-chronic vaginal discharge	Pale	Deep, weak, thready	K-3, Du-4, Ren-3, Ren-4, Ren-6, Sp-6, Ub-23, Ub-52	Jin Suo Gu Jing Wan, Su Quan Wan, Sang Piao Xiao San
Kidney Yang Deficiency	Aversion to cold, soreness of lower back, weak knees, impotence, premature ejaculation, lassitude, profuse clear urination, scanty clear urination, edema of the legs, infertility, poor appetite, loose stools, diarrhea, bright-white complexion, dizziness, tinnitus	Pale, swollen, wet	Deep, weak	Du-4, Du-20, K-3, K-7, Ren-4, Ren-6, Ren-8, Sp-6, Ub-23, Ub-52	You Gui Wan, Jin Gui Shen Qi Tang, Du Huo Ji Shen Tang, Si Shen Wan, Shen Fu Tang, Zhen Wu Tang, Shen Jie San, Ge Ji Da Bu Wan, Yao Tong Pian, Du Zhong Hu Gu Wan
Kidney Yin Deficiency	Dizziness, tinnitus, vertigo, insomnia, poor memory, deafness, night sweating, afternoon fever, dry mouth at night, 5 palm heat, malar flush, thirst, sore back, sore knees, nocturnal emissions, constipation, dark-scanty urine	Red, no coat, cracks	Floating, empty or thready and rapid	K-1, K-3, K-6, K-9, K-10, Ren-1, Ren-4, Sp-6, Ub-23	Liu Wei Di Huang Wan, Zuo Gui Wan, Tian Wang Bu Xin Dan, Er Zhi Wan, Bai He Gu Jin Tang, Ba Xian Chang Shou Wan, Gui Zhi Can Cao Long Gu Mu Li Tang, Mai Wei Di Huang Wan
Kidney Yin Deficiency Fire	Malar flush, mental restlessness, night sweating, low-grade fever, afternoon fever, insomnia, scanty-dark urine, hematuria, dry throat, soreness of the lower back, nocturnal emissions with dreams, excessive sexual desire, dry stools, constipation	Red, peeled, cracked, red tip	Floating, empty, rapid	K-1, K-2, K-3, K-6, K-9, K-10, Ren-4, Sp-6, Ub-23, Ht-5, Ht-7, Pc-7, Ub-15, Lu-7, Lu-10	Zhi Bai Di Huang Wan
Kidney Essence Deficiency	Soreness of lower back, weakness of lower back, weakness of knees, head hair loss, graying or whitening of hair, weak sexual function, atrophy, poor memory, senility, brittle bones, loose teeth, dizziness, tinnitus, hearing loss	Red, peeled	Floating, empty	K-3, K-6, K-7, K-10, Du-4, Ren-4, Gb-39, Ub-11, Ub-14, Ub-15, Ub-18, Sp-6, Ub-23, Du-20	Zuo Gui Wan, You Gui Wan, Er Long Zuo Ci Wan, Liu Wei Di Huang Wan, He Che Da Zao Wan
Kidney Failing to Receive Qi	Shortness of breath, difficult inhalation, cough, asthma, spontaneous sweating, cold limbs, swelling of the face, soreness of lower back	Pale	Deep, weak, tight	K-3, K-6, K-7, K-25, Lu-9, Du-4, Ren-4, Ren-6, Ren-17, St-36, Ub-13, Ub-23, Ub-43, Du-12	Bu Fei Tang, Ren Shen Ge Jie San, Ren Shen Hu Tao Tang
Kidney and Liver Yin Deficiency	Sallow complexion, dull headache, insomnia, dream-disturbed sleep, numbness of limbs, malar flush, dizziness, dry eyes, blurred vision, anger, soreness of the lower back, soreness of the knees, dry throat, tinnitus, night sweating, 5 palm heat, dry stools, nocturnal emissions, scanty menstruation, amenorrhea, infertility	Red, peeled, cracked	Thready, rapid, floating, empty or choppy	K-1, K-3, K-6, Liv-3, Liv-8, Ren-4, Sp-6, Ub-10, Ub-17, Ub-18, Ub-20, Ub-23, Du-20	Liu Wei Di Huang Wan, Yi Guan Jian, Da Bu Yin Wan, Zhi Bai Di Huang Wan

ZANG FU

ZANG FU

Zang Fu	Description	Tongue / Pulse	Points	Formulas
Kidney and Lung Qi Deficiency	Asthma, shortness of breath more on exhalation than inhalation, low voice, cold limbs, blue complexion, spontaneous sweating, incontinence of urine due to cough	Pale	Weak, deep	K-7, Du-4, Ht-7, Lu-9, Ren-9, Ren-17, Ub-13, Ub-15, Ub-23	Jin Gui Shen Qi Wan, Hei Xi Dan, Ren Shen Ge Jie San, Sheng Mai San + Ji Sheng Shen Qi Wang
Kidney and Lung Yin Deficiency	Dry cough that is worse in the evening, blood-tinged sputum, dry mouth, thin body, breathlessness on exertion, soreness of the lower back, weak limbs, afternoon fever, night sweating, nocturnal emissions, 5 palm heat	Red, peeled with transverse cracks in the lung area	Floating, empty, thready and rapid	K-3, K-6, Ren-4, Lu-7, Lu-9, Sp-6, Ub-43, Ub-23, Ub-13, Lu-1	Ba Xian Chang Shou Wan, Bai He Gu Jin Tang, Yang Yin Qing Fei Tang + Da Bu Yin Wan
Kidney and Spleen Yang Deficiency	Weakness, shortness of breath, abdominal distention, poor appetite, aversion to cold, cold limbs, profuse clear urination or scanty urination, loose stools, diarrhea, day break diarrhea, edema of the abdomen and legs, facial swelling, chronic diarrhea, borborygmus	Pale, swollen	Deep, weak, slow	K-3, K-7, Du-4, Ren-6, St-25, St-36, St-37, Ub-20, Ub-21, Ub-23, Ub-25	Fu Zi Li Zhong Wan, Si Shen Wan, Zhen Wu Tang, Shi Pi Yin
Kidney Yang Deficiency Water Flooding	Aversion to cold, edema of whole body particularly below the waist, soreness of lower back, pitting edema, abdominal distention with full sensations, cold limbs, congested gray or pale face, feeling nervous and cold with mental weariness, possible ascites	Pale, swollen, white coat	Deep, weak, slow	K-7, Du-4, Du-14, St-28, Ren-9, Sp-6, Sp-9, Ub-15,Ub-20, Ub-22, Ub-23	Ji Sheng Shen Qi Wan + Zhen We Tang, Jin Gui Shen Qi Wan
Gallbladder Heat Deficiency	Dizziness, blurred or impaired vision, possible phlegm	Greasy, yellow coat	Slippery, rapid	Pc-5, Pc-6, Ht-7, Gb-34, St-40, Ub-15, Ub-19, Ren-14	Wen Dan Tang
Liver Qi Stagnation	Distention of the hypochondrium and distention of the chest, hypochondriac pain, sighing, hiccups, depression, irritability, nausea, vomiting, diarrhea, epigastric pain, poor appetite, plum pit sensation in the throat, belching, sour regurgitation, abdominal distention, irregular periods, painful periods, distention of the breasts, PMS	Normal	Wiry on the left side	Liv-3, Liv-13, Liv-14, (Gb-34 & Sj-6), Gb-40, Gb-41, Pc-6, Sp-6, Ub-18	Xiao Yao San, Yu Ju Wan, Chai Hu Shu Gan Tang, Ban Xia Huo Po Tang- w/ Plumpit Qi, Tong Xie Yao Feng, Si Ni San, Shu Gan San, Si Qi Tang, Dan Zhi Xiao Yao San-w/Heat
Liver Blood Stagnation	Vomiting blood, epistaxis, painful periods, irregular periods, dark clotted menstrual blood, abdominal pain, abdominal masses	Purple especially on the sides, purplish spots	Wiry	Liv-3, Liv-13, Liv-14, Gb-34, Sp-6, Sp-10, Ren-6, Ub-17, Ub-18	Xue Fu Zhu Tang, Ge Xia Zhu Yu Tang

272

Zang Fu	Description	Tongue / Pulse	Points	Formulas
Liver and Gallbladder Damp-Heat	Bright yellow sclera and skin yang-type jaundice, pain and fullness in ribs on both sides, poor appetite, fever, bitter taste in mouth, nausea, bitter sour vomit, anorexia, dark urine, abdominal distension, yellow vaginal discharge, painful swollen and burning sensation in testicles	Thick, yellow, sticky coat	Liv-2, Liv-3, Liv-14, LI-11, Gb-34, Gb-24, Du-9, Pc-6, Sp-3, Sp-6, Sp-9, Ren-12, Ub-18, Ub-19, E-dannangxue	Long Dan Xie Gan Tang, Dai Chai Hu Tang, Yin Chen Hao Tang
Liver Blood Deficiency	Dizziness, vertigo, numbness of limbs, floaters, insomnia, blurred vision, night blindness, scanty menstruation or amenorrhea, dull, lusterless, pale complexion, pale lips, muscular weakness, muscle spasms, cramps, withered and brittle nails	Pale body, especially on the sides, dry	Liv-3, Liv-8, Ren-4, Pc-6, Sp-6, St-36, Ub-17, Ub-18, Ub-20, Ub-23	Si Wu Tang, Qi Ju Di Huang Wan, Hei Xiao Yao San, Ba Zhen Tang, Bu Gan Tang, Zou Gui Wan
Liver Yin Deficiency	Dizziness, blurred or impaired vision, headache, tinnitus, low-grade fever in the afternoon or evening, malar flush, night sweating, 5 palm heat, insomnia, dry mouth, dry throat, hoarse voice	Red, little	K-3, K-6, Liv-3, Ub-18, Ub-23	Yi Guan Jian, Qi Ju Di Huang Wan
Liver Blood Deficiency Transform to Wind	Blurry vision, dizziness, vertigo, numbness of limbs, tics or tremors, spasms or involuntary movements of the limbs or head, sallow complexion, dry skin, pale lips, insomnia, irregular menses, brittle fingernails	Pale body, deviated, little coat	Liv-3, Liv-8, LI-4, K-3, Sp-6, St-36, Du-14, Du-16, Du-20, Du-26, Gb-20, Ub-17, Ub-18, Ub-20	N/A
Liver Channel Cold Stagnation	Fullness and distention of the hypogastrium, pain that refers to the scrotum and testis and is alleviated by warmth, dysmenorrhea, infertility	Pale, wet, white coat	Liv-1, Liv-5, Liv-6, Ren-3, Ren-4, Sp-6, Ub-25, Ub-26, Ub-32	Nuan Gan Jian, Wu Zhu Yu Tang, Tian Tai Wu Yao San
Liver Fire	Irritability, anger, tinnitus, deafness, temporal headache, dizziness, red face, red, swollen and painful eyes, burning pain in the costal and hypochondriac regions, thirst, bitter taste, dream-disturbed sleep, constipation, dark-yellow urine, epistaxis, hematemesis, hemoptysis, dry mouth	Red especially on the sides, yellow dry coat	Liv-2, Liv-3, Gb-1, Gb-13, Gb-20, Du-20, E-taiyang	Long Dan Xie Gan Tang, Geng Yi Wan, Dang Gui Long Hui Wan-Most Severe Heat, Zuo Jin Wan W/ St Cramping Pain
Liver Fire Insulting the Lungs	Breathlessness, asthma, fullness and stuffiness of the chest and hypochondrium, burning pain in the costal and hypochondriac regions, cough, yellow or blood-tinged sputum, hemoptysis, headache, dizziness, red face, thirst, bitter taste, scanty dark urine, constipation, anger	Red, especially on the sides, swollen in the front part, yellow coat	Liv-2, Liv-14, Ren-17, Ren-22, Pc-6, Lu-7, LI-11, Ub-13, Ub-18	N/A
Liver Invading Spleen	Irritability, abdominal distention and pain, alternating constipation and diarrhea, loose stools, dry and bitty stools, flatulence, fatigue	Red on the sides or pale	Liv-3, Liv-13, Sp-6, Ren-6, Ren-12, St-25, St-36, St-37	Xiao Yao San, Tong Xie Yao Fang

(Weak on the right and wiry on the left — pulse for Liver Invading Spleen)

Zang Fu	Description	Tongue / Pulse	Points	Formulas
Liver Invading Stomach	Distention and pain in the costal, hypochondriac, and epigastric regions, belching, acid regurgitation, empty and uncomfortable feeling in the stomach, depression or irritability	*Thin coat*	*Wiry*	Liv-3, Liv-13, Liv-14, Gb-34, Pc-6, Sp-6, Ren-6, Ren-10, Ren-12, Ren-13, St-36, Ub-21	Zuo Jin Wan
Liver Yang Rising	Headache, dizziness, vertigo, red face, red eyes, tinnitus, deafness, dry mouth, dry throat, insomnia, dream-disturbed sleep, palpitations, poor memory, soreness and weakness of the low back and knees, irritability, anger	*Red, especially on the sides*	*Wiry, thready and rapid*	K-3, Liv-2, Liv-3, Liv-8, Gb-6, Gb-8, Gb-9, Gb-20, Gb-34, Gb-38, Gb-43, Sp-6, Sj-5, Ub-2, Ub-18, Ub-23, (Sedate): Du-20	Tian Ma Gou Teng Yin, Qi Ju Di Huang Wan, Zhen Gan Xi Feng Tang, Ling Jiao Gou Teng Tang, Tian Ma Shou Wu Pian
Liver Wind Due to Extreme Heat	High fever, convulsions, neck rigidity, upward staring of the eyes, tremors, opisthotonus, lock jaw, coma in severe cases	*Deep-red, stiff, thick yellow coat*	*Wiry, rapid, full*	Liv-2, Liv-3, LI-11, SI-3, Gb-20, Gb-43, Du-14, Du-16, Du-20, Du-26 or can bleed Liv-1 or LI-1	Da Ding Feng Zhu, Ling Jiao Gou Teng Tang, E Jiao Ji Zi Huang, Ling Yang Jiao Tang
Liver Wind Due to Liver Blood Deficiency	Numbness of limbs, tics, shaking of the head, tremors	*Pale, deviated*	*Choppy*	Ren-4, K-3, LI-4, Liv-3, Liv-8, Du-14, Du-16, Du-20, Du-26, St-36, Sp-6, Ub-17, Ub-18, Ub-20, Ub-23	Si Wu Tang, Da Ding Feng Zhu, Ling Yang Jiao Tang
Liver Wind Due to Liver Yang Rising	Unconsciousness, convulsions, deviation of the eyes and mouth, hemiplegia, numbness and tremors of the limbs, aphasia, dysphasia, dizziness, vertigo, headache, stiffness of the tongue	*Red, little or peeled coat, deviated*	*Floating and empty or wiry, fine and rapid depending on the degree of excess of deficiency*	K-3, K-1, Liv-2, Liv-3, Liv-8, Du-16, Du-20, Du-26, Gb-20, Pc-8, Sp-6, Ub-18	Tian Ma Gou Teng Yin, Zhen Gan Xi Feng Tang, Da Ding Feng Zhu, Ling Yang Jiao Tang
Liver Wind Due to Liver Yin Deficiency	Same as Liver Yin, but worse	*Red, narrow, dry, geographic*	*Thin*	(All Liv Yin Pts): Liv-3, Liv-8, Ren-4, Pc-6, Sp-6, St-36, Ub-17, Ub-18, Ub-20, K-3, K-10, Ub-23, Ren-3	San Jia Fu Mai Tang
Liver Yang Transform to Wind	Headache, dizziness, vertigo, numbness and tremors of the limbs, red face, red eyes, tinnitus, deafness, dry mouth, dry throat, insomnia, dream-disturbed sleep, palpitations, poor memory, irritability, anger	*Red*	*Wiry, thready*	K-1, K-3, Liv-2, Liv-3, Pc-6, Pc-8, Gb-20, Du-20, Du-26, Ub-18	Tian Ma Gou Teng Yin, Zhen Gan Xi Feng Tang, Da Ding Feng Zhu, Ling Yang Jiao Tang
Liver-Gallbladder Damp Heat	Fever, scanty dark urine, fullness, distention and pain of the chest and hypochondrium, jaundice, bitter taste, nausea, vomiting, loss of appetite, abdominal distention, vaginal discharge, red painful swelling of the scrotum, vaginal itching	*Red body, sticky yellow coat*	*Slippery, wiry, rapid*	Liv-3, Liv-14, Gb-34, Gb-24, LI-11, Pc-6, Sp-9, Ren-12, Ub-18, Ub-19, Ub-20	Long Dan Xie Gan Tang, Dai Chai Hu Tang

Abdominal obstruction	Tofu
Abdominal pain	Buckwheat, fennel seed, ginger, fresh green onion - white part only, hawthorn fruit, rosin, mutton or goat meat, sorghum, brown sugar, wild cabbage
Abdominal pain with chills	Grapefruit, lychee, black pepper, red or green pepper (chili pepper, cayenne pepper)
Acute gastroenteritis	Tea
Aging	Common button mushroom, royal jelly, walnut
Alcoholism	Freshwater clam
Alcoholism, chronic	Yam bean
Altitude sickness	Fenugreek seed
Anemia	Corn silk, longan
Angina pectoris	Bee venom, hawthorn fruit
Appendicitis	Purslane
Arrhythmia	Chicken egg yolk
Arsenic poisoning	Eggplant, radish leaf
Arteriosclerosis	Tea, tofu, eggplant, wheat bran, yam
Arthritis	Bee venom, loquat root, red vine spinach, royal jelly, sunflower disc or receptacle, vinegar
Asthma	Bamboo liquid oil, black sesame seed, cinnamon bark, cuttlebone, squash, grapefruit peel
Asthma, bronchial	Castor bean, pork testes, bee venom
Bleeding	Black fungus, day lily, white fungus, lotus rhizome, radish, shepherd's purse, water spinach
Bleeding after childbirth	Lotus rhizome
Bleeding gums	White sugar
Blocked urination	Prickly ash
Blood in stools	Black sesame seed, kumquat cake, lychee, longan, mung bean sprouts, chestnut, eggplant, kohlrabi, leaf or brown mustard
Blood in urine	Celery, lettuce towel gourd
	Food cure for blood in urine with diminished urination: Cut up 50g celery into small pieces. Place celery, 25g broad beans, and 100g rice in a saucepan and cover with water to about an inch above. Boil until soft. Eat at mealtime.
Blurred vision	Liver (beef, chicken, pork), matrimony vine leaf
Breast cancer	Crab, squash calyx
Breast lump	Cucumber, green onion (fibrous root), squash calyx
Bronchitis	Chicken, jellyfish, pork gallbladder, tangerine peel, water chestnut
Bronchitis, chronic	Fungus, white fungus, yam
	Food cure for bronchitis: Rinse 100g dried jellyfish. Place jellyfish and 100g fresh chestnuts in a saucepan and cover with water to about an inch above. Boil until soft. Eat at mealtime, once a day, until the symptoms disappear.
Burn	Cucumber, mung bean, mung bean powder, pork skin, watermelon

Cancer	Apricot, button mushroom, carrot, Chinese gooseberry, eggplant leaf, garlic, lily bulb leaf, ling, mulberry root bark, snail (river snail), wild cabbage
Canker, mouth	Watermelon
Cardiovascular diseases	Chinese chive
Cervical cancer	Shiitake mushroom, walnut twig (young branches)
Chicken pox	Potato
Childbirth, difficult	Pork
Cirrhosis	Azuki bean
Colon cancer	Chinese chive
Common cold	Coriander (Chinese parsley), duck egg, honeysuckle stem leaf, pine leaf, green onion - white part
	Food cure for the common cold: Combine 6 green onions, white part only, 50g maltose (or brown sugar if not available), and 2 cups (500mL) water. Bring to a boil for a few seconds. Discard the onions. Add an egg white into the soup and stir. Divide into three doses to drink morning, afternoon, and evening.
Concussion	Peanut plant
Conjunctivitis	Peanut oil, pork gallbladder
Constipation	Bamboo shoot, black sesame seed, carrots, green onion - white part, loquat leaf, potato, red vine spinach, small white cabbage, sweet potato, water spinach
	Food cure for constipation: Cut 250g carrots into cubes. Boil in water until soft. Eat at mealtime.
Constipation in the elderly	Walnut
Constipation with dry stools	Amaranth, banana, beef, black sesame seed, carrot, fungus, white fungus, honey, longevity fruit, mulberry, peach, pine-nut kernel, pork, spinach
	Food cure for constipation with dry stools: Boil 100g spinach in water until soft. Drain. Pour 1 teaspoon sesame oil over the spinach. Eat at mealtime.
Corns	Yellow soybean sprout
Coronary heart disease	Tofu, black fungus, chrysanthemum, hawthorn fruit
	Food cure for coronary heart disease: Immerse 6g black fungus in water for 20 minutes. Cut up 50g lean pork. Combine the pork and the black fungus with 30g cornstarch and add to 2 cups (500mL) water. Boil to make soup. Eat the soup at mealtime, once a day.
	Food cure for coronary heart disease with hypertension: Place 50g cornstarch, 10g rice, and 10g of tofu in a saucepan. Cover with water to about an inch above. Boil to make soup. Eat at mealtime, once a day.
Cough	Betel pepper, citron, crown daisy, goose meat, mandarin orange, olive, peanut, pear, squash
Cough, chronic	Chicken, lily bulb leaf
Cough (dry cough)	Apple, autumn bottle gourd, banana, fungus, white fungus, honey, peanut, pine-nut kernel, pork, sand pear, sugar cane
Cough due to weak lungs	Plum (prunes)
Cough with chills	Leaf or brown mustard

FOOD

Cough with copious phlegm	Apricot, bamboo shoot, chicken egg, ginkgo (cooked), grapefruit, towel gourd, water chestnut
Coughing up blood	Duck, loquat, persimmon
Cystitis	Magnolia vine fruit - Chinese, red vine spinach
Decreased vision	Matrimony vine leaf
Dehydration	Coconut meat
Depression	Red date, wheat
Dermatitis	Chicken egg, pork gallbladder, rice bran oil, safflower, tea, walnut, walnut twig (young branches)
Diabetes	Bottle gourd, black fungus, corn (sweet or Indian), eggplant, hyacinth bean, kiwi fruit, mulberry, palm seed, pear, pork pancreas, radish, sand pear, sheep or goat's pancreas, spinach, squash, sweet potato vine leaves, tangerine, orange, water spinach, wheat bran, wintermelon, yam
	Food cure for diabetes: Cut 150g squash and 100g yam into small pieces. Place in a saucepan and cover with water to about an inch above. Eat the soup at mealtime.
Diarrhea	Black pepper, brown sugar, buckwheat sprout, chestnut, chicken, garlic, grapefruit leaf, hyacinth bean, onion, papaya, purslane, rabbit liver, red bayberries, tangerine, orange, watermelon, yam
	Food cure for diarrhea: Place 30g hyacinth beans and 100g rice in a saucepan. Cover with water to about an inch above. Eat at mealtime.
Diarrhea, chronic	Apple, carrot, fig, gorgan fruit, guava, lychee, lotus rhizome, plum (prunes), pomegranate (sweet fruit), sword bean, wheat
	Food cure for chronic diarrhea: Peel 2 apples. Remove the seeds. Cut up and place in a saucepan. Cover with water to about an inch above. Boil until soft. Drink the liquid like tea.
Diarrhea, with indigestion	Pineapple
Diarrhea in infant	Tea
Digestive tract disorders	Black fungus
Diminished urination	Amaranth, asparagus, barley, bottle gourd, cantaloupe, carp, celery, Chinese cabbage, crown daisy, cucumber, grapes, green onion - white part, hami melon, kidney bean, lettuce, mandarin orange, mango, mulberry, red vine spinach, star fruit, string bean, wintermelon
Diphtheria	Pork gallbladder, walnut
Dizziness	Corn silk
Dog bite	Apricot seed (bitter)
Dry eyes	Liver (pork)
Dry throat	Apricot
Dysentery	Amaranth, bitter gourd (balsam pear), cantaloupe, chicken gallbladder, Chinese toon leaf, chrysanthemum, cucumber vine (stem), date tree bark, fig, garlic, ginger - fresh, grape, guava, hawthorn fruit, honeysuckle, hyacinth bean flower, lotus root, magnolia vine fruit - Chinese, olive, papaya, plum (prunes), pomegranate (sweet fruit and peel), purslane, radish leaf, red vine spinach, scallion bulb, smoked prunes, tea, tomato, towel gourd, walnut leaf

Earache (Otitis media)	Pork gallbladder
Eczema	Broad bean shell, chicken egg yolk, clam - freshwater, coconut shell, mung bean powder, olive, potato, soybean - black
Edema	Areca nuts, autumn bottle gourd, beef, bottle gourd, carp (common and gold), chicken, corn (Indian corn, maize), day lily, duck, grapes, kidney bean, kohlrabi, mulberry, radish leaf, shepherd's purse, sorghum root, wintermelon
	Food cure for edema: Cut 50g wintermelon into cubes. Place melon and 50g kidney beans in a saucepan. Cover with water to about an inch above. Boil until soft. Eat at mealtime.
Edema during pregnancy	Carp
Encephalitis	Banana rhizome, buffalo's horn, pine leaf
Enteritis	Chicken egg, Chinese toon leaf, date tree bark, ginkgo (cooked), kumquat, pork gallbladder, purslane, tea
Epilepsy	Castor bean root, green turtle, olive
Fatigue	Beef, goose meat, honey
Fatigue, chronic	Matrimony vine fruit, mutton
Food poisoning	Ginger - fresh
Forgetfulness	Longan
Fracture	Chicken egg shell inner membrane, mung bean powder
Frostbite	Cherry, cherry juice, chili rhizome, rosin, tangerine, orange peel
Fungus infections	Bee secretion
Gallstone	Radish
Gastroduodenal ulcer	Barley, green peel of unripe walnut, honey, potato, royal jelly
Gastric ulcer	Wild cabbage
Gastritis	Papaya, rice (polished)
Genital itch	Apricot seed (bitter), chicken egg yolk
Glaucoma	Areca nuts
Goiter	Kelp, laver
	Food cure for goiter: Place 50g kelp and 50g laver in a saucepan. Cover with water to about an inch above. Boil until soft. Eat at mealtime.
Headache	Buckwheat, carp, radish
Headache with the common cold	Green onion - white part
Heart disease	Ginkgo leaf, hawthorn fruit, loquat seed, pineapple, tea plant root
Hemophilia	Lotus rhizome, peanut
Hemorrhoid	Black fungus, clam - freshwater, chicken egg, eggplant, fig, leaf or brown mustard, pork, pork gallbladder, spinach, walnut leaf, water spinach, fig leaf
Hepatitis	Button mushroom, cotton root, garlic, glutinous rice stalk, honeysuckle stem leaf, loach, loquat root, magnolia vine fruit - Chinese, malt, muskmelon calyx receptacle, pork gallbladder, red and black date, rice straw, royal jelly, tea
Hernia	Green onion - white part/outer skin, pork
Herpes	Purslane, water spinach

Hiccups	Brown sugar, Chinese chive seeds, duck egg, ginger - fresh, persimmon calyx receptacle, rice (polished), sword bean and seed
	Food cure for hiccups: Grind 10 dried lychee nuts (shells removed) into a fine powder. Mix the powder in 1 cup (250mL) water with 2 tablespoons of brown sugar. Drink it as a tea.
Hiccups triggered by cold	Lychee
High cholesterol	Celery, corn (Indian corn, maize), cucumber, garlic, kiwi fruit, onion, shiitake mushroom, sunflower seed, tofu
Hookworm	Purslane
Hot sensations	Pear
Hyperglycemia	Black sesame seed, water spinach
Hypersensitive teeth	Tea
Hypertension	Apple, betel pepper, black sesame seed, broad bean flower, carrot, celery, chrysanthemum, corn (Indian corn, maize), cucumber vine (stem), eggplant, garlic, hawthorn fruit, jellyfish, matrimony vine root bark, onion, peanut, peanut plant, peony root bark, persimmon, persimmon calyx receptacle, royal jelly, sand pear, seaweed, spinach, sunflower sic or receptacle, sunflower leaf, tofu, tomato, watermelon
	Food cure for hypertension with high cholesterol: Crush 250g fresh celery to make celery juice. Drink in 1 day.
	Food cure for hypertension with heart disease: Immerse 50g hawthorn fruit in water for 15 minutes. Remove the fruit from the water and squeeze to obtain juice. Boil the juice over low heat to increase its concentration. Mix it with 50g rice to make soup. Drink the soup at mealtime.
Hyperthyroidism	Persimmon
	Food cure for hyperthyroidism: Crush 1kg unripe persimmons. Fry until soft. Add 3 teaspoons honey and continue to fry until very sticky. Take 1 teaspoon 3 times a day.
Hypothyroidism	Kelp, laver
Hysteria	Wheat
Impotence	Chinese chive, lobster, mutton, walnut
Indigestion	Apricot seed (bitter), chicken egg yolk, coriander - Chinese parsley, corncob, grapefruit, hawthorn fruit, lemon, papaya, pomegranate leaf, prickly ash, sorghum, tea, water chestnut
Indigestion in children	Coconut meat
Induced labor	Asparagus (lucid asparagus), sweet potato vine leaves
Infertility	Ginger - fresh
Inflammatory disease	Chili pepper (cayenne pepper)
Influenza	Garlic
Injury	Chili pepper (cayenne pepper), glutinous rice stalk, safflower
Lactation problems	Carp, button mushroom, day lily, fig, lettuce, papaya, towel gourd
Insomnia	Lotus (fruit, seed, root), grapes, lily bulb leaf, longan, peanut plant
	Food cure for insomnia: Place 15 longan nuts, 7 red dates, and 50g rice in a saucepan. Cover with water to about an inch above. Boil until soft and eat.

Intestinal obstruction	Brown sugar, ginger - fresh, green onion - white part, peanut oil, prickly ash, radish, rapeseed (canola) oil, soybean oil, tea oil
Intestinal parasites	Areca nuts
Intoxication	Apple, grapefruit, ling, mandarin orange, peanut, sand pear, tea, tea melon
Itch	Mung bean powder
Jaundice	Autumn bottle gourd, brown sugar, citron leaf, corn male flower, crab, eggplant, hawthorn fruit, jackfruit, kiwi fruit
	Food cure for jaundice: Cut 50g eggplant into cubes. Place eggplant, 100g rice and 5 pieces ginger into saucepan. Cover with water to about an inch above. Boil until soft. Eat at mealtime.
Kidney disease	Hami melon, watermelon
Laryngitis	Watermelon
Lead poisoning	Mung bean, water chestnut
Leukemia	Hairtail
Loss of voice	Fig, longevity fruit, loquat, mango, radish
Malaria	Areca nuts, black pepper, chicken egg
Malnutrition	Squash
Mastitis	Chicken egg yolk, eggplant, grapevine leaf, green onion - white part, honeycomb - wax cells, kumquat seed, pomegranate peel, sunflower disc or receptacle, tangerine, orange peel, seed
Mastitis, acute	Antler (deer horn)
Measles	Shepherd's purse, towel gourd
Measles, early stage	Cherry
Measles, delayed eruption	Bamboo shoot, coriander - Chinese parsley, shiitake mushroom, sugar cane
Meningitis	Garlic
Menorrhagia	Sorghum root
Menstrual cramps	Hawthorn fruit, lychee seed
Menstruation, irregular	Brown sugar, ginger - fresh, safflower
Migraine	Muskmelon calyx receptacle, radish
Miscarriage	Azuki bean sprout
Motion sickness	Mango
Mumps	Black pepper, mung bean, potato
Nervousness	Longan, wheat
Neurosis	Red date
Night blindness	Alfalfa root, carrot, liver (beef, chicken, pork), matrimony vine leaf, spinach
Night sweats	Duck, grapes, oyster shell, peach, rock sugar
	Food cure for night sweats: Peel and cut up 10g yam. Place yam, 50g rock sugar and 50g rice in a saucepan. Cover with water to about an inch above. Eat at mealtime.
Nipple, sore	Clove
Nosebleed	Chestnut, Chinese chive, green onion leaf, radish, spinach, vinegar
Numbness	Black fungus

Condition	Remedy
Numbness of four limbs	Cherry
Obesity	Wintermelon, yam
	Food cure for obesity: Boil 250g wintermelon in 3 cups (750mL) water until soft. Eat the soup as a daily tonic.
Osteoporosis	Chestnut
Pain in the arm	Carp (gold carp)
Pain in the leg	Chili pepper (cayenne pepper)
Pain in penis	Sunflower root
Pain in the testes	Kumquat seed
Pain in the tongue	Bee venom
Palpitations	Grapes, longan
	Food cure for palpitations: Place 50g longan nuts, 10g lotus fruit and seed, and 50g rice in a saucepan. Cover with water to about an inch above. Boil the three ingredients until soft. Eat at mealtime.
Penis swelling	Green onion leaf
Peptic ulcer	Banana, wild cabbage
Periodontal disease	Bee secretion
Perspiration	Radish
Pink eye (conjunctivitis)	Chicken egg, cucumber, shepherd's purse
Pneumonia	Garlic, honeysuckle (dried), jackfruit
	Food cure for pneumonia: Prepare an infusion of 30g dried honeysuckle and 6g peppermints to make tea. Drink the tea at mealtime.
Poor appetite	Black pepper, cantaloupe, honey, kiwi fruit, onion, shiitake mushroom, tangerine, orange, tomato
Poor memory	Tofu
Postnatal anemia	Liver, chicken
Postnatal spasm	Black fungus
Pregnancy, bleeding during	Chinese chive
Premature ejaculation	Lotus (fruit, seed, root)
Psoriasis	Chicken egg, smoked prunes, walnut
Pulmonary tuberculosis	Ginkgo (cooked), mutton
Rheumatoid arthritis	Bee venom, chili pepper (cayenne pepper), royal jelly
Rhinitis	Aloe vera, garlic, magnolia flower bud, peony root bark, sesame oil, sword bean seed
Ringing in the ears	Day lily
Scarlet fever	Burdock, garlic
Scrotum swelling	Lychee seed
Seminal emission	Duck, gorgan fruit, string bean, yam
Sinusitis	Peanut
Skin disease	Castor bean

Condition	Remedy
Skin inflammation	Green onion - white part
Sore throat	Chicken egg, cucumber, fig, longevity fruit, olive, radish, star fruit
Stomach cancer	Chinese chive, shiitake mushroom, sunflower stem and pith, walnut twig (young branches), wild cabbage
Stomachache	Green peel of unripe walnut, longan, papaya, potato, sorghum leaf, root
Stomachache with chills	Garlic, ginger - fresh, grapefruit, lychee
Sunstroke	Bitter gourd (balsam pear), hyacinth bean
Swallowing difficulty	Chinese chive
Swollen scrotum	Garlic
Swollen testes	Kelp
Tetanus	Green onion - white part, mulberry branch juices
Thirst	Apple, apricot, bitter gourd (balsam pear), kiwi fruit, lemon, loquat, mandarin orange, olive, pear, pineapple, plum (prunes), pomegranate (sweet fruit), red bayberries, sand pear, star fruit, tomato
Thrush	Sesame oil
Thyroid cyst	Seaweed
Toothache	Olive, prickly ash, star fruit, wax cells of honeycomb
Tuberculosis	Chicken egg yolk, garlic, ginkgo (fresh or cooked), honeysuckle, rabbit, radish, seaweed, sheep or goat's gallbladder
Tumors	Asparagus (lucid asparagus), sunflower disc or receptacle, kidney bean, sword bean seed
Tympanic membrane perforation	Ginger - dried
Ulcer	Chicken egg shell inner membrane, clam shell powder, cuttlebone, ginger - fresh, mung bean, onion, peanut oil, potato, safflower, soybean - yellow
Urinary infection	Watermelon
Urination difficulty	Arrowhead, autumn bottle gourd, garlic, kohlrabi, pear, white cabbage, wheat
Urination, frequent	Gorgan fruit, lotus (fruit, seed, root), mutton
Vaginal bleeding	Asparagus (lucid asparagus), cuttlefish ink sac, persimmon cake, sunflower disc or receptacle
Vaginal bleeding and discharge	Chicken
Vaginal bleeding during pregnancy	Liver, chicken
Vaginal discharge	Cuttlefish, ginkgo (cooked)
Vaginitis	Chinese toon leaf
Vertigo	Celery, day lily, liver - beef, mulberry, shepherd's purse
Vomiting	Ginger - fresh, loquat, lotus sprout, mango, red bayberries, sugar cane, sword bean and seed, orange
	Food cure for vomiting: Cut up fresh ginger into five pieces. Boil in water. Drink like tea.
Wart	Yellow soybean sprout
Whooping cough	Aloe vera, asparagus, chestnut, chicken egg yolk, purslane, celery, chicken egg, chicken gallbladder, cow's gallbladder, garlic, longevity fruit, pork gallbladder, sweet orange peel, tofu

Source: Henry Lu, *Traditional Chinese Medicine, How to Maintain Your Health and Treat Illness*, Basic Health Publications, 2005

FOOD AS MEDICINE

Categories	Cold	Cool	Neutral	Warm	Hot
Vegetables	Chinese cabbage, mung bean sprout, seaweed, snow pea, water chestnut	Alfalfa sprout, asparagus, bamboo shoot, beet, bokchoy, broccoli, burdock root, button mushroom, cabbage, carrot, celery, corn, cucumber, daikon radish, dandelion greens, eggplant, endive lettuce, lotus root, potato, pumpkin, romaine lettuce, soy bean sprout, spinach, summer squash, turnip, wintermelon, watercress winter squash, zucchini	Chard, lettuce, shitake mushroom, sweet potato, taro root, yam	Bell pepper, Chinese chive, ganoderma mushroom, green bean, kale, leek, mustard green, onion, parsley, parsnip	Garlic, scallion
Fruits	Banana, cantaloupe, grapefruit, mulberry, pear, pear-apple, watermelon	Apple, apricot, avocado, fig, lemon, orange, peach, kiwi, persimmon, strawberry, tomato, mandarin, mango	Chinese date, loquat, mango, olive, papaya, pineapple, plum, pomegranate, crabapple	Cherry, Chinese prune, coconut, dried papaya, grape, hawthorn berry, lychee, pineapple, raspberry, tangerine	
Grains	Millet, pearl barley, white rice, wheat		Buckwheat, brown rice, corn meal, rye	Oats, sweet rice, wheat bran, wheat germ	
Seeds & Beans	Pumpkin seed	Mung bean, soy bean, tofu, wintermelon seed	Almond, azuki bean, black sesame seed, kidney bean, louts seed, peanut, pea, sunflower seed	Black bean, brown sesame seed, chestnut, lentil, pine nut, walnut	
Meats	Pork	Chicken egg, clam, crab	Fish (ocean), gelatin, dairy products, oyster	Beef, chicken, fish (freshwater), shrimp, turkey	Lamb
Herbs	Bamboo shavings, cassia seeds, Chinese cucumber, chrysanthemum, goldenseal root, honeysuckle flower, lily bulb, motherwort leaf, mulberry leaf, oyster shell, reed root	American ginseng, cilantro, corn silk, kudzu, mint leaf, puearia root	Chinese yam, licorice root, lycium berries, poria mushroom	Anise seed, basil, cardamom seed, carb pod, citrus peels, coriander seed, dang gui, fennel seed, fresh ginger, Oriental ginseng	Black pepper, cinnamon bark, dry ginger
Miscellaneous	Salt, vitamin C, white sugar	Tea	Barley malt, rice malt, honey, black fungus, white fungus	Brown sugar, coffee, molasses, rice vinegar, wine	

Diagnosis	General Comments	Foods
Qi Deficiency	Foods which are easy to digest, warming and nourishing foods should be used. All cooked, warmed, slow-cooking foods are ideally suited for qi deficiency. Soups, broths, high-complex carbohydrates, vegetables, and small portions of meats are recommended. Avoid excessive fluids with meals, uncooked raw foods, cold damp foods, overeating, skipping meals, and eating while working.	Millet, garbanzo beans, pine nuts, figs, dates, squash, carrots, cabbage, small portions of meats, vegetables, grains, cooked squashed, leeks, oats, onion, pumpkins, sweet potatoes, sweet rice, yams, dried fruits, cherries, dry figs, peaches, strawberries, anchovies, chicken, turkey, spices, black pepper, cinnamon, ginger, nutmeg, barley malt, maple syrup
Qi Stagnation	Food choices similar to those of qi deficiency are good choices. Eat less and earlier in the day. Concentrate on light to mildly spicy foods, stir frying, poaching, and steaming your foods. Consider adding small amounts of strongly moving substances, such as black pepper to your foods. Avoid processed junk foods, cold foods, preservatives, eating while upset or under pressure, skipping meals, overeating, and eating too quickly.	Basil, cardamom, carrots, cayenne, chives, dill seeds, fennel, garlic, grapefruit, orange peels, peaches, peppermint, plum radish, squash, tangerine peels, turmeric, vinegar, watercress, onions, mint, asparagus
Yin Deficiency	Moistening and lubricating food are useful. Use plenty of water in cooking including soups and stews. A nourishing diet consists of seeds, beans, and high-quality protein.	Oats, rice, millet, barley, chicken, yogurt, tofu, nuts and seeds, oysters, mussels, clams, spirulina, potatoes, melons, black beans, apples, bananas, mung beans, flaxseed oil, almond oil
Dampness	Generally it is a result of long-term qi deficiency but may also arise quickly from a diet that contains too many cold, raw foods, excessive dairy products, or excessive amounts of greasy foods, animal products, or alcohol. Emphasize foods that are cooked and warm and have a low fat intake. Avoid dairy, sugar, deep fried, and junk foods. Bitter and pungent flavored foods are ideal for dampness.	Add foods which dry dampness, such as rye, scallions, turnips and limit the foods that contribute to dampness
Blood Deficiency	Generally foods which supplement the Spleen are considered good choices, including iron and protein-rich foods, folic acid and vitamin B12. Some vegetarians may need to supplement B12 from deficiency.	Dark leafy green vegetables, chlorophyll-rich foods, spinach, grapes, lotus root, cayenne pepper, and small amounts of meat products, especially liver, are beneficial additions to help the production and circulation of blood
Blood Stagnation	Foods similar to qi stagnation and blood deficiency in addition to those which strongly move the blood in the body. Avoid cold raw foods as they constrict blood circulation.	Turmeric, butter, leeks, onions, crab, red wine, cayenne, peaches, scallions, saffron, sweet rice, vinegar, chicken eggs, garlic, chives, egg plant, adzuki beans
Heat Condition	Shorten cooking times and add plenty of water to your foods, steaming, and stir frying. Heat may show up in a variety of ways depending on the underlying condition. Differentiate between "full heat" and "false heat" as it affects food choices. Avoid deep frying, BBQ, roasting, overeating and hot foods that contribute to excess conditions.	Apples, barley, chicken, cucumbers, mangoes, mung beans, pears, radishes, sesame seeds, strawberries, tangerines, turnips, wheat, bamboo shoots, bananas, chestnuts, crab, grapefruit, kelp, lettuce, oranges, salt, sea grass, seaweed, soft drinks, sour foods, watermelon, water chestnuts, fruits, raw vegetables, and salads
Cold Condition	Warming foods which emphasize movement are good choices. Avoid all raw food, including salads and vegetables. Differentiate between "full cold" and "false cold" conditions as it affects food choices. If necessary, warm or lightly steam foods.	Brown sugar, cayenne, chives, cinnamon twigs, cloves, coffee, egg yolks, fresh ginger, ham, leeks, lamb, nutmeg, peaches, raspberries, rosemary, shrimp, sunflower seeds, sweet basil, walnuts, wine

FOOD

Action	Food
Arrest bleeding	Black fungus, chestnut, chicken eggshell, guava, louts, spinach, vinegar
Calm shen	Licorice, lily flower
Check perspiration	Oyster shell, peach
Check urination	Raspberry
Check seminal emission	Lotus, oyster, walnut, black fungus
Counteract toxins	Abalone, banana, bead curd, black soybean, chicken egg white, clam, cucumber, date, fig, honey, radish, salt, sesame oil, red bean, vinegar
Disperse blood stagnation	Brown sugar, chive, crab, hawthorn, saffron vinegar
Disperse cold stagnation	Ginger, wine
Eliminate phlegm	Chinese wax gourd, clam, pear, radish, sea grass, seaweed
Facilitate measles eruptions	Cherry seed, sunflower seeds
Improve appetite	Green pepper, ham, red pepper
Induce bowel movement	Castor bean, sesame oil
Lubricate dryness	Bean curd, chicken egg, honey, maltose, mill, pear, pork, sesame oil, spinach, yellow soybean
Lubricate intestines	Apricot seed, banana, mill, peach, soybean oil, walnut, watermelon
Lubricate lung	Apple, apricot, ginseng, lily flower, orange, peanut, persimmon, strawberry, white fungus, white sugar
Produce fluids	Apricot, bean curd, coconut, ham, lemon, licorice, maltose, mil, peach, plum, strawberry, tomato, white fungus, white sugar
Promote blood circulation	Black soybean, brown sugar, chestnut, eel, peach, saffron, sweet basil, wine
Promote digestion	Apple, ginseng, green pepper, hops, nutmeg, papaya, pineapple, plum radish, red pepper, sweet basil, tomato
Promote energy circulation	Chive, dill seed, orange peel, fennel, garlic, kumquat, radish leaf, spearmint, sweet basil, tangerine, tobacco
Promote urination	Asparagus, barley, Chinese cabbage, carrot, Chinese wax gourd, coconut, coffee, corn, corn silk, cucumber, grape hops, kidney bean, lettuce, mango, mung bean, onion, pineapple, plum, sugar can juice, water chestnut, watermelon
Quench thirst	Crab apple, cucumber, mango, persimmon, pineapple
Reduce fever	Star fruit, water chestnut
Relieve asthma	Apricot seed
Relieve cough	Apricot seed, kumquat, orange, tangerine, thyme
Relieve diarrhea	Guava, sunflower seed
Relieve pain	Honey, spearmint, squash, tobacco
Sharpen vision	Abalone, bitter gourd, wild cucumber, clam, cuttlefish
Soften hardness	Clam, kelp, oyster shell, sea grass, seaweed
Tonify blood deficiency	Beef, chicken, egg, cuttlefish, mill, oyster, spinach
Tonify energy deficiency	Apricot seed, bean curd, beef, brown sugar, chicken, eel, licorice, maltose, lamb, rice, potato, sweet rice, sweet potato
Relieve drunkenness	Apple, ginseng, strawberry
Warm organs	Black pepper, chicken, clove, fennel, green pepper, lamb, nutmeg, red pepper, white pepper

FOOD

Source: Henry Lu, *Chinese System of Food Cures Prevention & Remedies,* Sterling Publishing, 1986

FOOD AS MEDICINE

Food Properties II

Meat	
Beef	Neutral, sweet, SP & ST qi & blood tonic
Lamb	Warm, sweet, ST, KD, qi tonic, warms interior
Ham	Warm, salty, ST qi tonic, produces fluids, subdues reb. qi
Pork	Neutral, sweet & salty, ST, ST, KD, lubricates dryness (sl. cold)

Seafood	
Shrimp	Warm, sweet, KD yang tonic
Eel	Warm, sweet, Liv, ST, KD, qi tonic, treats bi syndrome, strengthens bone
Mussel	Warm, salty, Liv & KD qi tonic, treats simple goiter
Abalone	Neutral, sweet & salty, detoxifies, sharpens vision
Shark	Neutral, sweet & salty, ST, tonifies qi, blood, & yin, lubricates dryness, reduces swelling, tonifies 5 zang
Carp	Neutral, sweet, ST & ST, facilitates water passage, promotes milk secretion, heals swelling
Cuttlefish	Neutral, salty, Liv & KD, blood tonic, sharpens vision
Oyster	Neutral, sweet & salty, blood tonic
Oyster shell	Cool, salty, Liv & KD, stops sweating, astringes jing, softens hardness
Saltwater clam	Cold, salty, ST, promotes water passage, eliminates phlegm, softens hardness
Freshwater clam	Cold, sweet & salty, Liv & KD, detoxifies, sharpens vision
Crab	Cold, salty, Liv & ST, activates blood, cools heat sensations, facilitates recovery of dislocations
Kelp	Cold, salty, ST, softens hardness, facilitates water passage
Seaweed	Cold, salty, softens hardness, eliminates phlegm, promotes water passage

Nuts	
Walnut	Warm, sweet, KD & LU, KD tonic, lubricates intestines, astringes jing
Chestnut	Warm sweet, ST, ST & KD tonic, circulates blood & stops bleeding
Peanut	Neutral, sweet, ST & LU, qi & blood tonic, lubricates LU, harmonizes stomach
Peanut oil	Neutral, sweet, qi & blood tonic, lubricates intestines, pushes accumulations downward
Almond	Neutral, sweet, LU, qi & blood tonic, lubricates LU, relieves cough, transforms phlegm, lowers reb. qi

Warm - Fruits	
Guava	Warm, sweet, (ST & LI) obstructive & constrictive, stops diarrhea & bleeding
Chinese Date	Warm, sweet, SP & ST, qi & blood tonic, produces fluids, detoxifies,
Longan	Warm, sweet, SP & HT, yang, qi & blood tonic, removes blood stag., calms Shen
Coconut milk & meat	Warm, sweet, produce fluids, promote urination, kills intestinal worms

Peach	Warm, sweet & sour, (LU & LI), activates blood, qi & yang tonic, produces fluid, lubricates intestines, stops cough, expels cold
Raspberry	Warm, sweet & sour, Liv & KD, Liv & KD tonic, controls urination, astringes jing
Litchi	Warm, sweet & sour, SP & Liv, yang, qi & blood tonic, regulates qi & blood, soothes Liv & calms Shen
Cherry	Warm, sweet & harsh, qi, yang, & blood tonic, activates qi & blood, expels cold, wind, & damp
Kumquat	Warm, pungent, sweet & sour, (LU & SP), circulates qi, relieves cough, transforms phlegm
Dried Mandarin orange peel	Warm, pungent & bitter, SP & LU, regulates qi, dries dampness, transforms phlegm
Hawthorn Fruit	Sl. Warm, sweet & sour, SP, ST & Liv, harmonizes middle jiao, removes qi, blood & food stagnation (esp. Meat), expels tapeworms

Neutral - Fruits	
Papaya	Neutral, sweet, (SP, ST, LU & LI), promotes digestion, destroys intestinal worms, lubricates LU, stops cough
Figs	Neutral, sweet, SP & LI, ST tonic, detoxifies
Grape	Neutral, sweet & sour, LU, SP & KD, qi & blood tonic, strengthens tendons & bones, promotes urination
Crab apple	Neutral, sweet & sour, HT, Liv & LU, quenches thirst, stops diarrhea, astringes jing
Olive	Neutral, sweet & sour, LU & ST, qi & blood tonic, clears LU, benefits throat, produces fluids, detoxifies
Loquat	Neutral, (sweet & sl. Bitter) (lu, st & liv), lubricates dryness, harmonizes st & soothes liv, descends reb. Qi, stops cough
Apricot	Neutral, sweet & sour, LU, lubricates LU, produces fluids
Pineapple	Neutral, sweet & sour, qi & blood tonic, promotes urination & digestion, quenches thirst, stops diarrhea, clears summer-heat
Plum	Neutral, sweet & sour, Liv & KD, produces fluids, promotes digestion & urination, soothes the Liv
Sour Plum	Neutral, sour, Liv, produces fluids, destroys worms

Cool - Fruit	
Lemon	Cool, sour, promotes fluids, harmonizes ST, relieves thirst
Mango	Cool, sweet & sour, (ST & LU), qi & blood tonic, benefits ST, relieves vomiting, quenches thirst, diuretic
Mandarin Orange	Cool, sweet & sour, (LU), diuretic, lubricates LU, relieves cough, transforms phlegm
Apple	Cool, sweet & sour, LU & ST, produces fluids, lubricates LU, promotes digestion, relieves intoxication

FOOD

Strawberry	Cool, sweet & sour, LU & SP, lubricates LU, produces fluids, detoxifies alcohol
Pear	Cool, sweet & sl. Sour, lu & st, produces fluids, lubricates dryness, transforms phlegm, clears heat
Persimmon	Cold, sweet, HT, SI, LU (& SP), qi, blood & yin tonic, quenches thirst, lubricates LU, benefits SP, clears heat
Watermelon	Cold, sweet, HT, ST & UB, promotes urination, lubricates intestines, quenches thirst, clears summer-heat, detoxifies
Banana	Cold, sweet, lubricates intestine, detoxifies
Grapefruit	Cold, sweet & sour, (ST & SP) harmonizes middle jiao, circulates qi, detoxifies alcohol.
Star Fruit (Carambola)	Cold, sweet & sour, (ST, KD & UB) clears heat, produces fluids, promotes urination (treats stone Lin), detoxifies
Muskmelon	Cold, sweet, HT & ST, clears heat, quenches thirst, promotes urination,
Lemon	Cool, sour, promotes fluids, harmonizes ST, relieves thirst

Poultry

Duck	Neutral, sweet & salty, LU, KD, facilitates water passage, reduces, swellings
Chicken	Warm, sweet, SP, ST, qi tonic, warms interior

Dairy

Milk	Neutral, sweet, HT, LU, ST, LU & ST tonic, produces fluids & lubricates the intestines
Butter	Warm, sweet, yang, qi & blood tonic, circulates blood

Grains

Glutinous rice	Warm, sweet, SP, ST, LU, SP qi tonic
Malt	Sl. warm, sweet, SP & ST, promotes digestion
White rice	Neutral, sweet, SP & ST, SP qi tonic
Rice bran	Neutral, sweet & pungent, ST, LI, descends energy
Rye	Neutral, bitter, dries dampness, diuretic
Whole wheat	Cool, sweet, HT, SP, KD, HT & KD tonic
Wheat bran	Cool, sweet, ST, cools ST fire,
Buckwheat	Cool, sweet, LI, ST, SP, qi & blood tonic, clears heat sedates yang
Job's tears	Cool, sweet, SP, LU, KD, detoxifies, SP & LU qi tonic, diuretic
Barley	Cool, sweet & salty, SP & ST, regulates ST, expands intestines, promotes urination
Millet	Cool, sweet & salty, ST, SP, KD, qi & blood tonic, clears heat, lubricates dryness, tonifies yin, benefits digestion detoxifies

Seeds

Cottonseed	Hot, pungent, SP & KD tonic, arrests bleeding, stops SP qi sinking
Sunflower seed	Warm & neutral, sweet & bland, Liv & LI, stops diarrhea, facilitates eruption of measles, subdues Liv
Pine nut	Warm, sweet, LU, LI & Liv, lubricates LU & LI, stops cough, qi, yang & blood tonic, promotes fluids, moves stagnant blood, expels cold & wind
Dill seed	Warm, pungent, SP & KD, qi & yang tonic, moves stagnant blood, regulates qi, expels cold
Fennel seed	Warm, pungent, ST, UB & KD, qi & yang tonic, moves stagnant blood, regulates qi, expels cold, harmonizes ST
Bitter apricot seed	Warm, pungent & bitter, toxic, LU & LI, stops cough, relieves asthma, lubricates intestines
Sweet apricot seed	Warm, pungent & sweet, LU, LI, SP, SP qi tonic, lubricates intestines, stops cough
Sesame seed	Sl. Warm, sweet, Liv & KD tonic, lubricates intestines, "blackens" gray hair, general tonic
Black sesame seed	Neutral, sweet, Liv & KD tonic
Cherry seed	Neutral, bitter & pungent, LI, promotes measles eruption, detoxifies
Lotus seed	Neutral, sweet & harsh, SP, HT & KD tonic, qi & blood tonic, constricts the intestines
Sesame oil	Cool, sweet, ST, detoxifies, lubricates dryness, promotes bowel movements, produces muscles

Miscellaneous foods

Brown sugar	Warm, sweet, Liv, SP & ST, qi tonic, circulates blood
Vinegar	Warm, sour & bitter, Liv & ST, disperses coagulations, detoxifies, arrests bleeding
Wine	Warm, sweet, bitter & pungent, HT, Liv, LU & ST, promotes blood circulation, expels cold, speeds up effects of herbs
Coffee	Warm, sweet & bitter, HT, heart tonic, stimulant, diuretic
Molasses	Warm, sweet, LU & SP, qi tonic, lubricates LU, stops cough
White sugar	Neutral, sweet, LU & SP, lubricates LU, produces fluids, qi tonic
Honey	Neutral, sweet, LU, ST & LI, detoxifies, lubricates dryness, relieves pain
Tea	Sl cold, bitter, sweet, HT, LU & ST, quenches thirst, promotes digestion & urination, awakens shen
Salt	Cold, salty, ST, KD, SI & LI, detoxifies, clears heat, lubricates dryness, yin tonic

FOOD

Warm - Vegetables

Leek	Warm, pungent, Liv & LU, qi & yang tonic, regulates qi, removes blood stagnation, expels cold, sedates yin, clears ST fire
Scallions	Warm, pungent, LU & ST, assists yang, tonifies & regulates qi, clears heat, sedates yang, dries damp, diuretic, removes blood stagnation, expels cold
Mustard Greens	Warm, pungent, LU, qi & yang tonic, circulates qi & blood, expels cold, sedates yin, expands LU, transforms phlegm
Squash	Warm sweet, SP & ST, qi, yang & blood tonic, circulates blood, heals inflammation, relieves pain

Cool - Vegetables

Alfalfa sprouts	Cool, bitter, ST & SP, benefits ST & SP, dispels dampness, lubricates intestines
Asparagus	Cool, sweet & bitter, LU & KD, qi, blood & yin tonic, clears heat & fire, dries damp, lubricates dryness, clears LU, diaphoretic
Lettuce (Iceberg)	Cool, bitter & sweet, ST & LI, qi & blood tonic, clears heat & yang, dries dampness & diuretic, aids lactation
Cucumber	Cool, sweet, SP, ST & LI, clears heat & yang, detoxifies, promotes urination & quenches thirst
Eggplant	Cool, sweet, SP, ST & LI, qi & blood tonic, clears heat & yang, removes blood stagnation, relieves pain, heals swelling
Mushroom (button)	Cool, sweet, LU, LI, ST & SP, qi & blood tonic, clears heat & yang, calms Shen, stimulates appetite, regulates qi, transforms phlegm
Spinach	Cool, sweet, LI & SI, qi & blood tonic, clears heat & yang, hemostatic, lubricates dryness
Winter Melon	Cool, sweet, LU, LI, UB, & SI, detoxifies, diuretic, transforms phlegm
Swiss Chard	Cool, sweet, LI, SP & ST, qi, yin & blood tonic, clears heat & yang, detoxifies, hemostatic, relieves coagulations
Watercress	Cool, sweet & pungent, LU & ST, qi, yang & blood tonic, circulates qi & blood, clears heat & yang, lubricates LU, quenches thirst, diuretic
Radish	Cool, pungent & sweet, LU & ST, qi, & blood tonic, clears heat & detoxifies, transforms phlegm-heat, lowers reb. Qi
Bamboo shoot	Cold, sweet, tonifies qi, blood & yin, clears heat, detoxifies (often used to balance warm energy of meat)
Kelp	Cold, salty, ST & SP, yin tonic, clears heat, lubricates dryness, softens hardness, promotes flow of water
Lotus Root	Cold, sweet, SP, ST & HT, qi, blood & yin tonic, cools blood (when raw), stimulates appetite, produces muscles, relieves diarrhea (when cooked)

Water Chestnut	Cold, sweet, LU & ST, clears heat, yin tonic, transforms phlegm, diuretic
Lettuce (Romaine)	Cold, bitter, LI & ST, qi & blood tonic, clears heat & yang, dries dampness, diuretic

Eggs

Chicken egg	Neutral, sweet, blood tonic, lubricates dryness
Egg white	Cool, sweet, detoxifies, lubricates LU, cools hot sensations, benefits throat
Egg yolk	Neutral, sweet, HT & KD, blood tonic, lubricates dryness
Eggshell	Checks gastric acid, arrests bleeding

Legumes

Soybean oil	Hot, pungent & sweet, lubricates intestines, warm, sweet, KD, ST, & LI, warms interior, tonifies KD, descends reb. qi.
String bean	Neutral, sweet, SP & KD, qi, blood & yin tonic
Yellow soybean	Neutral, sweet, SP & LI, qi tonic, lubricates dryness, eliminates edema
Black soybean	Neutral, sweet, SP & KD, circulates blood & fluids treats bi syndrome, detoxifies
Corn	Neutral, sweet, LI & ST, qi & blood tonic, diuretic
Hyacinth bean	Neutral, sweet, SP & ST, qi tonic, eliminates edema
Broad bean	Neutral, sweet, SP & ST, qi tonic, eliminates edema
Peas	Neutral, sweet, SP & ST, qi & blood tonic, descends reb. qi, diuretic, induces bowel movements
Kidney bean	Neutral, sweet & bland, diuretic, heals swellings
Adzuki bean	Neutral, sweet & sour, HT & SI, diuretic, heals swellings, detoxifies
Castor bean	Neutral, sweet & pungent, LU & LI, detoxifies & heals swellings, induces bowel movements
Mung bean	Cool, sweet, HT & ST, detoxifies, clears heat, diuretic
Soybean	Cool, sweet, LI & SP, qi & blood tonic, clears heat, lubricates dryness, eliminates edema
Tofu	Cool, sweet, SP, ST, LI, qi tonic, produces fluids, lubricates dryness, detoxifies

Spices & herbs

Dried ginger	Hot, pungent, LU, ST & SP, yang & qi tonic, circulates blood, warms middle jiao, opens the meridians
Pepper (black & white)	Hot, pungent, ST & LI, warms interior, descends reb. qi
Pepper (red & green)	Hot, pungent, ST, warms interior, harmonizes middle jiao, stimulates appetite
Cinnamon bark	Hot, sweet & pungent, SP, KD, UB, diaphoretic, strengthens ST, warms surface & interior
Fennel seed	Warm, pungent, KD, UB, ST, warms interior, circulates qi
Sweet basil	Warm, pungent, LU, LI, SP, ST, qi & yang tonic, circulates qi & blood, harmonizes ST

Dillseed	Warm, pungent, SP & KD, qi & yang tonic, circulates qi & blood
Garlic	Warm, pungent, SP, ST & LU, qi & yang tonic, circulates qi & blood, warms middle jiao, destroys worms
Clove	Warm, pungent, ST, SP & KD, yang tonic, warms interior
Fresh ginger	Warm, pungent, LU, ST & SP, diaphoretic, yang qi tonic, circulates blood, transforms phlegm, stops vomiting
Coriander	Warm pungent, LU & SP, diaphoretic, harmonizes middle jiao
Nutmeg	Warm pungent, SP & LI, qi & yang tonic, warms interior, circulates blood, warms middle jiao, lowers reb. qi
Cinnamon twig	Warm, pungent & sweet, UB, HT, LU, diaphoretic, warms upper jiao
Star anise	Warm, pungent & sweet, SP, KD, Liv, yang tonic, circulates qi, harmonizes ST, stops vomiting
Caraway seed	Warm, sl. pungent, KD & ST, circulates qi, descends reb. qi
Spearmint	Warm, pungent & sweet, (LU & SP), diaphoretic, circulates qi & blood
Ginseng	Warm, sweet, & sl bitter, SP, LU (HT), qi tonic, produces fluids, calms shen
Rosemary	Warm, pungent, (LU, ST), diaphoretic, activates blood, strengthens ST, calms shen
Saffron	Neutral, sweet, HT & Liv, circulates qi & blood, eliminates blood stagnation
Licorice	Neutral, sweet, SP, ST & LU, lubricates lungs, detoxifies, moderates effects of other herbs
Peppermint	Cool, pungent, LU & Liv, diaphoretic, regulates qi & blood
Marjoram	Cool, pungent, (LU & SP), diaphoretic, circulates qi, drains dampness
Neutral - Vegetables	
Chinese cabbage	Neutral, sweet, ST & LI, promotes digestion & urination, tonifies KD & Brain.
Carrot	Neutral, sweet, LU & ST, SP qi tonic, dries dampness & phlegm
Corn	Neutral, sweet, ST & LI, qi & blood tonic, regulates middle jiao, stimulates appetite, diuretic
Black Fungus	Neutral, sweet, ST & LI, qi & blood tonic, cools blood, stops bleeding
White Fungus	Neutral, sweet, LU, yin tonic, produces fluids, lubricates LU
Pumpkin	Neutral, sweet, (LU & SP), qi & blood tonic, dries damp, diaphoretic
Potato	Neutral, sweet, SP, SP qi tonic, heals inflammation
Sweet Potato	Neutral, sweet, LU, SP & KD, qi, blood & yin tonic, benefits KD, astringes jing
Shiitake Mushroom	Neutral, sweet, ST, qi & blood tonic, benefits ST
Celery	Neutral, sweet bitter, ST & Liv, qi & blood tonic, clears heat, sedates yang, dries damp, calms Liv, expels wind

Taro	Neutral, sweet & pungent, ST & LI, qi, yang & blood tonic, circulates qi & blood, clears heat, reduces swellings
Turnip	Neutral, sweet, pungent, bitter, qi, yang & blood tonic, circulates qi & blood, clears heat & yang, dries damp, diaphoretic, lowers reb. Qi, detoxifies yin tonic, clears heat & fire, dries damp, clears lu, lubricates dryness, diaphoretic

FOOD

Alfalfa sprouts	Vitamin A, C, B, E and K, calcium, silicon	The nervous system, bones and skin.
Apples	Carotenes, pectin, vitamin C, potassium, ellagic acid	The immune system, digestion, heart and circulation. Especially good for constipation, diarrhea and lowering of cholesterol.
Apricots	Beta-carotene, potassium, iron, soluble fiber	Skin and respiratory problems, protects against cancer. Dried apricots relieve constipation and high blood pressure.
Artichokes (Jerusalem and globe)	Inulin, phosphorus, iron	Digestion, as they stimulate liver and gallbladder function. Useful for gout, arthritis and rheumatism.
Asparagus	Vitamin C, riboflavin, folic acid, asparagines, potassium, phosphorus	Gentle diuretic treatment, hence it is excellent for cystitis and fluid retention. Good for rheumatism and arthritis, but not for gout.
Avocado	Potassium, vitamins E and A, essential fatty acids	Heart, circulation and skin. Relieves symptoms of PMS, and protects against cancer.
Bananas	Potassium, fiber, energy, magnesium, vitamin A, folic acid	Preventing cramps. Excellent for digestion, chronic fatigue syndrome and glandular fever.
Basil	Volatile oils: linalool, limonene, estragole	Stimulating the digestion and as a calming, stress-fighting herb.
Beans, dried	Protein, carbohydrates, fiber, B vitamins, minerals, folic acid, selenium, iron, zinc. Choose chickpeas for calcium, soy beans for cancer- and osteoporosis- fighting genistein	Maintaining a healthy heart and circulatory system, also fighting high blood pressure and lowering cholesterol. Offers excellent protection against cancer and regulates bowel function.
Beans, green	Vitamins A and C, potassium, folic acid	Skin, hair and digestive problems.
Beetroot	Vitamins B6 and C, beta-carotene, potassium, folic acid, iron, calcium	Anemia, chronic fatigue and convalescence.
Blackberries	Vitamins E and C, potassium, fiber, cancer-fighting phytochemicals	Heart, circulation and skin. Also good protection against cancer.
Blackcurrants	Vitamin C, carotenoids, anti-inflammatory and cancer-fighting phytochemicals	The immune system. Also protects against colds, flu and some cancers. Good for lowering blood pressure and reducing stress.
Blueberries	Vitamin C, carotenoids, antibacterial and cancer-fighting phytochemicals	See Blackberries.
Brazil nuts	Protein, selenium, vitamin E, B vitamins	One of the richest sources of selenium (five provide a day's dose), an essential mineral that protects against heart disease, breast cancer and prostate cancer.
Bread	Fiber, iron, B vitamins, vitamin E, protein	Everyone – except those with wheat intolerance. Especially valuable for combating stress, physically active people, and the prevention of constipation, Diverticulitis and piles.
Broccoli	Vitamins A and C, folic acid, riboflavin, potassium, iron, cancer-fighting phytochemicals	Anemia, chronic fatigue, before and during pregnancy, skin problems and protection against cancer.
Brussels	Especially rich in cancer-fighting phytochemicals, vitamin C and beta-carotene	Protection against cancer, skin problems.
Cabbage family	Vitamins A, C, E, folic acid, potassium, cancer-fighting phytochemicals	Protection against cancer, stomach ulcers, chest infections, skin problems, anemia.
Carrots	Vitamin A, carotenoids, folic acid, potassium, magnesium	Eyesight, circulation, and protection against heart disease and cancer. Also good for the skin and all mucous membranes.
Cauliflower	Vitamin C, folic acid, sulphur	Protection against cancer, natural immunity and skin problems.
Celeriac	Vitamin C, folic acid, potassium, fiber	Pre-pregnancy and pregnancy, constipation and lowering cholesterol levels.
Celery	Beta-carotene, potassium, vitamin C, coumarins, flavonoids, fiber	Fluid retention, constipation, rheumatism, gout, arthritis and stress.
Chard (Swiss)	Vitamins A and C, iron, calcium, phosphorus, carotenes, cancer-fighting phytochemicals	Protection against eye diseases such as macular degeneration. Also protection against cancer and good for anemia.
Cheese	Protein, calcium and vitamin B12. Also a valuable source of zinc, essential for normal growth, reproduction (especially sperm production) and immunity	Bones, teeth, and prevention/treatment of osteoporosis. Excellent pre-conceptual, pregnancy and breastfeeding food (avoid unpasteurized ones).
Cherries	Vitamin C, potassium, magnesium, flavonoids, cancer-fighting phytochemicals	Natural resistance, arthritis and rheumatism, protection against cancer. Especially good for gout.

Chestnuts	Fiber, vitamins E and B6, potassium	Energy. They are also easily digestible and make excellent gluten-free flour for those with wheat allergies.
Chicory	Folic acid, potassium, iron, vitamins C and A (the latter only if unblanched), liver-stimulating terpenoids	Before and during pregnancy. Has excellent detoxifying and cleansing properties and is mildly diuretic and liver stimulating.
Chilies	Vitamin C, carotenoids, capsaicin	Circulation, especially helpful for chilblains, sinus, digestion, chest problems. Fights stomach bugs.
Coriander	Flavonoids, coumarins, linalool	Digestion. Relieves gas, bloating, irritable bowel syndrome, stress.
Courgettes and other curcubits	Beta-carotene, vitamin C, folic acid, potassium	Skin problems, natural resistance and promotes weight loss.
Cranberries	Vitamin C, cancer-fighting phytochemicals, specific urinary antibacterial	Treatment/prevention of cystitis. Powerful cancer-fighter and immune system booster.
Cucumber	Tiny amounts of beta-carotene in the skin, also a little silica, potassium, and folic acid	Skin and eyes. The juice is useful for relieving fevers.
Dandelion leaves	Beta-carotene, other carotenoids, iron, diuretic, liver-stimulating phytochemicals	Fluid retention, bloating, liver problems, PMS.
Dates	Iron, potassium, folic acid, fiber, fruit, sugar	Anemia, fatigue, constipation, pregnancy. An excellent and easily digested energy source before and during sports.
Eggs	Protein, vitamin B12, iron, lecithin. Also a good source of zinc and vitamins A, D and E	Protection against cancer and heart disease, cholesterol stories are untrue. Also helps relieve anemia, rheumatoid arthritis, osteoarthritis and supports the male sexual function.
Fennel	Low in vitamins, but rich in volatile oils, including fenchone, anethole and anisic acid – all liver and digestive stimulants	Digestive problems, flatulence, and fluid retention.
Figs	Beta-carotene, iron, potassium, fiber ficin (a digestive aid), cancer-fighting phytochemicals	Energy, constipation, digestive problems, anemia and protection against cancer.
Fish	Protein, vitamin B, minerals – especially iron, zinc and iodine. Oily fish has the added bonus of vitamin D and essential fatty acids	Oily fish: joint diseases, brain development, pregnancy, and all inflammatory diseases. White fish: heart protection. Shellfish: male sexual function, heart protection.
Garlic	Antibacterial and anti-fungal sulphur compounds, cancer-fighting and heart-protective phytochemicals	Preventing heart disease, lowering cholesterol levels, and high blood pressure. Useful as an anti-fungal and antibacterial agent, and helps relieve sinus and chest infections.
Ginger	Circulatory-stimulating zingiberene and gingerol	Morning sickness in pregnancy, travel sickness, post-operative sickness, circulation, fevers and coughs.
Grapes	Vitamin C, natural sugars, powerful antioxidant flavonoids	Convalescence, anemia, fatigue, cancer protection and weight gain, especially after illness.
Grapefruit	Vitamin C, beta-carotene, potassium, bioflavonoids – especially naringin, which thins the blood and lowers cholesterol	Natural resistance, circulatory problems, sore throats and bleeding gums.
Kale	Beta-carotene, vitamin C, phosphorus, sulphur, iron, potassium, calcium, folic acid, cancer-fighting phytochemicals	Protection against cancer, provides a boost to immunity. Good for skin and eyes thanks to high content of beta-carotene.
Kiwi fruit	Vitamin C, beta-carotene, potassium, bioflavonoids, fiber	The immune system, skin, constipation and digestive problems.
Kohlrabi	Vitamin C, folic acid, potassium, cancer-fighting phytochemicals	Protection against cancer, immune fighter, and skin problems.
Lamb's lettuce	Vitamins A, C and B6, folic acid, iron, potassium, zinc. Contains calming phytochemicals	Anemia, stress and anxiety. Great before/ during pregnancy, and when breastfeeding.
Leeks	Vitamins A and C, folic acid, potassium, diuretic, anti-arthritic, anti-inflammatory, cancer-fighting phytochemicals	Chest and voice problems, especially sore throat. Helps reduce high blood pressure and cholesterol, and is particularly good for gout and arthritis.
Lemons	Vitamin C, bioflavonoids, potassium, limonene	This powerful immune booster is also good for digestive problems. Particularly beneficial for mouth ulcers and gum disease.
Lettuce	Vitamins A and C, folic acid, potassium, calcium, phosphorus, sleep- inducing phytochemicals	Insomnia, stress and bronchitis.

FOOD

Lime	Vitamin C, bioflavonoids, potassium, limonene	Immune fighter, terrific for the relief of coughs, colds and flu. Also highly cancer-fighting.
Mango	Vitamin C, beta-carotene, potassium, flavonoids, other antioxidants	Convalescence, skin problems, protection against cancer and a boost to the immune system.
Meats	Protein, iron, B vitamins, other minerals	Anemia, stress, and all-round nutrition, as meat contains a broad spread of essential nutrients.
Melon	Vitamins A, C, potassium, folic acid, some B vitamins	Mild constipation, gout, arthritis and urinary problems.
Milk	Calcium, riboflavin, zinc, protein	Growth, strong bones, and convalescence.
Mint	Antispasmodic volatile oils, menthol, flavonoids	Indigestion, irritable bowel syndrome, gastritis, bloating and flatulence.
Mushrooms	Some protein, vitamins B12 and E, zinc	Important nutrient for vegetarians and vegans. Valuable for depression, anxiety and fatigue.
Nuts and seeds	Protein, unsaturated fats, minerals (especially zinc and selenium), fiber, energy	Diabetes, male sexual function, fertility, constipation and varicose veins. Also cancer-fighting.
Oats	Calcium, potassium, magnesium, B-complex vitamins, some vitamin E	Reducing blood cholesterol, stress, digestion. Specifically protective against bowel cancer, heart disease and high blood pressure.
Olives	Protective antioxidants, vitamin E and monounsaturated oil	Skin, heart and circulation.
Onions	Vitamin C, sulphur-based phytochemicals similar to garlic	Reducing cholesterol, preventing blood clots, bronchitis, asthma, chest infections, gout, arthritis and chilblains.
Oranges (mandarins, satsumas, tangerines)	Vitamins C and B6, bioflavonoids, potassium, limonene, thiamine, folic acid, calcium, iron	Fighting infection and improving resistance, fighting heart disease and high blood pressure.
Pak choi	Vitamin C, beta-carotene, folic acid, B vitamins, cancer-fighting phytochemicals	Cancer protection, boosting immunity, anemia, pregnancy and skin problems.
Parsley	Vitamins A and C, iron, calcium, potassium	A strong diuretic and anti-inflammatory, relieves fluid retention, PMS, gout, rheumatoid and osteoarthritis. Also useful against anemia.
Parsnip	Vitamin E, folic acid, potassium, B vitamins, inulin	Fatigue, constipation, good for pregnancy and diabetes.
Pawpaw	Vitamin C, beta-carotene, flavonoids, magnesium, the digestive enzyme papain	Digestive problems, skin, improved immunity. Also for convalescence, particularly after gastric illness as they are extremely easy to digest.
Peaches	Beta-carotene, flavonoids, vitamin C, potassium	Good for pregnancy, people on low-salt diets, reducing cholesterol. Also good as a gentle laxative.
Pears	Soluble fiber, vitamin C	Energy, lowering cholesterol, convalescence and constipation.
Peas	Thiamine (B1), folic acid, beta-carotene, vitamin C, protein	Protein, stress, tension and all digestive problems.
Peppers	Vitamin C, beta-carotene, folic acid, potassium, phytochemicals that prevent blood clots, strokes and heart disease	All skin problems, mucus membranes, night and color vision. Also a good booster for the immune system.
Pineapple	Vitamin C, but most valuable for enzymes, especially bromelain	Angina, arthritis, constipation, fevers, sore throats and all soft tissue injuries.
Plums	Beta-carotene, vitamins C and E, malic acid	Heart, circulation, fluid retention and digestion.
Potatoes	Rich in vitamin C, fiber, B vitamins, contains some minerals	Anemia, digestive problems, fatigue, growth and natural resistance.
Poultry	Protein, vitamin B12, iron, zinc	Convalescence, anemia, natural resistance, PMS, good for pregnancy and growth.
Prunes	Beta-carotene, niacin, vitamin B6, potassium, iron, fiber, phytochemicals	High blood pressure, fatigue, exhaustion and constipation. Also contains high concentrations of cancer-fighting phytochemicals.
Pumpkin	Vitamins A, C, potassium, folic acid, some B vitamins	Protection against cancer, respiratory problems and skin disorders.
Radishes	Vitamin C, iron, magnesium, sulphur, potassium, phytochemicals	Protection against cancer, liver and gallbladder problems, indigestion and respiratory problems.
Raspberries	Vitamin C, soluble fiber, calcium, potassium, iron, magnesium	Immune system, protection against cancer and mouth ulcers.
Rhubarb	Calcium, potassium, manganese, some vitamin A and C	Relieving constipation.
Rice, brown	Protein, B vitamins	Good for people with diarrhea and celiac disease as it contains no gluten. Excellent source of energy.

FOOD AS MEDICINE

Spinach	Chlorophyll, folic acid, beta-carotene, lutein, iron, cancer-fighting phytochemicals	Skin, protection against cancer, prevention of vision loss in old age. Also good before and during pregnancy.
Spring greens	Vitamin C, beta-carotene, carotenoids, iron, cancer-fighting phytochemicals	Protection against cancer, skin problems and anemia.
Strawberries	Vitamins C and E, beta-carotene, anti-arthritic phytochemicals, soluble fiber	Protection against cancer, gout, arthritis, kidney problems and anemia.
Swede	Vitamin C, useful amounts of vitamin A, trace minerals	Protection against cancer, skin problems and an ideal weaning food for babies.
Sweet corn	Fiber, protein, some vitamins A and E, some B vitamins, folic acid	Energy and fiber.
Sweet potato	Vitamins C and E, beta-carotene and other carotenoids, protein, cancer-fighting phytochemicals	Eye problems, night vision and all skin problems. Also a powerful cancer-fighting food.
Tea	Vitamins E and K, protective phenolic compounds. Also trace minerals, tannin and powerful protective antioxidants	Mild stimulant for fatigue and exhaustion. Also cancer-fighting and heart protective.
Tofu and other soy products	Protein and enormous quantities of cancer-fighting genistein	Protection against cancer – especially breast and prostate. Good for vegetarians and diabetics. Good replacement for those with milk intolerance.
Tomatoes	Vitamins C and E, potassium, beta-carotene, lycopene	Protection against cancer, skin problems, fertility and heart protection.
Watercress	Vitamins C and E, beta-carotene, antibacterial mustard oils, phenethyl isothiocyanate, iron	Essential protection against lung cancer. Food poisoning, anemia, skin and underactive thyroid.
Wheat, wholegrain	B-complex vitamins, vitamin E, fiber, zinc, magnesium and (if North American or Canadian) selenium	A vital source of energy and essential nutrients.
Wine	Excellent source of heart-protective substances	The heart (in modest doses), improves circulation and helps mild depression.
Yogurt	Calcium, riboflavin, zinc, protein, beneficial bacteria	Diarrhea, natural resistance, prevention and treatment of osteoporosis, thrush and cystitis.

FOOD

Cranial Nerve Examination

Nerve	Test	Lesion
I-Olfactory	*Sensory:* smell; Can the patient smell coffee or soap with each nostril?	Anosmia (loss of smell)
II-Optic	*Sensory:* vision; Examine both retinas carefully with an ophthalmoscope and test for visual acuity, visual field, color vision, and optic disc appearance.	Visual field deficits
III-Oculomotor	*Motor & parasympathetic*: constrictor pupillae, cillary muscles (lens shape): rectus superior, inferior, medial; inferior oblique, levator palpebra; Record the pupil size and shape at rest. Next, note the *direct response*, meaning constriction of the illuminated pupil, as well as the *consensual response*, meaning constriction of the opposite pupil.	Dilated pupil, ptosis, eye turned down & lateral loss of pupillary light reflex on lesion side
IV-Trochlear	*Motor*: superior oblique; Check extraocular movements (eye movements) by having the patient look in all directions without moving their head and ask them if they experience any double vision.	Inability to look down when eye is adducted
V-Trigeminal	*Sensory:* V1(opthalmic), V2(maxillary), V3(mandibular), sensation anterior 2/3 tongue. *Motor:* V3-masseter, temporalis, lat & med pterygoid, anterior belly digastric, mylohyoid, tensor, tympani/veli palatini; Test facial sensation using a cotton wisp and a sharp object.	Paresthesia (pain & touch) mandible deviation to side of lesion when mouth is opened, masseter & temporalis do not contract
VI-Abducens	*Motor:* lateral rectus muscle; Test smooth pursuit by having the patient follow an object moved across their full range of horizontal and vertical eye movements. Test convergence movements by having the patient fixate on an object as it is moved slowly toward a point right between the patient's eyes. Also, observe the eyes at rest to see if there smooth tracking, nystagmus, or any abnormalities.	No abduction if ipsilateral eye medial strabismus, diplopia
VII-Facial	*Sensory:* taste – anterior 2/3 of tongue; Look for asymmetry in facial shape or in depth of furrows such as the nasolabial fold. Also look for asymmetries in spontaneous facial expressions and blinking. Ask patient to smile, puff out their cheeks, clench their eyes tight, wrinkle their brow, and so on. *Motor:* frontalis, occipitalis, orbicularis, buccinator, zygomaticus, mentalis, post. Belly digastric, stapedius, stylohyoid. *Parasympathetic:* lacrimal, nasal & palatine, sublingual, lingual submandibular, labial.	Loss of taste anterior 2/3 of tongue. Paralysis of facial muscles, hyperacousis (stapedius paralysis). ↓ salivation, lacrimation
VIII-Acoustic (vestibulocochlear)	*Sensory:* hearing & equilibrium; Can the patient hear fingers rubbed together or words whispered just outside of the auditory canal and identify which ear hears the sound?	Unilateral hearing loss of balance problems
IX-Glosso-pharyngeal	*Sensory:* sensation & taste posterior 1/3 of tongue, pharynx, tympanic cavity, carotid baro/chemo receptors; Say aah. Does the patient gag when the posterior pharynx is brushed? *Motor:* stylopharyngeus muscle. *Parasympathetic:* parotid gland.	Loss of taste on posterior 1/3 of tongue. Loss of sensation on affected side of soft palate. ↓ salivation
X-Vagus	See IX Test - *Sensory:* pinna of ear, GI distention. *Motor:* muscles of palate, pharynx & larynx. *Parasympathetic:* heart, esophagus, GI tract up to distal 2/3 of transverse colon.	Ipsilateral: uvula deviates to opposite side of lesion, dyspnea, hoarse voice
XI-Accessory	*Motor:* SCM, Trapezius; Ask the patient to shrug their shoulders, turn their head in both directions, and raise their head from the bed, flexing forward against the force of your hands.	Paralysis of SCM & superior fibers of trapezius → drooping of shoulder
XII-Hypoglossal	*Motor:* intrinsic muscle of tongue, genioglossus, styloglossus, hyoglossus; Ask the patient to stick their tongue straight out and note whether it curves to one side or the other. Ask the patient to move their tongue from side to side and push it forcefully against the inside of each cheek.	Tongue deviates toward side of lesion on protrusion (action of genioblossus)

Dermatomes are specific areas on the skin that represent sensory innervations from a specific root level. Dermatomes are useful in neurology for finding the site of damage to the spine. Abnormally functioning dermatomes provide important clues about injury to the spinal cord or specific spinal nerves. If a dermatome is stimulated but no sensation is perceived, it can be inferred that the nerve to that specific dermatome has been injured.

Refer to the dermatome chart on the following page for specific areas. Testing is usually done with a blunt object (paperclip) or a pin. Compare same area on opposite side and ask the patient if it is the same, increased (hypersensitive) or reduced (hyposensitive).

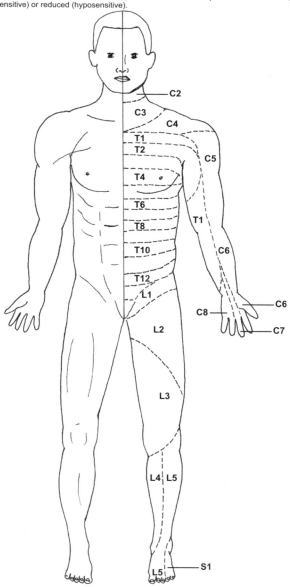

DERMATOMES

Posterior

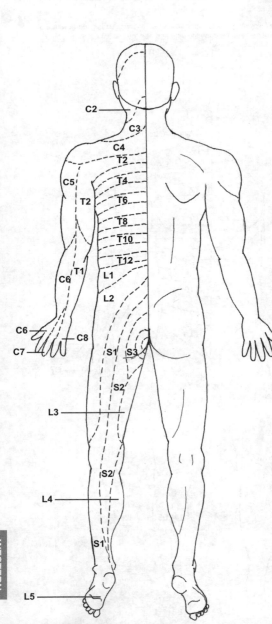

Nerve Root	Dermatome
C1	Vertex of skull
C2	Temple, forehead, occiput
C3	Entire neck, posterior cheek, temporal area, prolongation forward under mandible
C4	Shoulder area, clavicular area, upper scapular area
C5	Deltoid area, anterior aspect of entire arm to base of thumb
C6	Anterior arm, radial side of hand to thumb and index finger
C7	Lateral arm and forearm to index, long, and ring fingers
C8	Medial arm and forearm to long, ring, and little finger
T1	Medial side of forearm to base of little finger
T2	Medial side of upper arm to medial elbow, pectoral and midscapular areas
T3-T6	Upper thorax
T5-T7	Costal margin
T8-T12	Abdomen and lumbar region
L1	Back, over trochanter and groin
L2	Back, front of thigh to knee
L3	Back, upper buttock, anterior thigh and knee, medial lower leg
L4	Medial buttock, lateral thigh, medial leg, dorsum of foot, big toe
L5	Buttock, posterior and lateral thigh, lateral aspect of leg, dorsum of foot, medial half of sole, first, second, and third toes
S1	Buttock, thigh and leg posterior
S2	Buttocks, thigh and leg posterior
S3	Groin, medial thigh to knee
S4	Perinuem, genitals, lower sacrum

WESTERN

Manual Muscle Testing & Myotomes

Procedure: When conducting muscle tests, be sure to assess for asymmetry of the muscle groups (for example, atrophy on one side but not the other) and landmarks before testing.

General screening: check muscle in middle of range of motion (ROM) or through ADLs.

Specific muscle testing: estimate origin and insertion of muscle as accurately as possible.

Muscle testing is suggested for anyone with suspected or actual impaired muscle function, including strength, power or endurance. Impairments in muscle performance may be the effects of cardiovascular, pulmonary, musculoskeletal or neuromuscular disease or disorders. It is imperative to know how much resistance a **"normal"** muscle can endure to recognize when a muscle is not operating to its potential. All tests must be done bilaterally and the unaffected side should be tested before the other. This is crucial because the tester can then develop an accurate idea of the amount of resistance the unaffected side can take and what would be deemed normal for the patient. The scale below is composed of both subjective and objective factors.

Muscles should be tested on a regular basis in order to determine improvement or deterioration of function. It should be noted that the unaffected side should always be tested as well as the affected side for contrast. Identification of specific muscles or muscle groups with compromised function gives information for appropriate treatment, which may include strengthening exercises, functional drills, bracing, or compensatory muscle use.

1. Place patient in most pain-free and most favorable stance for testing
2. Use best testing position and body biomechanics
3. Show patient the motion you want him/her to oppose
4. Ask patient to hold position and rest when test is finished ("hold, hold, hold & relax")
   - Normally, s/he holds position for 3 seconds
   - If there is a high index of suspicion of injury or neurological compromise:
     - Hold for 5-10 seconds or,
     - Repeat for up to 10 repetitions (e.g. chart as 3/5 at 8x) or,
     - Test at various angles through ROM, eccentric, concentric, isometric
   - Joint should only be moved ~10° or through ~10% of range of motion
     - Typical mistake is to move joint too much, thereby examining many different muscles and affecting reliability & validity
     - Consider testing in positions or with actions that give patient mild discomfort to help get a true sense of specific limitations and actual muscle impairment or splinting
5. Compare results bilaterally and remember dominant vs. non-dominant extremity

Muscle strength grading system

Grade			
5	Normal	100%	Complete ROM against gravity with full resistance
4	Good*	75%	Complete ROM against gravity with some resistance (*reduced fine movements & motor control*)
3	Fair*	50%	Complete ROM against gravity but no resistance
2	Poor*	25%	Complete ROM with gravity eliminated
1	Trace	~5%	Evidence of slight contractility; *no joint motion or inability to achieve complete ROM with gravity eliminated*
0	Zero	0%	No evidence of contractility (*flaccid*)

% = % normal strength, ROM = range of motion, *Muscle spasm or contracture may limit ROM; Place question mark after grading a movement that is incomplete from this cause; Chart as a rating out of 5; e.g. 5/5, 4/5, 3/5, 2/5, 1/5, 0/5

WESTERN

Vital Signs

Pulse	
Descriptors: regular, irregular, strong or weak	
Adult	60 to 100 bpm
Children - age 1 to 8 years	80 to 100 bpm
Infants - age 1 to 12 months	100 to 120 bpm
Neonates - age 1 to 28 days	120 to 160 bpm

Blood pressure			
	Systolic	Diastolic	Average
Adult	90 to 130	60 to 90	80 to 120
Children	80 to 110	50 to 70	60 to 100
Infants	70 to 95	40 to 80	60 to 90
Neonates	>60		

Respirations	
Descriptors: normal, shallow, labored, noisy	
Adult (normal)	12 to 20 bpm
Children - 1 to 8 years	15 to 30
Infants - 1 to 12 months	25 to 50
Neonates - 1 to 28 days	40 to 60

Common Lab Values

There are some basic rules which hold true for nearly all laboratory tests

1. Different laboratories can get different results on the same sample of blood.
2. Laboratories can make mistakes. If your results have changed dramatically from your previous test, have it run again.
3. Most lab values need to be interpreted along with other clinical and laboratory data in order to develop a meaningful diagnosis. Very seldom will only one value give all of the answers.
4. Laboratory values differ according to age, sex, current medications, etc. Therefore, the interpretation of these values needs to be done with these other parameters in mind.

Clinical laboratory test are used by the practioner to aid in the diagnostic process; screen for early recognition of preventable health problems; and to monitor patient progress and outcomes. It is recommended that the practioner who used the services of a laboratory should be aware of laboratory's scope of services, recognition, and reputation. A listing of diagnostic labs can be found on page 397.

Test	Reference Range (conventional units)
17 Hydroxyprogesterone (Men)	0.06-3.0 mg/L
17 Hydroxyprogesterone (Women) Follicular phase	0.2-1.0 mg/L
25-hydroxyvitamin D (25(OH)D)	8-80 ng/mL
Acetoacetate	<3 mg/dL
Acidity (pH)	7.35 - 7.45
Alcohol	0 mg/dL (more than 0.1 mg/dL normally indicates intoxication) (ethanol)
Ammonia	15 - 50 µg of nitrogen/dL
Amylase	53 - 123 units/L
Ascorbic Acid	0.4 - 1.5 mg/dL
Bicarbonate	18 - 23 mEq/L (carbon dioxide content)
Bilirubin	Direct: up to 0.4 mg/dL Total: up to 1.0 mg/dL
Blood Volume	8.5 - 9.1% of total body weight
Calcium	8.5 - 10.5 mg/dL (normally slightly higher in children)
Carbon Dioxide Pressure	35 - 45 mm Hg
Carbon Monoxide	Less than 5% of total hemoglobin
CD4 Cell Count	500 - 1500 cells/µL
Ceruloplasmin	15 - 60 mg/dL
Chloride	98 - 106 mEq/L

Test	Reference Range (conventional units)	Test	Reference Range (conventional units)
Complete Blood Cell Count (CBC)	Tests include: hemoglobin, hematocrit, mean corpuscular hemoglobin, mean corpuscular hemoglobin concentration, mean corpuscular volume, platelet count, white blood cell count	Mean Corpuscular Hemoglobin Concentration (MCHC)	32 - 36% hemoglobin/cell
		Mean Corpuscular Volume (MCV)	76 - 100 cu μm
Copper	Total: 70 - 150 μg/dL	Osmolality	280 - 296 mOsm/kg water
		Oxygen Pressure	83 - 100 mm Hg
Creatine Kinase (CK or CPK)	Male: 38 - 174 units/L Female: 96 - 140 units/L	Oxygen Saturation (arterial)	96 - 100%
Creatine Kinase Isoenzymes	5% MB or less	Phosphatase, Prostatic	0 - 3 units/dL (Bodansky units) (acid)
Creatinine	0.6 - 1.2 mg/dL	Phosphatase	50 - 160 units/L (normally higher in infants and adolescents) (alkaline)
Electrolytes	Test includes: calcium, chloride, magnesium, potassium, sodium	Phosphorus	3.0 - 4.5 mg/dL (inorganic)
Erythrocyte Sedimentation Rate (ESR or Sed-Rate)	Male: 1 - 13 mm/hr Female: 1 - 20 mm/hr	Platelet Count	150,000 - 350,000/mL
		Potassium	3.5 - 5.0 mEq/L
Glucose	Tested after fasting: 70 - 110 mg/dL	Prostate-Specific Antigen (PSA)	0 - 4 ng/mL (likely higher with age)
Hematocrit	Male: 45 - 62% Female: 37 - 48%	**Proteins**	
Hemoglobin	Male: 13 - 18 gm/dL Female: 12 - 16 gm/dL	Total	6.0 - 8.4 gm/dL
		Albumin	3.5 - 5.0 gm/dL
Iron	60 - 160 μg/dL (normally higher in males)	Globulin	2.3 - 3.5 gm/dL
Iron-binding Capacity	250 - 460 μg/dL	Prothrombin (PTT)	25 - 41 sec
Lactate (lactic acid)	Venous: 4.5 - 19.8 mg/dL Arterial: 4.5 - 14.4 mg/dL	Pyruvic Acid	0.3 - 0.9 mg/dL
Lactic Dehydrogenase	50 - 150 units/L	Red Blood Cell Count (RBC)	4.2 - 6.9 million/μL/cu mm
Lead	40 μg/dL or less (normally much lower in children)	Sodium	135 - 145 mEq/L
Lipase	10 - 150 units/L	Thyroid-Stimulating Hormone (TSH)	0.5 - 6.0 μ units/mL
Zinc B-Zn	70 - 102 μmol/L	**Transaminase**	
Lipids		Alanine (ALT)	1 - 21 units/L
Cholesterol	Less than 225 mg/dL (for age 40-49 yr; increases with age)	Aspartate (AST)	7 - 27 units/L
Triglycerides	10 - 29 years; 53 - 104 mg/dL	Urea Nitrogen (BUN)	7 - 18 mg/dL
	30 - 39 years; 55 - 115 mg/dL	BUN/Creatinine Ratio	5 - 35
	40 - 49 years; 66 - 139 mg/dL	WBC (leukocyte count and white Blood cell count)	4.3-10.8 × 103/mm3
	50 - 59 years; 75 - 163 mg/dL	White Blood Cell Count (WBC)	4,300 - 10,800 cells/μL/cu mm
	60 - 69 years; 78 - 158 mg/dL	Vitamin A	30 - 65 μg/dL
	> 70 years; 83 - 141 mg/dL	Uric Acid	Male - 2.1 to 8.5 mg/dL (likely higher with age)
Liver Function Tests	Tests include bilirubin (total), phosphatase (alkaline), protein (total and albumin), transaminases (alanine and aspartate), prothrombin (PTT)		Female - 2.0 to 7.0 mg/dL (likely higher with age)
Magnesium	1.5 - 2.0 mEq/L		
Mean Corpuscular Hemoglobin (MCH)	27 - 32 pg/cell		

Complete Blood Count

Tests	Ranges	Calculations	Significance
RBC count	4.2 - 5.9 million cells/cmm	Absolute # of circulating RBCs per unit volume of blood • Indirect measure of the amount of circulating hemoglobin (i.e. oxygen carrying capacity of the blood) $\uparrow \rightarrow$ polycythemia vera; $\downarrow \rightarrow$ anemia	Decreased with anemia; increased when too many made and with fluid loss due to diarrhea, dehydration, burns
Hemoglobin Concentration	14.0-18.0 g/dl for men and 12.0-16.0 g/dl for women	Direct measure of weight of hemoglobin/unit volume of blood • Most sensitive measurement for existence of anemia • Used medically to judge need for transfusion $\uparrow \rightarrow$ dehydration, polycythemia vera; $\downarrow \rightarrow$ anemia, pregnancy	Hemoglobin measures the amount of oxygen-carrying protein in the blood.
HCT (Hematocrit)	Men are 40- 54% and for women 37-47%	PCV (Packed Cell Volume), ratio of the volume of the RBCs (after centrifugation) to that of whole blood $\uparrow \rightarrow$ polycythemia vera, Addison's disease, acute pancreatitis $\downarrow \rightarrow$ anemia, cystic fibrosis, CHF, pregnancy	Measures the amount of space red blood cells take up in the blood. It is reported as a percentage.
MCV (Mean Corpuscular Volume)	Normal range is 80 - 100	Calculated measure of the size of the average circulating RBC **MCV = HCT/RBC x 10** (Normocytic: 80 – 100 µm3 (fL); $\rightarrow$ iron deficiency anemia, leukocytosis; **Macrocytic:** > 100 µm3; $\rightarrow$ chronic alcoholism, methanol poisoning	Increased with B12 and folate deficiency; decreased with iron deficiency and thalassemia
MCH (Mean Corpuscular Hb Concentration)	Normal range is 27 - 32 picograms	Calculated weight of hemoglobin in the average circulating RBC **MCH = HGB/RBC x 10** (Normochromic: 27 – 32 pg) • **Hypochromic:** < 27 pg, **Hyperchromic:** > 32 pg	
MCHC (Mean Corpuscular Hb Concentration)	Normal range is 32 - 36%	Average concentration of Hb in a given volume of packed cells **MCHC = HGB/HCT x 100** (Normochromic: 330 – 370 g/L) • **Hypochromic:** < 330 g/L $\rightarrow$ hemolytic anemia; • **Hyperchromic:** > 370 g/L $\rightarrow$ polycythemia vera, malignancy, leukemia, rheumatoid arthritis	May be decreased when MCV is decreased; increases limited to amount of Hgb that will fit inside a RBC
RBC morphology		Microscope determinations from Wright's stained peripheral blood smear; **Microcytosis:** small MCV, **Macrocytosis:** large MCV, **Poikilocytosis:** different shapes	
WBC count (Leukocyte count)	4,300 and 10,800	Absolute quantification of total circulating WBC/unit volume blood • **Leukocytosis:** $\uparrow$ total WBC count $\rightarrow$ infection, inflammation, leukemia, bacterial infection • **Leukopenia:** $\downarrow$ total WBC count $\rightarrow$ aplastic anemia, pernicious anemia, severe infections, viral infections	May be increased with infections, inflammation, cancer, leukemia, decreased with some medications, some autoimmune conditions, some severe infections, bone marrow failure
WBC differential count -cytosis/-philia= $\uparrow$ -penia = $\downarrow$	Normal PMNs is 55-80%. Normal lymphocytes is 25-33% Normal for monocytes is 3-7%	**Neutrophilia** $\rightarrow$ Hodgkin's disease, infection **Lymphocytosis** $\rightarrow$ pertussis, mono, mumps, measles, TB **Monocytosis** $\rightarrow$ chronic infection, leukemia, protozoan infection **Eosinophilia** $\rightarrow$ allergies, parasitic infections, scarlet fever **Basophilia** $\rightarrow$ polycythemia vera, leukemia, chicken or small pox	
Platelet count	150,000-350,000/ cmm	Absolute quantification of circulating thrombocytes/volume	

$\rightarrow$ may indicate/suggests/seen in, $\uparrow$ = increase, $\downarrow$ = decrease, TB = tuberculosis

Test interpretation

CBC - The Complete Blood Count (CBC) is one of the most common tests ordered by most provider. It is a routine test used to evaluate the blood and general health.

RBC Count - The RBC count is the number of RBCs in a cubic millimeter of blood. The RBCs are the cells produced in the bone marrow that carry oxygen to your tissues. The normal range is 4.5 - 5.9 million/mm3 for men and 4.0-5.3 million/mm3 for women. A person with a significantly low RBC count can have symptoms of fatigue, shortness of breath, and appear pale in color. A low RBC count can be due to progression of illness or to certain medications, or both. A decrease in the RBC count usually causes a decrease in the hemoglobin and hematocrit values.

WBC Count - The WBC count is the number of WBCs in a cubic millimeter of blood. The primary function of these cells is to prevent and fight infections. There are many different types of white blood cells that play specific roles in fight infections. These specific types of WBCs can be measured in the white cell differential. Normal WBC count is from 4,300 to 10,800. The WBC count can be decreased for a variety of reasons: certain medications decease the production of WBCs in the bone marrow, minor viral infections which you may not even be aware of, stress, and opportunistic infections. Values markedly decreased should be cause for concern, since during this situation one is more susceptible to other infections.

Hemoglobin - Oxygen is carried to the tissues via hemoglobin in the RBC. A normal hemoglobin level is 14.0-18.0 g/dl for men and 12.0-16.0 g/dl for women. Any drug which causes a suppression of the bone marrow will decrease the hemoglobin level. In most cases it's a matter of balancing the effects of the drug with its potential side effects. When the side effects become too great, either the drug must be removed or the dose reduced to a tolerable level.

Hematocrit - The hematocrit (HCT) is the percent of the cellular components in your blood to the fluid or blood plasma. This test is one of the truest markers of anemia. Normal values for men are 40- 54% and for women 37-47%. A decrease in hematocrit is always seen with a decrease in the hemoglobin. These two values are linked to one another.

MCV - The mean cell volume or MCV is the most important of the RBC indices. It is a measure of the average size of the RBC. Normal MCV levels are 80-100. Vitamin B12 and Folic Acid deficiencies cause increases in MCV.

The other 2 indices are not so important. They are the MCH and the MCHC and are used to help diagnose various anemias and leukemias.

Platelets - Platelets are cellular fragments which are necessary for the blood to clot. When activated by "trauma," platelets migrate to the site of injury where they become "sticky," adhering to the injured site and subsequently used in the developing fibrin clot (scab). Normal platelet values are 150,000-350,000.

White Cell Differential - The white cell differential counts 100 white cells and differentiates them by type. This gives a percent of the different kinds of white cells in relation to one another. The three main types are: polymorphonuclear cells (or PMNs), lymphocytes, and monocytes. PMNs are increased during bacterial infections while lymphocytes are decreased with viral infections. Increased monocytes are sometimes seen in chronic infections. Normal percent of PMNs is 55-80%, 25-33% is the normal number of lymphocytes, and 3-7% is normal for monocytes.

Liver function Tests - Liver Function Tests include 5-6 individual tests which collectively can help determine the status of ones liver, detect liver damage or disease. Elevated liver enzymes are most often caused by certain medications or hepatitis. Therefore compound factors can be at work. The names of these liver function tests include SGOT, SGPT, alkaline phosphate, total bilirubin and LDH.

Kidney Function Tests - Two tests which measure kidney function are the BUN and creatinine. The usefulness of these tests usually relates to toxicity of the kidneys. Hence kidney function is monitored in this way. Normal BUN levels are 10-20 mg/dl. Normal levels of creatinine are 0.6-1.2 mg/dl.

ALT - the enzyme mainly found in the liver and is the ideal test for detecting hepatitis and evaluating patient who has symptoms of a liver disorder.

ALP - an enzyme related to the bile ducts; often increased when they are blocked. It helps check for liver disease or damage to the liver.

AST - an enzyme found in the liver and a few other places, particularly the heart and other muscles in the body. AST test is requested with several other tests to help evaluate a patient who has symptoms of a liver disorder.

Test Intepretation (cont.)

Amylase - amylase is an enzyme that is secreted in the mouth by the salivary glands and also in the pancreas. It can be an early warning sign of acute Pancreatitis when elevated. DDL can cause problems with the pancreas in a small number of patients taking the drug. Normal amylase levels are 25-125 milliunits/ml.

Cholesterol - Normal cholesterol levels are 150-250 mg/dl.

CPK - CPK or CK is an enzyme that's found in the brain and the muscles of the body. Strenuous exercise as well as a heart attack can cause increases in CPK. This makes clear the point of evaluating an abnormal test result in the context of other factors. Myopathy, dysfunction/distress with the muscles, can sometimes be confirmed with an elevated CPK. Normal levels of this enzyme are 12-80 milliunits/ml (30 degrees) or 55-170 milliunits/ml (37 degrees). Values will be slightly lower for women.

Total bilirubin - measures all the yellow bilirubin pigment in the blood. Another test, direct bilirubin, measures a form made in the liver and is often requested with total bilirubin in infants with jaundice.

Albumin – measures the main protein made by the liver and tells how well the liver is making this protein.

Blood Enzyme Tests

Enzyme	Source	Significance	
ALP Alkaline phosphatase	Bone Liver Placenta Intestine Malignant tissue	↑ALP Primary biliary tract disorders Bone disorders (osteoblastic) Healing fractures Paget's disease	↓ALP Malnutrition Hypophosphatasia Hypothyroidism
ALT - alanine aminotransferase **SGPT** - serum glutamate-pyruvate transaminase	Liver (99%) Heart Muscle Kidney	↑ALT Liver disease Myocardial Infarction (MI) Skeletal muscle disease	
AST - aspartate aminotransferase	Liver, Heart, Skeletal Muscle	↑AST Hepatobiliary inflammation Myocardial pathology Cirrhosis; Neoplasm Skeletal muscle condition	
CGT - gamma glutamyl transferase	Liver Kidney	↑CGT Liver disorders: all forms Hepatotoxic drugs - ETOH (alcoholics), Acetaminophen; Diabetes mellitus, Renal disease, Neurological disorders	
LDH or LD - lactate dehydrogenase	LDH₁ Heart, RBCs LDH₂ Heart, RBCs LDH₃ Lungs LDH₄ Liver, Sk. Muscle LDH₅ Liver, Sk. Muscle	↑LDH Hematological conditions, liver inflammation or disorders, disseminated cancer, cardiopulmonary conditions, muscular pathology	
CK - creatine kinase **CPK** - creatine phosphokinase	CK₁ Brain, smooth muscle, GI, genitourinary CK₂ Cardiac muscle CK₃ Cardiac, Sk. Muscle	↑CK Myocardial Infarction, skeletal muscle abnormalities, trauma, severe exercises, cholesterol lowering medication, brain trauma	

Selected Conditions Labs

Allergic Reactions
- Eosinphilia, increased total IgG
- RAST testing - sneezing, itchy eyes, runny/ congested nose, swollen sinuses, coughing, and wheezing

Atherosclerosis
- Cholesterol (HDL, LDL, VLDL)
- Triglycerides, glucose, uric acid, thyroxine

Bacterial Infections
- Neutrophilia, high total WBC

Bone Cancer
- Anemia is usually normocytic anemia
- Elevated serum ALP; also indicative of osteomalacia or celiac sprue

Hepatitis
- AST, ALT, ALP; leukopenia, bilirubinuria
- Specific serological viral markers for individual types
- Anti-HAV (IgM), HbsAg (surface antigen), Anti-HCV, Anti-HBc (core antigen)

Kidney Function
- BUN, albumin, globulins, uric acid, creatine

Metastatic Cancer
- Check with levels of enzymes are highest
- Increase WBC, ALP, pancytopenia
- Consider bone scan

Mononucluceis
- Leukocytosis, lymphocytes comprise > 50%
- (+) HA monspot, anti-VCA IgM, IgG

Multiple Myeloma
- IgG (monoclonal antibody), Rouleaux formation, Bence-Jones proteins
- Increased total protein, increase globulin, decreased A/G ratio
- Definitive bone marrow aspiration

Myocardial Infarction
- SGOT, LDH, CPK

Obstructive Liver Disease
- Bilirubin (best) - total, indirect, or direct
- ALP (best)
- ALT (mild increase) AST (mild increase)
- CGT/GGTP (increase), LDH if severe

Prostate Cancer
- Digital Rectal Exam (DRE)
- PSA - may also be increased in benign prostatic hypertrophy (BPH)
- May be falsely elevated post-prostatic massage/ exam

Rheumatoid Arthritis
- Rheumatoid factor - IgM type
- N/N anemia
- ESR, CRP, & other acute phase reactant proteins may be increased
- Involves PIP joint & MCP joints

SLE (Lupus)
- ANA or FANA (Anti-Nuclear Antibodies)
- Anti-DNA (only do this if ANA/FANA is positive)
- CBC - N/N anemia, leukocytopenia, lymphocytopenia
- Possible thrombocytopenia
- UA - hematuria, proteinuria, casts

Thyroid Disease
- Free T4, T3
- TSH - best test for general screen
- THBR (thyroid hormone binding ratio)
- Serum calcium, PTH

Viral Infections
- Lymphocytosis (normal 20-40%)
- Possible decreased WBC count or neutrophils (neutropenia)

Warning Signs of Cancer (General)
- Insidious onset with no known mechanism of injury
- A change in bowel or bladder habits
- A sore that does not heal
- Unusual bleeding or discharge from any place
- A lump in the breast or other parts of the body
- Chronic indigestion or difficulty in swallowing
- Obvious changes in a wart or mole
- Persistent coughing or hoarseness

Prostate
- A need to urinate frequently, especially at night
- Difficulty starting urination or holding back urine
- Inability to urinate
- Weak or interrupted flow of urine
- Painful or burning urination
- Painful ejaculation
- Blood in urine or semen
- Frequent pain or stiffness in the lower back, hips, or upper thighs

Bladder
- Blood in the urine
- Burning with urination
- Bladder spasms/pain
- Intense urge to urinate

Skin
- A sore that does not heal
- A new growth
- Spread of pigment from the border of a spot to surrounding skin
- Redness or a new swelling beyond the border
- Change in sensation—itchiness, tenderness or pain
- Change in the surface of a mole - scaliness, oozing, bleeding or the appearance of a bump or nodule

Breast
- Lump or mass in breast(s)
- Enlarged lymph nodes (lumps) in the armpit(s)
- Nipple symptoms: bleeding or discharge, retraction, elevation, eczema
- Skin symptoms: dimpling, redness, edema (swelling), ulceration

Lung
- Nagging cough
- Coughing up blood
- Recurrent attacks of pneumonia or bronchitis
- Chest and arm pain
- Unexplained weight loss
- Increased shortness of breath upon exertion
- Increase in the amount of sputum
- Swelling of the face and arms

Liver
- Pain in the upper abdomen on the right side; the pain may extend to the back and shoulder
- Swollen abdomen (bloating)
- Weight loss
- Loss of appetite and feelings of fullness
- Weakness or feeling very tired
- Nausea and vomiting
- Yellow skin and eyes and dark urine from jaundice
- Fever

Leukemia
- Fevers or night sweats
- Frequent infections
- Feeling weak or tired
- Headache
- Bleeding and bruising easily
- Pain in the bones or joints
- Swelling or discomfort in the abdomen
- Swollen lymph nodes, especially in the neck or armpit
- Weight loss

Ovarian
- General abdominal discomfort and/or pain (gas, indigestion, pressure, swelling, bloating, cramps)
- Nausea, diarrhea, constipation, or frequent urination
- Loss of appetite
- Feeling of fullness even after a light meal
- Weight gain or loss with no known reason
- Abnormal bleeding from the vagina

Colon and Rectal
- A change in bowel habits
- Diarrhea, constipation or feeling that the bowel does not empty completely
- Blood (either bright red or very dark) in the stool
- Stools that are narrower than usual
- General abdominal discomfort (frequent gas pains, bloating, fullness and/or cramps)
- Weight loss with no known reason
- Constant tiredness
- Vomiting

Thyroid
- A lump in the front of the neck near the Adam's apple
- Hoarseness or difficulty speaking in a normal voice
- Swollen lymph nodes, especially in the neck
- Difficulty swallowing or breathing
- Pain in the throat or neck

Stomach
- A loss of appetite
- Difficulty swallowing, particularly difficulty that increases over time
- Vague abdominal fullness
- Nausea and vomiting
- Vomiting blood
- Abdominal pain
- Excessive belching
- Breath odor
- Excessive gas (flatus)
- Weight loss
- A decline in general health
- Abdominal fullness prematurely after meals

Uterine
- Unusual vaginal bleeding or discharge, including in women older than 40: extremely long, heavy or frequent episodes of bleeding
- Difficult or painful urination
- Pain during intercourse
- Lower abdominal pain or cramping in the pelvic area

The ABCD Rule for Early Detection of Melanoma
Almost everyone has moles. The vast majority of moles are perfectly harmless. A change in a mole's appearance is a warning sign to your patient to get it checked by their general practitioner. Here is the simple ABCD rule to help you remember the important signs of melanoma and other skin cancers.

- **A is for ASYMMETRY:** One-half of a mole or birthmark does not match the other.
- **B is for BORDER:** The edges are irregular, ragged, notched or blurred.
- **C is for COLOR:** The color is not the same all over, but may have differing shades of brown or black, sometimes with patches of red, white or blue.
- **D is for DIAMETER:** The area is larger than 6 millimeters (the size of a pencil eraser) or is growing larger.

Source: National Cancer Institute; www.cancer.gov and the American Cancer Society; www.cancer.org

WESTERN

Red Flag Cases to Refer to a Physician

Here is a list of the more common conditions that require immediate or prompt referral to a Western medical doctor or treatment facility. Remember that when urgently referring a patient to a hospital, a practitioner must make direct voice-to-voice contact with the person who will receive the patient.

- **Sudden chest pain** (coronary artery occlusion, spontaneous pneumothorax, pulmonary embolism, dissecting thoracic aneurysm)
- **Persistent cough** (could be benign, such as postnasal drip or even acid reflux, but might be lung cancer, lymphoma, heart failure, pleural effusion, etc.)
- **Severe abdominal pain** (appendicitis, ruptured duodenal or gastric ulcer, acute pancreatitis, Chrohn's disease or ulcerative colitis with intestinal rupture or abscess, acute cholecystitis, acute diverticulitis, or many other conditions)
- **Upper GI or lower GI bleeding** (bleeding duodenal or gastric ulcer, ulcerative colitis, gastrointestinal cancer, bleeding from intestinal polyps or vascular malformations, esophageal or gastric varices, or many other conditions)
- **New onset of severe headaches** (always worrisome; could be any number of severe neurological conditions, possibly a brain tumor)
- **Impending or actual gangrene of a finger, toe or foot in a patient** (advanced arteriosclerosis, diabetes mellitus, Raynaud's disease or syndrome, or many other possible causes)
- **Tender swelling in a calf or thigh** (impending or actual deep thrombophlebitis, with the risk of potentially fatal pulmonary embolism)

- **Redness in the whites of the eye**, especially with pain and alteration of vision (may be benign, but could be uveitis, glaucoma, or a foreign body in the eye)
- **Change in level of consciousness** (impending or actual stroke, diabetic coma, intracerebral bleeding from ruptured cerebral aneurysm or trauma, brain tumor, hydrocephalus, others)
- **Pain with weight loss** (possible cancer, often missed by practitioners in the early stages when it can still be cured)
- **Suspicious breast lumps; abdominal masses; axillary, neck or groin masses** (may be cancer)
- **Vaginal bleeding after menopause, or excessive bleeding before menopause** (may be benign, but might be cancer, large fibroids, endometriosis)
- **New onset of neurological symptoms** such as weakness, numbness, visual changes, sudden mood swings, irrational or reckless behavior (could be a degenerative disease, brain infection, stroke, cancer, etc.)
- **Fever of unknown origin**
- **Frequent episode of dizziness or light-headedness** (may be benign, but might be an impending stoke, heart trouble, or possible brain tumor)
- **Unexplained weight loss** or failure to thrive in a normal fashion

This list is necessarily incomplete and cannot take into account every conceivable urgent clinical situation you might encounter. Cancer in any form is best treated in conjunction with a Western physician or hospital, and a TCM practitioner who takes on the role of primary provider of a cancer patient can expose himself or herself to medical liability. Of course, there is much that Chinese medicine can do to improve the outcome of Western medical cancer treatments and reduce the morbidity of such modalities as chemotherapy and radiation.

More Red Flags According to Body Systems

Cancer
- Persistent night pain
- Constant pain anywhere in body
- Unexplained weight loss
- Loss of appetite
- Unusual lumps or growth

Cardiovascular
- Shortness of breath
- Dizziness
- Pain or feeling of heaviness in the chest
- Pulsating pain anywhere in the body
- Constant and severe pain in lower leg or arm
- Discolored or painful feet
- Swelling (without history of injury)

Gastrointestinal / Genitourinary
- Frequent or severe abdominal pain
- Frequent heartburn or indigestion
- Frequent nausea or vomiting
- Change in or problems with bladder function
- Unusual menstrual irregularities

Miscellaneous
- Fever or night sweats
- Recent severe emotional disturbances
- Swelling or redness in any joint (without history of injury)
- Pregnancy

Neurological
- Changes in hearing
- Frequent or severe headaches (without history of injury)
- Problems with swallowing or changes in speech
- Changes in vision (blurriness, loss of sight)
- Problems with balance, coordination, or falling
- Fainting spells
- Sudden weakness

It's good to remember the old adage, "If in doubt, check it out." Talk with a Western doctor if you are uncertain about what is going on with one of your patients and are concerned it might be serious or even potentially life-threatening.

Source: Bruce Robinson, Acupuncture Today.com and Stith, J. S, S. A. Sahrmann, K.K Dixion, and B.J. Norton, *Ciurriculum to prepare diagnostics in physical therapy.* J. Phys. Ther. Educ. 9:50, 1995

WESTERN

The ABC's of CPR

Establish responsiveness: Gently shake the victim and shout, "Are you OK?" If the person answers;

Call 911 or have someone with you call 911; If the person is unresponsive or conscious and showing signs of a stroke or heart attack;

Immediately initiate the ABCs of life support:

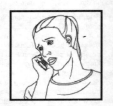

A-Airway – Open Airway: If the person is unresponsive, open the airway as soon as you've called 911. If the victim has no head or neck injuries, gently tilt the head back by lifting the chin with one hand and pushing down on the forehead with the other. Place your ear near the mouth and listen and feel for breath while looking at the chest to see if it is rising and falling.

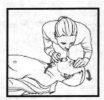

B-Breaths – Check Breath: If the person is not breathing normally, **give two rescue breaths**. Keeping the victim's head tilted, pinch the nose closed and place your mouth around their mouth. Give two slow, full breaths (about two seconds each), while watching to see that the chest rises with each breath. After delivering two breaths, check for signs of circulation, such as breathing, coughing, movement or responsiveness. Keeping the head tilted, once again place your ear near the mouth and listen, feel, and look for signs of breathing while you watch for movement.

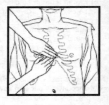

C-Chest – Compressions: If no pulse is detected, begin chest compressions immediately. Place the heel of one hand in the center of the chest (right between the nipples), with the heel of the second hand on top. Position your body directly over your hands, elbows locked. **Give 15 compressions** by pushing the breastbone down about two inches, allowing the chest to return to normal between compressions. Use the full weight of your body and DO NOT bend your elbows. **After 15 compressions, make sure the victim's head is tilted, and give two more rescue breaths**. Repeat this "pump and blow" cycle three more times, for a total of 60 compressions.

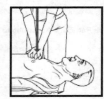

Reassess for signs of circulation

If no signs of circulation, repeat the pump-and-blow cycle until circulation resumes or help arrives.

When performing CPR, keep in mind that the person you are working on is clinically dead: You cannot make the situation any worse. Don't be afraid to put your whole weight behind each compression - a cracked rib can be repaired, dead brain cells cannot.

Where to find a course
Call 1-877-AHA-4CPR or visit www.americanheart.org/cpr. Or, call your local American Heart Association office for a list of training sites. Some states require current CPR card for licensing or renewal.

PHYSICAL EXAMINATION

Dr. Fred Lerner and Lerner Education provides a 300 hour Acupuncture Orthopaedics program to acupuncturists with advanced training in clinical skills and education regarding primary care as it relates to neuromusculoskeletal disorders. The program is accredited by the National Board of Acupuncture Orthopaedics. For more information www.lernereducation.com.

Head Examination

Patient Name: _____ Date: _____

Diagnosis: _____ Examiner: _____

Vital Signs: Pulse: _____ Blood Pressure: ___ / ___ L R Respiration: _____ Temperature: _____

Inspection/Palpation:

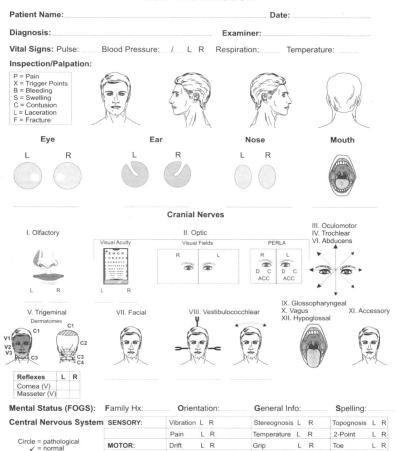

P = Pain
X = Trigger Points
B = Bleeding
S = Swelling
C = Contusion
L = Laceration
F = Fracture

Eye   Ear   Nose   Mouth

L   R   L   R   L   R

Cranial Nerves

I. Olfactory   II. Optic   III. Oculomotor
                                      IV. Trochlear
                                      VI. Abducens

        Visual Acuity   Visual Fields   PERLA

L   R   L   R

V. Trigeminal   VII. Facial   VIII. Vestibulococchlear   IX. Glossopharyngeal
Dermatomes   X. Vagus   XI. Accessory
                                                                        XII. Hypoglossal

Reflexes	L	R
Cornea (V)		
Masseter (V)		

Mental Status (FOGS): Family Hx: _____ Orientation: _____ General Info: _____ Spelling: _____

Central Nervous System

Circle = pathological
✓ = normal

SENSORY:	Vibration L R	Stereognosis L R	Topognosis L R
	Pain L R	Temperature L R	2-Point L R
MOTOR:	Drift L R	Grip L R	Toe L R
COORDINATION:	Finger to Nose	Rapid Movement	Balance
PATHOLOGICAL:	Babinski L R	Hoffman: L R	Ankle Jerk L R

WESTERN

PHYSICAL TESTS

Test Name	Structures	Description of Test	Positive Test
ANKLE			
Anterior Drawer Test	Anterior Talofibular Ligament, Medial Deltoid ligament	Patient in sitting or supine position, knee flexed and relaxed, examiner stabilizes the tibia and fibula and grasps the foot or calcaneus, examiner draws the foot anteriorly.	Anterior shift of the foot relative to the stabilized tibia/fibula, if lateral side of ankle translates forward, lateral ligament damage is suspected, if both medial and lateral sides of the ankle translate forward, damage is suspected to the deltoid ligament as well.
External Rotation Test	Distal tibiofibular joint (syndesmosis)	Patient seated, knee hanging from edge of bed, examiner holds foot with ankle in slight dorsiflexion, examiner passively externally rotates the lower leg slowly but forcefully.	Pain between tibia and fibula either anteriorly or posterior.
Distal Tibiofibular Compression Test	Distal Tibiofibular joint	Patient in seated, leg hanging over edge of bed, examiner applied a compression force to both malleoli of the same ankle (squeezing them together), Examiner may ALSO apply an anterior force to one and a posterior force on the other malleolus, shearing them gently.	Compression Test-pain on compression, indicating a problem with the syndesmosis at the distal tibiofibular joint, Shear Test-Pain on shear and/or significant displacement, indicating possible ligament rupture.
Homan's sign (Test for DVT)	DVT	Examiner passively dorsiflexes ankle with knee extended.	Pain in calf suggests possible DVT. Other signs and symptoms must be taken into consideration, history, coloration, pulses and swelling.
Posterior Drawer Test	Posterior talofibular ligament, medial deltoid ligament (posterior elements)	Patient in sitting or supine position, knee flexed and relaxed, examiner stabilizes the tibia and fibula and grasps the foot or calcaneus, examiner pushes the foot posterior, examining for change of position of the ankle relative to the tibia and fibula.	Posterior shift of the foot relative to the stabilized tibia/fibula, if lateral side of ankle translates backward, lateral ligament damage is suspected, if both medial and lateral sides of the ankle translate backward, damage is suspected to the deltoid ligament as well.
Talar Tilt Test	Calcaneofibular ligament, medial deltoid ligament (middle element)	Patient in side lying or supine, foot and ankle relaxed, knee bent. Foot is placed into 90° relative to the tibia; talus is tilted from side to side into adduction and abduction. If foot is plantar flexed, the ATF is more likely to be tested.	Laxity and elicited pain.
Thompson's Sign	Achilles Tendon rupture	Patient lies prone or kneels in a chair, foot and ankle relaxed, examiner squeezes calf muscle.	Absence of plantar flexion when calf is squeezed.
Tinel's Sign	Anterior branch of deep peroneal nerve, Posterior tibial nerve	Examiner taps on the peripheral nerve being tested, anterior branch of the deep peroneal nerve-anterio portion of ankle (dorsum of foot), slightly lateral to the EHL tendon, posterior tibial nerve-behind medial malleoli, tap for 30 sec.	Anterior branch of deep peroneal nerve-parasthesia on dorsum of foot, posterior tibial nerve-parasthesia on plantar aspect of foot.

Source: David J. Magee, *Orthopedic Physical Assessment Enhanced Edition, 4th Edition*, 2006, W.B. Saunders Company, NY, NY.

PHYSICAL EXAMINATION

Ankle & Foot Examination

Patient Name: _____ **Date:** _____

Diagnosis: _____ **Examiner:** _____

Vital Signs: Pulse: ____ Blood Pressure: ___/___ L R Respiration: ____ Temperature: ____

Inspection/Palpation:

P = Pain
X = Trigger Points
B = Bleeding
S = Swelling
C = Contusion
L = Laceration
H = Hot

Range of Motion:

Activity	Normal	Active	Passive
Plantar Flexion	50		
Dorsiflexion	20		
Inversion	45-60		
Eversion	15-30		
Great Toe Extension	70		
Great Toe Flexion	45		

Nerve Supply (Skin):

Anterior   **Posterior**

L4, L5, Saphenous, S1, L5, Superficial Peroneal, Sural, Deep Peroneal, Saphenous, S2, S1, Tibial, L5

Pulses	L	R
Dorsalis Pedis		
Post. Tibial		

Muscle Testing/Myotomes:

Muscle	Strength L	R
Hamstrings (L5):		
Medial		
Lateral		
Quadriceps (L2-4):		
Rectus Femoris		
Vastus Lateralis		
Vastus Medialis		
Sartorius (L2-3)		
Gracilis (L3)		
Tensor Fascia Lata (L5)		
Gluteus Min/Med (L5)		
Adductors (L4)		
Tibialis Anterior (L4)		
Tibialis Posterior (L4)		
Peroneus Long/Brev (L5)		
Peroneus Tertius (L5)		
Gastrocnemius (S1)		
Soleus (S1)		

Circumferential	L	R
Thigh		
Calf		

Functional Assessment	✓
Squatting	
Squatting on Toes	
Squatting & Bouncing	
Standing on One Foot At A Time	
Standing on Toes, 1 Foot At A Time	
Going Up & Down Stairs	
Walking on Toes	
Running Straight Ahead	
Running & Twisting	
Jumping	
Jumping & Full Squatting	

Orthopedic: _____

Neurological: _____

Antalgia: _____ **Special:** _____

WESTERN

PHYSICAL TESTS

Test Name	Structures	Description of Test	Positive Test
CERVICAL			
Cranial Nerve Tests	*Cranial Nerves*	**CN1:** (olfactory): Smell coffee or a similar substance with eyes closed. **CN2:** (optic): Read something with one eye closed. **CN3, 4, 6:** Eye movements - note any ptosis. **CN5:** (trigeminal): Contract muscles of mastication (masseter and temporalis). **CN7:** (facial): Move eyebrows up and down, purse lips, bare teeth; Bell's Palsy common - esp. if patient unable to whistle or wink on one side. **CN8:** (auditory): Have patient repeat what you say with eyes closed. **CN9:** Patient swallows. **CN10:** (vagus): Patient swallows. **CN11:** (spinal accessory): Have patient contract SCM. **CN12:** Patient sticks out tongue & moves left/right.	Inability to perform actions above.
Distraction Test	*IVF, IV Disc, Spinal nerve root*	Patient in sitting, lying or standing position. Examiner places one hand under chin, the other under the occiput and provides an axial traction to the head. If symptoms are referred to the shoulder, a further reduction in symptoms can be achieved by abducting the arms while traction is applied.	Reduction of radicular symptoms.
Spurling's Test	*Cervical Foramen, IVF*	Patient seated. First stage, examiner provides a compression force on the head in neutral. Second stage, patient extends head and examiner applies axial compression. Third stage, patient extends head and rotates to unaffected side first, then affected side while examiner applies axial compression. Spurling's version simply applies axial compression with side flexion, first to the unaffected side, then to the affected side.	Radicular pain which peripheralizes on the side when the head is flexed sideways or rotated. Traction should alleviate the peripheral symptoms.
Hautant's Test	*Vertebral artery*	Patient sits, forward flexes both arms to 90°, closes eyes and examiner watches for any loss of arm position, Patient rotates or extends and rotated neck while holding arm position and eyes are closed again, hold each position for 10-30 sec.	If arms move when neck is NOT rotated, cause is non-vascular. If wavering of arms occurs with cervical motion (rotation), likely vascular problem to brain.
Hoffman's Sign	*Upper Motor Neuron Lesion*	Patient lying, sitting or standing position. Examiner holds patient's middle finger and gently "flicks" the distal phalanx.	IP joint of thumb on hand flexes.
Romberg's Test	*Upper Motor Neuron Lesion*	Patient standing. Ask patient to close eyes and remain still for 30 seconds.	Patient begins to sway excessively or loses balance.
Stability -Lateral Shear Test- Coronal Stability	*Dens integrity*	Patient in supine position. Supporting the occiput, examiner places radial side of 2nd MCP on transverse processes of atlas, on one side and on axis on other side, Examiner stabilizes the axis while providing a lateral force on the Atlas and occiput.	Soft end feel, cord signs, lump-in-throat feeling, excessive movement or reproduction of patient symptoms. **Pain is a normal sensation and does not indicate a positive test**
Stability- Alar Ligament Rotational Test	*Alar Ligament*	Patient sitting, clinician fixes C2 using a grip over the lamina. Clinician rotates the head.	More than 20-30 degrees of rotation indicates damaged contra lateral alar ligament. If excessive rotation occurs ipsilaterally to the side of excessive lateral flexion in the lateral flexion test, this points to alar ligament damage. If the excessive motions are in opposite directions, this suggests joint instability at C0-C1.
Stability- Anterior translation- atlas on axis	*Atlanto-axial joint*	With the patient supine, the clinician fixes C2. (using thumb pressure over the anterior aspect of the transverse processes) and then lifts the head and atlas vertically.	Excessive movement. cord signs, symptom reproduction.
Stability- Sharp-Purser Test- Saggital Stability	*Transverse Ligament of C1-2*	Patient flexes head and neck in seated position. Examiner places on hand over patient's forehead and stabilizes C2 posteriorly at the spinous process with thumb of other hand, examiner applies a gentle posterior force to patient's forehead.	Relief of patient's symptoms, relief of cord signs, Clunk of posterior slide of occiput (less reliable).
Stability-Alar Ligament Side Flexion Test	*Alar ligament*	Patient supine head in neutral, examiner stabilizes C2 with wide pinch grip around spinous process and lamina, Examiner attempts to side flex head away from side being stabilized (ie. contralateral side flexion). REPEAT test in flexion and extension of upper C-spine.	Significant side flexion possible in ALL three positions.

Test Name	Structures	Description of Test	Positive Test
Stability-Anterior-atlanto-occipital joint	*Atlanto-occipital joint*	Patient supine, clinician applies a posterior force bilaterally to the anterolateral aspect of the transverse processes of the atlas and axis on occiput.	Excessive movement, cord signs.
Stability-Distraction Test-Longitudinal Stability	*Tectoral membrane, Upper cervical ligaments.*	Patient supine, examiner applies traction to the occiput, if no symptoms, reposition head in flexion and reapplies traction.	Pain or parasthesia, cord signs.
Stability-Posterior Test-Atlanto-occipital joint	*Atlanto-Occipital Joint*	Patient supine, clinician applies an anterior force bilaterally to the atlas and axis on the occiput.	Excessive Movement, cord signs.
Upper Limb Tension Test (Genera)	*Median Nerve, C5, C6, C7, Anterior Interosseous Nerve*	Patient in supine lying position. Scapular depression and shoulder abduction to 110° without rotation. Forearm supination and wrist extension are applied. The fingers and thumb are also extended. Finally, the elbow is moved into full extension. An additional sensitizing motion that can be used is cervical side flexion to the contralateral side.	Reproduction of patient's symptoms, significant differences between sides.
Upper Limb Tension Test (Median Nerve)	*Median Nerve, Musculocutaneous Nerve, Axillary Nerve*	Patient lying supine. Shoulder depression and slight abduction (10°) with full medial rotation. Position forearms into supination with wrist extension and extend the thumb and fingers. Elbow is then moved into extension. The test can be sensitized further by side flexing the cervical spine to the contralateral side.	Reproduction of patient's symptoms, significant differences between sides.
Upper Limb Tension Test (Radial Nerve)	*Radial Nerve*	Patient lying supine. Shoulder depression and slight abduction (10°) with full medial rotation. Position forearm into pronation with wrist flexion and ulnar deviation and flex the thumb and fingers. Elbow is then moved into extension. The test can be sensitized further by side flexing the cervical spine to the contralateral side.	Reproduction of patient's symptoms, significant differences between sides.
Upper Limb Tension Test (Ulnar-ULTT4)	*Ulnar Nerve, C8, T1*	Patient lying supine. Shoulder depression and abduction (90°) in lateral rotation with elbow flexion, as though they were placing their hand on their ear. Position forearms into pronation with wrist extension and radial deviation and extend the thumb and fingers. The test can be sensitized further by side flexing the cervical spine to the contralateral side.	Reproduction of patient's symptoms, significant differences between sides.
Cervical kineasthesia	*Proprioceptors in cervical spine*	Use ROM measure at start to measure position then move patient out of position and ask them to go back to the start position. Record amount of change from initial and final measure.	N/A

Neck Examination

Patient Name: _____ Date: _____

Diagnosis: _____ Examiner: _____

Vital Signs: Pulse: ____ Blood Pressure: ____/____ L R Respiration: ____ Temperature: ____

Inspection/Palpation:

P = Pain
X = Trigger Points
B = Bleeding
S = Swelling
C = Contusion
L = Laceration
H = Hot

Range of Motion:

Activity	Normal	Active
Flexion	50	
Extension	60	
Right Lateral Bend	45	
Left Lateral Bend	45	
Right Rotation	80	
Left Rotation	80	

Nerve Supply (Skin):

SUPRACLAVICULAR N.
MEDIAL BRACHIAL CUTANEOUS N.
AXILLARY NERVE
RADIAL N.
LATERAL ANTEBRACHIAL CUTANEOUS N.
MEDIAL ANTEBRACHIAL CUTANEOUS N.
ULNAR NERVE
MEDIAN N.

C1 C2 C3 C4 C5 C6 C7 C8 T1

Grip (JAMAR)	L	R
Trial #1		
Trial #2		
Trial #3		

Reflexes:	L	R
Biceps (C5)		
Brachioradialis (C6)		
Triceps (C7)		

Muscle Testing/Myotomes:

Muscle	Strength	
	L	R
Scalenes (C4-8)		
SCM (C2)		
Trapezius (C3-4)		
Upper		
Middle		
Lower		
Rhomboid (C5)		
Levator Scapula (C4-5)		
Serratus Anticus (C6)		
Latissimus Dorsi (C6-8)		
Pectoralis Major:		
Clavicular (C5-7)		
Sternal (C6-8)		
Deltoid: (C5-6)		
Anterior		
Middle		
Posterior		
Supraspinatus (C5)		
Teres Minor (C5-6)		
Infraspinatus (C5-6)		
Subscapularis (C5-6)		
Teres Major (C6)		
Coracobrachialis (C6-7)		
Biceps (C5-6)		
Triceps (C7-8)		
Wrist Extensors (C7)		
Finger Flexors (C8)		
Interossei (T1)		

Orthopedic: _____

Neurological: _____

Gait: _____ Special: _____

© 2003 LERNER EDUCATION. Permission granted to reproduce.

Source: Reproduced with the permission of Lerner Education. Forms can be downloaded at www.lernereducation.com

308

Test Name	Structures	Description of Test	Positive Test
ELBOW			
Lateral Epicondylitis Test 1 (Cozen's Test)	*Lateral Epicondylitis*	Patient seated. Examiner stabilizes elbow with one hand, thumb resting on lateral epicondyle. Patient actively makes a fist, pronates the forearm, radially deviates, and then extends the wrist. Examiner applies a force to the wrist, resisting the above motions.	Pain at the lateral epicondyle.
Lateral Epicondylitis Test 2 (Mill's Test)	*Lateral Epicondylitis, Radial Nerve*	Patient seated. Examiner palpates the lateral epicondyle while passively pronating the forearm, flexing the wrist fully and extending the elbow.	Pain at the lateral epicondyle is positive for lateral epicondylitis or radial nerve compression.
Lateral Epicondylitis Test 3 (Tennis Elbow Test)	*Lateral Epicondylitis*	Patient seated. Examiner resists extension of the 3rd digit distal to the PIP joint, stressing extensor carpi digitorum.	Pain over the lateral epicondyle.
Medial Epicondylitis Test	*Medial Epicondylitis*	Patient seated. Examiner palpates medial epicondyle while the forearm is passively supinated and the elbow and wrist are extended.	Pain over medial epicondyle.
Pinch Grip Test	*Anterior interosseous nerve*	Patient is asked to pinch tip of the index finger together with the tip of the thumb.	Patient is unable to touch tip-to-tip and instead touches the pad of each digit together. May indicate median nerve or anterior interosseous nerve pathology. May also be indicative of pronator teres syndrome or entrapment.
Posterolateral Pivot-shift Apprehension Test	*Olecranon dislocation, subluxation, Posterolateral stability*	Patient in supine position lying with arm overhead. Examiner grasps forearm at the elbow and proximal to the wrist. A slight supination force is applied to the forearm. Examiner flexes elbow while applying a valgus force and axial compression force.	Subluxation or clunk between 40-70° as elbow is flexed.
Pronator Teres Syndrome Test	*Pronator Teres*	Patient sits with elbow flexed 90° and supinated. Examiner strongly resists active pronation while the elbow is actively extended.	Tingling or parasthesia in a median nerve distribution.
Wartenberg's Sign	*Ulnar nerve*	Patient sitting with hands resting on table. Examiner passively spreads fingers apart and asks the patient to actively bring them together.	Unable to adduct little finger indicates positive test for ulnar neuropathy.

Elbow Examination

Patient Name: _____ **Date:** _____

Diagnosis: _____ **Examiner:** _____

Vital Signs: Pulse: _____ Blood Pressure: _____/_____ L R Respiration: _____ Temperature: _____

Inspection/Palpation:

| P = Pain |
| X = Trigger Points |
| B = Bleeding |
| S = Swelling |
| C = Contusion |
| L = Laceration |
| F = Fracture |

Range of Motion:

Activity	Normal	Active	Passive
Flexion	140-150		
Extension	0-10		
Supination	90		
Pronation	80-90		

Muscle Testing/Myotomes:

Muscle	Strength	
	L	R
Triceps/Anconeus (C7-8)		
Biceps/Brachialis (C5-6)		
Brachioradialis (C5-6)		
Supinator (C6)		
Pronator Teres (C6-7)		
Forearm Extensors (C7-8)		
Forearm Flexors (C7-T1)		

Nerve Supply (Skin):

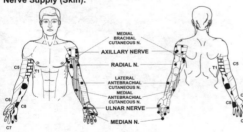

MEDIAL BRACHIAL CUTANEOUS N.
AXILLARY NERVE
RADIAL N.
LATERAL ANTEBRACHIAL CUTANEOUS N.
MEDIAL ANTEBRACHIAL CUTANEOUS N.
ULNAR NERVE
MEDIAN N.

C5 T1 C6 C8 C7

Orthopedic: _____

Neurological: _____

Antalgia: _____ **Special:** _____

WESTERN

Source: Reproduced with the permission of Lerner Education. Forms can be downloaded at www.lernereducation.com

310

PHYSICAL TESTS

Test Name	Structures	Description of Test	Positive Test
HIP			
90-90° SLR	Hamstrings length	Patient lies supine and flexes hips to 90° and holds both legs up with arms. Patient actively extends knees one at a time to full extension, maintaining hip flexion, then relaxes and attempts the other side.	Knee should extend to at least 20° from full extension, if not, indicates hamstring tightness.
Anatomical Leg Length Test	Femoral, tibial leg length	Patient lies supine. Examiner has patient perform a Weber-Barstow maneuver, measure with tape measure from ASIS to lateral malleolus, compare bilaterally.	Should be no more than 1.5 cm difference between legs.
Craig's Test	Femoral Neck position	Patient lies prone, knee flexed to 90°. Examiner palpates posterior aspect of greater trochanter, then rotates it medially and laterally until the greater trochanter is parallel with the examining table. Degree of retro or ante version can be estimated based on the angle of the lower leg from vertical.	Ante version is indicated by internal hip rotation in the final position (tibia falls laterally due to 90 degrees of knee flexion in prone).
FABER (Patrick) Test	Sacroiliac joint, hip flexor muscles, hip joint	Patients lie supine. Examiner places patient's leg with foot of test leg on top of the knee of opposite leg, examiner slowly lowers knee toward examining table.	Test leg knee remains above opposite straight leg.
Functional Leg Length Test	Pelvis effect on leg position	Patient lies supine. Examiner has patient perform a Weber-Barstow maneuver, measure with tape measure from umbilicus or xyphoid process to lateral malleolus, compare bilaterally.	Should be no more than 1.5 cm difference between sides
Modified Ober's Test	Iliotibial band, tensor fascia latae	Patient in side lying position. Examiner stands behind patient, flexes hip slightly with the knee nearly straight and abducts fully, stabilizing pelvis. Examiner then extends hip, allowing no internal or external rotation, examiner then slowly lowers leg into adduction while patient relaxes.	Leg "hangs" in abduction or does not fall below horizontal.
Quadrant (Scouring) Test	Hip Joint Play	Patient lies supine. Examiner flexes hip and adducts so that knee points to opposite shoulder, examiner maintains slight resistance while the hip is moved passively towards abduction forming an arc of motion, examiner notes any lack of smoothness in the motion, pain or apprehension. Test is done with hip in internal rotation (tests anterior femoral head and superior acetabulum), then external rotation (tests superior acetabulum and posterior femoral head). Also repeat test in extension.	Pain, irregular motion pattern, "bump" in the movement pattern, apprehension, crepitus.
Rectus Femoris Test	Rectus femoris	Patient lies supine with legs hanging over edge of table. Examiner flexes one hip and knee similar to Thomas Test, patient holds bent knee towards chest (not all the way), examiner observes the "hanging" knee. Knee flexion should not change (remain at 90°), if knee straightens, examiner should passively flex the knee to see if it will remain in flexion.	Knee straightens, indicating tight rectus femoris.
Sign of the Buttock	Hip pathology versus neurological tissue lesion or hamstring Tension	Patient lies supine. Examiner performs a Straight Leg Raise. Once maximum SLR is reached, examiner flexes knee and attempts to further flex the hip.	If hip continues to flex once knee is flexed (stretch taken off hamstrings and dura), pathology is likely in the neurological structures or the hamstrings. If the hip will not flex further, the pathology is likely in the hip structures.
Thomas Test	Hip flexors, rectus femoris	Patient lies supine. Examiner checks for excessive lordosis, examiner raises one hip and flexes that knee, bringing the knee towards the chest (but not all the way) to flatten the lordosis, patient holds this leg with both hands locked, the straight leg is examined.	Straight leg lifts off table, when leg is pushed down, increased pelvic tilt or lordosis becomes evident.
Trendelenburg	Gluteus medius, gluteus minimus, superior gluteal nerve, L4, L5, S1 nerve roots	Patient in standing position. Examiner behind patient, patient lift leg on test side off ground, examiner assesses PSIS for symmetry.	Pelvis drops on side of test leg.
Weber-Barstow Maneuver	Reset pelvic position while lying supine	Patient lies in supine position, knees bent so feet are flat on treatment bed, patient pushes down with heels to raise buttocks off of bed, patient then drops buttocks down onto the table, allowing a natural position to be assumed, examiner then passively straightens legs and pulls gently to "take up slack".	Examine medial malleolus for asymmetry.

Hip Examination

Patient Name: _____ Date: _____

Diagnosis: _____ Examiner: _____

Vital Signs: Pulse: _____ Blood Pressure: ___/___ L R   Respiration: _____ Temperature: _____

Inspection/Palpation:

P = Pain
X = Trigger Points
B = Bleeding
S = Swelling
C = Contusion
L = Laceration
H = Hot

Muscle Testing/Myotomes:

Muscle	Strength	
	L	R
Psoas (L2,3)		
Iliacus (L2,3)		
Piriformis (S1,2)		
Abdominals		
Hamstrings (L5):		
Medial		
Lateral		
Quadriceps (L2-4):		
Rectus Femoris		
Vastus Lateralis		
Vastus Medialis		
Sartorius (L2-3)		
Gracilis (L3)		
Tensor Fascia Lata (L5)		
Gluteus Min/Med (L5)		
Adductors (L4)		
Gluteus Maximus (S1)		

Range of Motion:

Activity	Normal	Active	Passive
Flexion	110-120		
Extension	10-15		
Abduction	30-50		
Adduction	30		
Internal Rotation	30-40		
External Rotation	40-60		

Nerve Supply (Skin):

Anterior   Posterior

L1 Ilioinguinal Lumboinguinal
L2
L3   Posterior
              Femoral
              Cutaneous
L4 Obturator   Lateral
                Femoral
                Cutaneous
L5   Anterior
                Femoral
                Cutaneous

S1
L5

L1
L3
L5 L2
S1 L4
S2
S3

Circumferential	L	R
Thigh		

Orthopedic: _____

_____

Neurological: _____

Antalgia: _____   Special: _____

WESTERN

Source: Reproduced with the permission of Lerner Education. Forms can be downloaded at www.lernereducation.com

312

Test Name	Structures	Description of Test	Positive Test
KNEE			
Anterior Drawer Test	Anterior Cruciate Ligament, posterolateral capsule, posteromedial capsule, MCL, Iliotibial Band, posterior oblique ligament, arcuate-popliteus complex	Patient lying supine, with knee bent to 90°, foot flat on testing surface. Examiner palpates posterior aspect of tibia and fibula, grasps tibia posteriorly and draws it anteriorly. Test is done in neutral, then repeated in lateral tibial rotation, then medial tibial rotation to test two-plane instability.	Greater than 6 mm of anterior tibial translation, soft "mushy" end feel.
Apley's Compression Test	Lateral and medial menisci	Patient lies prone on the examining table, knees flexed 90°, and soles of his feet are parallel to the ceiling. Examiner places hands on the foot or heel, presses down firmly on the lower limb, axially loading it, and rotate it back and forth thus applying a compressive grinding force to the meniscus.	More pain on compression than on distraction indicates a meniscal injury rather than a ligament tear. The location of injury can be hard to determine.
Apley's Distraction Test	LCL, MCL, ACL, PCL, ITB, Patellar tendon	Patient lies prone on the examining table, knees flexed 90°, and soles of his feet are parallel to the ceiling. Examiner places hands on the ankle and stabilizes the patient's thigh with their knee. Examiner then lifts the tibia upwards, distracting the joint, and rotates the tibia internally and externally.	More pain on distraction than on compression indicates a ligamentous injury rather than a meniscal tear. The location of injury is determined by location of pain.
Lachman Test	Anterior Cruciate Ligament, Posterior Oblique Ligament, Arcuate-popliteus complex	Patient lying supine. Examiner holds patient's knee and passively bends to 20-30° of flexion. Examiner stabilizes the anterior femur with outside hand and applies a P-A force to the posterior tibia with the inside hand.	Soft end feel, significant anterior translation.
McMurray Test- Lateral Meniscus	Lateral Meniscus	Patient in supine lying position, knee completely flexed (heel to butt), examiner applies a varus stress to the knee, medially rotates the tibia fully and extends knee slowly looking for any snapping or clicking, indicating a lateral meniscal tear.	Clunk, snapping, or reproduction of patient's typical pain. Popping or snapping is NOT necessary for a positive sign.
McMurray Test- Medial Meniscus	Medial meniscus	Patient in supine lying position, knee completely flexed (heel to butt), examiner applies a valgus stress to the knee, laterally rotates the tibia fully and extends knee slowly looking for any snapping or clicking, indicating a medial meniscal tear.	Clunk, snapping, or reproduction of patient's typical pain. Popping or snapping is NOT necessary for a positive sign.
Patellar Tap Test	Knee Effusion	Patient in supine position. Knee positioned in extension and relaxed. Examiner applies a thumb and forefinger lightly to each side of the patella, the examiner then strokes downward on the suprapatellar pouch with the other hand.	Separation of the thumb and forefinger due to fluid expanding the area.
Posterior Drawer Test	Posterior Cruciate Ligament	Patient lies supine, knee bent to 90°, foot flat on testing surface. Examiner palpates anterior aspect of tibia and fibula, grasps tibia anteriorly and draws it posteriorly. Test is done in neutral, then repeated in lateral tibial rotation, then medial tibial rotation to test two-plane instability.	Greater than 6 mm of posterior translation, soft "mushy" end feel.
Posterior Sag sign	Single Plane Posterior Instability, PCL, Posterior oblique ligament, ACL	Patient lies supine, hip flexed 45° and knee flexed to 90°, foot flat on table. Examiner observes position of tibia relative to femur.	Tibia "sags" backward on femur with gravity. Normally, the medial tibial plateau extends 1cm anteriorly beyond the femoral condyle when the knee is flexed 90°. If this step-off is lost, the test is considered positive.
Q Angle Measurement	Femoral/tibial alignment	Examiner ensures that the lower limbs are at a right angle to a line drawn through both ASIS. On a single side, draw a line from ASIS through the mid-point of the patella. Then draw a line from the midpoint of the patella through the tibial tuberosity. The angle between the two lines is the Q angle.	In Males, Q angle is approximately 10° (13° in Magee) and in females, approximately 15° (18° in Magee). Increased Q angle may be indicative of femoral neck ante version and lateral tibial torsion and may lead to lateral tracking of the patella (common). Decreased Q angle may be indicative of femoral neck retroversion and medial tibial torsion and this tends to centralize patellar tracking.
Quadriceps Active Test	PCL, joint capsule	Subject is supine with knee flexed to 90° in the drawer-test position. The foot is stabilized by the examiner, and the subject is asked to slide the foot gently down the table.	Contraction of the quadriceps muscle in the PCL-deficient knee results in an anterior shift of the tibia of >2mm.
Reverse Lachman	Posterior Cruciate Ligament	Patient lying prone, knee flexed to 30°. Examiner grasps tibia with one hand and stabilizes femur with the other. Examiner pulls tibia posteriorly.	Soft end feel and/or significant posterior translation.

WESTERN

PHYSICAL TESTS

Test Name	Structures	Description of Test	Positive Test
Slocum Test (Anterolateral/ medial Instability)	*Anterolateral instability, Anteromedial instability, ACL, Posterolateral capsule, Arctuate-Popliteus complex, PCL, LCL, ITB*	Patient in supine lying, hip flexed 45° and knee bend 90°, test starts with 30° internal tibial rotation with examiner sitting on foot to stabilize, examiner performs an anterior drawer test. This assesses anterolateral instability. If positive, foot is moved into 15° external tibial rotation and the test is repeated.	First test-positive is movement occurring primarily on the lateral portion of the knee. Second test-positive is movement primarily on the medial side of the knee.
Valgus (MCL) Stress Test	*MCL*	Patient supine on the examination table. Flex the knee to 30° over the side of the table, place 1 hand about the lateral aspect of the knee, and grasp the ankle with the other hand. Apply abduction (valgus) stress to the knee. The test must also be performed in full extension.	Excessive motion, joint gapping on medial side.
Varus (LCL) Stress Test	*LCL*	Patient supine on the examination table. Flex the knee to 30° over the side of the table, place 1 hand about the medial aspect of the knee, and grasp the ankle with the other hand. Apply adduction (varus) stress to the knee. The test must also be performed in full extension.	Excessive movement, pain reproduction.

Knee Examination

Patient Name: _____   **Date:** _____

Diagnosis: _____   **Examiner:** _____

Vital Signs: Pulse: ____   Blood Pressure: ___ / ___ L R   Respiration: ____   Temperature: ____

Inspection/Palpation:

P = Pain
X = Trigger Points
B = Bleeding
S = Swelling
C = Contusion
L = Laceration
H = Hot

Muscle Testing/Myotomes:

Muscle	Strength	
	L	R
Hamstrings (L5):		
Medial		
Lateral		
Quadriceps (L2-4):		
Rectus Femoris		
Vastus Lateralis		
Vastus Medialis		
Sartorius (L2-3)		
Gracilis (L3)		
Tensor Fascia Lata (L5)		
Gluteus Min/Med (L5)		
Adductors (L4)		
Tibialis Anterior (L4)		
Tibialis Posterior (L4)		
Peroneus Long/Brev (L5)		
Peroneus Tertius (L5)		
Gastrocnemius (S1)		
Soleus (S1)		

Range of Motion:

Activity	Normal	Active	Passive
Flexion	135		
Extension	0 - 15		
Medial Rotation	20 - 30		
Lateral Rotation	30 - 40		

Circumferential	L	R
Thigh		
Calf		

Nerve Supply (Skin):

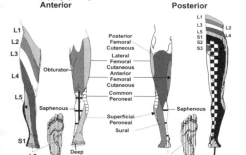

Functional Assessment	✓
Squatting	
Squatting & Bouncing	
Ascend Stairs	
Descend Stairs	
Running Straight Ahead	
Running & Twisting	
Jumping	
Jumping & Full Squatting	

Orthopedic: _____

_____

Neurological: _____

Antalgia: _____   **Special:** _____

WESTERN

Source: Reproduced with the permission of Lerner Education. Forms can be downloaded at www.lernereducation.com

ACUPUNCTURE DESK REFERENCE   315

PHYSICAL TESTS

Test Name	Structures	Description of Test	Positive Test
LUMBAR			
Anterior Lumbar Stability Test	*Anterior Spinal Stability*	Patient in side lying position, hips flexed 70°, knees flexed to 90°. Examiner palpates Spinous process at desired level and stabilizes SP above, examiner pushes patient's knees posteriorly along the line of the femur, lower segment moves posteriorly with stabilized segment remaining (flexion).	Reproduction of symptoms, significant motion compared to other segments.
Bowstring Test	*Sciatic Nerve*	Perform a Straight Leg Raise, once dural stretch has been attained, the hip is maintained in position and the knee is slightly flexed until stretch disappears, examiner then pushes their thumb in to the popliteal fossa against the sciatic nerve to re-establish dural tension.	Reproduction of symptoms.
Crossed Straight Leg Raise	*Sciatic nerve, L5, S1, and S2 nerve roots*	Performed in similar manner to straight leg raising, except the non-symptomatic leg is raised.	Reproduction of symptoms in contralateral leg.
Farfan Test	*Facet joints, joint capsule, supraspinous and interspinous ligaments, neural arch, longitudinal ligaments, intervertebral disc*	Patient in prone lying, examiner stabilizes ribs and spine at T12, examiner places other hand on anterior aspect of ilium, examiner pulls ilium backwards, rotating spine.	Reproduction of symptoms.
H and I Stability Test	*Hypo/ Hypermobility, Disc, Z-joints*	H Test-Patient in standing position, pain-free side tested first, patient flexes to side as far as possible, then move into flexion, then extension (or reverse if flexion is painful), patient returns to neutral and attempts on opposite side. I Test-Patient in standing position, pain-free side tested first, patient fully flexes as far as possible (or reverse if flexion painful). Examiner stabilizes while patient side bends to right and left, patient returns to neutral and repeats in extension.	Hypo-mobility indicated by 2 movements into the same quadrant would be limited. If hypermobility (instability) one quadrant will be affected with only one of the movements (H or I but not both).
Lateral Lumbar Stability Test	*Lateral Spinal Stability*	Patient in side lying position. Examiner places forearm over the side of thorax at L3, examiner applies downward pressure to L3 Transverse process.	Reproduction of symptoms.
Posterior Lumbar Stability Test	*Posterior Spinal Stability*	Patient in sitting position at edge of table. Examiner stands in front, patient places pronated forearms on examiner's shoulders; examiner puts both hands around the patient below the desired level (ie. place on sacrum if L5 being assessed), patient is asked to push through their forearm while maintaining lordosis.	Reproduction of symptoms, excessive movement.
Prone Knee Bend (Nachlas) Test	*L2 or L3 nerve root, femoral nerve*	Patient lying prone. Examiner passively flexes the knee as far as possible so patients heel rests against the buttocks. Ensure patient's hip is not rotated. Test may also be performed by passive extension of the hip while the knee is flexed as much as possible.	Unilateral pain in the lumbar, buttock, and/or posterior thigh may indicate an L2 or L3 nerve root lesion. Pain in anterior thigh may indicate femoral nerve or quadriceps lesion/tightness.
Quadrant Test	*Intervertebral foramen, Z joints*	Patient in standing position. Examiner stands behind. Patient extends spine while examiner stabilizes (can also support head on their shoulder), overpressure is applied while the patient sideflexes and rotates to the side of pain.	Reproduction of symptoms.
Repeated Extension movements	*Z-joints (Facet joints), anterior longitudinal ligament, pars interarticularis, Spinous processes of vertebrae and intervertebral foramen*	Patient in standing position. Examiner stands near to assist if needed, patient places hands on buttocks or hips and bends backward, keeping knees straight, repeat up to 10 times, examiner asks what symptoms are doing during test.	Increased localized pain, increased peripheralization, peripheral parasthesia, crepitus.
Repeated Flexion movements	*Intervertebral Disc, posterior longitudinal ligament, ligamentum flavum, erector spinae, thoracolumbar fascia*	Patient in standing position. Examiner stands near to assist if needed, patient slowly bends forward with knees straight to fully flex as far as tolerated, then return to start position, repeat up to 10 times, examiner asks patient what symptoms are doing during the test, repeat in lying position after standing extension is performed.	Peripheralization of pain, increase in localized pain (weaker indicator).
Slump Test	*Spinal cord, cervical and lumbar nerve roots, sciatic nerve*	Patient in short sitting position. Patient slumps lumbar and thoracic spine, examiner pushes down on shoulders, patient flexes head, examiner applies over pressure to cervical spine, examiner extends patient's knee, examiner dorsiflexes foot, patient extends head.	If symptoms are reproduced further movements are not attempted.

Test Name	Structures	Description of Test	Positive Test
Specific Lumbar Spine Torsion Test	Rotary torsion of specific spinal levels, Z-joints	Patient in side lying position and in slight extension. Examiner "winds" up the patient by pulling bottom arm towards them (rotates patient's chest towards ceiling until movement is felt at the tested segment), thus locking all vertebrae above, examiner stabilizes segment while rotating pelvis forward to detect motion.	Minimal movement and normal capsular end feel.
Straight Leg Raise	Sciatic nerve, L5, S1, S2 nerve roots	Patient in supine position. Hip medially rotated and adducted, knee fully extended. Examiner passively flexes hip until radicular symptoms are precipitated. Leg is lowered slowly until pain is relieved, examiner then dorsiflexes foot, cervical spine can also be flexed.	Radicular symptoms with straight leg raise, and return of symptoms with foot dorsiflexion. Most important is to compare findings bilaterally to determined if a difference exists.
Pelvic Stability	Pelvic and spinal stability, musculature	Patient lying prone. Examiner palpates PSIS first and asks patient to extend arm overhead, then other arm followed by each leg in turn, therapist feels for any rotation of pelvis with movement, repeat test, palpating ASIS.	Movement which cannot be controlled by patient. Posterior rotation/side flexion indicates possible weakness of the opposite back extensors or hip flexor tightness. Drop in ASIS may indicate hip flexor tightness or abs weakness or same side back extensor weakness .
SACROILIAC			
Gillett Test	Sacroiliac mobility	Patient standing. Examiner behind. Examiner palpates PSIS and sacral spine at level of PSIS, patient is asked to flex ipsilateral hip, PSIS should move inferiorly at the start, then the SI will lock and the PSIS and sacrum move together. Following this, patient is asked to flex the contralateral hip while maintaining the same landmarks, in this case, the sacrum should not move until the end of hip flexion, at which time it will move inferiorly while the ipsilateral PSIS remains fixated.	No PSIS movement individually, or on contralateral leg, no sacral movement.
Long Sitting Test (Supine to Sit)	Sacroiliac joint-clearing test	Patient lying supine. Examiner notes symmetry of medial malleoli relative to one another, patient sits up into long sitting position, examiner re-examines levels of malleoli.	Change in symmetry of malleoli from supine lying position to long sitting position.
Prone Knee Flexion Test	Sacroiliac joint-clearing test	Patient lying prone. Examiner compares position of medial malleoli. Examiner passively flexes both knees and compares height of medial malleoli.	Asymmetry of malleolus when knees are extended indicates either femoral or pelvic involvement regarding leg length. Asymmetry when knees are bent indicates tibial or foot shortening.
PSIS in Sitting	Sacroiliac joint-clearing test	Patient in sitting. Examiner palpates and compares PSIS bilaterally.	PSIS asymmetry.
Sacral Apex Pressure (Sacral P-A)	Anterior & Posterior ligaments, A-P joint stability, Rotational shift of SI, Sacral shearing force	Patient Prone, examiner applies anteriorly directed force directly to sacrum.	Elicited pain over SI joint.
SI Compression (Transverse Anterior Stress) Test	Anterior joint gapping, posterior joint compression	Patient supine. Examiner applies a cross arm pressure to the ASIS bilaterally, examiner pushes down and out with his arms.	Unilateral gluteal or posterior leg pain.
SI Distraction (Approximation Test)	Anterior joint compression, posterior ligament stretch	Patient side-lying. Examiner stabilizes and ensures no rotation of pelvis, examiner applies a downward force on the upper portion of the topmost iliac crest, force is directly straight downward towards lower iliac crest.	Increase pain or pressure feeling in SI area.
Standing Flexion Test	Sacroiliac joint-clearing test	Patient standing. Examiner palpates PSIS, examines for symmetry, patient flexes, examiner re-examines symmetry.	Asymmetry between PSIS.

WESTERN

Lumbosacral Examination

Patient Name: _____ **Date:** _____

Diagnosis: _____ **Examiner:** _____

Vital Signs: Pulse: _____ Blood Pressure: ____ / ____ L R   Respiration: _____ Temperature: _____

Inspection/Palpation:

| |
| P = Pain |
| X = Trigger Points |
| B = Bleeding |
| S = Swelling |
| C = Contusion |
| L = Laceration |
| H = Hot |

Muscle Testing/Myotomes:

Muscle	Strength	
	L	R
Quadratus Lumborum		
Psoas (L2,3)		
Iliacus (L2,3)		
Piriformis (S1,2)		
Abdominals		
Hamstrings (L5):		
Medial		
Lateral		
Quadriceps (L2-4):		
Rectus Femoris		
Vastus Lateralis		
Vastus Medialis		
Sartorius (L2-3)		
Gracilis (L3)		
Tensor Fascia Lata (L5)		
Gluteus Min/Med (L5)		
Adductors (L4)		
Gluteus Maximus (S1)		
Tibialis Anterior (L4)		
Tibialis Posterior (L4)		
Peroneus Long/Brev (L5)		
Peroneus Tertius (L5)		
Gastrocnemius (S1)		
Soleus (S1)		

Range of Motion:

Activity	Normal	Active
Flexion	60	
Extension	25	
Left Lateral	25	
Right Lateral	25	
Right Rotation	0	
Left Rotation	0	

Nerve Supply (Skin):

Anterior   Posterior

Reflexes:	L	R
Patella (L4)		
Achilles (S1)		

Circumferential	L	R
Thigh		
Calf		

Orthopedic: _____

_____

Neurological: _____

Antalgia: _____ **Special:** _____

WESTERN

PHYSICAL TESTS

Test Name	Structures	Description of Test	Positive Test
SHOULDER			
AC Crossover Test/Horizontal Adduction Test	AC Joint	Patient in standing or sitting position. Examiner passively flexes the shoulder to 90° and horizontally adducts it across body as far as possible.	Localized pain over AC joint indicates AC joint problem. Localized pain over sternoclavicular joint indicates pathology there.
AC Sheer Test	AC Joint	Patient in sitting position. Examiner clasps hands over the anterior and posterior aspects of the AC joint, one hand on the clavicle and the other on the spine of the scapula. Examiner slowly squeezes the heels of the hands together, providing a sheer force on the AC joint.	Pain or abnormal movement at the AC joint.
Active Compression Test of O'Brian	SLAP lesions in labrum	Patient in standing position. Patient forward flexes arm to 90° with elbow straight and shoulder adducted 15° from midline, thumb pointed down. Examiner applies a downward force on the forearm. The test is then repeated with the palm facing up, fully supinated.	Pain during the first portion of the test with reduced symptoms during the second portion.
Apprehension (Crank) Test	Joint capsule, G-H ligaments, rotator cuff	Patient in supine lying position. Examiner passively abducts arm to 90°. Examiner then slowly laterally rotates patient's arm watching for facial grimacing or apprehension. Examiner can add sensitivity by placing the hand or fist under the posterior humeral head to increase the postero-anterior force. This is termed the Fulcrum test. Conversely, the examiner can also place an antero-posterior force on the humeral head to reduce it back into the glenoid fossa. This is termed the relocation test and should reduce the patient's symptoms.	Apprehension and Fulcrum tests- apprehension or pain before 90° of lateral rotation. Relocation test-able to move further into lateral rotation without apprehension than during the Apprehension or Fulcrum tests.
Biceps Tension Test (Biceps Load Test I and II)	Biceps Tendon, SLAP lesion	Patient in standing or sitting position actively abducts to 90° and laterally rotates fully with the elbow extended and forearm supinated. If apprehension occurs, patient is asked to flex elbow against resistance (examiner supports arm and isolated elbow flexion is performed by patient). The test may be repeated in 120° of abduction (Biceps Load Test II).	Reproduction of typical symptoms may indicate a SLAP lesion. Use Speed's Test to rule out biceps tendon pathology. If patient becomes MORE apprehensive with resisted elbow flexion occurs, SLAP lesion can be suspected.
Clunk Test	Labrum	Patient lying supine. Examiner places hand on posterior aspect of shoulder over humeral head. Examiner's other hand grasps the humerus above the elbow. Examiner provides a P-A force on the humeral head while the other hand rotates the shoulder into lateral rotation. Examiner may alter the position of the shoulder to test various areas of the labrum.	Clunking or grinding sound through movement.
Coracoclavicular Ligament Test	Coracoclavicular Ligament	Patient in side lying position facing therapist. Examiner stabilizes clavicle while pulling the inferior angle of the scapula away from the chest wall. This tests the coracoid portion of the ligament. The trapezoid portion of the ligament may be tested by pulling the medial border of the scapula away from the chest wall.	Pain under the anterior clavicle between outer one-third and inner two-thirds of the clavicle.
Crank Ligament Test	GH Ligaments- Superior, middle, inferior	Patient sitting with arms at side and elbow bent to 90°. Examiner passively externally rotates humerus at 0° (superior GH Ligament), 45-60° (middle GH Ligament), over 90° (inferior GH ligament).	Significant GH joint laxity or pain.
Drop Arm Test	Rotator Cuff	Patient in standing position. Examiner passively abducts the patients arm to 90°. Patient is instructed to slowly lower the arm actively to the side.	Patient unable to lower arm slowly, significant pain.
Empty Can/Full Can Test	Supraspinatus	Patient in sitting or standing position. Patient abducts arm to 90° and resistance is applied by examiner. Shoulder is then medially rotated fully and angled forward 30° from the saggital plane, the patient's thumbs pointing to the floor. Resistance is applied again. Finally, the shoulder is laterally rotated so the thumbs are pointing up and resistance is applied again.	Pain or weakness unilaterally.
Faegin Test (Sulcus)	Glenohumeral joint, joint capsule	Patient in sitting or standing position. Examiner passively abducts shoulder to 90°, elbow extended and resting on top of the examiner's shoulder. Examiner clasps hands over the patient's humerus at the upper third and applies inferiorly and anteriorly.	Appearance of a sulcus above the corocoid process, apprehension.
Hawkins-Kennedy Test for Impingement	Supraspinatus, biceps tendon	Patient standing while examiner forward flexes the arm to 90° and medially rotates the humerus. Test may also be performed.	Pain or apprehension in superior/ anterior aspect of shoulder.
Infraspinatus Spring Back Test	Infraspinatus, Teres minor	Patient in sitting or standing position with arm at side and elbow flexed to 90°. Examiner passively abducts the arm to 90° in scapular plane and laterally rotates shoulder to end range.	Patient cannot hold the position and hand "springs back" out of lateral rotation.

WESTERN

ACUPUNCTURE DESK REFERENCE ■ 319 ▶

PHYSICAL TESTS

Test Name	Structures	Description of Test	Positive Test
Load and Shift Test	*Glenohumeral instability, joint capsule*	Patient in sitting position. Examiner stands slightly behind patient and stabilizes the scapula and clavicle from the top. Examiner grasps the head of the humerus with thumb over the posterior aspect and fingers over the anterior humeral head. Examiner feels for the seating of the humeral head in the glenoid to determine postural position. Examiner then moves the humeral head anteriorly and posteriorly to determine proper seating position within the glenoid, ie. the "start" position. This is the LOAD part of the test to seat the head fully in the glenoid fossa. To complete the SHIFT part of the test, the examiner glides the humeral head anteriorly or posteriorly, noting the amount of displacement from the seated position.	Translation greater than 25% of the humeral head width either posteriorly or anteriorly from the seated position.
Neer's Test for Impingement	*Supraspinatus, biceps tendon*	Patient in sitting or standing position. Examiner passively elevates shoulder in the scapular plane (scaption) with arm medially rotated. Examiner controls scapular and clavicular movement. The test is repeated in lateral rotation, which should be negative.	Pain in superior or anterior aspect of the shoulder. If positive in lateral rotation, suspect an AC joint problem.
Norwood Test for Posterior Instability	*Posterior Capsule, Infraspinatus, Teres Minor*	Patient lying supine with shoulder abducted 60-100° and laterally rotated 90° with elbow flexed to 90°. Examiner stabilizes the scapula at the AC joint, palpating the posterior humerus head with fingers. The examiner then passively moves the arm into horizontal adduction until the forward flexed position is reached.	Humeral head translating posteriorly in relation to the glenoid.
Posterior Apprehension Test	*Posterior Capsule, Infraspinatus, Teres Minor*	Patient in supine lying (can be done in sitting) position with elbow bent 90° and shoulder flexed to 90°. Examiner applies an axial load along the arm and passively medially rotates and horizontally adducts the arm, feeling on the posterior aspect of the GH joint for posterior dislocation or excessive translation. This should be repeated in 90° of abduction with one hand palpating the head of the humerus and the other hand providing a posterior force to the humeral head.	More than 50% of the humeral head width translation is considered positive.
Posterior Inferior Glenohumeral Ligament Test	*Posterior Inferior Glenohumeral Ligament, Posterior joint capsule*	Patient in sitting position. Examiner flexes shoulder to 90° then horizontally adducts the shoulder 40° with medial rotation. Examiner palpates the posteroinferior region of the glenoid during movement.	Humerus protrudes or pain in posteroinferior glenoid area. Restriction in motion indicates tight posterior capsule.
Posterior Internal Impingement Test	*Infraspinatus*	Conducted similarly to the Crank test. Patient in supine lying position. Examiner passively abducts shoulder to 90° with 15-20° of forward flexion and full external rotation.	Posterior shoulder pain.
Push-Pull Test	*Posterior Capsule*	Patient lying supine. Examiner holds patient's arm at wrist and abducts shoulder to 90° and flexes to 30°. Examiner places other hand over the humeral head. Examiner then pulls up on wrist while pushing down on the humeral head, placing a posterior force on the humerus.	Greater than 50% translation of the humeral head width is considered positive.
Reverse Impingement Sign	*Supraspinatus, biceps tendon*	Conduct impingement, test then provide an inferior force on the humeral head.	Relief of symptoms with the inferior force indicates that supraspinatus impingement is relieved with the application of force.
Speed's Test	*Biceps tendon, possible Labral involvement if SLAP lesion is present*	Patient in sitting or standing position, elbow fully extended. Patient flexes arm to 90° and examiner provides an eccentric force on the forearm. Testing is done both in full pronations, followed by full supination.	Increased symptoms in the bicipital groove when the forearm is supinated.
Lift Off Test	*Subscapularis*	Patient in standing position, hand behind back against mid-lumbar spine. Patient lifts hand away from low back. Examiner can apply an external load to further test subscapularis.	Inability to lift hand off low back. Abnormal scapular motion may indicate scapular instability.
Sulcus Sign	*Glenohumeral joint, joint capsule*	Patient stands with arm by their side and muscles relaxed. Examiner grasps patient's forearm below the elbow and pulls inferiorly.	Appearance of a sulcus above the corocoid process or below the AC joint.
Wall Pushup Test	*Scapular stability*	Patient in standing arms length from wall. Patient is asked to do a push-up against the wall 15-20 times.	Weakness of the scapular stabilizers may occur with 5-10 push ups and presents as winging or changes in elevation or depression.
Yergason's Test	*Transverse Humeral Ligament*	Patient in sitting or standing position. Patient's elbow flexed to 90°, arm stabilized against the side, forearm pronated. Examiner provides resistance against supination while the patient laterally rotates. Examiner palpates the biceps tendon in the bicipital groove to feel if the tendon "pops out."	Biceps tendon is felt to "pop out" of the groove.

WESTERN

PHYSICAL EXAMINATION

Shoulder Examination

Patient Name: _____ **Date:** _____

Diagnosis: _____ **Examiner:** _____

Vital Signs: Pulse: _____ Blood Pressure: ____/____ L R Respiration: _____ Temperature: _____

Inspection/Palpation:

P = Pain X = Trigger Points B = Bleeding S = Swelling C = Contusion L = Laceration F = Fracture	

Range of Motion:

Activity	Normal	Active	Passive
Flexion	170		
Extension	50		
Abduction	170		
Adduction	45		
External Rotation	110		
Internal Rotation	80		

Muscle Testing/Myotomes:

Muscle	Strength	
	L	R
Trapezius (C3-4)		
Upper		
Middle		
Lower		
Rhomboid (C5)		
Levator Scapula (C4-5)		
Serratus Anticus (C6)		
Latissimus Dorsi (C6-8)		
Pectoralis Major:		
Clavicular (C5-7)		
Sternal (C6-8)		
Pectoralis Minor (C7-8)		
Subclavius (C5-6)		
Deltoid: (C5-6)		
Anterior		
Middle		
Posterior		
Supraspinatus (C5)		
Teres Minor (C5-6)		
Infraspinatus (C5-6)		
Subscapularis (C5-6)		
Teres Major (C6)		
Coracobrachialis (C6-7)		
Biceps (C5-6)		
Triceps (C7-8)		

Nerve Supply (Skin):

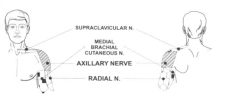

SUPRACLAVICULAR N.

MEDIAL
BRACHIAL
CUTANEOUS N.

AXILLARY NERVE

RADIAL N.

Orthopedic: _____

Neurological: _____

Antalgia: _____ **Special:** _____

WESTERN

PHYSICAL TESTS

Test Name	Structures	Description of Test	Positive Test
THORACIC			
Adson's Test	*Thoracic Outlet Syndrome*	Patient in sitting position. Examiner palpates the radial pulse. Patient rotates the head to the test side, and then extends head while examiner laterally rotates and extends the shoulder. Patient is instructed to take a deep breath and hold it.	Disappearance of the radial pulse.
Allen Maneuver	*Thoracic Outlet Syndrome*	See Wright test.	
EAST (Roos) Test	*Thoracic Outlet syndrome*	Patient in sitting or standing position. Patient abducts both arms to 90°, laterally rotates fully, flexes the elbows to 90° and horizontally extends the shoulder so the elbows are slightly behind the frontal plane. The patient is asked to slowly open and close the hands for up to 3 min.	Fatigue or distress is NOT positive tests. Profound weakness, ischemic symptoms, whitening of the arms or numbness/tingling of the hand are considered positives.
Halstead Test	*Thoracic Outlet Syndrome*	Examiner palpates radial pulse and applies an inferior traction on the test extremity while the patient's neck is extended and rotated AWAY from the test side.	Disappearance of the radial pulse.
Wright Test (Allen Maneuver)	*Thoracic Outlet Syndrome*	Patient in sitting position. Examiner flexes the elbow to 90° and horizontally extends the shoulder and fully rotates it laterally. Patient then rotates the head AWAY from the test side. Examiner then palpates the radial pulse. Examiner may also have the patient take a deep breath and hold it or extend the cervical spine.	Radial pulse disappears.
WRIST/HAND			
Allen Test	*Ulnar and radial arteries*	Patient in sitting or lying position. Examiner palpates the radial and ulnar arteries and provides a firm compression while the patient makes a fist and releases 3-4 times, driving blood out of the hand. Examiner releases the arterial compression on one artery while watching for blood refill in the hand.	Reduced blood re-fill from a singular artery may indicate a blockage.
Finkelstein Test	*DeQuervain's Tenosynovitis*	Patient makes a fist with thumb inside the fingers. Examiner stabilizes the forearm and deviates the wrist toward the ulnar side.	Unilateral pain over the abductor pollicis longus and brevis may indicate paratenonitis. Test can produce symptoms in normal populations, so test should be compared to other side. Test is positive only if patient's typical symptoms are produced.
Fromont's Sign	*Adductor Pollicis Brevis/Longus, Ulnar nerve*	Patient grasps a piece of paper between the index finger and the thumb. Examiner pulls paper away while patient attempts to resist this action.	Distal phalanx of thumb flexes when paper is pulled. If, at the same time, the MCP joint hyperextends, the ulnar nerve may be suspected.
Grind Test	*Thumb MCP or metacarpo-trapezial joint*	Examiner holds patient's hand with one hand and grasps the patient's thumb distal to the MCP joint. Examiner then applies an axial compression and rotates the MCP joint. This test may be repeated with any of the MCP joints.	Localized pain and/or grinding may indicate degenerative joint disease.
Phalen's Test	*Carpal Tunnel*	Examiner flexes patient's wrists fully and holds this position for 1 minute by pushing patient's wrists together.	Tingling or numbness in a median nerve distribution (thumb, index and middle finger and radial half of ring finger).
Reverse Phalen's Test	*Carpal Tunnel*	Examiner extends patients hand while asking patient to grip the examiner's hand. Examiner then applies pressure directly over the carpal tunnel for 1 minute. The test may also be performed by placing both hands in a prayer position and pulling back towards the body while keeping the palms in direct contact, although the reliability is reduced using this method.	Tingling or numbness in a median nerve distribution (thumb, index and middle finger and radial half of ring finger).
Supination Lift Test	*TFCC (Triangular fibrocartilage complex)*	Patient in sitting position, forearm supinated, and elbows flexed to 90°. Patient is asked to place hands palms up on the underside of a heavy table, or flat against the examiner's hands (which are palm down). Patient is then asked to lift upward.	Localized pain on the ulnar side of the wrist or difficulty applying the force unilaterally.
Sweater Finger Sign	*Flexor digitorum profundus*	Patient attempts to make a fist.	Distal phalanx of one of the fingers does not flex, may indicate a rupture of the tendon of flexor digitorum profundus.
Tinel's Sign	*Nerve regeneration, Median nerve (in wrist)*	Examiner taps over the carpal tunnel (also can be performed at elbow and shoulder by tapping on various nerve locations).	Tingling or parasthesia distal to the site of pressure.

Thoracic Examination

Patient Name: _____ **Date:** _____

Diagnosis: _____ **Examiner:** _____

Vital Signs: Pulse: _____ Blood Pressure: ____ / ____ L R Respiration: _____ Temperature: _____

Inspection/Palpation:

P = Pain
X = Trigger Points
B = Bleeding
S = Swelling
C = Contusion
L = Laceration
H = Hot

Range of Motion:

Activity	Normal	Active	Passive
Flexion	50		
Extension	0		
Right Rotation	30		
Left Rotation	30		

Neurology

Nerve Supply (Skin):

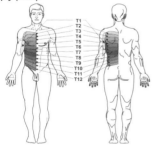

T1
T2
T3
T4
T5
T6
T7
T8
T9
T10
T11
T12

Muscle Testing/Myotomes:

Muscle	Strength	
	L	R
Abdominals (T7-L1)		
Serratus Anterior (C5-7)		

Reflexes:	L	R
Upper Abdominals (T7-10)		
Lower Abdominals (T10-L1)		

Orthopedic: _____

Neurological: _____

Antalgia: _____ **Special:** _____

© 2003 LERNER EDUCATION. Permission granted to reproduce.

WESTERN

Source: Reproduced with the permission of Lerner Education. Forms can be downloaded at www.lernereducation.com

ACUPUNCTURE DESK REFERENCE   323

Wrist & Hand Examination

Patient Name:_____ **Date:** _____

Diagnosis: _____ **Examiner:** _____

Vital Signs: Pulse: ____ Blood Pressure: ___/___ L R Respiration:_____ Temperature: _____

Inspection/Palpation:

P = Pain
X = Trigger Points
B = Bleeding
S = Swelling
C = Contusion
L = Laceration
F = Fracture

Wrist Range of Motion:

Activity	Normal	Active	Passive
Flexion	80-90		
Extension	70-90		
Radial Deviation	15		
Ulnar Deviation	30-45		

Muscle Testing/Myotomes:

Muscle	Strength	
	L	R
Pronator Quadratus (C8-T1)		
Finger Flexors (C7-T1)		
Finger Extensors (C7-8)		
Thumb Flexors (C8-T1)		

Grip (JAMAR)	L	R
Trial #1		
Trial #2		
Trial #3		

Nerve Supply (Skin):

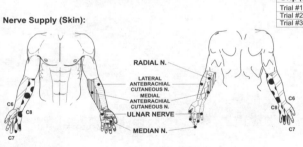

RADIAL N.

LATERAL
ANTEBRACHIAL
CUTANEOUS N.
MEDIAL
ANTEBRACHIAL
CUTANEOUS N.

ULNAR NERVE

MEDIAN N.

C6 C8 C7 C6 C8 C7

Orthopedic: _____

Neurological: _____

Antalgia: _____ **Special:** _____

WESTERN

Source: Reproduced with the permission of Lerner Education. Forms can be downloaded at www.lernereducation.com

324

TOP 50 MEDICATIONS & USAGE

Top 50 Drugs of 2004

1	Lipitor	Lowers cholesterol levels in the blood. Helps prevent certain heart and blood vessel diseases in people who are at higher risk for these diseases.
2	Synthroid	Treats hypothyroidism and other associated thyroid disorders.
3	Norvasc	A calcium channel blocker that treats high blood pressure and chest pain.
4	Toprol XL	A beta-blocker that treats high blood pressure and angina and lowers the risk of repeated heart attacks.
5	Zoloft	A selective serotonin reuptake inhibitor (SSRI) that treats depression, OCD, posttraumatic stress disorder (PTSD), PMS, social anxiety disorder (SAD), and panic disorder.
6	Zocor	Lowers cholesterol levels to prevent heart attack or other circulatory problems. Used in combination with a diet program to lower cholesterol.
7	Zithromax	An antibiotic that treats infections caused by certain bacteria.
8	Ambien	Treats insomnia.
9	Lexapro	A selective serotonin reuptake inhibitor (SSRI) that treats severe depression and generalized anxiety disorder (GAD).
10	Prevacid	Treats stomach ulcers, GERD, esophagitis, and other conditions caused by too much stomach acid.
11	Nexium	Treats GERD and conditions associated with stomach acids. Also used with antibiotics to treat certain types of ulcers. Prevents stomach ulcers and stomach irritation in patients taking pain and arthritis drugs, such as aspirin or ibuprofen, for long periods of time.
12	Singulair	Helps prevent and control asthma attacks and treats seasonal allergies.
13	Levoxyl	Treats hypothyroidism, enlarged thyroid gland, goiter and thyroid associated problems.
14	Celebrex	An NSAID that treats pain, including pain caused by arthritis, ankylosing spondylitis, or menstrual cramps.
15	Fosamax	Treats and prevents osteoporosis and other bone disorder.
16	Effexor XR	A selective serotonin reuptake inhibitor (SSRI) that treats depression, panic disorder, social anxiety disorder, and generalized anxiety disorder.
17	Premarin	Treats menopausal symptoms including hot flashes, severe dryness, itching, and burning, in and around the vagina area and to help reduce your chances of getting osteoporosis.
18	Allegra	An antihistamine used to relieve the symptoms of hay fever and hives of the skin.
19	Plavix	A blood thinner that Helps reduce strokes, heart attacks, and other heart problems caused by atherosclerosis.
20	Protonix	Decreases stomach acid. Treats inflammation and ulcers of the esophagus and acid regurgitations.
21	Zyrtec	An antihistamine that treats hay fever and allergy symptoms, hives, and itching.
22	Advair Diskus	A steroid and a bronchodilator that prevents the symptoms of asthma or COPD and chronic bronchitis.
23	Neurontin	Controls certain types of seizures in people who have epilepsy and also treats pain caused by infections such as shingles.
24	Flonase	A corticosteroid that treats stuffy nose caused by hay fever and other allergies.
25	Viagra	Treats erectile dysfunction and also treats a lung condition and pulmonary arterial hypertension.
26	Levaquin	An antibiotic that treats infections that are caused by certain kinds of bacteria.
27	Pravachol	Lowers high levels of cholesterol, and helps prevent heart attack and stroke in people who have heart disease.
28	Lotrel	An ACE inhibitor and a calcium channel blocker that treats high blood pressure.
29	Diovan	Treats high blood pressure and heart failure. May also prolong life after a heart attack.
30	Vioxx	An NSAID that treats pain caused by arthritis, menstruation, or recent medical surgery or dental surgery. Treats pain caused by migraine headaches and certain kinds of arthritis. Withdrawn from the U.S. market in September 2004.
31	Altace	An ACE inhibitor that treats high blood pressure. Treats congestive heart failure after a heart attack. Reduces risk of heart attack, stroke, and death in people 55 years of age or older who have heart disease.
32	Klor-Con	A diuretic that treats potassium loss from the body.
33	Bextra	An NSAID that treats symptoms of osteoarthritis and rheumatoid arthritis, and also treats painful menstrual periods.
34	Celexa	A selective serotonin reuptake inhibitor (SSRI) that treats depression.
35	Ortho Evra	A birth control patch that prevents pregnancy.
36	Diovan HCT	A diuretic that treats high blood pressure.
37	Accupril	An ACE inhibitor that treats high blood pressure and heart failure.
38	Paxil CR	A selective serotonin reuptake inhibitor (SSRI) that treats depression, OCD, panic disorder, social anxiety disorder, PMS, and generalized anxiety disorder.
39	Actonel	Treats and prevents osteoporosis in women who have gone through menopause.
40	Actos	Treats type 2 diabetes and used together with diet and exercise to help control your blood sugar.
41	Wellbutrin XL	An antidepressant that treats depression and aids in quitting smoking.
42	Cozaar	Used alone or with other medicines to treat high blood pressure. Reduces the risk of stroke in patients with high blood pressure and enlargement of the heart. Treats kidney disease in patients with Type 2 diabetes and a history of high blood pressure.
43	Zetia	A statin drug that lowers cholesterol in your blood.
44	Yasmin	Prevents pregnancy.
45	Avandia	Treats type 2 diabetes and used together with proper diet and exercise to help control your blood sugar.
46	Aciphex	Treats stomach ulcers, GERD, Zollinger-Ellison syndrome, and other conditions caused by excess stomach acid.
47	Zithromax	An antibiotic that fights bacteria in the body.
48	Adderall XR	A stimulant that treats attention deficit hyperactivity disorder (ADHD).
49	Concerta	Treats attention deficit hyperactivity disorder (ADHD) and narcolepsy.
50	Flomax	An alpha-blocker that treats problems with urination caused by an enlarged prostate or BPH.

Source: Verispan, 2005.

DRUGS

DRUG EFFECTS & PRECAUTIONS

Drugs	Effects and Precautions
Antibiotics	
Cephalosporins, penicillin	Take on an empty stomach to speed absorption of the drugs.
Erythromycin	Don't take with fruit juice or wine, which decrease the drug's effectiveness.
Sulfa drugs	Increase the risk of Vitamin B-12 deficiency.
Antifungal	Best taken with food. Can cause skin rash and increase sun sensitivity.
Tetracycline	Dairy products reduce the drug's effectiveness. Lowers Vitamin C absorption.
Anticonvulsants	
Dilantin, phenobarbital	Increase the risk of anemia and nerve problems due to deficiency of folate and other B vitamins.
Antidepressants	
Fluoxetine	Reduce appetite and can lead to excessive weight loss.
Lithium	A low-salt diet increases the risk of lithium toxicity; excessive salt reduces the drug's efficacy.
MAO Inhibitors	Foods high in tyramine (aged cheeses, processed meats, legumes, wine, beer, among others) can bring on a hypertensive crisis.
Antipsychotic	Do not take if you have blood problems and liver damage.
Tricyclics	Many foods, especially legumes, meat, fish, and foods high in Vitamin C, reduce absorption of the drugs.
Antihypertensive, Heart Medications	
ACE inhibitors	Take on an empty stomach to improve the absorption of the drugs.
Alpha blockers	Take with liquid or food to avoid excessive drop in blood pressure.
Antiarrhythmic drugs	Avoid caffeine, which increases the risk of irregular heartbeat.
Beta blockers	Take on an empty stomach; food, especially meat, increases the drug's effects and can cause dizziness and low blood pressure.
Digitalis	Avoid taking with milk and high fiber foods, which reduce absorption, increasing potassium loss.
Diuretics	Increase the risk of potassium deficiency. Do not take if you have any known allergies to sulfa drugs, or oral diabetes medicine. Avoid sudden changes in posture and use caution when driving or operating machinery that requires alertness.
Nitrates	Not usually used on their own, but may be added with other medications.
Potassium sparing diuretics	Unless a doctor advises otherwise, don't take diuretics with potassium supplements or salt substitutes, which can cause potassium overload.
Thiazide diuretics	Increase the reaction to MSG.
Asthma Drugs	
Pseudoephedrine	Avoid caffeine, which increases feelings of anxiety and nervousness.
Bronchodilators	Do not use if solution turns brown or contains sold particles and follow inhaler instructions closely.
Steroids	May be risky in cases of serious infections.
Theophylline	Charbroiled foods and high protein diet reduce absorption. Caffeine increases the risk of drug toxicity.
Cholesterol Lowering Drugs	
Cholestyramine	Increases the excretion of folate and vitamins A, D, E, and K.
Gemfibrozil	Avoid fatty foods, which decrease the drug's efficacy in lowering cholesterol.
Heartburn and Ulcer Medications	
Antacids	Interfere with the absorption of many minerals; for maximum benefit, take medication 1 hour after eating.
Cimetidine, Fanotidine, Sucralfate	Avoid high protein foods, caffeine, and other items that increase stomach acidity.

DRUGS

Drugs	Effects and Precautions
Hormone Preparations	
Oral contraceptives	Salty foods increase fluid retention. Drugs reduce the absorption of folate, vitamin B-6, and other nutrients; increase intake of foods high in these nutrients to avoid deficiencies.
Steroids	Salty foods increase fluid retention. Increase intake of foods high in calcium, vitamin K, potassium, and protein to avoid deficiencies.
Thyroid drugs	Iodine-rich foods lower the drug's efficacy.
Digestives Drugs	
Stomach acid reducers	Higher doses can cause constipation, diarrhea, headaches, dizziness, and rashes.
Kaolin-pectin	Takes 1 to 4 hours to work.
Loperamide	Do not use if you have blood in diarrhea or excess temperature and use caution if you have ulcerative colitis.
Antiemetic	Do not use if you have breathing problems, emphysema, bronchitis, and difficult urination due to enlarged prostrate.
Saline laxative	Do not take if you have kidney disease, abdominal pain, nausea or vomiting.
Stool softeners	Long-term usage should be avoided.
Mineral Oils	Overuse can cause a deficiency of vitamins A, D, E, and K.
Painkillers	
Acetaminophen	Excessive amounts can cause liver disease.
Aspirin and stronger NSAIDs	Always take with food to lower the risk of gastrointestinal irritation; avoid taking with alcohol, which increases the risk of bleeding. Frequent use of these drugs lowers the absorption of folate and vitamin C.
Codeine	Increase fiber and water intake to avoid constipation.
Sleeping Pills, Tranquilizers	
Benzodiazepines	Never take with alcohol. Caffeine increases anxiety and reduces drug's effectiveness.
Cold and Allergy Drugs	
Antihistamine	Use caution if you have glaucoma, cardiovascular disease, high blood pressure, or asthma. Can have a sedative effect.
Decongestant	Take 30 minutes to 1 hour prior to work and use caution if you have heart disease or high blood pressure.
Suppressants	Drink plenty of fluids while taking these drugs.

MEDICATIONS & USAGE

Brand	Generic	Usage	Brand	Generic	Usage
Accupril	quinapril	ACE inhibitor Rx: HTN - CHF	Amikin	amikacin	Antibiotic
Accurbron	theophylline	Bronchodilator - Rx: COPD - asthma	Amiloride	midamor	Potassium-sparing diuretic - Rx: CHF - hypertension
Accutane	isotretinoin	Rx: severe cystic acne	Aminophylline	mudrane	Bronchodilator - Rx: COPD - asthma
Acebutolol	sectral	B-blocker - Rx: HTN - angina - arrhythmias	Amitril	amitriptyline	Tricyclic antidepressant
Acetaminophen	tylenol	Non-narcotic analgesic	Amitriptyline	elavil	Tricyclic antidepressant
Acetazolamide	diamox	Diuretic / anticonvulsant - Rx: glaucoma - CHF - epilepsy - mountain sickness	Amoxicillin	amcill	Antibiotic
Acetylcysteine	mucomyst	Mucolytic - Rx: asthma	Amoxil	amoxicillin	Antibiotic
Achromycin V	tetracycline	Antibiotic	Amphotericin B	fungizone	Antifungal agent
Aclovate	alclometasone	Steroid anti-inflammatory	Amytal	amobarbital	Barbiturate sedative / hypnotic
Actibine	yohimbine	Alpha-2 blocker - Rx: male impotence	Anadrol-50	oxymetholone	Androgen / steroid - Rx: anemia
Actidil	triprolidine	Antihistamine - Rx: allergies	Anafranil	clomipramine	Tricyclic antidepressant
Actifed	triprolidine + pseudoephedrine	Antihistamine /decongestant - Rx: allergies	Anaprox -	naproxen	NSAID analgesic / anti-inflammatory agent
Actigall	ursodiol	Bile acid - Rx: dissolves gall stones	Ancobon	flucytosine	Antifungal agent
Adalat	nifedipine	Calcium blocker - Rx: angina - hypertension	Android	methyltestosterone	Androgen / steroid - Rx: hypogonadism
Adapin	doxepin	Cyclic antidepressant	Anexsia	hydrocodone - apap	Narcotic analgesic
Adipex-P	phentermine	Appetite suppressant / stimulant	Anhydron	cyclothiazide	Antihypertensive / diuretic
Adrenalin	epinephrine	Bronchodilator - Rx: asthma	Ansaid	flurbiprofen	NSAID analgesic - Rx: arthritis
Advil	ibuprofen	NSAID analgesic	Antabuse	disulfiram	Inhibits metabolism of alcohol - Rx: alcohol addiction
Aerobid	flunisolide	Steroid anti-inflammatory inhaler - Rx: asthma - bronchitis	Antivert	meclizine	Anti-nausea - Rx: vertigo
Aerolate - Aerolate Iii - Aerolate Jr.	theophylline	Xanthine bronchodilator - Rx: asthma - COPD	Anturane	sulfinpyrazone	Uricosuric - Rx: gouty arthritis
Aerolone	isoproterenol	B-2 -bronchodilator - Rx: asthma	Apap	acetaminophen	Non-narcotic analgesic
Aerosporin	polymycin	Antibiotic	Apresazide	hydralazine - hctz	Antihypertensive / diuretic
Akineton	biperiden	Antiparkinsonian - Rx: prophylaxis of EPS	Apresoline	hydralazine	Antihypertensive / diuretic
Albuterol	proventil	B-2 bronchodilator - Rx: asthma - COPD	Aquatensen	methyclothiazide	Antihypertensive / diuretic
Aldactazide	hctz - spironolactone	Antihypertensive /diuretic	Aralen	chloroquine	Anti-malarial agent
Aldactone	spironolactone	Potassium-sparing diuretic	Aristocort	triamcinolone	Steroid anti-inflammatory
Aldochlor	methyldopa + chlorothiazide	Antihypertensive / diuretic compound	Artane	trihexyphenidyl	Anti-parkinsonian - Rx: prophylaxis of EPS
Aldomet	methyldopa	Antihypertensive	Asa	acetylsalicylic acid	Aspirin - NSAID analgesic
Aldoril	methyldopa + hctz	Antihypertensive compound	Asbron-G	theophylline - guaifenesin	Xanthine bronchodilator - expectorant compound Rx: asthma - copd
Alfenta	alfentanil	Narcotic analgesic / anesthetic	Asendin	amoxapine	Tricyclic antidepressant
Allopurinol	zyloprim	Reduces serum uric acid - Rx: gout	Astramorph Pf	morphine	Narcotic analgesic
Alprazolam	xanax	Benzodiazepine hypnotic	Atarax	hydroxyzine	Tranquilizer / antihistamine - Rx: urticaria - anxiety
Altace	ramipril	ACE inhibitor - Rx: hypertension	Ativan	lorazepam	Benzodiazepine hypnotic
Alupent	metaproterenol	B-2 bronchodilator - Rx: COPD - asthma	Atromid-S	clofibrate	Antilipidemic. Rx: hyperlipidemia
Alurate	aprobarbital	Barbiturate - Rx: insomnia	Atrovent	ipratropium	Anticholinergic bronchodilator - Rx: copd
Ambenyl Cough Syrup	codeine - bromodiphenhydramine	Narcotic antitussive / antihistamine - Rx: colds - allergies	Augmentin	amoxicillin - clavulanate potassium	Antibiotic
Ambien	zolpidem	Hypnotic - Rx: insomnia	Aventyl	nortriptyline	Tricyclic antidepressant
Amcill	ampicillin	Antibiotic	Axid	nizatidine	Histamine-2 antagonist - which inhibits gastric acid secretion - Rx: ulcers

MEDICATIONS & USAGE

DRUGS

Brand	Generic	Usage	Brand	Generic	Usage
Axotal	butalbital - asa	Anxiolytic / analgesic Rx: Tension H/A	Bronkaid Tablets	ephedrine - theophylline - guaifenesin	Bronchodilator / expectorant compound
Azdone	hydrocodone - asa	Narcotic analgesic compound	Bronkephrine	ethylnorepinephrine	Bronchodilator - Rx: asthma
Azmacort	triamcinolone	Steroid anti-inflammatory - Rx: asthma - bronchitis	Bronkodyl	theophylline	Bronchodilator - Rx: COPD - asthma
Azo Gantanol	sulfamethoxazole phenazopyridine	Antibiotic/analgesic - Rx: urinary tract infection	Bronkolixir	ephedrine - guaifenesin - theophylline - phenobarbital	Xanthine bronchodilator / expectorant
Azt	zidovudine	Antiviral agent - Rx: HIV AIDS virus	Bronkometer	isoetharine	B-2 bronchodilator - Rx: COPD - asthma
Azulfidine	sulfasalazine	Anti-infective - Rx: colitis	Bronkosol	isoetharine	B-2 bronchodilator - Rx: COPD - asthma
Bactocill	oxacillin	Antibiotic	Bronkotabs	ephedrine - theophylline - phenobarbital - guaifenesin	Bronchodilator / expectorant - Rx: COPD - asthma
Bactrim - Bactrim Ds	trimethoprim - sulfamethoxazole	Antibacterial - Rx: UTI - ear infection - bronchitis	Bucladin-S	buclizine	Piperazine antiemetic
Bancap Hc	hydrocodone - apap	Narcotic analgesic	Bumex	bumetanide	Diuretic - Rx: CHF - edema
Beclovent	beclomethasone	Steroid anti-inflammatory agent - Rx: COPD - asthma	Buprenex	buprenorphine	Narcotic analgesic
Beconase	beclomethasone	Steroid anti-inflammatory	Butalbital	fiorinal	Barbiturate muscle relaxant / sedative
Beepen-Vk	penicillin	Antibiotic	Butazolidin	phenylbutazone	NSAID analgesic - Rx: arthritis
Belladonna	belladenal	Antispasmodic - Rx: irritable bowel syndrome	Buticaps	butabarbital	Barbiturate sedative - Rx: insomnia
Bellergal	phenobarbital - ergotamine - belladonna	Rx: menopause - headaches - uterine cramps	Butisol	butabarbital	Barbiturate sedative - Rx: insomnia
Benadryl	diphenhydramine	Antihistamine - Rx: allergies	Clidinium	librex	Antispasmodic - Rx: peptic ulcers
Benemid	probenecid	Uricosuric - Rx: gout. Also prolongs effects of penicillin	Cafergot	ergotamine - caffeine	Cranial vasoconstrictor - Rx: migraine & vascular headaches
Bentyl	dicyclomine	GI tract antispasmodic	Cafergot P-B Suppository	ergotamine - caffeine - belladonna - pentobarbital	Cranial vasoconstrictor /antiemetic / sedative - Rx: migraine & vascular H/A
Benylin	diphenhydramine	Antihistamine	Calan - Calan Sir	verapamil	Calcium blocker - Rx: angina - hypertension - PSVT prophylaxis - headache
Benzamycin	erythromycin - benzoyl peroxide	Topical antibiotic / keratolytic compound - Rx: acne	Calcidrine	codeine - calcium iodide	Narcotic antitussive /expectorant compound
Benzthiazide	exna	Antihypertensive / diuretic	Caldecort	hydrocortisone	Steroid anti-inflammatory
Bepadin	bepridil	Calcium channel blocker - Rx: angina	Capital W/ Codeine	apap - codeine	Narcotic analgesic
Bepridil	bepadin	Calcium channel blocker - Rx: angina	Capoten	captopril	Ace inhibitor - Rx: HTN - CHF
Betaloc	metoprolol	B -blocker - Rx: HTN - angina - arrhythmias	Capozide	captopril - hctz	Antihypertensive / diuretic
Betapace	sotalol	B-blocker - Rx: angina - HTN - arrhythmias	Carafate	sucralfate	Anti-ulcer agent
Betaseron	interferon	Immunologic agent - Rx: Multiple Sclerosis	Carbamazepine	tegretol	Anticonvulsant - Rx: epilepsy
Betaxolol	kerlone	Beta blocker - Rx: HTN	Carbidopa & Levodopa	sinemet	Dopamine precursors - Rx: Parkinson's disease
Bethanechol	urecholine	Vagomimetic agent which increases bladder tone - Rx: urinary retention	Cardene	nicardipine	Calcium blocker - Rx: angina - HTN
Betoptic	betaxolol	Beta-1 blocker eye drops - Rx: glaucoma	Cardilate	erythrityl tetranitrate	Vasodilator - Rx: angina
Biaxin	clarithromycin	Antibiotic	Cardioquin	quinidine	Antiarrhythmic - Rx: cardiac dysrhythmias
Bicillin	penicillin	Antibiotic	Cardizem - Cardizem Cd - Cardizem Sr	diltiazem	Calcium blocker - Rx: angina - HTN - PSVT
Biphetamine	dextroam-phetamine - amphetamine	Stimulants	Cardura	doxazosin	Ace inhibitor alpha blocker - Rx: HTN
Blocadren	timolol	O-blocker - Rx: angina - HTN	Carisoprodol	soma	Muscle relaxant / analgesic
Brethaire	terbutaline	B-2 bronchodilator - Rx: asthma - COPD	Carteolol	cartrol	Beta blocker - Rx: HTN - angina
Brethine	terbutaline	B-2 bronchodilator - Rx: asthma - COPD	Cartrol	carteolol	Nonselective b-blocker - Rx: HTN - angina
Brevicon		Oral contraceptive	Cataflam	diclofenac	NSAID analgesic
Bricanyl	terbutaline	B-2 bronchodilator - Rx: asthma - COPD	Catapres	clonidine	Antihypertensive agent
Bronitin Mist	epinephrine	B-2 bronchodilator - Rx: asthma			
Bronkaid Mist	epinephrine	B-2 bronchodilator - Rx: asthma			

MEDICATIONS & USAGE

Brand	Generic	Usage
Catapres Tts	transdermal clonidine	Antihypertensive
Ceclor	cefaclor	Antibiotic
Ceftin	cefuroxime	Antibiotic
Cefzil	cefprozil	Antibiotic
Celestone	betamethasone	Steroid anti-inflammatory
Celontin	methsuximide	Anticonvulsant - Rx: absence SZ
Centrax	prazepam	Benzodiazepine hypnotic
Cephalexin	keflex	Antibiotic
Cephradine	anspor	Antibiotic
Chardonna-2	belladonna alkaloids - phenobarbital	Antispasmodic compound - Rx: ulcers
Chlor-Trimeton	chlorpheniramine	Antihistamine
Chlordiazepoxide	librium	Benzodiazepine hypnotic
Cipro	ciprofloxacin	Antimicrobial agent
Claforan	cefotaxime	Antibiotic
Claritin	loratadine	Non-sedating antihistamine - Rx: allergies
Cleocin	clindamycin	Antibiotic
Clindamycin	cleocin	Antibiotic
Clomipramine	anafranil	Tricyclic antidepressant
Clonidine	catapres	Antihypertensive agent
Cloxapen	cloxacillin	Antibiotic
Clozaril	clozapine	Psychotropic - Rx: schizophrenia
Codalan	codeine - apap - salicylamide - caffeine	Narcotic analgesic compound
Codeine	codeine	Narcotic analgesic / antitussive
Codiclear Dh	hydrocodone - guaifenesin	Narcotic antitussive/expectorant - Rx: coughs
Codimal Dh	hydrocodone - phenylephrine - pyrilamine	Narcotic antitussive / decongestant - Rx: colds - allergies
Codimal Expectorant	phenypropanolamine - guaifenesin	Decongestant / expectorant - Rx: colds - allergies
Codimal La	chlorpheniramine - pseudoephedrine	Antihistamine / decongestant compound - Rx: colds - allergies
Codimal Ph	codeine - phenylephrine - pyrilamine	Narcotic antitussive / decongestant compound - Rx: colds - allergies
Cogentin	benztropine	Antiparkinsonian - Rx: EPS
Cogesic	hydrocodone - apap	Narcotic analgesic compound
Cognex	tacrine	Cholinomimetic / Ach-ase inhibitor - Rx: Alzheimer's disease
Colace	docusate	Stool softener
Colbenemid	probenecid - colchicine	Uricosuric - Rx: gout
Colchicine	colbenemid	Reduces incidence of gout attacks
Colestid	colestipol	Reduces serum cholesterol
Combipres	clonidine - chlorthalidone	Antihypertensive/diuretic
Compazine	prochlorperazine	Phenothiazine antiemetic
Congess Jr/Sr	guaifenesin - pseudoephedrine	Expectorant / decongestant compound - Rx: colds - asthma

Brand	Generic	Usage
Conjugated Estrogens	premarin	Rx: menopause
Constant-T	theophylline	Bronchodilator - Rx: asthma - COPD
Cordarone	amiodarone	Ventricular antiarrhythmic
Corgard	nadolol	Beta blocker - Rx: angina - hypertension
Corzide	nadolol - bendroflumethiazide	B-blocker / antihypertensive / diuretic compound
Cotrim	sulfamethoxazole - trimethoprim	Antibacterial
Coumadin	warfarin	Anticoagulant - Rx: thrombosis prophylaxis
Cromolyn	intal	Antiallergenic - Rx: asthma prophylaxis
Crystodigin	digitoxin	Cardiac glycoside - Rx: CHF - SVT
Cutivate	fluticasone	Topical steroid anti-inflammatory - Rx: dermatoses
Cyanocobalamin	vitamin b-12	Rx: anemia
Cyclacillin	none	Antibiotic
Cyclobenzaprine	flexeril	Skeletal muscle relaxant
Cyclospasmol	cyclandelate	Vasodilator - Rx: cerebral & peripheral ischemia
Cycrin	medroxyprogesterone	Hormone - Rx: uterine bleeding
Cylert	pemoline	Stimulant - Rx: attention deficit disorder in children
Cyproheptadine	periactin	Antihistamine
Cystospaz - Cystospaz-M	hyoscyamine	Urinary tract antispasmodic
Cytotec	misoprostol	Prevents gastric ulcers caused by nsaids
Cytovene	ganciclovir	Antiviral - Rx: cytomegalovirus - ARC - AIDS
Dalgan	dezocine	Narcotic analgesic
Dallergy	chlorpheniramine - phenylephrine - methscopolamine	Antihistamine / decongestant - Rx: allergies
Dalmane	flurazepam	Hypnotic - Rx: insomnia
Damason-P	hydrocodone - asa - caffeine	Narcotic analgesic
Dantrium	dantrolene	Skeletal muscle antispasmodic - Rx: multiple sclerosis - cerebral palsy
Daranide	dichlorphenamide	Carbonic anhydrase inhibitor-lowers intraocular pressure - Rx: glaucoma
Darvocet-N	propoxyphene - apap	Narcotic analgesic
Darvon	propoxyphene	Narcotic analgesic
Darvon Compound	propoxyphene - asa - caffeine	Narcotic analgesic compound
Darvon W/Asa	propoxyphene - aspirin	Narcotic analgesic
Daypro	oxaprozin	NSAID - Rx: arthritis.
Ddavp	desmopressin	Antidiuretic hormone - Rx: nocturia - diabetes insipidus
Decadron	dexamethasone	Steroid anti-inflammatory
Declomycin	demeclocycline	Antibiotic
Deconamine	chlorpheniramine - pseudoephedrine	Antihistamine / decongestant compound - Rx: colds - allergies
Delsym	dextromethorphan	Cough suppressant
Deltasone	prednisone	Steroid anti-inflammatory agent
Demadex	torsemide	Diuretic - Rx: HTN - edema - CHF - kidney disease - liver disease.

DRUGS

Brand	Generic	Usage	Brand	Generic	Usage
Demerol	meperidine	Narcotic analgesic	Diltiazem	cardizem	Calcium blocker - Rx: angina - HTN - PSVT
Demerol Apap	meperidine - apap	Narcotic analgesic	Dimetane-Dc	codeine - brompheniramine - phenylpropanol- amine	Narcotic antitussive - antihistamine - decongestant
Demi-Regroton	chlorthalidone - reserpine	Antihypertensive / diuretic compound	Dimetapp	brompheniramine - phenylpropanolamine	Antihistamine / decongestant - Rx: allergies
Demser	metyrosine	Antihypertensive - Rx: pheochromocytoma	Diphenhydramine	benadryl	Antihistamine
Depakote	divalproex	Antiepileptic - Rx: absence seizures	Dipyridamole	persantine	Vasodilator - Rx: angina
Depen	penicillamine	Chelating agen - Rx: Wison's disease, RA	Disalcid	salsalate	NSAID - Rx: arthritis
Deponit	nitroglycerin	Transdermal nitrate Rx: angina	Disopyramide	norpace	Antiarrhythmic - Rx: pvc's
Deprol	meprobamate - benactyzine	Antidepressant/ tranquilizer compound	Disulfiram	antabuse	Inhibits metabolism of alcohol - Rx: alcohol addiction
Desoxyn	methamphetamine	Stimulant	Ditropan	oxybutynin	Anticholinergic / antispasmodic - Rx: urinary frequency - incontinence - dysuria
Desyrel	trazodone	Antidepressant	Diucardin	hydroflumethiazide	Antihypertensive / diuretic
Detensol	propranolol	B-blocker - Rx: HTN - angina - arrhythmias	Diuchlor-H	hydrochlorothiazide	Antihypertensive / diuretic
Dexamethasone	decadron	Steroid anti-inflammatory agent	Diupres	chlorothiazide - reserpine	Antihypertensive / diuretic
Dexedrine	dextroamphetamine	Stimulant	Diuril	chlorothiazide	Antihypertensive / diuretic
Dextromethorphan	delsym	Cough suppressant	Diutensen	cryptenamine - meclothiazide	Antihypertensive / diuretic compound
Diabeta	glyburide	Oral hypoglycemic - Rx: diabetes	Diutensen-R	methyclothiazide - reserpine	Antihypertensive / diuretic compound
Diabinese	chlorpropamide	Oral hypoglycemic agent - Rx: diabetes	Dizac	diazepam	Anxiolytic - antianxiety agent
Dialose	docusate	Stool softener	Docusate	dialose	Stool softener
Diamox	acetazolamide	Diuretic / anticonvulsant - Rx: glaucoma - CHF - epilepsy - mountain sickness	Dolene	propoxyphene	Narcotic analgesic
Diazepam	valium	Benzodiazepine hypnotic	Dolobid	diflunisal	NSAID analgesic
Dibenzyline	phenoxybenzamine	Alpha blocker - Rx: HTN - sweating	Dolophine	methadone	Narcotic analgesic
Dicloxacillin	dynaden	Antibiotic	Dolprn # 3	codeine - apap - asa - mgoh2 - aioh3	Buffered narcotic analgesic compound
Dicumarol	bishydroxycoumarin	Anticoagulant	Donnagel	kaolin - pectin - belladonna alkaloids	Antispasmodic / stool binder - Rx: diarrhea
Dicyclomine	bentyl	Anticholinergic - Rx: colitis	Donnagel Pg	kaolin - pectin - belladonna alkaloids - opium	Narcotic antispasmodic / stool binder - Rx: diarrhea
Didrex	benzphetamine	Stimulant - Rx: obesity	Donnatal	phenobarbital - belladonna alkaloids	Barbiturate sedative - antispasmodic - Rx: ulcers
Diethylpropion	tepanil	Stimulant	Doral	quazepam	Benzodiazepine hypnotic - Rx: insomnia
Diflucan	fluconazole	Antifungal agent	Doryx	doxycycline	Antibiotic
Diflunisal	dolobid	NSAID analgesic	Dovonex	calcipoprine	Topical agent Rx: psoriasis
Digitoxin	crystodigin	Cardiac glycoside - Rx: CHF - supraventricular dysrhythmias	Doxepin	sinequan	Tricyclic antidepressant
Digoxin	lanoxin	Cardiac glycoside - Rx: CHF - supraventricular dysrhythmias	Doxidan	docusate - danthron	Stool softener
Dihydrocodeine	synalgos-dc	Narcotic analgesic	Doxycycline	vibramycin	Antibiotic
Dilacor	diltiazem	Calcium blocker - Rx: angina - HTN - PSVT	Dramamine	dimenhydrinate	Anti-nausea
Dilacor Xr	diltiazem	Calcium blocker - Rx: HTN	Drixoral	dexbrompheniramine - pseudoephedrine	Antihistamine / decongestant - Rx: allergies
Dilantin	phenytoin	Anticonvulsant	Dss	docusate	Stool softener
Dilatrate Sr	isosorbide dinitrate	Long-acting nitrate - Rx: angina prophylaxis	Dulcolax	bisacodyl	Laxative
Dilaudid	hydromorphone	Narcotic analgesic	Duo-Medihaler	isoproterenol - phenylephrine	Bronchodilator - decongestant - Rx: asthma - COPD
Dilor - Dilor-200 - Dilor-400 - Dilor Elixir	dyphylline	Xanthine bronchodilator - Rx: asthma - COPD	Duocet	hydrocodone - apap	Narcotic analgesic compound
Dilor-G	dyphylline - guaifenesin	Bronchodilator / expectorant	Duotrate	pentaerythritol tetranitrate	Long-acting nitrate - Rx: angina prophylaxis

MEDICATIONS & USAGE

DRUGS

Brand	Generic	Usage	Brand	Generic	Usage
Duradyne	hydrocodone - apap	Narcotic analgesic	Equanil	meprobamate	Tranquilizer
Duragesic	fentanyl	Narcotic analgesic	Ergo-Stat	ergotamine	Cerebral vasoconstrictor - Rx: migraines
Duramorph	morphine	Narcotic analgesic	Ery-Tab	erythromycin	Antibiotic
Duraquin	quinidine	Rx: cardiac dysrhythmias	Eryc	erythromycin	Antibiotic
Duratuss	hydrocodone - pseudoephedrine - guaifenesin	Antitussive - decongestant - expectorant - Rx: colds - allergies	Erythrityl Tetranitrate	cardilate	Long-acting nitrate
Duretic	methyclothiazide	Antihypertensive / diuretic	Erythrocin	erythromycin	Antibiotic
Duricef	cefadroxil	Antibiotic	Esgic	apap - caffeine - butalbital	Analgesic / muscle relaxant / antianxiety compound - Rx: headache
Dyazide	hctz - triamterene	Antihypertensive / diuretic - Rx: HTN	Esgic C Codeine	apap - caffeine - butalbital - codeine	Analgesic / muscle relaxant / anxiolytic compound
Dycill	dicloxacillin	Antibiotic	Esidrix	hctz	Antihypertensive / diuretic
Dymelor	acetohexamide	Oral hypoglycemic	Esimil	guanethidine - hctz	Antihypertensive / diuretic
Dynacirc	isradipine	Calcium blocker - Rx: HTN - angina	Eskalith	lithium	Tranquilizer - Rx: mania - depression
Dynapen	dicloxacillin	Antibiotic	Esp	erythromycin - sulfisoxazole	Antibiotic compound
Dyphylline	lufyllin	Bronchodilator - Rx: COPD - asthma	Estrace	estradiol	Estrogen - Rx: menopause
Dyrenium	triamterene	Potassium-sparing diuretic - Rx: CHF	Estraderm	estradiol	Topical estrogen - Rx: menopause
E-Mycin	erythromycin	Antibiotic	Estropipate	ogen	Estrogens - Rx: menopause
Easprin	asa	NSAID analgesic - Rx: arthritis	Ethatab	ethaverine	Smooth muscle relaxant / vasodilator - Rx: vascular insufficiency - GI & GU tract spasm.
Ecotrin	aspirin	Enteric coated aspirin - NSAID analgesic	Ethmozine	moricizine	Antiarrhythmic - Rx: severe ventricular dysrhythmias
Edecrin	ethacrynic acid	Diuretic - Rx: CHF	Etrafon	perphenazine - amitriptyline	Major tranquilizer - tricyclic antidepressant - Rx: anxiety with depression
Ees	erythromycin	Antibiotic	Eutonyl	pargyline	MAO inhibitor - Rx: hypertension
Effexor	venlafaxine	Antidepressant	Eutron	pargyline - methyclothiazide	MAO inhibitor / antihypertensive / diuretic - Rx: hypertension
Elavil	amitriptyline	Tricyclic antidepressant	Exna	benzthiazide	Antihypertensive/diuretic
Eldepryl	selegiline	MAO inhibitor - Rx: Parkinson's disease	Extendryl	phenylephrine - methscopolamine - chlorpheniramine	Antihistamine - decongestant - Rx: allergies
Elimite	permethrin	Topical scabicidal agent - Rx: scabies - lice	Famvir	famciclovir	Antiviral - Rx: shingles
Elixophyllin	theophylline	Bronchodilator - Rx: asthma - COPD	Fastin	phentermine	Stimulant - Rx: appetite suppression
Elocon	mometasone	Topical steroid anti-inflammatory	Felbatol	felbamate	Antiepileptic Rx: seizures
Emetrol	glucose - fructose - phosphoric acid	Anti-nausea	Feldene	piroxicam	NSAID analgesic
Empirin W/ Codeine	asa - codeine	Narcotic analgesic	Felodipine	renedil	Calcium blocker - Rx: HTN - angina
Endep	amitriptyline	Tricyclic antidepressant	Femcet	apap - butalbital - caffeine	Analgesic / anxiolytic - Rx: tension headaches
Enduron	methyclothiazide	Antihypertensive / diuretic	Feosol	ferrous sulfate	Iron supplement
Enduronyl	methyclothiazide - daserpidine	Antihypertensive / diuretic compound	Fergon	ferrous gluconate	Iron supplement
Enkaid	encainide	Ventricular antiarrhythmic	Fevernol	apap	Antipyretic/analgesic suppository
Enovid	norethynodrel - mestranol	Oral contraceptive	Fioricet	butalbital - apap - caffeine	Analgesic - Rx: h/a
Entex La	phenylpropanolamine - guaifenesin	Decongestant / expectorant compound	Fiorinal	butalbital - asa - caffeine	Non-narcotic analgesic
Ephed li	ephedrine	Bronchodilator - decongestant	Fiorinal W/ Codeine	butalbital - asa - caffeine - codeine	Narcotic analgesic compound
Ephedrine	tedral	Bronchodilator - Rx: asthma - COPD	Flagyl	metronidazole	Antimicrobial agent
Epi-Pen	epinephrine	Bronchodilator - vasoconstrictor - Rx: allergic reaction	Flatulex	simethicone - activated charcoal	Anti-flatulent
Epinephrine	bronkaid-mist	Bronchodilator - Rx: asthma	Flexeril	cyclobenzaprine	Skeletal muscle relaxant
Equagesic	meprobamate - asa	Tranquilizer / analgesic	Florone	diflorasone	Steroid anti-inflammatory agent

MEDICATIONS & USAGE

DRUGS

Brand	Generic	Usage	Brand	Generic	Usage
Floropryl	isoflurophate	Topical miotic - Rx: glaucoma	Hydralazine	apresoline	Antihypertensive agent
Floxin	ofloxacin	Antibiotic	Hydrex	benzthiazide	Antihypertensive / diuretic
Flumadine	rimantadine	Antiviral - Rx: influenza A	Hydro Diuril	hctz	Antihypertensive / diuretic
Fortaz	ceftazidime	Antibiotic	Hydro-Chlor	hydrochlorothiazide	Antihypertensive / diuretic
Fulvicin	griseofulvin	Antifungal agent	Hydro-D	hydrochlorothiazide	Antihypertensive / diuretic
Furadantin	nitrofurantoin	Antibacterial agent - Rx: UTI	Hydrocet	hydrocodone - apap	Narcotic analgesic compound
Furosemide	lasix	Diuretic - Rx: CHF - hypertension	Hydrochlorothiazide	hctz	Antihypertensive / diuretic
Gantanol	sulfamethoxazole	Antibacterial agent - Rx: UTI	Hydrocodone	vicodin	Narcotic analgesic / antitussive
Gantrisin	sulfisoxazole	Antibacterial agent - Rx: UTI	Hydrocodone W! Apap	t-gesic	Narcotic analgesic
Garamycin	gentamicin	Antibiotic	Hydrocortisone	cortef	Steroid anti-inflammatory agent
Gemnisyn	apap - asa	Non-narcotic analgesic	Hydroflumethiazide	salutensin	Antihypertensive / diuretic
Genora	ethinyl estradiol	Oral contraceptive	Hydromorphone	dilaudid	Narcotic analgesic / antitussive
Gentamicin	garamycin	Antibiotic	Hydromox	quinethazone	Diuretic - Rx: hypertension
Geocillin	carbenicillin	Antibiotic	Hydropres	hctz - reserpine	Antihypertensive / diuretic
Geopen	carbenicillin	Antibiotic	Hydroxyzine	atarax	Antiemetic / antitussive agent
Glucagon	glucoagon	Hormone which releases glucose from the liver - Rx: hypoglycemia	Hygroton	chlorthalidone	Antihypertensive / diuretic
Glucophage	metformin	Oral hypoglycemic - Rx: diabetes	Hylorel	guanadrel	Sympatholytic antihypertensive
Glucotrol	glipizide	Oral hypoglycemic - Rx: diabetes	Hyoscyamine	cystospaz	Antispasmodic - Rx: lower UTI & GI tract spasm
Glynase	glyburide	Oral hypoglycemic - Rx: diabetes	Hytrin	terazosin	Antihypertensive agent
Grifulvin V	griseofulvin	Antifungal - Rx: ringworm	Iletin	insulin	Insulin preparations - Rx: diabetes mellitus
Grisactin	griseofulvin	Antifungal agent	Ilosone	erythromycin	Antibiotic
Guaifed - Guaifed-Pd	guaifenesin - pseudoephedrine	Expectorant / decongestant	Imdur	isosorbide mononitrate	Long-acting nitrate - Rx: angina prophylaxis.
Guanethidine	ismelin	Sympatholytic antihypertensive agent	Imipramine	tofranil	Tricyclic antidepressant
Gyne-Lotrimin	clotrimazole	Antifungal agent	Imitrex	sumatriptan	Auto-injectible drug - Rx: migraine H/A
Halcion	triazolam	Benzodiazepine hypnotic - Rx: insomnia	Imodium	loperamide	Slows peristalsis - Rx: diarrhea
Haldol	haloperidol	Major tranquilizer	Imuran	azathioprine	Immunosuppressant - Rx: organ transplants - ulcerative colitis - lupus - severe arthritis
Harmonyl	daserpidine	Sedative / antihypertensive	Inapsine	droperidol	Major tranquilizer
Hctz	hydrochlorothiazide	Antihypertensive / diuretic - Rx: HTN	Inderal	propranolol	Beta blocker - Rx: HTN - prophylaxis of: angina - cardiac dysrhythmias - AMI - migraine H/A
Hexadrol	dexamethasone	Steroid anti-inflammatory	Inderal La	propranolol	Long-acting B-blocker - Rx: HTN; prophylaxis of: angina - cardiac dysrhythmias - AMI - & migraine H/A
Hismanal.	astemizole	Antihistamine - Rx: allergies	Inderide	propranolol - hctz	Beta blocker - antihypertensive / diuretic compound - Rx: hypertension
Hivid	zalcitabine	Antiviral - Rx: AIDS	Indocin	indomethacin	NSAID analgesic - Rx: arthritis
Humorsol	demecarium	Topical miotic - Rx: glaucoma	Indomethacin	indocin	NSAID analgesic - Rx: arthritis
Hycodan	hydrocodone - homatropine	Narcotic antitussive	Inn	isoniazid	Antibiotic - Rx: TB
Hycomine Compound	hydrocodone - chlorpheniramine - apap - caffeine - phenylephrine	Narcotic antitussive / antihistamine / decongestant - Rx: colds - URI	Intal	cromolyn	Antiallergic - Rx: asthma prophylaxis
Hycomine Syrup	hydrocodone - phenylpropanolamine	Narcotic antitussive /decongestant - Rx: cough - nasal congests.	Inversine	mecamylamine	Antihypertensive agent
Hycotuss	hydrocodone - guaifenesin	Narcotic antitussive / expectorant	Ionamin	phentermine	Stimulant - Rx: appetite suppression
Hydergine	ergoloids	Rx: improves mentation in the elderly	Ismelin	guanethidine	Sympatholytic antihypertensive agent
			Iso-Bid	isosorbide dinitrate	Long-acting nitrate - Rx: angina

MEDICATIONS & USAGE

Brand	Generic	Usage	Brand	Generic	Usage
Isoclor Expectorant	codeine - pseudoephedrine - guaifenesin	Narcotic antitussive / decongestant / expectorant compound - Rx: cough - colds	Levsin	hyoscyamine	Antispasmodic - Rx: ulcers
Isocom	isometheptene - dichloralphenazone - apap	Cerebral vasoconstrictor - sedative - analgesic - Rx: headaches	Librax	chlordiazepoxide - clidinium	Benzodiazepine hypnotic - antispasmodic compound - Rx: ulcers
Isoniazid	inh	Antibiotic - Rx: TB	Libritabs	chlordiazepoxide	Benzodiazepine hypnotic
Isoproterenol	isuprel	B-bronchodilator - Rx: asthma - COPD	Librium	chlordiazepoxide	Benzodiazepine hypnotic
Isoptin - Isoptin Sr	verapamil	Calcium blocker - Rx: angina - hypertension - PSVT prophylaxis - headache	Limbitrol - Limbitrol Ds	chlordiazepoxide - amitriptyline	Benzodiazepine hypnotic / tricyclic antidepressant - Rx: depression with anxiety
Isordil	isosorbide dinitrate	Long-acting nitrate - Rx: angina	Lithane	lithium	Anti-manic agent - Rx: depression - mania
Isosorbide Dinitrate	isordil	Long-acting nitrate - Rx: angina	Lithium Carbonate	lithobid	Anti-manic - Rx: depression - mania
Isoxsuprine	vasodilan	Beta vasodilator - Rx: cerebral & peripheral ischemia	Lithobid	lithium	Anti-manic agent - Rx: depression - mania
Isuprel	isoproterenol	Bronchodilator - Rx: asthma	Lithonate	lithium	Anti-manic agent - Rx: depression - mania
K-Dur	kcl	Potassium supplement	Lithotabs	lithium	Anti-manic agent - Rx: depression - mania
K-Lor	kcl	Potassium supplement	Lo-Ovral	ethinyl estradiol	Oral contraceptive
K-Lyte	kcl	Potassium supplement	Lodine	etodolac	NSAID - analgesic
K-Norm	kcl	Potassium supplement	Lomotil	diphenoxylate - atropine	Narcotic anti-diarrhea / antispasmodic compound
Kaolin - Pectin	kaopectate	Stool binder - Rx: diarrhea	Loniten	minoxidil	Vasodilator - Rx: hypertension - baldness
Kaopectate	kaolin-pectin	Stool binder - Rx: diarrhea	Lopid	gemfibrozil	Lowers serum lipids
Kenalog	triamcinolone	Steroid anti-inflammatory agent	Lopressor	metoprolol	Beta-1 blocker - Rx: hypertension
Kerlone	betaxolol	Beta-1 blocker - Rx: HTN	Lopurin	allopurinol	Reduces uric acid in gout
Ketoprofen	orudis	NSAID - Rx: arthritis	Lorazepam	ativan	Benzodiazepine hypnotic
Klonopin	clonazepam	Benzodiazepine hypnotic	Lorcet Hd - Lorcet Plus	hydrocodone - apap	Narcotic analgesic compound
Klor-Con	kcl	Potassium supplement	Lorelco	probucol	Reduces serum cholesterol
Klorvess	kcl	Potassium supplement	Lortab	hydrocodone - apap	Narcotic analgesic
Klotrix	kcl	Potassium supplement	Lortab Asa	hydrocodone - asa	Narcotic analgesic
Kolyum	potassium chloride	Potassium supplement	Lotensin	benazepril	Ace inhibitor - Rx: HTN
Labetalol	normodyne	Beta blocker - Rx: HTN - angina	Lotrimin	clotrimazole	Antifungal agent
Lamictal	lamotrigine	Antiepileptic - Rx: absence seizures	Lotrisone	clotrimazole - betamethasone	Topical antifungal / steroid anti-inflammatory compound
Lanoxicaps	digoxin	Cardiac glycoside - Rx: CHF - supraventricular dysrhythmias	Loxitane	loxapine	Tranquilizer
Lanoxin	digoxin	Cardiac glycoside - Rx: CHF - dysrhythmias	Lozol	indapamide	Antihypertensive / diuretic
Larodopa	levodopa - carbidopa	Dopamine precursors - Rx: Parkinson's disease	Ludiomil	maprotiline	Tetracyclic antidepressant
Lasix	furosemide	Diuretic - Rx: CHF - hypertension - edema	Lufyllin	dyphylline	Bronchodilator - Rx: COPD - asthma
Laudanum	tincture of opium	Narcotic analgesic	Luminal	phenobarbital	Barbiturate sedative / anticonvulsant
Ledercillin	penicillin	Antibiotic	Lurline PMS	apap - pamabrom - pyridoxine	Analgesic / diuretic / vitamin B-6 - Rx: premenstrual syndrome
Lescol	fluvastatin	Cholesterol reducer	Luvox	fluvoxamine	Rx: obsessive compulsive disorder
Levatol	penbutolol	Beta blocker - Rx: hypertension	Macrobid	nitrofurantoin	Antibacterial - Rx: UTI
Levo-Dromoran	levorphanol	Narcotic analgesic	Macrodantin	nitrofurantoin	Antibacterial - Rx: UTI
Levorphan	levorphanol	Narcotic analgesic	Magan	magnesium salicylate	NSAID - Rx: arthritis
Levorphanol	levorphan	Narcotic analgesic	Magonate	magnesium gluconate	Electrolyte sedative - Rx: alcoholism - HTN - asthma
Levothroid	levothyroxine	Thyroid hormone	Mandelamine	methylamine	Antibacterial - Rx: UTI
Levoxine	levothyroxine	Thyroid hormone	Marax	ephedrine - theophylline - hydroxyzine	Bronchodilator compound - Rx: asthma

MEDICATIONS & USAGE

DRUGS

Brand	Generic	Usage	Brand	Generic	Usage
Marinol	dronabinol	Appetite stimulant - Rx: weight loss in AIDS - chemotherapy	Midamor	amiloride	Potassium-sparing diuretic
Marplan	isocarboxazid	Mad inhibitor - Rx: depression	Midol 200	ibuprofen	NSAID - Rx: menstrual cramps
Materna	prenatal vitamin	Vitamin supplement	Midol PMS	apap - pamabrom - pyrilamine	Analgesic - diuretic - antihistamine/ sedative - Rx: premenstrual syndrome
Maxair	pirbuterol	Beta-2 stimulant - Rx: asthma - COPD	Milontin	phensuximide	Anticonvulsant - Rx: absence Sz
Maxzide	triamterene - hctz	Anti-hypertensive / diuretic	Miltown	meprobamate	Tranquilizer
Mebaral	mephobarbital	Barbiturate sedative / anticonvulsant	Minipress	prazosin	Alpha-1 blocker - Rx: hypertension
Meclizine	antivert	Anti-nausea - Rx: vertigo	Minizide	prazosin - polythiazide	Antihypertensive
Meclomen	meclofenamate	NSAID - Rx: arthritis - pain - dysmenorrhea - heavy menstrual blood loss	Minocin	minocycline	Antibiotic
Medihaler-Epi	epinephrine	B-bronchodilator - Rx: asthma	Minoxidil	loniten	Vasodilator / antihypertensive / topical hair growing agent - Rx: HTN - baldness
Medrol	methylprednisolone	Steroid anti-inflammatory	Moban	molindone	Tranquilizer
Mefoxin	cefoxitin	Antibiotic	Moduretic	amiloride - hctz	Antihypertensive / diuretic
Megace	megestrol	Appetite stimulant - Rx: anorexia with AIDS	Monistat 7	micronazole	Antifungal agent
Mellaril	thioridazine	Major tranquilizer	Monitan	acebutolol	B-blocker - Rx: HTN - angina - arrhythmias
Menrium	chlordiazepoxide - estrogens	Anxiolytic / hormone compound - Rx: menopause symptoms	Mono-Gesic	salsalate	NSAID - Rx: arthritis
Mepergan	meperidine - promethazine	Narcotic analgesic - phenothiazine sedative/antiemetic	Monoclate-P	factor viii	Antihemophilic factor
Meperidine	demerol	Narcotic analgesic	Monoket	isosorbide mononitrate	Nitrate - Rx: angina
Meprobamate	meprospan	Tranquilizer	Monopril	fosinopril	Ace inhibitor - Rx: HTN
Mepron	atovaquone	Antibiotic - Rx: pneumocystis carinii pneumonia in AIDS	Morphine Sulfate	morphine	Narcotic analgesic
Meprospan	meprobamate	Tranquilizer	Motofen	difenoxin - atropine	Narcotic antidiarrheal agent
Mesantoin	mephenytoin	Anticonvulsant	Ms Contin	morphine	Narcotic analgesic
Mestinon	pyridostigmine	Anticholinesterase - Rx: myasthenia gravis	Msir	morphine	Narcotic analgesic
Metahydrin	trichlormethiazide	Antihypertensive / diuretic	Mucomyst	acetylcysteine	Mucolytic - Rx: asthma
Metaprel Inhaler	metaproterenol	Bronchodilator - Rx: COPD - asthma	Myambutol	ethambutol	Chemotherapeutic - Rx: TB
Metastron	strontium	Non-narcotic analgesic - Rx: bone ca	Mycobutin	rifabutin	Antibiotic - Rx: AIDS
Metatensin	trichlormethiazide - reserpine	Antihypertensive / diuretic	Mycolog li	nystatin - triamcinolone	Antifungal / steroid
Methadone	dolophine	Narcotic analgesic	Mycostatin	nystatin	Antifungal agent
Methergine	methylergonovine	Uterotonic - Rx: postpartum hemorrhage	Mykrox	metolazone	Antihypertensive / diuretic
Methocarbamol	robaxin	Skeletal muscle antispasmodic	Mysoline	primidone	Anticonvulsant - Rx: epilepsy
Methyclothiazide	aquatensen	Antihypertensive / diuretic	Nadolol	corgard	B-blocker - Rx: HTN - angina - arrhythmias
Methyldopa	aldomet	Antihypertensive	Naftin	naftifine	Topical antifungal agent
Methylprednisolone	medrol	Steroid anti-inflammatory	Naldecon	phenylpropanolamine - phenylephrine - phenyltoloxamine - chlorpheniramine	Antihistamine / decongestant compound - Rx: colds - allergies
Metoclopramide	reglan	Improves gastric emptying - Rx: heartburn - ulcers	Nalfon	fenoprofen	NSAID analgesic
Metoprolol	lopressor	Cardio selective beta blocker - Rx: HTN - angina - arrhythmias	Naprosyn	naproxen	NSAID analgesic
Metronidazole	flagyl	Antimicrobial agent	Naproxen	anaprox	NSAID analgesic
Mevacor	lovastatin	Lowers serum cholesterol	Naqua	trichlormethiazide	Antihypertensive / diuretic
Mexitil	mexiletine	Antiarrhythmic	Naquavil	trichlormethiazide - reserpine	Antihypertensive / diuretic
Micro-K	kcl	Potassium supplement	Nardil	phenelzine	MAO inhibitor - Rx: depression
Micronase	glyburide	Oral hypoglycemic - Rx: diabetes	Nasalcrom	cromolyn	Antiallergic - Rx: allergic rhinitis

DRUGS

Brand	Generic	Usage	Brand	Generic	Usage
Nasalide	flunisolide	Steroid anti-inflammatory agent	Norlestrin	ethinyl estradiol	Oral contraceptive
Naturetin	bendroflumethiazide	Antihypertensive / diuretic	Normodyne	labetalol	Beta blocker - Rx: HTN - angina
Navane	thiothixene	Major tranquilizer	Noroxin	norfloxacin	Urinary tract antibiotic
Nebupent	pentamidine	Anti-protozoal agent - Rx: pneumocystis carinii infection in AIDS	Norpace	disopyramide	Antiarrhythmic - Rx: pvc's
Nembutal	pentobarbital	Barbiturate sedative / hypnotic	Norpramin	desipramine	Tricyclic antidepressant
Neo-Codima	hydrochlorothiazide	Antihypertensive / diuretic	Norvasc	amlodipine	Calcium blocker - Rx: HTN - angina
Neosporin	polymycin - bacitracin - neomycin	Antibiotic	Novahistine Dh	codeine - pseudoephedrine - chlorpheniramine	Narcotic antitussive / decongestant / antihistamine
Neothylline	dyphylline - guaifenesin	Xanthine bronchodilator compound - Rx: COPD - asthma	Novahistine Expectorant	codeine - pseudoephedrine - guaifenesin	Narcotic antitussive / decongestant / expectorant
Neptazane	methazolamide	Reduces intraocular pressure - Rx: glaucoma	Novo-Hydrazide	hydrochlorothiazide	Antihypertensive /diuretic
Neurontin	gabapentin	Antiepileptic	Novolin	insulin	Rx: diabetes mellitus
Neutrexin	trimetrexate	Antineoplastic - Rx: Ca & pneumocystis pneumonia in AIDS.	Novopranol	propranolol	Beta blocker - Rx: HTN - angina - arrhythmias
Nia-Bid	niacin	Reduces serum cholesterol	Novosalmol	albuterol	B-2 bronchodilator - Rx: asthma - COPD
Niacels	nicotinic acid	Reduces serum cholesterol niacin	Nubain	nalbuphine	Narcotic analgesic
Nicobid	niacin	Reduces serum cholesterol	Nucofed	codeine. pseudoephedrine	Narcotic antitussive / decongestant
Nicolar	niacin	Reduces serum cholesterol	Numorphan	oxymorphone	Narcotic analgesic
Nifedipine	procardia	Calcium blocker - Rx: angina - HTN	Nuprin	ibuprofen	NSAID analgesic
Nilstat	nystatin	Antifungal agent	Nylidrin	arlidin	Beta vasodilator - Rx: peripheral ischemia
Nimotop	nimodipine	Calcium channel blocker - improves neurological deficits after subarachnoid hemorrhage	Nystatin	mycostatin	Antifungal agent
Nisentil	alphaprodine	Narcotic analgesic	Octamide	metoclopramide	Improves gastric emptying - Rx: heartburn - ulcers
Nitro-Bid	nitroglycerin	Long-acting nitrate - Rx: angina prophylaxis	Ogen	estropipate	Estrogen - Rx: menopause
Nitro-Dur	nitroglycerin	Long-acting nitrate - Rx: angina prophylaxis	Omnipen	ampicillin	Antibiotic
Nitrodisc	nitroglycerin	Long-acting nitrate - Rx: angina prophylaxis	Optimine	azatadine	Antihistamine - Rx: urticaria - rhinitis
Nitrofurantoin	furadantin	Antibacterial agent - Rx: UTI	Oramorph	morphine sulfate	Narcotic analgesic
Nitrogard	nitroglycerin	Long-acting nitrate - Rx: angina prophylaxis	Orap	pimozide	Antipsychotic - Rx: meter & phonic tics
Nitroglycerin	nitrostat	Vasodilator - Rx: angina	Oretic	hydrochlorothiazide	Antihypertensive / diuretic
Nitrol	nitroglycerin	Nitrate ointment - Rx: angina	Oreticyl	hctz - deserpidine	Antihypertensive
Nitrolingual Spray	nitroglycerin	Nitrate - Rx: angina	Orinase	tolbutamide	Oral hypoglycemic - Rx: diabetes
Nitrong	nitroglycerin	Nitrate - Rx: angina prophylaxis	Orlaam	levomethadyl	Opiate agonist - Rx: narcotic addition
Nitrostat	nitroglycerin	Vasodilator - Rx: angina	Ornade	chlorpheniramine - phenylpropanolamine	Antihistamine/ decongestant compound
Nix	permethrin	Parasiticide - Rx: head lice			
Nizoral	ketoconazole	Antifungal agent - Rx: yeast infections	Ortho-Novum	ortho	Oral contraceptive
Nolamine	phenindamine - chlorpheniramine - phenylpropanolamine	Antihistamine / decongestant	Orudis	ketoprofen	NSAID - Rx: arthritis
Nolvadex	tamoxifen	Anticancer agent - Rx: breast ca	Oruvail	ketoprofen	NSAID analgesic
Nordette	ethinyl estradiol	Oral contraceptive	OsCal	calcium carbonate	Calcium & Vitamin D supplement
Norflex	orphenadrine	Non-narcotic analgesic	Ovcon	ethinyl estradiol	Oral contraceptive
Norgesic	orphenadrine	Non-narcotic analgesic	Ovide	malathion	Organophosphate insecticide - Rx: lice
Norinyl	ethinyl estradiol	Oral contraceptive	Ovral	ethinyl estradiol	Oral contraceptive
Norisodrine Aerotrol	isoproterenol	B-bronchodilator -Rx: asthma - COPD	Oxacillin	antibiotic	Antibiotic

DRUGS

Brand	Generic	Usage	Brand	Generic	Usage
Oxazepam	serax	Benzodiazepine hypnotic	Peritrate	pentaerythritol tetranitrate	Long-acting nitrate - Rx: angina prophylaxis
Oxistat	oxiconazole	Topical antifungal agent	Permax	pergolide	Dopamine receptor stimulator - Rx: Parkinson's disease
Oxprenolol	trasicor	B-blocker - Rx: HTN - angina - arrhythmias	Perphenazine	trilafon	Phenothiazine major tranquilizer
Oxycodone	percodan	Narcotic analgesic	Persantine	dipyridamole	Cerebral & coronary vasodilator - Rx: CVA - angina
Oxycodone W/Apap	tylox	Narcotic analgesic compound	Pertofrane	desipramine	Tricyclic antidepressant
Pabalate	salicylate - aminobenzoate	Analgesic	Phazyme	simethicone	Anti-gas agent
Pamelor	nortriptyline	Tricyclic antidepressant	Phenaphen With Codeine	apap - codeine	Narcotic analgesic
Panmycin	tetracycline	Antibiotic	Phenergan	promethazine	Phenothiazine sedative / antiemetic
Pantopon	opium alkaloids	Narcotic analgesic	Phenobarbital	luminal	Barbiturate sedative / anticonvulsant
Panwarfarin	warfarin	Anticoagulant	Phenurone	phenacemide	Antiepileptic
Panwarfin	warfarin	Anticoagulant	Phenylbutazone	butazolidin	NSAID - Rx: arthritis
Papaverine	pavabid	Vasodilator - Rx: cerebral & peripheral vascular ischemia	Phenylpropanolamine W/ Guaifenesin	entex la	Decongestant / expectorant compound
Paradione	paramethadione	Antiepileptic agent - Rx: absence seizures	Phenytoin	dilantin	Anticonvulsant - Rx: epilepsy
Paraflex	chlorzoxazone	Skeletal muscle antispasmodic - Rx: sprains - strains	Phrenilin	butalbital - apap	Analgesic compound
Parafon Forte	chlorzoxazone - acetaminophen	Muscle relaxant / analgesic compound	Pindolol	visken	Bata blocker - Rx: HTN - angina
Paregoric	tincture of opium	Narcotic - Rx: diarrhea	Placidyl	ethchlorvynol	Hypnotic - Rx: insomnia
Parepectolin	opium - pectin	Narcotic analgesic / stool binder compound - Rx: diarrhea	Plaquenil	hydroxychloroquine	Antimalarial agent
Parlodel	bromocriptine	Ergot - Rx: Parkinson's disease; also decreases milk production in the postpartum female	Plendil	felodipine	Calcium blocker - Rx: HTN - angina
Parnate	tranylcypromine	MAO inhibiter - Rx: depression	Pmb 200 & 400	estrogens - meprobamate	Rx: s/s menopause
Pavabid	papaverine	Vasodilator - Rx: cerebral & peripheral vascular disease	Polaramine	dexchlorpheniramine	Antihistamine - Rx: allergies
Paxil	paroxetine	Antidepressant.	Poly-Vi-Flor	multivitamin	Vitamins with fluoride
Paxipam	halazepam	Benzodiazepine hypnotic	Polycillin	ampicillin	Antibiotic polymycin
Pce	erythromycin	Antibiotic	Pondimin	fenfluramine	Stimulant - Rx: appetite suppression
Pediaprofen	ibuprofen	NSAID analgesic / antipyretic	Ponstel	mefenamic acid	NSAID analgesic
Pediazole	erythoromycin	Antibiotic compound	Potassium	potassium supplement	K-tab
Peganone	ethotoin	Antiepileptic - Rx: seizures	Pravachol	pravastatin	Cholesterol reducer
Pen-Vee K	penicillin	Antibiotic	Prazosin	minipress	Alpha-1 blocker - vasodilator - Rx: HTN
Penbutolol	levatol	Beta blocker - Rx: HTN - angina	Prednisolone	prelone	Steroid anti-inflammatory agent
Penicillin	penicilin	Antibiotic	Prednisone	deltasone	Steroid anti-inflammatory agent
Pentam 300	pentamidine	Antimicrobial - Rx: pneumocystis carinii pneumonia	Prelone Syrup	prednisolone	Steroid anti-inflammatory agent
Pentasa	mesalamine	For ulcerative colitis	Preludin	phenmetrazine	Stimulant - Rx: appetite suppression Rx: ulcers - esophagitis
Pentids	penicillin	Antibiotic	Primatene Mist	epinephrine	Bronchodilator - Rx: asthma
Pentritol	pentaerythritol tetranitrate	Long-acting nitrate - Rx: angina prophylaxis	Primatene Tablets	theophylline - ephedrine - phenobarbital	Xanthine bronchodilator - Rx: asthma
Pepcid	famotidine	Histamine-2 blocker which inhibits gastric acid production - Rx: ulcers	Primidone	mysoline	Anticonvulsant - Rx: epilepsy
Percocet	oxycodone - apap	Narcotic analgesic	Principen	ampicillin	Antibiotic
Percodan	oxycodone - aspirin	Narcotic analgesic	Prinivil	lisinopril	Ace inhibitor - Rx: HTN - CHF
Percodan-Demi	oxycodone - aspirin	Narcotic analgesic	Prinzide	lisinopril - hctz	Antihypertensive compound
Periactin	cyproheptadine	Antihistamine	Pro-Banthine	propantheline	Anticholinergic - Rx: ulcers

MEDICATIONS & USAGE

Brand	Generic	Usage	Brand	Generic	Usage
Probenecid	benemid	Increases uric acid secretion in gout; also slows the elimination of penicillin from the body	Renese	polythiazide	Antihypertensive / diuretic
Procainamide	procan	Antiarrhythmic - Rx: pvc's	Renese-R	polythiazide - reserpine	Antihypertensive / diuretic compound - Rx: hypertension
Procan	procainamide	Antiarrhythmic - Rx: pvc's	Renormax	spirapril	Ace inhibitor - Rx: hypertension
Procardia - Procardia Xl	nifedipine	Calcium channel blocker - Rx: angina - hypertension	Rescudose	morphine	Oral narcotic analgesic
Prochlorperazine	compazine	Phenothiazine antiemetic	Reserpine	serpasil	Antihypertensive / tranquilizer
Proglycem	diazoxide	Increases blood glucose - Rx: hypoglycemia	Respbid	theophylline	Bronchodilator - Rx: asthma - COPD
Prograf	tacrolimus	Immunosuppressant - Rx: liver transplant	Restoril	temazepam	Benzodiazepine hypnotic
Prolixin	fluphenazine	Major tranquilizer	Retin-A	tretinoin	Anti-acne - anti-wrinkle agent
Proloid	thyroglobulin	Thyroid hormones	Retrovir	zidovudine	Antiviral agent - Rx: HIV/AIDS
Promet	promethazine	Phenothiazine antiemetic	Rid	pyrethrins	Parasiticide - Rx: lice
Promethazine	phenergan	Phenothiazine sedative/ antiemetic	Ridaura	auranofin	Gold compound - Rx: arthritis
Pronestyl	procainamide	Antiarrhythmic - Rx: pvc's	Rifadin	rifampin	Antibiotic - Rx: TB - meningitis
Propacet	propoxyphene - apap	Narcotic analgesic compound	Rifamate	rifampin - isoniazid	Antibiotics - Rx: TB
Propagest	phenylpropanolamine	Nasal decongestant	Rifater	isoniazid - rifampin - pyrazinamide	Antibiotic - Rx: TB
Propoxyphene	darvon	Narcotic analgesic	Risperdal	risperidone	Antipsychotic - Rx: schizophrenia
Propranolol	inderal	Beta blocker - Rx: HTN - prophylaxis of: angina - cardiac dysrhythmias - AMI - migraine H/A	Ritalin - Ritalin-Sr	methylphenidate	Stimulant - Rx: attention deficit disorder in children
Propulsid	cisapride	Increases gastric emptying	Rms	morphine sulfate	Narcotic analgesic suppositories
Proscar	finasteride	Rx: prostatic hypertrophy	Robaxin	methocarbamol	Skeletal muscle antispasmodic
Prosom	estazolam	Hypnotic - Rx: insomnia	Robaxisal	methocarbamol - aspirin	Skeletal muscle antispasmodic / analgesic compound
Prostigmin	neostigmine	Anticholinesterase - Rx: myasthenia gravis	Robitet	tetracycline	Antibiotic
Protropin	somatrem	Human growth hormone	Rocephin	ceftriaxone	Antibiotic
Proventil	albuterol	Beta-2 bronchodilator - Rx: asthma	Roferon-A	interferon	Immunoadjuvant - Rx: hairy cell leukemia - AIDS-related Karposi's sarcoma
Provera	medroxyprogesterone	Hormone - Rx: amenorrhea	Rogaine	minoxidil	Topical hair growing agent - Rx: baldness
Prozac	fluoxetine	Heterocyclic antidepressant	Roxanol 100	morphine	Narcotic analgesic
Pulmozyme	domase alfa or dnase	Lyric enzyme which dissolves infected lung secretions - Rx: cystic fibrosis	Roxicet	oxycodone - apap	Narcotic analgesic compound
Pyridium	phenazopyridine	Urinary tract analgesic	Roxicodone	oxycodone	Narcotic analgesic
Quadrinal	ephedrine - phenobarbital - theophylline - potassium iodide	Bronchodilator / sedative / expectorant - Rx: COPD	Rynatan	phenylephrine - chlorpheniramine - pyrilamine	Antihistamine / decongestant compound
Questran	cholestyramine	Lowers serum cholesterol	Rynatuss		Antitussive / decongestant / antihistamine
Quibron	theophylline - guaifenesin	Xanthine bronchodilator compound - Rx: COPD - asthma	Rythmol	propafenone	Antiarrhythmic - Rx: severe ventricular dysrhythmias such as ventricular tachycardia
Quinaglute	quinidine	Antiarrhythmic - Rx: supraventricular & ventricular dysrhythmias	Sabril	vigabatrin	Anticonvulsant
Quinidex	quinidine	Antiarrhythmic - Rx: supraventricular & ventricular dysrhythmias	Salbutamol	albuterol	Bronchodilator - Rx: asthma - COPD
Quinidine Gluconate	quinidine	Antiarrhythmic - Rx: supraventricular & ventricular dysrhythmias	Salflex	salsalate	NSAID analgesic - Rx: arthritis
Quinidine Sulfate	quinidine	Antiarrhythmic - Rx: supraventricular & ventricular dysrhythmias	Saluron	hydroflumethiazide	Antihypertensive / diuretic
Rauzide	rauwolfia - bendroflumethiazide	Antihypertensive / diuretic compound	Salutensin - Salutensin Demi	hydroflumethiazide - reserpine	Antihypertensive / diuretic compound
Reglan	metoclopramide	Improves gastric emptying - Rx: heartburn - ulcers	Sandimmune	cyclosporine	Immunosuppressant agent - Rx: prophylaxis of rejection of transplanted organs
Regroton	chlorthalidone - reserpine	Antihypertensive / diuretic compound	Sansert	methysergide	Serotonin inhibitor - Rx: headaches
Relafen	nabumetone	NSAID - Rx: arthritis	Scopolamine	plexonal	Antispasmodic / sedative
Renedil	felodipine	Calcium channel blocker - Rx: HTN - angina			

MEDICATIONS & USAGE

DRUGS

Brand	Generic	Usage	Brand	Generic	Usage
Secobarbital	seconal	Barbiturate sedative / hypnotic	Spt	pork thyroid hormone	Rx: hypothyroidism
Seconal	secobarbital	Barbiturate sedative / hypnotic	Sski	potassium iodide	Expectorant
Sectral	acebutolol	B-blocker - Rx: HTN - cardiac dysrhythmias	Stadol	butorphanol	Narcotic analgesic
Sedapap # 3	codeine - apap - butalbital	Narcotic analgesic	Stelazine	trifluoperazine	Major tranquilizer
Sedapap - Sedapap # 10	butalbital - apap	Sedative / analgesic compound - Rx: tension headaches	Sublimaze	fentanyl	Narcotic analgesic
Seldane	terfenadine	Antihistamine - Rx: allergies	Sufenta	sufentanil	Narcotic analgesic / anesthetic
Selenium	selsun blue	Trace mineral - Rx: seborrhea - dandruff	Sulfamethoxazole	gantanol	Bacteriostatic - Rx: UTI
Senokot	senna fruit extract	Laxative	Sulfisoxazole	gantrisin	Bacteriostatic agent - Rx: UTI
Septra	trimethoprim - sulfamethoxazole	Antibacterial compound - Rx: UTI - ear infection - bronchitis	Sulindac	clinoril	NSAID analgesic - Rx: arthritis
Ser-Ap-Es	reserpine - hydralazine - hctz	Antihypertensive / diuretic compound	Sumycin	tetracycline	Antibiotic
Serax	oxazepam	Benzodiazepine hypnotic	Supac	apap - asa - caffeine - calcium	Analgesic compound - Rx: colds - headache - arthritis
Serentil	mesoridazine	Major tranquilizer	Suprax	cefixime	Broad spectrum antibiotic
Serevent	salmeterol	B-2 bronchodilator - Rx: asthma - COPD	Surfak	docusate	Stool softener
Seromycin	cycloserine	Antibiotic - Rx: TB - UTI	Surmontil	trimipramine	Tricyclic antidepressant
Serpasil	reserpine	Antihypertensive / tranquilizer	Symmetrel	amantadine	Antiparkinsonian / antiviral
Serpasil-Apresoline	reserpine - hydralazine	Antihypertensive compound	Synalgos	aspirin - promethazine - caffeine	Analgesic - sedative/ antiemetic compound
Serpasil-Esidrix	reserpine - hctz	Antihypertensive	Synalgos-Dc	dihydrocodeine - aspirin - caffeine	Narcotic analgesic compound
Serzone	nefazodone	Antidepressant - Rx: depression	Synthroid	levothyroxine	Thyroid hormone
Silvadene	silver sulfadiazine	Topical antimicrobial agent - Rx: infection prophylaxis for bums of the skin	T-Gesic	apap - hydrocodone	Narcotic analgesic
Sinemet	carbidopa - levodopa	Dopamine precursors - Rx: Parkinson's disease	T-Phyl	theophylline	Bronchodilator - Rx: asthma - COPD
Sinequan	doxepin	Tricyclic antidepressant	Tagamet	cimetidine	Histamine-2 blocker which inhibits gastric acid secretion - Rx: ulcers
Sinubid	apap - phenylpropanolamine - phenyltoloxamine	Analgesic / decongestant compound	Talacen	pentazocine + apap	Narcotic analgesic
Sinulin	apap - phenylpropanolamine - chlorpheniramine	Analgesic / decongestant / antihistamine - Rx: colds - allergies	Talwin	pentazocine	Narcotic analgesic
Slo-Bid	theophylline	Bronchodilator - Rx: COPD - asthma	Talwin Compound	pentazocine - asa	Narcotic analgesic
Slo-Phyllin	theophylline	Bronchodilator - Rx: COPD - asthma	Talwin Nx	pentazocine - naloxone	Narcotic analgesic
Slow-Trasicor	oxprenolol	Beta blocker - Rx: HTN - angina - arrhythmias	Tambocor	flecainide	Ventricular antiarrhythmic
Sofarin	warfarin	Anticoagulant	Tamoxifen	nolvadex	Anticancer agent - Rx: breast ca
Solfoton	phenobarbital	Barbiturate sedative/hypnotic	Taractan	chlorprothixene	Major tranquilizer
Soma	carisoprodol	Sedative / antispasmodic	Tavist	clemastine	Antihistamine - Rx: allergies
Soma Compound	carisoprodol - aspirin	Sedative / antispasmodic / analgesic - Rx: muscle spasm	Tavist-D	clemastine - phenylpropanolamine	Antihistamine /decongestant - Rx: allergies
Sorbitrate	isosorbide dinitrate	Nitrate - Rx: angina	Tazicef	ceftazidime	Antibiotic
Sotacor	sotalol	B-blocker - Rx: HTN - angina - arrhythmias	Tazidime	ceftazidime	Antibiotic
Sotalol	betapace	B-blocker - Rx: HTN - angina - arrhythmias	Tedral	theophylline - ephedrine - phenobarbital	Bronchodilator compound - Rx: asthma - bronchitis
Sparine	promazine	Major tranquilizer	Tegretol	carbamazepine	Anticonvulsant - Rx: epilepsy
Spectazole	econazole	Antifungal agent	Teldrin	chlorpheniramine	Antihistamine
Spectrobid	bacampicillin	Antibiotic	Temaril	trimeprazine	Phenothiazine antipyretic / antihistamine - Rx: urticaria
Spironolactone	aldactone	Potassium-sparing diuretic	Ten-K	potassium	Potassium supplement
Sporanox	itraconazole	Antifungal	Tenex	guanfacine	Antihypertensive agent

MEDICATIONS & USAGE

DRUGS

Brand	Generic	Usage	Brand	Generic	Usage
Tenodmin	atenolol	Beta-1 blocker - Rx: dysrhythmias - HTN - angina - MI prophylaxis	Trandate Hct	labetalol - hctz	Alpha & beta blocker/ antihypertensive / diuretic compound - Rx: hypertension
Tenuate	diethylpropion	Stimulant / appetite suppressant	Transderm Nitro	nitroglycerin	Nitrate vasodilator - Rx: angina prophylaxis
Terazol	terconazole	Antimicrobial - Rx: candidiasis	Transderm-Scop	scopolamine	Anticholinergic antiemetic - Rx: motion sickness prophylaxis
Terazosin	hytrin	Alpha-1 blocker antihypertensive	Tranxene T-Tab - Tranxene-Sd	clorazepate	Benzodiazepine hypnotic - Rx: anxiety - seizures
Terpin Hydrate	codeine	Expectorant	Trasicor	oxprenolol	B-blocker - Rx: HTN - angina - arrhythmias
Terramycin	oxtetracycline	Antibiotic	Trazodone	desyrel	Antidepressant
Teslac	testolactone	Antineoplastic - Rx: breast cancer	Trecator-Sc	ethionamide	Bacteriostatic - Rx: TB
Tessalon	benzonatate	Non-narcotic cough suppressant	Trental	pentoxifylline	Reduces blood viscosity - improves circulation in peripheral vascular disease
Tetracycline	achromycin	Antibiotic	Trexan	naltrexone	Opioid antagonist - Rx: maintenance of narcotic-free state for detoxified addicts
Thalitone	chlorthalidone	Antihypertensive / diuretic - Rx: HTN - CHF	Tri-Levlen		Oral contraceptive
Theo-24	theophylline	Bronchodilator - Rx: asthma - COPD	Trialodine	trazodone	Antidepressant
Theo-Dur	theophylline	Bronchodilator - Rx: asthma - COPD	Triamcinolone	azmacort	Steroid anti-inflammatory
Theo-Organidin	theophylline - glycerol	Bronchodilator/ expectorant compound - Rx: asthma - COPD	Triamterene C Hctz	dyazide	Antihypertensive / diuretic
Theobid	theophylline	Bronchodilator - Rx: asthma - COPD	Triavil	amitriptyline - perphenazine	Tricyclic antidepressant / major tranquilizer combination
Theochron	theophylline	Bronchodilator - Rx: asthma - COPD	Trichlorex	trichlormethiazide	Antihypertensive / diuretic
Theoclear	theophylline	Bronchodilator - Rx: asthma - COPD	Trichlormethiazide	metahydrin	Antihypertensive / diuretic
Theolair	theophylline	Bronchodilator - Rx: asthma - COPD	Tridione	trimethadione	Antiepileptic - Rx: absence seizures
Theophyl-Sr	theophylline	Bronchodilator - Rx: asthma - COPD	Trifluoperazine	stelazine	Major tranquilizer
Theophylline	theodur	Bronchodilator - Rx: asthma - COPD	Trihexyphenidyl	artane	Antispasmodic - Rx: Parkinson's disease
Theox	theophylline	Bronchodilator - Rx: asthma - COPD	Trilafon	perphenazine	Major tranquilizer
Thiosulfil-A	phenazopyridine - sulfamethizole	Urinary tract analgesic / antibiotic	Trilisate	salicylate	Anti-inflammatory / analgesic
Thorazine	chlorpromazine	Major tranquilizer	Trimethoprim	bactrim	Antibiotic
Thyrolar	liotrix	Thyroid hormone	Trimethoprim-Sulfamethoxazole	bactrim	Antibacterial - Rx: UTI - ear infection - bronchitis
Tigan	trimethobenzamide	Antiemetic	Trimox	amoxicillin	Antibiotic
Timentin	ticarcillin / clavulanate	Antibiotic compound	Trinalin	azatadine - pseudoephedrine	Antihistamine / decongestant compound
Timolide	timolol - hctz	B-blocker / antihypertensive / diuretic	Triphasil	ethinyl estradiol	Oral contraceptive
Timoptic	timolol	Beta blocker - Rx: glaucoma	Triprolidine	actidil	Antihistamine - Rx: allergies
Tobrex	tobramycin	Antibiotic	Tuinal	secobarbital - amobarbital	Barbiturate/sedative
Tofranil	imipramine	Tricyclic antidepressant	Tussar -Sf	codeine - chlorpheniramine - guaifenesin	Narcotic antitussive / antihistamine / expectorant - Rx: colds
Tolazamide	tolinase	Oral hypoglycemic - Rx: diabetes	Tussar-2	codeine - chlorpheniramine - guaifenesin	Narcotic antitussive / antihistamine / expectorant - Rx: colds
Tolbutamide	orinase	Oral hypoglycemic - Rx: diabetes	Tussend	hydrocodone	Narcotic antitussive agent
Tolectin	tolmetin	NSAID analgesic	Tussi-Organidin	glycerol - codeine	Narcotic antitussive / expectorant compound
Tolinase	tolazamide	Oral hypoglycemic - Rx: diabetes	Tussi-Organidin Dm	dextromethorphan - iodinated glycerol	Antitussive / mucolytic - Rx: COPD - asthma - colds
Tonocard	tocainide	Ventricular antiarrhythmic	Tussigon	hydrocodone - homatropine	Narcotic antitussive
Toprol-Xl	metoprolol	Cardio selective beta blocker - Rx: HTN - angina - arrhythmias	Tussionex	hyde - chlorpheniramine	Narcotic antitussive / antihistamine compound
Toradol	ketorolac	NSAID analgesic	Tylenol W/ Codeine	apap - codeine	Narcotic analgesic
Torecan	thiethylperazine	Phenothiazine antiemetic	Tylox	oxycodone - acetaminophen	Narcotic analgesic
Trancopal	chlormezanone	Anxiolytic agent	Ultracef	cefadroxil	Antibiotic
Trandate	labetalol	Beta blocker - Rx: hypertension			

340

DRUGS

Brand	Generic	Usage	Brand	Generic	Usage
Uniphyl	theophylline	Bronchodilator - Rx: asthma - COPD	Virazole	ribavirin	Antiviral drug - Rx: chronic hepatitis C
Unipres	hydralazine - hctz - reserpine	Antihypertensive / diuretic compound	Visken	pindolol	Beta blocker - Rx: HTN - angina
Unitensen	cryptenamine	Antihypertensive	Vistaril	hydroxyzine	Antiemetic / antihistamine / sedative
Urecholine	bethanechol	Vagomimetic agent which increases bladder tone - Rx: urinary retention	Vivactil	protriptyline	Tricyclic antidepressant
Uridon	chlorthalidone	Antihypertensive / diuretic	Voltaren	diclofenac	NSAID analgesic - Rx: arthritis
Urispas	flavoxate	Urinary tract antispasmodic - Rx: urinary incontinence	Vontrol	diphenidol	Antiemetic - Rx: N&V - vertigo
Urozide	hydrochloro-thiazide	Antihypertensive / diuretic	Wellbutrin	bupropion	Antidepressant
V-Cillin	penicillin	Antibiotic	Westcort	hydrocortisone	Topical steroid - Rx: dermatoses
Valisone	betamethasone	Steroid anti-inflammatory	Wigraine	ergotamine - caffeine	Alpha blocker / cranial vasoconstrictor - Rx: migraine headache
Valium	diazepam	Benzodiazepine hypnotic	Winstrol	stanozolol	Anabolic steroid / androgen - Rx: hereditary angioedema
Valmid	ethinamate	Sedative	Wycillin	penicillin	Antibiotic
Valrelease	diazepam	Benzodiazepine hypnotic	Wygesic	propoxyphene - apap	Narcotic analgesic
Valtrex	valaciclovir	Antiviral - Rx: herpes	Wymox	amoxicillin	Antibiotic
Vancenase - Vancenase Ac	beclomethasone	Steroid anti-inflammatory agent - Rx: allergic rhinitis - nasal polyps	Wytensin	guanabenz	Antihypertensive
Vanceril Inhaler	beclomethasone	Steroid - Rx: asthma	Xanax	alprazolam	Benzodiazepine hypnotic
Vancocin	vancomycin	Antibiotic	Yocon	yohimbine	Sympatholytic / cholinergic agent - Rx: male erectile impotence
Vantin	cefpodoxime	Antibiotic	Yodoxin	iodoquinol	Amebicide - Rx: intestinal amebiasis
Vapo-Iso	isoproterenol	B-bronchodilator - Rx: asthma - COPD	Yohimex	yohimbine	Sympatholytic / cholinergic agent - Rx: male erectile impotence
Vaponephrine	racepinephrine	Bronchodilator - Rx: asthma	Yutopar	ritodrine	Beta-2 stimulant which decreases uterine activity - prevents labor & prolongs gestation
Vascor	bepridil	Calcium blocker - Rx: angina	Zantac	ranitidine	Histamine-2 blocker which inhibits gastric acid secretion - Rx: ulcers
Vaseretic	enalapril - hctz	Antihypertensive / diuretic	Zarontin	ethosuximide	Anticonvulsant - Rx: absence SZ
Vasodilan	isoxsuprine	Beta vasodilator - Rx: peripheral & cerebral ischemia	Zaroxolyn	metolazone	Antihypertensive/diuretic
Vasotec	enalapril	Ace inhibitor - Rx: hypertension - CHF	Zebeta	bisoprolol	Beta blocker antihypertensive
Veetids	penicillin	Antibiotic	Zefazone	cefmetazole	Antibiotic
Velosef	cephradine	Antibiotic	Zerit	stavudine	Anti-HIV antibiotic
Venlafaxine	effexor	Antidepressant	Zestoretic	lisinopril - hctz	Ace inhibitor / diuretic - Rx: HTN
Ventolin	albuterol	B-2 bronchodilator - Rx: asthma - COPD	Zestril	lisinopril	Ace inhibitor - Rx: HTN - CHF
Verapamil	calan	Calcium blocker - Rx: angina - PSVT - HTN - H/A	Ziac	bisoprolol - hctz	Antihypertensive/diuretic - Rx: HTN.
Verelan	verapamil	Calcium blocker - Rx: angina - hypertension - PSVT - prophylaxis - headache	Zidovudine	azt	Antiviral agent - Rx: HIV aids virus
Vermox	mebendazole	Anthelminthic - Rx: intestinal worms	Zithromax	azithromycin	Antibiotic
Versed	midazolam	Benzodiazepine hypnotic	Zocor	simvastatin	Cholesterol reducer
Vesprin	triflupromazine	Major tranquilizer	Zoladex	goserelin	Gonadotropin-releasing hormone agonist - Rx: endometriosis.
Vibramycin	doxycycline	Antibiotic	Zoloft	sertraline	Antidepressant
Vibratabs	doxycycline	Antibiotic	Zorprin	aspirin	NSAID analgesic
Vicodin	hydrocodone - apap	Narcotic analgesic	Zostrix	capsaicin	Topical analgesic - Rx: herpes
Vicodin Es	hydrocodone - apap	Narcotic analgesic	Zovirax	acyclovir	Antiviral agent - Rx: herpes - shingles
Vicon-C	multivitamin	Vitamins	Zydone	apap - hydrocodone	Narcotic analgesic
Videx	didanosine	Antiviral - Rx: aids	Zyloprim	allopurinol	Reduces serum uric acid - Rx: gout

DRUGS

Herb	Interaction
Astragalus	**Immunosuppressants** - astragalus ↓ the efficacy of these medications
Bilberry	**Warfarin, aspirin, anti-platelet drugs** - bilberry (at very high doses) ↑ the risk of bleeding
Black cohosh	**Chemotherapeutic agents** - black cohosh may affect the cytotoxicity of some drugs used in breast cancer treatment
	Tamoxifen - evidence regarding the effect of black cohosh on tamoxifen efficacy and breast cancer cell growth is conflicting
Celery	**Thyroid hormone** - celery ↓ blood levels of this medication
Coleus	**Antihypertensive medication** - coleus may have additive hypotensive effects
Cranberry	**Warfarin** - cranberry juice ↑ or ↓ the anticoagulant effect of this medication
Dong quai	**Warfarin** - dong quai ↑ the risk of bleeding
Echinacea	**Immunosuppressants** - echinacea ↓ the efficacy of these medications
Evening primrose oil	**Phenothiazines** - EPO ↑ the risk of seizures in patients receiving phenothiazines
Fenugreek	**Hypoglycemic therapy** - fenugreek ↓ blood glucose levels
Garlic	**Protease inhibitors** - garlic ↓ blood levels of protease inhibitors
	Warfarin, aspirin, anti-platelet drugs - garlic ↑ the risk of bleeding with these medications
Ginkgo	**Haloperidol, olanzapine** - ginkgo may enhance the therapeutic effect of these medications in the treatment of schizophrenia
	Hypoglycemic therapy - ginkgo may affect blood glucose levels
	Nifedipine - ginkgo ↑ blood levels and side effects of this medication
	Warfarin, aspirin, anti-platelet drugs - ginkgo ↑ the risk of bleeding with these medications
Ginseng (Korean)	**Digoxin** - Korean ginseng may affect digoxin assays
	Hypoglycemic therapy - Korean ginseng may affect blood glucose levels
	Phenelzine - Korean ginseng ↑ side effects of phenelzine or other MAOIs
	Warfarin - Korean ginseng ↓ the anticoagulant effect of warfarin
Ginseng (Siberian)	**Digoxin** - Siberian ginseng may affect digoxin assays
	Phenelzine - Siberian ginseng ↑ side effects of phenelzine or other MAOIs
Hawthorn	**Antihypertensive medication** - hawthorn may have an additive hypotensive effect with these medications
Kelp	**Thyroid hormone** - kelp (at very high doses) may precipitate or exacerbate hyper- or hypothyroidism

Herb	Interaction
Licorice	**Antihypertensive medication** - licorice may have a hypertensive effect
	Digoxin - licorice ↑ the risk of digoxin toxicity (possibly via hypokalaemia)
	Diuretics, laxatives - licorice (at high doses) ↑ the risk of electrolyte disturbances, especially hypokalemia, with the use of these medications
	Prednisolone - licorice ↑ blood levels of prednisolone
Milk thistle/ St. Mary's thistle	**Metronidazole** - milk thistle ↓ blood levels of this medication
	Paracetamol and other hepatotoxic medications - milk thistle protects and stimulates the regeneration of normal liver cells
Pau d'arco	**Warfarin, aspirin, anti-platelet drugs** - pau d'arco (at very high doses) ↑ the risk of bleeding with these medications
Psyllium husk	**Lithium, other orally administered drugs** - psyllium ↓ the absorption of lithium and other oral drugs unless doses are taken at least one hour before
Red clover/ isoflavones	**Tamoxifen** - evidence regarding the effect of red clover on tamoxifen efficacy and breast cancer cell growth is conflicting
St John's wort	**St John's wort has been noted to increase the action of the hepatic enzyme system, which ↓ the efficacy of these medications**: oral contraceptives, warfarin, protease inhibitors, reverse transcriptase inhibitors, simvastatin, verapamil, irinotecan, imatinib, methadone, cyclosporin, tacrolimus, midazolam, omeprazole
	Digoxin - St John's wort ↓ blood levels of this medication
	Prescription antidepressants - tricyclics & SSRIs - St John's wort may cause serotonergic syndrome with SSRIs; St John's wort ↓ blood levels of tricyclic antidepressants
Slippery elm	**Orally administered drugs** - slippery elm may reduce the absorption of some medications unless doses are separated by 2-3 hours
Soy/ isoflavones	**Tamoxifen** - evidence regarding the effect of soy on tamoxifen efficacy and breast cancer cell growth is conflicting
	Thyroid hormone - soy protein ↓ absorption and efficacy of this medication unless doses are separated by at least 2 hours
	Warfarin - soy protein ↓ the anticoagulant effect of this medication
Willow	**Warfarin, aspirin, anti-platelet drugs** - willow ↑ the risk of bleeding with these medications

DRUGS

Nutrient	Interaction
L. acidophilus	**Antibiotics** - probiotics such as L. acidophilus restore gut flora and reduce diarrhea secondary to antibiotic therapy
Calcium	**Bisphosphonates, tetracycline and quinolone antibiotics, thyroid hormones** - calcium ↓ the absorption and efficacy of these medications unless doses are separated by at least 2 hours
	Calcium channel blockers - calcium ↓ the hypotensive and antiarrhythmic effects of verapamil
	Thiazide diuretics - calcium ↑ the risk of hypercalcaemia with these medications
Co-enzyme Q10	**HMG-CoA reductase inhibitors (statins)** - CoQ10 levels may be depleted by statin medications
	Hypoglycemic therapy - CoQ10 ↓ blood glucose levels
	Warfarin - CoQ10 ↓ the anticoagulant effect of warfarin
Fish oil	**Hypoglycemic therapy** - fish oils (at high doses) ↑ blood glucose levels and/or affect insulin levels
Flaxseed oil	**Warfarin, aspirin, anti-platelet drugs** - flaxseed oil ↑ the risk of bleeding with these medications
Folic acid	**Anticonvulsant medication** - folic acid ↓ the efficacy of phenytoin. Phenytoin and folic acid should be commenced at the same time
	Co-trimoxazole, sulphasalazine, phenytoin, phenobarbital, primidone and methotrexate - ↓ efficacy of folic acid supplements
	Fluorouracil - folic acid ↑ the toxicity of fluorouracil
Glucosamine	**Hypoglycemic therapy** - glucosamine may affect blood glucose levels in diabetics
Iodine	**Lithium carbonate** - iodine (at high doses) ↑ the hypothyroid activity of lithium carbonate
	Thyroid hormone - iodine (at very high doses) may precipitate or exacerbate hyper- or hypothyroidism
Iron	**Bisphosphonates, tetracycline and quinolone antibiotics, thyroid hormone, methyldopa, carbidopa, levodopa and penicillamine** - iron ↓ the absorption and efficacy of these medications unless doses are separated by at least 2 hours
Magnesium	**Tetracycline and quinolone antibiotics** - magnesium ↓ the absorption and efficacy of these medications unless doses are separated by at least 2 hours
L-Methionine	**Levodopa** - L-Methionine ↓ the efficacy of levodopa in Parkinson's disease
Nicotinic acid	**Antihypertensive medication** - nicotinic acid may have additive hypotensive effects with antihypertensive
	HMG-CoA reductase inhibitors (statins) - nicotinic acid ↑ the risk of rhabdomyolysis and myopathy with statins
	Hypoglycemic therapy - nicotinic acid ↓ the efficacy of these medications
Para-aminobenzoic acid (PABA)	**Sulphonamides** - PABA ↓ the efficacy of these medications
	Dapsone - PABA ↓ activity of dapsone
Policosanol	**Aspirin** - policosanol (at very high doses) ↑ the risk of bleeding with aspirin
	Beta blockers - policosanol ↑ the hypotensive effect of beta blockers. Only systolic BP is affected, not diastolic BP or heart rate. Not usually clinically significant
Potassium	**ACE inhibitors** - potassium ↑ the risk of hyperkalemia
	Potassium-sparing diuretics - potassium ↑ the risk of hyperkalemia
Vitamin B6	**Anticonvulsant medication** - vitamin B6 ↓ blood levels of phenytoin and phenobarbitone
Vitamin C	**Aluminum-containing antacids** - vitamin C increases aluminum absorption
	Desferrioxamine - vitamin C may cause transient deterioration of cardiac function with desferrioxamine
	Indinavir - vitamin C ↓ blood levels of indinavir
Vitamin D3	**Thiazide diuretics** - vitamin D3 ↑ the risk of hypercalcemia if taken with calcium supplements and/or thiazide diuretics (note: cod liver oil contains 85 IU vitamin D per 1 g)
Vitamin E	**Warfarin, aspirin, anti-platelet drugs** - vitamin E (at doses over 400 IU) daily ↑ the risk of bleeding with these medications
Vitamin K	**Warfarin** - vitamin K decreases the activity of warfarin and other coumarin (oral) anticoagulants. Avoid changes in vitamin K intake whilst taking these medications
Zinc	**Tetracycline and quinolone antibiotics** - zinc ↓ the absorption and blood levels of these medications unless doses are separated by at least 2 hours

INTERACTIONS

DRUGS

Drug	Interaction
Aluminum-containing antacids	**Vitamin C** - increases aluminum absorption
Antibiotics/antimicrobials	
Cotrimoxazole and sulphasalazine	↓ the efficacy of folic acid supplements
Dapsone	**Para-aminobenzoic acid -** ↓ the efficacy of dapsone
General	**Probiotics therapy such as L. acidophilus -** helps restore gut flora and reduces diarrhea secondary to antibiotic therapy
Metronidazole	**Milk thistle** - ↓ blood levels of metronidazole
Sulphonamides	**Para-aminobenzoic acid -** ↓ the efficacy of sulphonamides
Tetracyclines & quinolones	**Calcium, iron, magnesium and zinc -** ↓ absorption and blood levels unless doses are separated by at least 2 hours
Anticonvulsants	**Folic acid -** ↓ the efficacy of phenytoin. Phenytoin and folic acid should be commenced at the same time to avoid risk of adverse effects
	Phenytoin, phenobarbital and primidone - ↓ the efficacy of folic acid
	Vitamin B6 - ↓ blood levels of phenytoin and phenobarbitone
Antidepressants	
Monoamine oxidase inhibitors (MAOIs)	**Korean or Siberian ginseng -** ↑ side effects of phenelzine or other MAOIs
SSRIs (selective serotonin reuptake inhibitors)	**St John's wort -** may cause serotonergic syndrome with SSRIs
Tricyclics	**St John's wort -** ↓ blood levels of tricyclic antidepressants
Antihypertensives/ Cardiovascular medications	
ACE inhibitors	**Potassium -** ↑ the risk of hyperkalemia
Antihypertensives	**Coleus -** may have additive hypotensive effects with these medications
	Hawthorn - may have an additive hypotensive effect with these medications
	Licorice - may have a hypertensive effect
	Nicotinic acid - may have an additive hypotensive effect with these medications
Beta blockers	**Policosanol -** ↑ the hypotensive effect of beta blockers. Only systolic BP is affected, not diastolic BP or heart rate. Not usually clinically significant
Calcium channel blockers	**Calcium -** ↓ the hypotensive and antiarrhythmic effects of verapamil
Digoxin	**Licorice -** ↑ the risk of digoxin toxicity (possibly via hypokalemia)
	Korean or Siberian ginseng - may affect digoxin assays
	St John's wort - ↓ blood levels of digoxin
Methyldopa	**Iron -** ↓ absorption and blood levels unless doses are separated by at least 2 hours
Verapamil	**St John's Wort -** ↓ blood levels of verapamil
Antineoplastic agents	
Antineoplastic agents	**Black cohosh -** may affect the cytotoxicity of some drugs used in breast cancer treatment
Cisplatin	**Vitamin E -** ↓ the incidence and severity of neurotoxicity caused by cisplatin
Fluorouracil	**Folic acid -** ↑ the toxicity of fluorouracil
Imatinib mesylate	**St John's wort -** ↓ blood levels of imatinib mesylate
Irinotecan	**St John's wort -** ↓ blood levels of irinotecan
Methotrexate	**Folic acid -** ↓ the efficacy of methotrexate. Efficacy of methotrexate may be reduced by folic acid
Tamoxifen	Evidence regarding the effect of black cohosh on tamoxifen and breast cancer cell growth is conflicting
	Evidence regarding the effect of red clover on tamoxifen efficacy and breast cancer cell growth is conflicting
	Evidence regarding the effect of soy on tamoxifen efficacy and breast cancer cell growth is conflicting
Anti-platelet drugs Anticoagulants	
Aspirin	**Policosanol** (at very high doses) - ↑ the risk of bleeding with aspirin
Aspirin, warfarin	**Bilberry** (at very high doses) - ↑ the risk of bleeding with these medications
	Flaxseed oil - ↑ the risk of bleeding with these medications
	Garlic - ↑ the risk of bleeding with these medications
	Ginkgo - ↑ the risk of bleeding with these medications
	Pau d'arco (at very high doses) - ↑ the risk of bleeding with these medications
	Vitamin E (at doses over 400 IU daily) - ↑ the risk of bleeding with these medications
	Willow - ↑ the risk of bleeding with these medications
Warfarin	**CoQ10 -** ↓ the anticoagulant effect of warfarin
	Cranberry - ↑ or ↓ the anticoagulant effect of warfarin
	Dong quai - ↑ the risk of bleeding with warfarin
	Korean ginseng - ↓ the anticoagulant effect of warfarin
	Soy protein - ↓ the anticoagulant effect of warfarin
	St John's wort - ↓ blood levels and efficacy of warfarin
	Vitamin K - ↓ the activity of warfarin and other coumarin (oral) anticoagulants. Avoid changes in vitamin K intake whilst taking these medications

DRUGS

Drug	Interaction
Anti-psychotics	
Haloperidol, olanzapine	**Ginkgo** - may enhance the therapeutic effects of haloperidol and olanzapine in the treatment of schizophrenia
Lithium	**Iodine** (at high doses) - ↑ the hypothyroid activity of lithium carbonate
	Psyllium - ↓ the absorption of lithium unless doses are separated by at least 1 hour
Phenothiazines	**Evening primrose oil** - ↑ the risk of seizures in patients receiving phenothiazines
Anti-rheumatoids	
Methotrexate	**Folic acid** - ↓ the efficacy of methotrexate. Efficacy of methotrexate may be reduced by folic acid
Penicillamine	**Iron** - ↓ absorption and efficacy of penicillamine unless doses are separated by at least 2 hours
Antiviral agents	
Protease inhibitors	**Garlic** - ↓ blood levels of protease inhibitors
	Vitamin C - ↓ blood levels of protease inhibitors
Protease inhibitors, reverse transcriptase inhibitors	**St John's wort** - ↓ blood levels of protease inhibitors and reverse transcriptase inhibitors
Bisphosphonates	**Calcium** - ↓ absorption of alendronate and clodronate unless doses are separated by at least 30 minutes
	Iron - ↓ absorption of bisphosphonates unless doses are separated by at least 2 hours
Corticosteroids	**Licorice** - ↑ blood levels of prednisolone
Desferrioxamine	**Vitamin C** - may cause transient deterioration of cardiac function with desferrioxamine
Diabetic medication	See 'Hypoglycemics'
Diuretics	
Loop and thiazide (potassium-depleting) diuretics	**Licorice** - ↑ the risk of electrolyte disturbances, especially hypokalemia
Potassium-sparing diuretics	**Potassium** - ↑ the risk of hyperkalemia
Thiazide diuretics	**Calcium** - ↑ the risk of hypercalcemia with thiazide diuretics
	Vitamin D3 - ↑ the risk of hypercalcemia if taken with calcium and/or thiazide diuretics
HIV medications	See 'Antiviral agents'
HMG-coa reductase inhibitors	See 'Statins'
Hypoglycemics - oral and insulin	**CoQ10** - ↓ blood glucose levels
	Fenugreek - ↓ blood glucose levels
	Fish oil (at high doses) - ↑ blood glucose levels and/or affect insulin levels
	Ginkgo - may affect blood glucose levels
	Glucosamine - may affect blood glucose levels in diabetics
	Korean ginseng - may affect blood glucose levels
	Nicotinic acid - ↓ the efficacy of these medications
Hypolipidamics	See 'Statins'
Immunomodifiers	**Astragalus** - ↓ the efficacy of immunosuppressants
	Echinacea - ↓ the efficacy of immunosuppressants
	St John's wort - ↓ the efficacy of cyclosporin, and other immunosuppressants
Methadone	**St John's wort** - may reduce blood levels of methadone and cause withdrawal symptoms
Midazolam	**St John's wort** - ↓ blood levels of midazolam
Omeprazole	**St John's wort** - ↓ blood levels of omeprazole
Paracetamol	**Milk thistle** - protects and stimulates the regeneration of normal liver cells
Oral contraceptives	**St John's wort** - ↓ the efficacy of oral contraceptives
Parkinson's medications	**Iron** - ↓ the absorption and efficacy of levodopa and carbidopa unless doses are separated by at least 2 hours
	L-methionine - ↓ the efficacy of levodopa
Penicillamine	See 'Anti-rheumatoids'
Statins	**CoQ10** - levels may be depleted by statins
	Nicotinic acid - ↑ the risk of rhabdomyolysis and myopathy if taken with HMG-CoA reductase inhibitors
	St John's wort - ↓ levels of simvastatin (but not pravastatin)
Thyroid hormone	**Calcium** - ↓ absorption and efficacy of thyroid hormone unless doses are separated by at least 2 hours
	Celery - ↓ blood levels of this medication by at least 2 hours
	Kelp and iodine supplements (at very high doses) - may precipitate or exacerbate hyper- or hypothyroidism
	Soy protein - ↓ absorption and efficacy unless doses are separated by at least 2 hours

Vitamin	Major Functions	Reported Usage	Deficiency Signs and Symptoms	Toxicity Signs and Symptoms	Top Food Sources	Therapeutic Research
Vitamin A (retinol) RDA 5000 IU RDA males 1000 IU RDA females 800 IU	Strengthens mucus membranes, the immune system immune response; required for normal vision, healthy epithelial membranes and skin; high doses have been used for acne and to prevent immune compromise during radiation and chemotherapy	Acne, AIDS, cancer prevention, circulation, colds/flu, Chrohn's disease, eczema, glaucoma, hemorrhoids, measles, menorrhagia, PMS, psoriasis, rosacea, sore throat, ulcerative colitis, UTI	Poor night vision, Bitot's spots, eye problems, fatigue, anemia, poor growth, frequent infections, impaired wound healing, follicular hyperkeratosis (rough, dry, scaly skin), brittle nails, loss of appetite, kidney stones, reduced sweat glands, birth defects; deficiencies may result from low dietary intake, malabsorption or depletion caused by infection	Vomiting, headaches, malaise, loss of appetite/weight, difficult sleep, birth defects, abortion, rough skin, hair loss, bone/joint pain, eye irritation, blurred vision, constipation	Retinol form: Liver, beef, egg yolks, butter, cream, cod liver oil, cheese	Vitamin A plays a major role in wound and bone fracture healing. Has cancer prevention effects 15,000 IU. Can improve menstrual pain. Topical and oral application can improve skin and scalp conditions.
Beta carotene No RDA	Converted to vitamin A by the liver; diabetics have a decreased ability to make this conversion; although not technically a vitamin, it is the only source of vitamin A in many multi formulas	Asthma, cancer prevention, immune support	Low dietary levels are associated with higher rates of several types of cancer	Orange skin (palms, soles, nasolabial folds) are seen with high levels of ingestion but pose no health risks; large supplemental amounts in heavy smokers can increase lung cancer rates	Carotenoid form: carrot, sweet potatoes, red peppers, yams, mangos, apricots, spinach, dark greens vegetables, most orange and yellow fruits	It also acts as an antioxidant and an immune system booster. Ingestion of large dosages can result in orange coloring of the skin.
Vitamin D (cholecalciferol) RDA 400 IU RDA 70+ is 600 IU	Supports bone and tooth formation and muscle function; aids in calcium, phosphorus, and magnesium absorption, thus, critical for healthy bones; supports healthy functioning of the thyroid glands; inhibits proliferation of several types of cancer; may slow the progression of multiple sclerosis	Chrohn's disease, epilepsy, hearing loss, osteoporosis, psoriasis, rickets, scleroderma	(Rickets in children, i.e. bent and bowed legs), late teeth development, osteoporosis, osteomalacia, osteopenia, impaired immune response, muscle weakness around hip/pelvis.	Most toxic; weakness, tiredness, excessive thirst, loss of appetite, nausea, vomiting, headache, constipation, mental retardation, hypercalcuria (which can lead to decreased kidney function and calcium deposits), liver damage, high cholesterol and blood pressure, fetal abnormalities, slow growth	Fortified milk products, liver, seafood, salmon, sunflower seeds, cod liver oil, eggs, mushrooms, herring	Treatment of bone disorders can slow or prevent bone loss with calcium. Can decrease hyperproliferation of skin cells in psoriasis. Stimulates white blood cells and increases resistance to infection. May reduce the risk of colorectal and breast cancer. 4000-5000 IU provides protection for multiple sclerosis and autoimmune conditions.

VITAMINS

Vitamin	Major Functions	Reported Usage	Deficiency Signs and Symptoms	Toxicity Signs and Symptoms	Top Food Sources	Therapeutic Research
Vitamin E (tocopherols) "d" natural form "dl" synthetic form RDA males 15mg RDA females 12mg for d alpha tocopherol	Helps the formation of red blood cells, neurological and lung tissue; slows the aging of cells; helps maintain normal enzyme function, aids in tissue healing	Acne, Alzheimer's disease, atherosclerosis, BPH, cataracts, cancer, diabetes, heart attacks, increase immune function, lupus, osteoarthritis, peptic ulcer, peripheral circulation, PMS, rheumatoid arthritis, sunburn	Rare: peripheral neuropathy, fluid in arms and legs; increased RBC fragility (hemolytic anemia), ataxia, muscle weakness	Generally safe; can cause stomach upset, fatigue, muscle weakness, breast tenderness, emotional problems; may increase blood pressure in hypertensives; may augment anticoagulant activity in persons with clotting disorders; women with heart disease on hormone-replacement therapy should avoid high doses.	Wheat germ, vegetable oil, nuts, seeds, cabbage, liver, wheat flour	Cardiovascular diseases 300-1600 IU for 3 months. Enhances immunity, age-related eye disease; may help reduce nocturnal leg cramps and PMS. May slow progression of Parkinson's & Alzheimer's disease. May be beneficial for osteoarthritis and rheumatoid arthritis. May decrease oxidative damage and enhance use of insulin in diabetics. Use with caution in individuals with history of bleeding.
Vitamin K (phylloquinone) RDA males 80 mcg females 65 mcg	Critical for blood clotting; activates proteins essential for bone mineralization and calcium binding.	Blood clotting, osteoporosis	Easy bruising, GI bleeding, nose bleeds, heavy periods	Natural forms are safe; persons on warfarin or other anti-coagulants should avoid supplements	Green, leafy vegetables, Brussels sprouts, broccoli, cabbage, spinach, cauliflower, liver, oats, cheddar cheese	Counteracts anticoagulant overdoses. May help optimize bone mineralization and remodeling. Deficiency may be dietary, malabsorption, or loss of storage sites (liver disease).
Vitamin B1 (thiamin) RDA males 1.5 mg RDA females 1.2 mg	Energy production from carbohydrates; required for healthy nervous tissue and brain cells	Alcoholism, Alzheimer's disease, anemia, CHF, diabetes, fibromyalgia, insomnia, psychiatric patients	Fatigue, weakness, depression, neuropathy, loss of appetite, depression, nervous system problems, severe deficiency is seen in beriberi, heart weakness, decreased reflex activity, edema, heart enlargement	Non-toxic	Brewer's yeast, wheat germ, whole grains, nuts, beans, oats, bran, pork, sunflower seeds, lean beef or pork, soybeans, peanuts	Used to treat chronic alcoholics. May ease chronic pain, trigeminal neuralgia, diabetic neuropathy in many nervous system disorders. May improve outcome of myocardial infarction.
Vitamin B2 (riboflavin) RDA males 1.8 mg RDA females 1.2 mg	Energy production from carbohydrates, fats, and proteins; antioxidant effects by regeneration of glutathione; supports the production of adrenal hormones; helps the body utilize other vitamins	Cataracts, depression, migraines	Usually not seen alone; cheilosis (chapped, swollen, fissured lips), angular stomatitis (sores at the corner of the mouth), glossitis (swollen, fissured, sore tongue), photophobia, seborrheic dermatitis (crusty, scaly skin) especially around nasolabial folds, scrotum, and labia	Non-toxic; high doses over long periods may cause diarrhea; harmless coloring of urine (orange/yellow) appears a few hours following ingestion	Liver, lean beef or pork, chicken, spinach, brewer's yeast, almonds, wild rice, mushrooms, egg yolks	Substantial intake may reduce the risk of developing cataracts. Maintains healthy skin and may help prevent stomatitis and cheilosis. May help fatigue and depression if symptoms are due to riboflavin deficiency.

Vitamin	Major Functions	Reported Usage	Deficiency Signs and Symptoms	Toxicity Signs and Symptoms	Top Food Sources	Therapeutic Research
Vitamin B3 Niacin, niacinamide (nicotinic acid and nicotinamide) RDA 20 mg	Involved with over 200 reactions in the body; supports healthy function of the nervous and digestive systems; involved in the production of sex hormones; helps maintain healthy skin	Acne, cataracts, circulation, diabetes, high cholesterol, glucose intolerance, heart attack prevention, osteoarthritis, Raynaud's disease, rheumatoid arthritis, schizophrenia	Dermatitis, diarrhea, inflamed tongue and mouth, psychiatric changes; pellagra includes the above symptoms with irreversible dementia and is seen with acute deficiency	Burning flush on hands and face, hypersensitivity which may be accompanied with upset stomach, cramps, nausea, vomiting, itching, dizziness, palpitations, and sweating; severe toxicity from time release forms can cause liver damage, elevated blood glucose, peptic ulcers, rash on large areas, gouty arthritis	Lean beef, white meat, tuna, salmon, milk, eggs, legumes, chicken, rice bran, wheat bran, peanuts, rabbit, peanut butter	May help prevent headaches associated with PMS and migraines. Niacin may be beneficial for osteoarthritis especially involving the knee. May lower LDL and serum triglycerides and increase HDL levels.
Vitamin B5 (pantothenic acid, pantothenate) RDA 7 mg	A component of coenzyme A, it is used for energy production from carbohydrates, proteins, and fats; it is also involved in the synthesis of acetyl choline, adrenal hormones, heme, and cholesterol; supports the sinuses; supports normal growth and development	Adrenal support, allergies, arthritis, constipation, hyperlipidemia, surgery and wound healing	Symptoms are rare. Nausea, numbness and tingling of the hands and feet, muscle cramps of the arms and legs, sleep disturbances, headache, GI disturbances, fatigue, depression, irritability	Non-toxic; megadoses may cause diarrhea	Lobster, beef, pork, chicken, fish, nuts, mushrooms, eggs, corn, peas, soybeans, sunflower seeds	May decrease morning stiffness in both RA & OA sufferers. Improves wound healing after trauma or surgery. B5 supports adrenal function. May decrease serum cholesterol and triglycerides.
Vitamin B6 (pyridoxine, pyridoxal) RDA 2 mg	Protein and amino acid metabolism; it is involved in over 100 enzyme reactions; involved in the production of red blood cells and antibodies; helps maintain healthy skin	Arthritis, asthma, autism, cardiovascular disease, carpal tunnel syndrome, depression, diabetes, epilepsy, kidney stones, MSG, nausea and vomiting, PMS	Symptoms are rare. Cheilosis, glossitis, stomach irritability, depression, anemia	Non-toxic; high dosage (2,000 to 6,000 mg) can cause peripheral neuropathy, insomnia	Lean beef and pork, fish, beans, walnuts, eggs, bananas, sunflower seeds	May help a variety of conditions including carpal tunnel syndrome, anemia, arthritis, epilepsy, depression, osteoporosis, PMS, and kidney stones.
Vitamin B9 (folic acid (folate, folacin) RDA 400 mcg RDA pregnancy 600 mcg	Purine and pyrimidine synthesis, heme production converts homocysteine to methionine and helps in the formation of tyrosine, serine, and glutamic acid; deficiency while pregnant can cause neural tube defects	Alcoholism, anemia, atherosclerosis, cancer prevention, coronary heart disease, Chrohn's disease, dementia, depression, osteoporosis, pregnancy and lactation, ulcer	Megaloblastic anemia can cause fatigue, weakness, headache, sleeping difficulty, irritability, depression, restless leg syndrome, facial color loss; anemia is similar to that of vitamin B12 deficiency and include increased MCV, MCH, and MCHC	Safe unless there is a B12 deficiency; high doses will correct the hematological symptom complex, thus masking inadequate B12 which will result in neurological damage	Black-eyed peas, wheat germ, bran, beans, green, leafy vegetables, nuts	May reduce premature birth defects, cleft lip and neural tube defects. Diabetics may improve circulation and visual acuity in elderly diabetics.

VITAMINS

Vitamin	Major Functions	Reported Usage	Deficiency Signs and Symptoms	Toxicity Signs and Symptoms	Top Food Sources	Therapeutic Research
Vitamin B12 (cobalamin, cyanocobalamin) RDA 2 mcg	Red blood cell production; healthy myelin; DNA and RNA synthesis; converts homocysteine to methionine; helps the body use folic acid; supports healthy function of the nervous system	AIDS, atherosclerosis, bronchial asthma, depression, diabetes, male infertility, memory loss, multiple sclerosis, pernicious anemia	Pernicious anemia, loss of reflexes and nerve sensation, tingling hands and feet, fatigue, shortness of breath, pallor; neuropathy, especially over age 60; hematological signs are very similar to folic acid; age-related loss of hearing, memory, and concentration; loss of bladder, bowel control; impotence, glossitis, weight loss, insomnia	Non-toxic; GI upset, urticaria, rash, and pruritus have been reported; megadoses can lead to kidney stones and gout	Most animal products, meats, fish, shellfish, dairy, oysters, egg yolks, sardines, liver	May decrease dementia. May inhibit HIV replication. May decrease pain and symptoms of trigeminal neuralgia and accelerate healing time in nerve injuries.
Biotin RDA 300 mcg	Energy production, fatty acid synthesis, healthy hair and nails, sweat glands, nerves and bone marrow	Diabetes, brittle nails, diabetic peripheral neuropathy, dermatitis	Dermatitis around orifices (mouth, nose, ears, eyes, perianal), hair loss, depression, gray skin	Non-toxic	Soy, liver, organ meats, oatmeal, egg yolk, soy, mushrooms, bananas, peanuts, brewer's yeast, egg yolk, peanuts, walnuts	May be supportive for people with diabetes by lowering blood glucose levels and by preventing diabetic neuropathy.
Vitamin C (ascorbic acid, ascorbyl palmitate, ascorbate) RDA males 90 mg RDA females 75 mg	Most important water-soluble antioxidant in the body; reduces several species of free radicals; regenerates vitamin E; involved in the formation of collagen formation, which is crucial for healthy intervertebral discs, teeth, bones, gums, ligaments and blood vessels; involved in the synthesis of the neurotransmitters and adrenal gland hormones; plays an important role in immune response to infection and support wound healing	AIDS, allergies, asthma, atherosclerosis, cancer, cervical dysplasia, Chrohn's disease, common cold, diabetes, gingivitis, immunity Parkinson's disease, peptic ulcer, wound healing	Fatigue, shortness of breath, bleeding gums, easy bruising, slow wound healing, frequent infections; severe deficiency is seen in scurvy which has the above symptoms along with weakness, inability to stand, pain, shrunken black tendons, depression, anemia, hemorrhage, purple spots on skin, loose teeth	Rare; high amounts can cause diarrhea, nausea, bloating	Rose hips, red peppers, broccoli, citrus fruit, guavas, collard, parsley, turnip, mustard), spinach, kiwis, strawberries, black currants	May act as an anti-inflammatory, and helps the body fight inflammatory diseases, including arthritis, fibromyalgia, chronic fatigue and angina. May reduce the toxicity and improve effectiveness of chemotherapy and radiation of cancer patients

Mineral	Major Functions	Reported Usage	Deficiency Signs and Symptoms	Toxicity Signs and Symptoms	Top Food Sources	Therapeutic Research
Calcium RDA 1000 mg RDA 50+ and pregnancy 1200 mg	Calcium is crucial to building and maintaining strong bones, teeth, and connective tissue; it is helpful for muscle contraction, nerve impulse stimulation, blood clotting, enzyme activation, ion transport in cell membranes, cardiac rhythm, hormone secretion; helps regulate insulin secretion	Blood pressure regulation, cancer prevention, hypertension, kidney stones, osteoporosis, poison IV, PMS, pregnancy	Nocturnal cramps; chronic deficiency results in rickets, osteomalacia, osteopenia, osteoporosis. Excess dietary fiber, fat, vitamin A, caffeine along with high stress and low activity reduces the absorption and/or increases the excretion of calcium. Epidemiological association between low intake and obesity	Non-toxic; constipation, may reduce absorption of biphosphate drugs; kidney stones may develop in severe cases	Cheese (except cottage cheese) milk, yogurt, bran, carob, almonds, sesame seeds, tofu, sardines	May help with osteoporosis; suggested dose is 1000 mg and 1500 mg for postmenopausal women. Reduces hypertension in some patients and may reduce risk of colon cancer. Can reduce irritability and depression for PMS sufferers.
Magnesium RDA males 350 mg RDA females 280 mg	Reputed to be the "antistress" mineral and part of enzymatic reactions including muscle contractions, nerve impulse relaxation, cardiac rhythm, ATP phosphate transfer, vascular tone, glycolysis, protein and fatty acid synthesis; essential for healthy teeth and bones; decreases platelet stickiness, helps thin the blood, blocks calcium uptake, and relaxes blood vessels	ADD, PMS, asthma, cardiovascular disease, circulation, CHF, diabetes, dysmenorrhea, epilepsy, fatigue, fibromyalgia, gallbladder, heart disease, hypertension, insomnia, kidney stones, migraine headaches, multiple sclerosis, muscle cramps, osteoporosis	Muscle spasticity, cramping, fasciculations, tremors, twitches, weakness, arrhythmias; cerebral vasospasm, confusion, irritability, insomnia, decreased appetite, osteoporosis	Rare toxicity; diarrhea, nausea, abdominal cramping, reduced heart and breathing rate; persons with renal failure should avoid large doses	Whole grains, molasses, fish, nuts, green, leafy vegetables, soybeans, shellfish, almonds, cocoa, most processed foods are low in magnesium	The adequate intake of magnesium may help to control blood pressure, kidney stone prevention, muscle cramps, migraine headaches, asthma and PMS. Dosages over 1000 mg can cause diarrhea, drowsiness, weakness and lethargy.
Phosphorus RDA adults 800 mg RDA teens 1250 mg	Components of bone, teeth, and energy molecules, ATP, ADP, AMP, and creatine phosphate; required for phospholipid synthesis; regulates extracellular pH; plays a role in cell growth and repair; supports kidney function	No reported use	Rare; loss of appetite, weight, and strength, and bone demineralization	Diarrhea, hypocalcemia, vomiting, nausea, abdominal pain	Found in almost all foods, fish, pumpkin seeds, dairy, almonds, soft drinks, fast food, grains, beef, chicken, beans	May increase endurance performance in athletes and increase libido.

Mineral	Major Functions	Reported Usage	Deficiency Signs and Symptoms	Toxicity Signs and Symptoms	Top Food Sources	Therapeutic Research
Sodium DV 2000 mg EMR 500 mg	Involved in muscle contraction, nerve function, carbohydrate absorption, and fluid balance as the principle extracellular ion; supports blood and lymph system	No reported use	Most often seen in athletes during competition in the heat; symptoms include muscle cramps, dehydration, heat exhaustion, and heat stroke caused by excessive loss of sweat w/insufficient replacement	Hypertension, water retention, bloating and increase in urinary calcium excretion	Processed foods including canned, frozen, fast, chips, cheeses, sauces, condiments, and restaurant foods	We consume most of our sodium through normal table salt. Most often excess sodium can be a factor in high blood pressure.
Potassium DV 3500 mg EMR 2000 mg	Muscle contraction, nerve transmission and steady flow of the nervous system; supports the heart, muscles, kidneys and blood; important for fluid balance and acid-base balance	Cardiac arrhythmias, CHF, hypertension, kidney stones	Rapid and/or irregular heart beat, abnormal EKG	Muscle pain and weakness; hyperkalemia which may lead to life-threatening cardiac dysfunction	Almost all fruits and vegetables, beef	May help a variety of conditions including lowering blood pressure, constipation, cardiac arrhythmias, and exercise.
Iron RDA males 10 mg RDA females 15 mg RDA 50+ 10 mg RDA pregnancy 30 mg	A component of both hemoglobin and myoglobin, it is involved in oxygen transportation; required for collagen synthesis, and immune function; helps build resistance to disease; necessary for energy production	Anemia, menorrhagia, pregnancy, restless leg syndrome	Microcytic anemia, fatigue, shortness of breath, pallor, angular stomatitis, decreased cold tolerance (esp. hands and feet), restless leg Syndrome	One percent of people of European descent have hemochromatosis, a genetic error that causes excessive iron absorption which can lead to liver disease and coma; vomiting; cramps, diarrhea, weak pulse, exhaustion; frequent cause of poisoning in children who mistakenly take their parent's supplements	Red meat, oysters, beans, raisins, egg yolks, molasses, sunflower seeds	Mainly used to prevent iron deficiency anemia.
Zinc RDA males 15 mg RDA females 12 mg	Involved in over 100 enzymatic reactions; important for growth, development, wound healing, and immune response; has antioxidant activity, sperm production, normal fetal growth; needed for proper functioning of insulin and Vitamin A transport	Acne, athletes foot, BPH, common cold, Chrohn's disease, diabetes, diaper rash, immune function, osteoporosis, skin conditions, ulcers, wound healing	Poor wound healing, frequent infections, decreased libido, stunted growth in children, white spots on nails, multiple dermatological problems (eczema, acne, skin ulcer, rashes, seborrhea)	Diarrhea, delayed growth development, vomiting, GI pain, kidney failure, poor coordination	Red meat, lamb, crab, seafoods, nuts, seeds, beans, oysters, egg yolks, dark meat, poultry	May help a variety of conditions including acne, wound healing, male infertility, diabetes, gastric ulcers.

VITAMINS

Mineral	Major Functions	Reported Usage	Deficiency Signs and Symptoms	Toxicity Signs and Symptoms	Top Food Sources	Therapeutic Research
Selenium RDA males 70 mcg RDA females 55 mcg	A component of glutathione peroxidase, a powerful antioxidant; required for thyroid hormone conversion (T_4 to T_3); works synergistically with vitamin E; detoxification of heavy metal; has antiviral activity, increase T lymphocytes and enhance natural killer cell activity	Acne, AIDS, atherosclerosis, cancer prevention, cataracts, chemotherapy, circulation, eczema, epilepsy, hemorrhoids, herpes simplex virus, hypothyroidism, ulcerative colitis	Low dietary levels are associated with increased risk of heart disease and several types of cancer including prostate and colorectal	Tooth decay, nerve problems; doses over 1000 mcg may in time cause brittle hair, brittle nails with white horizontal streaks, skin rash, and garlic breath	Wheat (germ, bran, and unprocessed flour), butter, organ meats, scallops, lobster, shrimp, crab	May help a variety of conditions including cancer prevention, RA, hypothyroidism, heavy metal accumulation in the body, and act as an immune stimulant.
Copper ESSADI 1.5–3.0 mg	A component of enzymes required for collagen cross linking, melanin, hemoglobin, phospholipids, and norepinephrine synthesis; has antioxidant activity; plays a role in mental and emotional processes	Anemia, osteoporosis, rheumatoid arthritis	Elevated cholesterol, triglyceride, and glucose levels; depigmentation of skin and hair; anemia and osteoporosis	Nausea, vomiting, muscle aches, diarrhea, GI pain; persons with liver and kidney disease should use with extreme caution; Wilson's disease is a genetic disorder which results in excessive copper accumulation	Oysters, soy lecithin, potatoes w/skin, beans, almonds, walnuts, sunflower seeds, brazil nuts, pecans, split peas	May help reduce symptoms of RA and certain types of anemia. Use in Wilson's disease is contraindicated.
Chromium ESSADI 50–200 mcg	Helps control blood glucose by activating insulin membrane receptors enabling insulin to promote glucose, amino acid, and triglyceride uptake by cells; influences the metabolism of carbohydrates and fats	Atherosclerosis, diabetes, glaucoma, hypothyroidism, PMS, weight loss	Glucose intolerance, hypoglycemia, craving for simple sugar and protein metabolism; carbohydrates, fatigue, and irritability	Rare toxicity; disturbances in fat, sugar and protein metabolism; there have been a few reports where the picolinate form was taken in large amounts by people who developed renal failure, however, there was no proof chromium picolinate was the cause	Oysters, brewer's yeast, beef, whole wheat, chili, potatoes, wheat bran, wheat germ, milk	May help improve glucose tolerance, reduce serum cholesterol and increase lean body masses during weight training.
Iodine RDA 150 mcg	Synthesis of thyroid hormones are involved in basal metabolic rate, heart rate, endocrine secretion, respiration, digestion, carbohydrate and fat metabolism	Fibrocystic breast disease, goiter prevention, hypothyroidism	Causes reduced levels of T_3 and T_4 which cause increases in thyroid stimulating hormone (TSH); this results in goiter, hypothyroidism, cretinism, and myxedema	Metallic taste, paresthesias, arrhythmias, rashes, acne, hyperthyroidism, nervousness and anxiety	Iodized salt, kelp, seafood, seaweed or sea plants, milk	Mainly used to prevent or reduce iodine deficiency and hypothyroid deficiency.
Manganese ESSADI 2-5 mg	Participates in formation connective tissue, fats, cholesterol, bones, blood clotting factors, proteins and glucose transport; functions as antioxidant cofactor for enzymes	Diabetes, epilepsy, osteoporosis	Poor growth of hair and nails, both demineralization which may lead to fracture and osteoporosis	Psychiatric and nerve disorders; persons with liver failure may accumulate high levels in the basal ganglia which leads to Parkinson-like symptoms	Whole grains, nuts, especially pecans, brazil and almonds; fruits, barley, rye, buckwheat, wheat, and split peas	May help a variety of conditions including osteoarthritis, diabetes, and schizophrenia.

Mineral	Major Functions	Reported Usage	Deficiency Signs and Symptoms	Toxicity Signs and Symptoms	Top Food Sources	Therapeutic Research
Boron No established value	Appears to influence intracellular and extracellular calcium transport; helps the kidney in the synthesis of the active form of vitamin D; helps regulatory effect on the production of estrogens and testosterone	Osteoarthritis, osteoporosis, rheumatoid arthritis	Increased urinary losses of calcium and magnesium, bone demineralization, osteoarthritis	Huge doses (100 mg plus) may cause nausea, diarrhea, abdominal pain, appetite and weight loss	Most fruits and vegetables	May help levels of estrogen and testosterone in the body and this has belief that boron can enhance lean muscle mass for bodybuilding purposes and can also be used to treat menopausal symptoms by raising estrogen levels.
Molybdenum RDA 75 mcg	Component of enzymes used to detoxify alcohol, sulfites, and uric acid	No reported use	Headache, tachycardia (caused by sulfate buildup)	Gout-like symptoms	Meats, lentils, peas, brown rice, whole grains	Too much molybdenum is not a good thing, and can cause painfully swollen joints and deplete the body of copper.

Source: *Natural Medicines Comprehensive Database, 4th Edition*, Therapeutic Research Faculty; *Vitamins Herb, Minerals & Supplments, The Complete Guide*, H.Winter Griffith, Da Capo Press; Doug Andersen, Andersen Chiropractic at www.andersenchiro.com

VITAMINS

Condition	Supplements / Vitamins	Nutrition
Acne	1. Multivitamins and minerals daily. 2. Vitamin C, 500 to 1,000 mg tid is essential for healthy collagen. 3. Vitamin E, 200 to 400 IU daily enhances healing. 4. Chromium, 400 to 600 mcg daily aids in reducing infections of the skin. 5. Zinc, 45 to 60 mg daily is important for healthy skin. 6. Selenium, 100 to 200 mg daily encourages tissue elasticity and is a powerful antioxidant. 7. Vitamin B6 is helpful for premenstrual acne. Take 50 mg B-Complex before and during premenstrual flare-ups. 8. Homeopathic silica reduces pus formation. 9. Vitex and saw palmetto alleviates hormone-related acne. 10. Kombucha tea, which has antibacterial and immune-boosting properties, has been found by many people to be beneficial for acne.	1. Make sure the diet contains an adequate amount of fruits, vegetables, whole grains, and dietary fiber. 2. Other foods: squash, cucumbers, watermelon, winter melon, celery, carrots, cabbage, beet tops, dandelions, aloe vera, mulberry leaves, carrot tops, lettuce, potatoes, cherries, papayas, pears, persimmons, raspberries, buckwheat, alfalfa sprouts, millet, brown rice, mung beans, and plenty of water. 3. Increase intake of raw foods especially foods that contain oxalic acid, including almonds, beets, cashews, and Swiss chard. 4. Avoid high fat foods, junk foods, fried foods, processed foods, saturated fats, refined carbohydrates, sugar, caffeine, chocolate, citrus fruits, oily foods, spicy foods, alcohol, smoking, ice cream, soft drinks, and emotional stress.
Allergy	1. Multivitamins and minerals daily. 2. Nutrients that give immune systems an extra boost include: Vitamin A, C, E, B-complex, zinc, quercetin, pycnogenol, EFAs and gamma linolenic acid. 3. Vitamin A, 10,000 IU daily is a great immune supporter. 4. Vitamin C, 1,000 mg tid detoxifies, strengthens the immune system, and reduces histamine levels in the blood. 5. Vitamin D, 600 IU daily. 6. Quercetin, 1,000 mg tid. 7. Take EFAs, which include 1 to 2 tablespoons of flaxseed oil or 3 grams of fish oil daily. 8. Coenzyme Q10, 100 mg daily improves cellular oxygenation. 9. L-Tyrosine, 500 mg daily has an important function in protein synthesis. 10. MSM, 1,000 mg tid improves allergies, asthma, headache and skin problems.	1. Make sure the diet contains an adequate amount of vitamin A and C. Vitamin A is essential for healthy mucus lining of the respiratory tract. Vitamin C is well recognized for its effect to prevent and treat infection. 2. Reduce or eliminate intake of dairy products, as they increase mucus production. 3. Drink plenty of distilled water throughout the day to help drainage.
Alopecia	1. Cysteine, 2,000 mg daily. 2. Vitamin B-complex, 150 mg daily with niacin, 50 mg daily. 3. Zinc, 75 mg daily prevents hair loss. 4. EFAs, in the form of flaxseed oil, fish oil, and evening primrose oil are rich in fatty acids and are essential for healthy hair. 5. Natural silica is the building block that boosts hair growth. 6. MSM, 700 mg daily is a vital substance to the life of hair and skin. 7. L-Cysteine and L-methionine improve quality, texture, and growth of hair. 8. Kelp 500 mg daily, supplies needed minerals for proper hair growth. 9. Consider Aangamik DMG from Food Science Labs or Ultra Hair Plus from Nature's Plus for good circulation to the scalp.	1. Biotin, found in green peas, oats, soybeans, sunflower seeds, and walnuts, is essential for healthy hair and skin. Kelp and seaweed are also excellent choices to include in the daily diet. 2. Protein is the essential make-up of hair. Therefore, the intake of food high in protein such as milk, fish, eggs, and beans is recommended. 3. Foods that are high in collagen will improve the elasticity and shine of hair, such as wild yams, taro, lotus root, and beans. 4. Intake of vitamins A and B are also recommended, as they can improve circulation to the scalp and promote hair growth. 5. Increase intake of water, vegetables, fruits, seeds, and nuts for patients with dry skin.
Alzheimer's	1. Multivitamins and minerals daily. 2. Vitamin C, 500 to 1,000 mg tid. 3. Vitamin E, 400 to 800 IU daily is a beneficial antioxidant. 4. EFAs, Flaxseed oil, 1 tablespoon daily. 5. Thiamin, 3 to 8 grams daily. 6. Phosphatidylserine, 100 mg tid. 7. Methylcobalamin (active vitamin B12), 1,000 mcg bid. 8. Melatonin, one to three time-release tablets before sleep. 9. SAMe, 400 to 1,600 mg daily. 10. CoQ10, 50 mg daily augments the supply of oxygen to the brain. 11. DHEA supplementation during the later years can aid mental abilities and alleviate stress. 12. Huperzine A, 200 mcg bid, slows disease progression, improves memory, and inhibits destruction of acetylcholine.	1. Consume adequate amounts of vegetables for vitamins A, B1, B2, C, and E. 2. Encourage a diet with a diverse source of all nutrients, including raw fruits, vegetables, whole grains, nuts, and seeds. B vitamins are important to maintain nerve health. 3. Small frequent meals are recommended, instead of a few large meals. Weight loss is recommended if obese. 4. Avoid fried foods, smoked or barbecued foods, meat, alcohol, hot sauces, spicy foods, rich foods, salty foods, coffee, caffeine, sweet foods, and sugar. 5. Encourage more white meat and less red meat.
Amenorrhea		1. Adequate intake of calcium is important to prevent menstrual cramps. Calcium level in the body is decreased about 10 days before a period. 2. Increase the intake of vegetable oil and fish. They are rich resources of prostaglandin, which relieves cramping and pain associated with painful menstruation. 3. Soy products are also beneficial as they help to regulate hormone imbalance. 4. Increase the intake of foods that are warm in nature, such as onions, garlic, mutton, chili, or chives.
Angina	1. L-carnitine, 1,000 to 3,000 mg daily helps improve functioning of the heart. 2. Vitamin E, 200 to 800 IU daily is a powerful antioxidant and reduces clotting. 3. Selenium, 200 mcg daily keeps tissue elastic. 4. Multivitamins and minerals daily that include vitamins A, C, and E. 5. EFAs, in the form of fish oils help reduce chest pain. 6. Melatonin, 500 to 3,000 mcg prevents free-radical damage. 7. CoQ10, 90 to 180 mg daily prevents heart disease. 8. Magnesium, 500 to 1,000 mg daily helps reverse heart disease.	1. Increase the intake of fresh fruits and vegetables, including broccoli, Brussels sprouts, carrots, pumpkin, and cantaloupe. 2. Avoid MSG, meat, fat, aged foods, alcohol, diet soft drinks, preservatives, sugar substitutes, meat tenderizers, and soy sauce. 3. Garlic is effective to lower blood pressure, lower bad LDL, and increase good HDL.

Condition	Supplements / Vitamins	Nutrition
Ankle Pain		1. Glucosamine sulfate and chondroitin sulfate are well recognized for their nutritional support, as they are important for the formation of bones, tendons, ligaments, and cartilage. 2. Sulfur helps the absorption of calcium. Consume foods high in sulfur such as asparagus, eggs, fresh garlic, and onions. 3. Sea cucumber is very beneficial for synovial joints and joint fluids. 4. Fresh pineapples are recommended as they contain bromelain, an enzyme that is excellent in reducing inflammation. 5. Avoid spicy foods, caffeine, citrus fruits, sugar, milk, dairy products, and red meat.
Anxiety	1. EFAs, flaxseed oil, 1 tablespoon daily. 2. Calcium, 500 to 1,000 mg daily. 3. Magnesium, 250 to 500 mg daily. 4. Niacin, 250 to 500 mg daily. 5. Zinc, 15 mg bid. 6. Consider Liquid kyolic with B12 from Wakunaga. 7. Consider Floradix Iron. 8. 5-HTP, 50 to 100 mg tid, but do not take with any pharmaceutical antidepressant or anti-anxiety medication. 9. B-complex, 50 mg bid. 10. GABA, 500 mg tid between meals, has a calming effect.	1. A diet high in calcium, magnesium, phosphorus, potassium, and vitamins B and E is recommended. These nutrients are easily depleted by stress. 2. Encourage the consumption of fruits and vegetables such as apricots, wintermelon, asparagus, avocados, bananas and broccoli in addition to brown rice, dried fruit, figs, salmon, garlic, green leafy vegetables, soy products, and yogurt. 3. Avoid caffeine (coffee, tea, soda, chocolate), tobacco, alcohol, and sugar whenever possible.
Arthritis	1. Bioflavonoids, 500 mg daily. 2. Chondroitin sulfate, 1,000 to 2,000 mg daily, holds cartilage together, prevents damage, and stimulates repair. 3. Digestive enzymes. 4. Glucosamine sulfate, 700 to 1,000 mg daily repairs joint cartilage and tissue damage, reduces symptoms of osteoarthritis. 5. Omega-3 fatty acids (fish oil capsules), 50 mg tid. 6. MSM, 500 to 1,000 mg tid reduces inflammation. 7. Sea cucumber. 8. Silica. 9. Vitamin E, 400 to 800 IU daily reduces symptoms. 10. NSAIDs.	1. Consume more foods containing iron, such as broccoli, Brussels sprouts, cauliflower, fish, lima beans, and peas. 2. Eat more sulfur-containing foods, such as asparagus, eggs, garlic, and onions. 3. Eat fresh pineapple, which contains bromelain, an enzyme that reduces inflammation. 4. Avoid nightshade vegetables, greasy foods, and NSAIDs. 5. Avoid iron supplements because they are suspected of being involved in pain, swelling, and joint destruction. 6. Avoid all forms of hydrogenated oils, which include peanut butter, cooking oils, snack chips, margarine, and processed foods.
Asthma	1. Multivitamins and minerals daily. 2. Vitamin C, 10 to 30 mg for every two pounds of body weight, daily. 3. Vitamin E, 200 to 400 IU daily. 4. EFAs, Flaxseed oil, 1 tablespoon daily. 5. Magnesium, 200 to 400 mg tid prevents bronchial spasm attacks. 6. Adrenal cortex extract, 250 mg tid. 7. Asthma-X5, 500 to 1,000 mg tid, from Olympian Labs is an herbal combination for chronic sufferers of asthma. 8. B6, 50 to 200 mg daily decreases frequency of attacks. 9. Quercetin, 500 to 1,000 mg tid acts as an antihistamine.	1. Eat a diet with a wide variety of raw vegetables and fruits, and whole-grain cereals to ensure a complete supply of nutrients for the bones, nerves, and muscles. 2. Adequate intake of calcium is essential for the repair and rebuilding of bones, tendons, cartilage, and connective tissues. 3. Fresh pineapples are recommended for reducing inflammation. 4. To relieve cramps and spasms, eat plenty of fruits and vegetables, especially those high in potassium, such as bananas and oranges. 5. Avoid red meat and seafood as they contain high levels of uric acid, which strain the kidneys. 6. Avoid cold beverages, ice cream, caffeine, sugar, tomatoes, milk, and dairy products.
Back pain	1. Multivitamins and minerals daily. 2. Calcium, 1,500 to 2,000 mg daily. 3. DLPA (dl-phenylalanine), 375 mg capsule pm 4/24 for discomfort. 4. Glucosamine sulfate, 700 to 1,200 mg daily. 5. Chondroitin sulfate, 1,200 mg daily. 6. Magnesium, 700 to 1,000 mg daily. 7. Zinc, 50 mg daily. 8. Consider Arth-X from Trace Minerals Research containing herbs, sea minerals, calcium and other nutrients for bones and joints. 9. Consider horsetail, alfalfa, burdock, oat straw, slippery elm, white willow bark in capsules or extract, tea form to reduce inflammation. 10. MSM, 3,000 to 8,000 mg daily in divided dosages for inflammation. 11. Bromelain, 500 mg tid between meals. 12. Consider bovine cartilage and shark cartilage as added support for back pain.	1. Always drink plenty of water, juice, soup, and tea as they can help flush out the body and prevent dehydration. 2. Vitamin C is well recognized for its effect to prevent and treat common colds and influenza. Foods high in vitamin C, such as oranges, are strongly recommended. 3. Vitamin A, a vital nutrient for the mucus membranes throughout the respiratory system, should also be consumed in adequate quantity. Foods rich in vitamin A include raw fruits and vegetables, such as carrots. 4. To avoid infection, a diet high in garlic and onions is recommended as these two foods contain a natural antibiotic effect.
Bronchitis	1. Selenium, 200 mg daily. 2. Vitamin C, 500 to 1,000 mg daily neutralizes free-radicals and aids mucus lining. 3. Goldenseal root extract and bromelain at a dosage of 400 mg of each, tid on an empty stomach decrease bronchial secretions. 4. Vitamin E, 400 to 800 IU daily protects lung tissue and increases oxygen supply. 5. Vitamin A, 25,000 IU daily protects lung tissue. 6. Carnitine, 2,000 mg bid eases breathing during exercises. 7. EFAs, in the form of flaxseed oil and fish oil daily are helpful anti-inflammatory. 8. Magnesium, 300 to 500 mg daily strengthens muscles and relaxes the bronchi. 9. Colloidal silver is a natural antibiotic that destroys bacteria, viruses, and fungi and promotes healing.	1. Always drink plenty of water, juice, soup, and tea as they can help flush out the body and prevent dehydration. 2. Vitamin C is well recognized for its effect to prevent and treat common colds and influenza. Foods high in vitamin C, such as oranges, are strongly recommended. 3. Vitamin A, a vital nutrient for the mucus membranes throughout the respiratory system, should also be consumed in adequate quantity. Foods rich in vitamin A include raw fruits and vegetables, such as carrots. 4. To avoid infection, a diet high in garlic and onions is recommended as these two foods contain a natural antibiotic effect.
Bursitis	1. Calcium, 400 mg tid, and magnesium 200 mg tid are essential to help relax muscles. 2. Manganese, first 2 weeks, 50 to 200 mg daily in divided dosages; thereafter, 15 to 30 mg daily. 3. Quercetin, 1,000 mcg tid with extra bromelain. 4. DLPA, mg as needed. 5. Probiotics can help improve digestive function and eliminate bacterial buildups. 6. Omega 3 flax oil, 1 teaspoon tid. 7. Chondroitin sulfate, 500 mg bid. 8. Inositol, 500 mg tid. 9. Proteolytic enzymes work to decrease inflammation and help relieve pain.	1. Eat organically grown foods with no chemical treatments or additives, including vegetarian and alkaline foods like celery, avocados, pineapple, potatoes, wheat germ sweet fruits, sprouts, leafy green vegetables, brewers yeast, oats and sea greens. 2. Eat foods high in magnesium like green and yellow vegetables, broccoli, and cauliflower. 3. Avoid acid-forming foods, such as caffeine, salts, refined foods, red meats and nightshade plants like tomatoes, potatoes and eggplant. 4. Consider carrot or beet juice twice a week to cleanse sediment residues.

VITAMINS

Condition	Supplements / Vitamins	Nutrition
Cancer Pain	1. Multivitamins and minerals daily. 2. Vitamin C, 3,000 to 12,000 mg daily in divided dosages protects the immune system. 3. Vitamin E, 400 to 800 IU daily. 4. EFAs, Flaxseed oil, 1 to 2 tablespoons daily. 5. Carotene complex, 50,000 to 100,000 IU daily. 6. Thymus extract, 750 mg crude polypeptide fraction once or bid. 7. Coenzyme Q10, 150 to 300 mg daily during chemotherapy treatment.	1. Consider a raw diet, or whenever possible, eat organically grown food. 2. Foods that are helpful to strengthen the body and fight infection include garlic, citrus fruits, and green vegetables. 3. Limit the intake of sweet foods and refined white sugar because they impair the body's ability to kill bacteria. 4. Eat more fiber, including whole grain, oats and brown rice. 5. Eat lean protein from beans, eggs, tofu, poultry or fish to help up your strength and energy. 6. Fermented soy products such as tofu, tempeh, and miso appear to have anticancer properties.
Carpal Tunnel	1. Multivitamins and minerals daily. 2. Vitamin C, 500 to 1,000 mg tid. 3. Vitamin E, 200 to 400 IU daily. 4. EFAs, flaxseed oil, 1 to 2 tablespoons daily. 5. Vitamin B6, 50 to 100 mg daily relieves symptoms, followed by Vitamin B complex to enhance effectiveness of B6. 6. St. John's Wort and Skullcap relieve muscle spasms and pain. 7. Bromelain, take 500 mg tid between meals, has natural anti-inflammatory effect. 8. Calcium and magnesium help reduce muscle tightness and nerve irritation.	1. Deficiency of B6 may be the cause of CTS, so consume plenty of beans, brewer's yeast, and wheat germ. Green leafy vegetables are good sources. 2. Food for SJ and PC related children problems include: Olives, rye, lima beans, rice bran, bananas, sprouts, watercress, and apples. 3. Drink plenty of water. 4. Reduce intake of salty foods, oranges, tomatoes and wheat which have been shown to exacerbate problems.
Chronic Fatigue	1. Multivitamins and minerals daily. 2. Vitamin C with bioflavonoids, 500 to 1,000 mg tid, plus an additional 3,000 to 8,000 IU daily has a powerful antiviral effect and increases the energy level. 3. Vitamin E, 200 to 400 IU daily is a powerful free-radical scavenger that protects cells and enhances immune function to fight viruses. 4. EFAs, Flaxseed oil, 1 tablespoon daily. 5. Thymus extract, 750 mg once or bid. 6. Magnesium, 250 mg tid, which is critical for energy production. 7. Vitamin B-complex, 50 mg bid increases energy. 8. CoQ10, 100 mg tid enhances the effectiveness of the immune system. 9. Probiotics can help improve digestive function and eliminate bacterial buildup. 10. Consider proteolytic enzymes or Infla-Zyme Forte from American Biologics or Wobenzym N from Marlyn Nutraceuticals to reduce inflammation and improve absorption.	1. Increase the consumption of foods rich in Zinc, Vitamins C, and B-complex including: Fresh fruits, vegetables, grains, seeds, and nuts. 2. Eat more fish, fish oils, onions, garlic, olives, olive oil, herbs, beans, spices, soy products, tofu, yogurt, and fiber. 3. Foods with antioxidant effects such as vitamin A, C, and E are beneficial as they neutralize the free-radicals and minimize damage to cells. 4. Sea vegetables, such as kelp and seaweeds, replenish the body with minerals like magnesium, potassium, calcium, iodine, and iron. 5. Ensure adequate intake of vitamin B complex to process and utilize energy. 6. Eat frequent, small meals and drink more liquids. 7. Avoid the use of stimulants, such as coffee, caffeine, and high-sugar products. 8. Avoid meat, processed foods, junk food, alcohol, greasy food, and dairy products.
Common Cold	1. Selenium, 100 to 200 mcg daily. 2. Vitamin C, 500 to 1,000 mg every hour with a glass of water boosts the immune system function. 3. Thymus extract, 750 mg once or bid. 4. Vitamin A, 5,000 to 10,000 IU daily, helps heal the inflamed mucus membranes and strengthens the immune system. 5. Vitamin E, 400 to 500 IU daily. 6. Zinc lozenges, 15 to 25 mg every 2 hours for 4 days. 7. Consider echinacea and goldenseal as they build immune system and fights microbes. 8. Zinc lozenges enhance and stimulate immune function to fight the virus.	1. For treatment of the common cold or influenza, always drink plenty of water, juice, soup, and tea as they can help flush out the body and prevent dehydration. 2. Vitamin C is well recognized for its effect to prevent and treat common colds and influenza. Foods high in vitamin C, such as oranges, are strongly recommended. 3. Vitamin A foods, a vital nutrient for the mucus membranes throughout the respiratory system, should also be consumed in adequate quantity. 4. To avoid infection, a diet high in garlic and onions is recommended as these two foods contain a natural antibiotic effect. 5. Phlegm-producing foods such as sweets, dairy products, and heavy or greasy foods are not recommended.
Constipation	1. Magnesium, 250 to 500 mg daily helps muscle contraction. 2. Probiotics can help improve digestive function and eliminate bacterial buildup. 3. Vitamin C, 500 to 1,000 mg daily encourages regular bowel movements. 4. Dietary fiber, 1 to 3 grams bid. 5. EFAs, flaxseed oil, 1 to 2 tablespoons daily are needed for proper digestion and stool formation. 6. Psyllium, 1 teaspoon or 5 grams of psyllium husks bid. 7. Consider Triphala from Planetary Formulas aids in the formation of odor-free, firm, and healthy stools. 8. Kombucha tea which has detoxifying and immune-boosting properties may be beneficial for relieving constipation and other digestive disorders. 9. Garlic destroys harmful bacteria in the colon.	1. Eat plenty of foods with high-fiber, such as fresh fruits, green leafy vegetables, cabbage, peas, sweet potatoes, and whole grains. 2. Drink plenty of water, at least 8 glasses daily. 3. Avoid fried foods, fatty foods, and spicy foods that may irritate the mucus membranes of the intestines. 4. Prunes or prune juice are very effective to regulate bowels and relieve dry stool or constipation. 5. A combination of wild honey with fresh grapefruit will also relieve dry stool or constipation. 6. Black sesame with wild honey or flaxseed oil is a helpful combination to soften stool and facilitate bowel movements.
Depression	1. Multivitamins and minerals daily. 2. Vitamin C, 500 to 1,000 mg tid. 3. Vitamin E, 200 to 400 IU daily. 4. EFAs, flaxseed oil, 1 tablespoon daily. 5. SAMe, 200 mg bid for the first two days, 400 mg bid for three to nine days, 400 mg tid on days ten through twenty, full dosage of 400 mg qid after twenty days if needed. SAMe raises dopamine and serotonin levels and improves binding of neurotransmitters to reception sites. 6. Folic acid and vitamin B12, 1,000 mcg of each daily. 7. 5-HTP, 100 to 200 mg daily at bedtime acts as a mild anti-depressant.	1. Eat plenty of fresh fruits, leafy green vegetables, and whole grains. 2. Avoid greasy and fried foods. A diet high in saturated fat may cause sluggishness, fatigue and slow thinking. 3. Depression may be due in part to nutritional deficiency. Foods such as white bread, flour, saturated animal fats, hydrogenated vegetable oils, sweets, soft drinks, and canned goods deprive the body of vitamin B and increase the probability of depression. 4. Avoid a diet too low in complex carbohydrates as it may cause serotonin depletion and depression. 5. Stay away from wheat products, sugar, alcohol, caffeine, dairy products, and processed foods.

Condition	Supplements / Vitamins	Nutrition
Diabetes	1. Multivitamins and minerals daily. 2. Vitamin C, 500 to 1,000 mg tid improves glucose tolerance reducing insulin needs, fights infections, and strengthens blood vessels. 3. Vitamin E, 400 to 800 IU daily improves glucose tolerance. 4. EFAs, Flaxseed oil, 1 tablespoon daily. Do not take excessive EFAs, fish oil capsules or supplements that contain large amounts of PABA. 5. Chromium picolinate, 400 to 600 mcg daily, improves insulin's efficiency, which lowers blood-sugar levels. 6. Magnesium, 250 mg bid to tid may improve insulin production. 7. Methylcobalamin (active vitamin B12), 1,000 mcg daily. 8. Alpha-lipoic acid, 150 mg daily improves diabetic neuropathy and reduces pain.	1. Eat a high-complex-carbohydrate, low-fat, high-fiber diet focused on whole, unprocessed foods, whole grains, legumes, vegetables, fruits, nuts, and seeds. 2. Get protein from vegetable sources, such as grains and legumes, fish and low-fat dairy products. 3. Eliminate alcohol, caffeine, and sugar. Avoid the consumption of simple sugars, which have an adverse effect on glucose tolerance. 4. Supplement your diet with spirulina which helps stabilize blood-sugar levels. 5. Other foods that help normalize blood-sugar include berries, brewer's yeast, dairy products (especially cheese), egg yolks, fish, garlic, kelp, sauerkraut, soybeans, and vegetables.
Diarrhea	1. Probiotics can help improve digestive function and eliminate bacterial buildup. 2. Calcium, 500 to 1,000 mg daily. 3. Digestive enzyme, 1 to 3 capsules with each meal. 4. Kelp, 150 mcg daily replaces minerals lost through diarrhea. 5. Potassium, 100 mg tid. 6. Colostrum has been shown to reduce acute and chronic diarrhea. 7. Activated charcoal, four to six 250 mg capsules every 2 hours until symptom relief helps remove toxins from the body. 8. Kombucha tea, which has detoxifying and immune-boosting properties, may be beneficial for diarrhea and other digestive disorders.	1. Patients with diarrhea should keep taking in plenty of pure water and appropriate foods to prevent dehydration and malnutrition. Eat oat bran, rice bran, raw foods, yogurt, and soured products daily. A high-fiber diet is important. 2. During the recovery phase of diarrhea, eat foods that are easy to digest early in the meal, such as soup, yogurt, toast, and porridge, and cooked fruits and vegetables. 3. Avoid foods that may trigger diarrhea or are hard to digest, such as sorbitol, dairy products, spicy food, alcohol, and caffeine. 4. Avoid eating raw, cold or unsanitary food and beverages.
Dysmenorrhea	1. Free-form amino acid complex daily. 2. Calcium, 1,500 mg daily and magnesium, 1,000 mg daily to replace minerals lost with correction of edema. 3. Consider SP-6 Cornsilk Blend from Solaray that aids the body in expelling excess fluids. 4. Kelp, 1,000 to 1,500 mg daily supplies needed minerals and improves thyroid function. 5. Bromelain aids digestion and metabolism. 6. Vitamin E, 400 IU daily aids circulation.	1. Foods and fruits that are cold or sour in nature should be avoided one week prior to or during menstruation. Cold and sour foods create more stagnation, and may worsen the pain. 2. Decrease the consumption of salt, red meats, processed foods, junk foods, and foods with high sodium content. Caffeine should be avoided as it acts as a stimulant to excite the central nervous system and as a diuretic. The overabundant consumption of whole-grain foods, and broiled chicken, turkey, and fish. 4. Menstrual cramps due to calcium deficiency should be treated calcium-rich foods, such as green vegetables, legumes, and seaweeds.
Edema	1. Free-form amino acid complex daily. 2. Calcium, 1,500 mg daily and magnesium, 1,000 mg daily to replace minerals lost with correction of edema. 3. Consider SP-6 Cornsilk Blend from Solaray that aids the body in expelling excess fluids. 4. Kelp, 1,000 to 1,500 mg daily supplies needed minerals and improves thyroid function. 5. Bromelain aids digestion and metabolism. 6. Vitamin E, 400 IU daily aids circulation.	1. A high-fiber diet is important, eat plenty of apples, beets, garlic, grapes, and onions. 2. Avoid drinking ice-cold beverages, or eating cold or raw foods that are cold in nature such as watermelon, salads, tomatoes and cucumbers. 3. Avoid eating fried, greasy or food high in fat content. 4. Reduce the intake of dairy and sugar. 5. A low-sodium diet is recommended, as sodium may cause fluid retention. 6. Consume an adequate amount of vitamin B complex, which helps to reduce water retention.
Elbow Pain	1. Multivitamins and minerals daily. 2. B-complex vitamins, 50 mg bid, are involved in estrogen metabolism. 3. Vitamin E, 400 IU bid. 4. EFAs, flaxseed oil, 1 to 2 tablespoons or fish oil 3,000 to 5,000 daily. 5. Vitex, 160 to 250 mg daily, balances estrogen and progesterone ratio. 6. Natural progesterone, apply 20 mg to your skin bid from days 6 to 26 of your cycle, and stopping during the week of your menstrual flow. Use under the care of your health care professional. 7. Beta-carotene, 150,000 to 200,000 IU decreases related cramping, fluid retention and fatigue. 8. Calcium, 1,000 to 1,500 mg daily helps to maintain muscle tone and lower chance of cramping.	1. Eat plenty of whole grains, seafood, dark-green vegetables, and nuts. These foods are rich in Vitamin B complex and magnesium, which are essential for nerve health and relaxation of tense muscles, respectively. 2. Adequate intake of minerals, such as calcium and potassium, are essential for pain management. A deficiency of these minerals will lead to spasms, cramps, and tense muscles.
Endo-metriosis	1. Multivitamins and minerals daily. 2. B-complex vitamins, 50 mg bid, are involved in estrogen metabolism. 3. Vitamin E, 400 IU bid. 4. EFAs, flaxseed oil, 1 to 2 tablespoons or fish oil 3,000 to 5,000 daily. 5. Vitex, 160 to 250 mg daily, balances estrogen and progesterone ratio. 6. Natural progesterone, apply 20 mg to your skin bid from days 6 to 26 of your cycle, and stopping during the week of your menstrual flow. Use under the care of your health care professional. 7. Beta-carotene, 150,000 to 200,000 IU decreases related cramping, fluid retention and fatigue. 8. Calcium, 1,000 to 1,500 mg daily helps to maintain muscle tone and lower chance of cramping	1. Foods and fruits that are cold or sour in nature should be avoided, especially one week prior to or during menstruation. Cold and sour foods create more stagnation, and may worsen the pain. 2. Decrease the consumption of salt, red meats, processed foods, junk foods, and foods with high sodium content. Caffeine should be avoided as it acts as a stimulant to excite the central nervous system and as a diuretic to deplete many important nutrients. 3. Increase the consumption of whole-grain foods, and broiled chicken, turkey, and fish.
Energy / Fatigue	1. Multivitamins and minerals daily. 2. Vitamin C, 500 to 1,000 mg tid, plus an additional 3,000 to 8,000 mg. 3. Vitamin E, 200 to 400 IU daily. 4. EFAs, Flaxseed daily. 5. Thymus extract, 750 mg once or bid. 5. Magnesium, 250 mg tid, which is critical for energy production. 6. Vitamin B-complex, 50 mg bid. Brewer's yeast is a good source of B vitamins. 7. CoQ10, 100 mg tid. 8. DHEA, 25 to 50 mg daily. 9. Pregnenolone, 10 mg daily. 10. Selenium, 100 to 200 mcg daily. 11. Glutamate, 400 mg with each meal helps stabilize blood-sugar levels. 12. Royal Jelly increases energy levels. 13. Shiitake or reishi mushrooms help build immunity and boost energy levels.	1. Increase the consumption of fresh fruits, vegetables, grains, seeds, and nuts. 2. Eat more fish and fish oils, onions, garlic, olives, olive oil, herbs, spices, soy products, tofu, yogurt, and fiber. 3. Foods with antioxidant effects such as vitamin A, C, and E are beneficial as they neutralize the free-radicals and minimize damage to cells. 4. Sea vegetables, such as kelp and seaweeds, replenish the body with minerals like magnesium, potassium, calcium, iodine, and iron. 5. Ensure adequate intake of vitamin B complex to process and utilize energy. 6. Eat frequent, small meals and drink more liquids. 7. Avoid the use of stimulants, such as coffee, caffeine, and high-sugar products.

CONDITIONS, VITAMINS & NUTRITION

Condition	Supplements / Vitamins	Nutrition
Fever	1. Vitamin C, 500 to 1,000 mg qid, supports immune system. Reduce the dosage if diarrhea occurs. 2. Echinacea, 500 mg qid. 3. Yarrow, 300 mg capsule form or 2 ml tincture qid or until fever breaks.	1. Eat lightly, steamed vegetables, soups, broths, and herbal tea which will let your body focus on healing. 2. Stay hydrated and drink plenty of clean water. 3. Increase consumption of ginger, onions, and garlic. 4. Avoid sugar and be cautious about fruit juices, especially orange juices that contain more sugar than vitamin C. 5. Avoid milk and dairy products while you're sick as they tend to suppress immunity.
Fibromyalgia	1. Coenzyme Q10, 60 mg tid, improves oxygenation of tissues. 2. Arginine, 1,500 mg bid. 3. EFAs, evening primrose oil capsules, 500 to 1,000 mg daily helps to reduce pain and fatigue. 4. Vitamin E, 400 to 500 IU daily protect the body's cells and enhance immune function. 5. Consider chlorophyll tablets form or in "green drinks" such as Kyo-Green from Wakunaga of America to cleanse the bloodstream. 6. Consider Spiratein from Nature's Plus which is a good protein drink. 7. Magnesium, 250 mg tid relaxes muscles. 8. 5-HTP, 50 to 100 mg tid, which reduces pain, improves sleep and mood. 9. SAMe, 400 mg bid, improves detoxification and helps with cartilage formation. 10. Multivitamins and minerals daily. 11. Vanadyl sulfate protects the muscles and reduces overall body fatigue.	1. Eat a well balanced diet of 50 percent raw foods and fresh live juices. 2. Increase the consumption of fresh fruits, vegetables, grains, seeds, soy products, skinless turkey or chicken, deep-water fish, and nuts. 3. Eat more fish and fish oils, onions, garlic, olives, olive oil, herbs, spices, soy products, tofu, yogurt, and fiber. 4. Sea vegetables, such as kelp and seaweeds, replenish the body with minerals like magnesium, potassium, calcium, iodine, and iron. 5. Eat four to five small meals daily and drink plenty of liquids to help flush out toxins. 6. Limit the consumption of green peppers, eggplant, tomatoes and white potatoes, as these foods contain solanin, which interfere with enzymes in the muscle and may cause pain and discomfort.
Flu	1. Selenium, 100 to 200 mcg daily. 2. Vitamin C, 500 to 1,000 mg every hour with a glass of water boosts the immune system function. 3. Thymus extract, 750 mg once or bid. 4. Vitamin A, 5,000 to 10,000 IU daily, helps heal the inflamed mucus membranes and strengthens the immune system. 5. Vitamin E, 400 to 500 IU daily. 6. Zinc lozenges, 15 to 25 mg every 2 hours for 4 days. 7. Consider echinacea and goldenseal as they build immune system and fights microbes. 8. Zinc lozenges enhance and stimulate immune function to fight the virus.	1. For treatment of the common cold or influenza, always drink plenty of water, juice, soup, and tea as they can help flush out the body and prevent dehydration. 2. Vitamin C is well recognized for its effect to prevent and treat common colds and influenza. Foods high in vitamin C, such as oranges, are strongly recommended. 3. Vitamin A, a vital nutrient for the mucus membranes throughout the respiratory system, should also be consumed in adequate quantity. Foods rich in vitamin A include raw fruits and vegetables, such as carrots.
Focus	1. Choline, 500 to 100 mg daily. 2. DMAE, 75 mg bid boosts neurotransmitters, elevates mood, and increases energy. 3. Folic acid, 400 to 800 mg daily. 4. L-Carnitine, 50 to 500 mg daily. 5. Pantothenic acid, 30 to 100 mg daily. 6. High potency multivitamins and minerals that include: Vitamin B, B12, and Zinc for daily nutrients and enhanced memory function.	1. Make sure the diet contains an adequate amount of lecithin, which is essential for transmission of nerve impulses that control memory. Good sources of lecithin include flax seed oil, walnut oil, sesame oil, egg yolk, soybean, and raw wheat germ. 2. The B vitamins are also important for energy and proper brain function. 3. Avoid smoking and drinking alcohol.
Fungal Infection	1. Berberine, has an anti-fungal function. Goldenseal, a berberine-containing herb, works against fungi, including candida. 2. Korlorex from Nature's Sources is an herbal product that has been shown to be effective in treating ringworm and tinea fungi infections. 3. Pau d' arco, 3 cups daily has strong anti-fungal properties. 4. Tea tree oil is a natural anti-fungal treatment for external use.	1. Eat a raw diet. Eat plenty of fresh vegetables and moderate amounts of broiled fish and skinless chicken. 2. Do not eat foods containing sugar or refined carbohydrates, soda drinks, grains, processed foods, greasy and fried foods. 3. Probiotics can help improve digestive function and eliminate bacterial buildup.
Goiter		1. Recommended foods high in iodine, silicon, and phosphorus: Kelp, dulse, swiss chard, turnip greens, egg yolks, wheat germ, cod roe, lecithin, sesame seed butter, seed, nuts, and raw goat milk.
Gout	1. Vitamin C, 500 to 1,000 mg tid increases excretion of uric acid and reduces the levels in the blood. 2. Vitamin E, 200 to 400 IU daily. 3. Flaxseed oil, 1 tablespoon daily. 4. EFAs are beneficial for gout, as they are needed to repair tissues and healing of joint disorders. 5. Vitamin B6, 50 mg daily helps distribute water in the body to keep tissues hydrated. 6. Magnesium, 400 mg daily. 7. AE Mulsion Forte from Biotics SE aids in reducing uric acid in the blood and is a potent antioxidant. 8. Kelp, 1,000 to 1,500 mg daily contains complete protein and vital minerals to reduce serum uric acid.	1. Low purine diet is highly recommended. 2. Since gout attack is caused by excessive deposit of uric acid in the joints, increased intake of food rich in uric acid will increase the risk of gout attacks. Purine-rich food should be avoided, including meat, soup (bone broth), gravies, meat extracts, seafood, anchovies, fish, herring sardine, mussels, shellfish, internal organ meats (liver and kidneys), alcoholic beverages, spinach, asparagus, mushrooms, and cauliflower. 3. Increase intake of cherries, blueberries and strawberries, all of which are excellent in neutralizing uric acid.
Hair Loss	1. Cysteine, 2,000 mg daily. 2. Vitamin B-complex, 150 mg daily with niacin, 50 mg daily. 3. Zinc, 75 mg daily prevents hair loss. 4. EFAs, in the form of flaxseed oil, fish oil, and evening primrose oil which are rich in fatty acids are essential for healthy hair. 5. Natural silica is the building block that boosts hair growth.	1. Biotin, found in green peas, oats, soybeans, sunflower seeds, and walnuts, is essential for healthy hair and skin. Kelp and seaweed are also excellent choices to include in the daily diet. 2. Protein is the essential make-up of hair. Therefore, the intake of food high in protein such as milk, fish, eggs, and beans are recommended. 3. Foods that are high in collagen will improve the elasticity and shine of hair, such as wild yams, taro, lotus root, and tendons.

Condition	Supplements / Vitamins	Nutrition
Headache	1. Calcium, 500 to 1,000 mg daily. 2. Magnesium, 250 to 500 mg daily may relieve and reduce migraines in young women and individuals with low tissue or low magnesium levels. 3. Pantothenic acid, 30 to 100 mg daily. 4. Vitamin C, 500 to 1,000 mg daily. 5. Vitamin E, 500 IU daily can help stabilize estrogen levels and prevent migraines. 6. Vitamin D, 400 IU daily. 7. SAMe may relieve symptoms. 8. Vitamin B6, 50 mg daily helps stabilize the brain's serotonin levels. 9. Riboflavin, 400 mg daily can reduce menstrual related migraines.	1. Encourage the patient to consume an adequate amount of fruits, vegetables, grains, raw nuts, and seeds. 2. Drink plenty of water throughout the day to avoid dehydration. 3. Caffeine withdrawal is one of the most common causes of headache. 4. Avoid intake of ice drinks or cold food, as they constrict vessels, channels and collaterals. 5. Avoid foods containing tyramine and MSG, which can trigger headaches, such as alcohol, chocolate, bananas, citrus fruits, avocados, smoked fish, aged cheese, figs, fermented foods, sour cream, lima beans, yeast, red wine, and potatoes.
Hemorrhoids	1. Vitamin E oil or cream to apply to hemorrhoids. 2. Rutin, 50 mg tid reduces swelling, bleeding, and itching. 3. Probiotics can help improve digestive function and eliminate bacterial buildup. 4. Water-soluble fiber, 1 to 2 grams tid. 5. Bromelain, 1,500 mg daily is an effective anti-inflammatory. 6 Vitamin K, 100 mcg bid helps rebuild the colon and rectum. 7. Consider Aerobic Bulk Cleanse (ABC) from Aerobic Life keeps the colon clean, relieving pressure on the colon and rectum. 8. Consider Key-E Suppositories from Carlson Labs which are good for relief of itching and pain.	1. Increase fluids and high-fiber to protect against hemorrhoids, increase cellulose and hemi-cellulose foods in diet. 2. Recommend cooling foods, lubricating foods, and Qi-tonifying foods: Cranberries, black fungus, wheat chestnut, buckwheat, tangerines, figs, plums, fish, prunes, guavas, bamboo shoots, mung beans, winter melon, black sesame seeds, persimmons, bananas, squash, cucumbers, and tofu.
Herpes (Genital)	1. Vitamin E, 200 to 400 IU daily. 2. EFAs, Flaxseed oil, 1 tablespoon daily. 3. Thymus extract, 750 mg once or bid. 5. Lysine, 500 mg qid at the outbreak or bid reduces symptoms and recurrence, especially during first 72 hours of the outbreak. 6. Zinc, 15 mg bid internally or zinc sulfate applied topically prevents viral replication. 7. Vitamin C and bioflavonoids, 600 mg tid at first sign of appearance, reduces blister formation and symptoms. 8. Vitamin A, 25,000 IU tid. 9. B-complex, 50 mg bid. 11. Selenium, 200 mcg daily. 12. MSM, 500 mg tid proven relief from herpes outbreak.	1. Consume a diet that focuses on whole, unprocessed foods, whole grains, legumes, vegetables, and fruits. 2. Consume foods that naturally contain lysine including yogurt, cheese, fish, potatoes, eggs, and brewer's yeast since it has been shown to reduce outbreak. 3. Avoid high arginine-containing foods, chocolate, peanuts, almonds, other nuts, and seeds. 4. Eliminate alcohol, caffeine, and sugar.
Herpes (Oral)	1. Lysine, 500 to 1,000 mg daily inhibits herpes virus growth. 2. Consider Oxy C-2 Gel from American Biologics applied topically which is a useful antiviral, antifungal, and bactericide. 3. Vitamin A, 50,000 IU daily prevents spreading of infection. 4. Vitamin B complex, 50 mg tid combats the virus and helps to keep it from spreading. 5. Vitamin C, 5,000 to 10,000 mg daily prevents sores and inhibits the growth of the virus. 6. Vitamin E, 600 IU daily assists in healing sores. 7. Maitake, shiitake, and reishi mushrooms that have immune-boosting and antiviral properties.	1. Patients with oral herpes should avoid heat, UV rays, over-exertion, stress, spicy or greasy foods, seafood, or anything that may trigger an attack. 2. Conversely, they are advised to eat plenty of vegetables or fruits that are cold in nature (cucumbers, pears, watermelon, tomatoes and yogurt). 3. Replacement of their toothbrush is also recommended as some herpes virus may linger on the bristles.
Herpes Zoster	1. Try using essential oils that include bergamot, calophyllum, eucalyptus, geranium, goldenseal, and lemon oil. 2. DMSO has been used with success to relieve the pain of shingles and promote healing of lesions. 3. French Green Clay and tea tree oil can be used topically to dry herpes blisters. 4. Activated charcoal made into a paste with cornstarch or grounded flaxseed can dry healing blisters. 5. Hydrogen peroxide applied topically can speed up shingle healing. 6. Multivitamins and minerals daily. 7. Vitamin C, 1,000 mg daily supports the immune system. 8. Lysine, 1,000 mg daily can help decrease the recurrence of outbreaks.	1. There are many nutrients that are essential for preventing, fighting, and healing of shingles. Some examples include garlic, L-lysine, calcium, magnesium, and vitamins A, B, C, and E. 2. The following foods are also beneficial: Brewer's yeast, brown rice, garlic, raw fruits and vegetables, whole grains, and foods rich in vitamin C. 3. Avoid foods that are spicy, fried or greasy. Refrain from foods that are high in L-carnitine, such as peanuts, chocolate, and corn. Shellfish and seafood are also contraindicated. 4. Avoid alcohol and tobacco products.
Hyper-tension	1. Vitamin E, 400 to 800 IU daily. 2. EFAs, Flaxseed oil, 1 tablespoon daily. 3. Magnesium, 800 to 1,200 mg daily. 4. Coenzyme Q10, 150 to 300 mg daily.	1. Eliminate salt from the diet in cases of hypertension. Avoid MSG, baking soda, meat, fat, aged foods, alcohol, diet soft drinks, preservatives, sugar substitutes, meat tenderizers, and soy sauce. Increase the intake of fresh fruits and vegetables. 2. Aspartame should also be avoided, since a high level may increase blood pressure. 3. Increase the intake of fresh, raw vegetables and fruits to control blood pressure. Nuts and seeds should be consumed daily for a source of protein. 4. Garlic is effective to lower blood pressure and thin the blood.
Hyper-thyroidism	1. EFAs help your immune system function properly and provide effective anti-inflammatory. 2. Bromelain, 250 to 500 mg bid reduces swelling. 3. Vitamin C, 250 to 500 mg bid supports immune function and decreases inflammation. 4. Calcium, 1,000 mg and magnesium, 200 to 600 daily are cofactors for many metabolic processes. 5. Vitamin E, 400 IU bid can help protect the heart. 6. CoQ10, 50 mg bid can help protect the heart.	1. Consume plenty of the following foods: Broccoli, Brussels sprouts, cabbage, cauliflower, kale, mustard greens, peaches, pears, soybeans, spinach, and turnips. These foods may help to suppress thyroid hormone production. 2. Short-term consumption of foods rich in iodine will provide temporary relief of hyperthyroidism due to a negative feedback mechanism. Foods rich in iodine include sea salt, iodized salt, kelp, and sargassum.

CONDITIONS, VITAMINS & NUTRITION

Condition	Supplements / Vitamins	Nutrition
Hypo-thyroidism	1. Iodine, 150 mcg daily. 2. Tyrosine, 500 mg daily is an important amino acid that helps stimulate thyroid function. 3. Vitamin B complex, 25 to 50 mg daily is necessary for regulation of the endocrine system. 4. Thyroid glandular extract, 60 mg daily. 5. Consider ginseng to reduce fatigue and restore energy. 6. Consider natural progesterone. 7. Selenium, 200 to 600 mcg daily assists in the removal of toxins from the body. 8. CoQ10, 100 mg daily is an effective antioxidant and prevents thyroid destruction.	1. Add to your diet rich sources of natural iodine, including seafood, sea vegetables, kelp, dulse, hijiki, and kombu. 2. Avoid eating raw foods, and foods that contribute to sluggish thyroid action, among them cabbage, Brussels sprouts, and broccoli. 3. Avoid tap water because it contains fluorine and chlorine, two chemicals that inhibit the ability to absorb iodine.
Impotence	1. Vitamin C, 500 to 1,000 mg tid. 2. Vitamin E, 400 to 800 IU daily. 3. EFAs, Flaxseed oil, 1 tablespoon daily. 4. Zinc, 30 to 45 mg daily. 5. Arginine, 1,500 mg, bid and 3,000 mg about an hour prior to having sex. 6. DHEA, 50 mg daily for men 40+. 7. Selenium, 100 to 200 mcg daily.	1. Eliminate alcohol from the diet as it decreases the body's ability to produce testosterone. 2. Intake of vitamin E should be increased. Foods high in vitamin E include wheat germ oil, almonds, sunflower seeds or oil, peanuts, soybeans, whole wheat products and asparagus. Kiwi and fresh oysters can also be taken together as an aphrodisiac. 3. Shellfish, oysters, shrimp, cashews, beef and mushrooms are all foods that either contain high protein or zinc that many increase libido. 4. Increase the consumption of niacin foods (eggs, peanut butter, avocado, and fish) and vitamin E (raw wheat germ and vegetable oil) for circulatory problems.
Incontinence	1. Kidney Bladder Formula from Nature's Way and SP-6 Cornsilk Blend from Solaray are herbal formulas that have a diuretic effect and reduce spasms. Take 2 capsules twice daily.	1. Avoid caffeine, alcohol, carbonated beverages, coffee, chocolate, refined and processed foods, and simple sugars. Caffeine acts as an irritant to the bladder and as a diuretic.
Indigestion	1. Probiotics can help improve digestive function and eliminate bacterial buildup.	
Infertility	1. High potency multivitamin and mineral supplement. 2. Vitamin C, 500 to 1,000 mg tid. 3. Vitamin E, 400 to 800 IU daily may improve sperm's impregnating ability. 4. EFAs, Flaxseed oil, 1 tablespoon daily. 5. Beta-carotene, 100,000 to 200,000 IU daily. 6. Folic acid, 400 mg daily helps normalize blood chemistry. 7. Zinc, 30 to 60 mg daily helps with impotence in men. 8. Panax-ginseng tid. 9. Ginseng-root, 1,500 to 2,000 mg tid. 10. Iron, 35 mg daily helps normalize blood chemistry.	1. Foods that are cold (sushi, uncooked vegetables, salad, tomatoes, watermelon, cucumbers, winter melon, strawberries, tofu, crabs, bananas, pear, soy milk, kiwi, ice cream, cold beverages) or sour (all citrus) in nature should be avoided one week before and during menstruation. Cold and sour foods create stagnation and cause pain. 2. Eat more nuts and seeds in their diet. 3. Avoid overly spicy and pungent food as they may cause excessive bleeding. 4. Decrease processed food and increase organic food. 5. Avoid alcohol, coffee, and cigarette smoking.
Insomnia	1. Melatonin, 0.1 to 3 mg, 30 to 45 minutes before retiring, particularly for the elderly. 2. Magnesium, 500 mg, 30 to 45 minutes before retiring. 3. Valerian root extract, 300 mg, 30 to 45 minutes before retiring. 4. Niacin, 100 mcg, 30 to 45 minutes before retiring. 5. Vitamin B6, 50 mg daily. 6. 5-HTP, 50 to 200 mg before bed to rebalance serotonin. 7. Calcium, 1,500 to 2,000 mg daily has a calming effect.	1. Increase consumption of foods that contain high levels of trytophan such as turkey, bananas, figs, dates, yogurt, milk, tuna, and whole grain crackers as they help promote sleep. 2. A diet high in calcium, magnesium, phosphorus, potassium, and vitamins B and E is recommended. These vitamins and minerals are easily depleted by stress. 3. Encourage the consumption of fruits and vegetables such as apricots, wintermelon, asparagus, avocados, bananas and broccoli in addition to brown rice, dried fruit, figs, salmon, garlic, green leafy vegetables, soy products, and yogurt. 4. Avoid caffeine (coffee, tea, cola, chocolate), tobacco, alcohol, and sugar whenever possible.
IBS	1. Multivitamins and minerals daily. 2. Consider Probiotics can help improve digestive function and eliminate bacterial buildups. 3. Consider digestive enzymes, gentian root, skullcap, or ginger root with each meal to help with food combinations. 4. Aloe vera juice, ¼ cup bid is soothing and healing to the digestive tract and helps fight intestinal infection. 5. Garlic aids in digestion and destruction of toxins in the colon. 6. EFAs, in primrose oil or flaxseed oil are needed to protect the intestinal lining. 7. Vitamin B12, 200 mcg bid for proper absorption of foods. 8. Vitamin B complex, 50 to 100 mg tid, is needed for proper muscle tone in the gastrointestinal tract.	1. Correct nutrient deficiencies with adequate calories. Consider probiotics or acidophilus before meals to help assimilate nutrients. A high-fiber diet based on vegetables and whole grains is essential. Consider eating raw vegetables and fruits. 2. Be careful with food combinations: Especially avoiding starch, sugar, and protein combinations (for example, cheesecake). 3. Avoid, dairy products, caffeine, saturated fats, fried foods, red meat, alcohol, wheat and eating too many types of foods at one time. Minimize intake of gas producing foods such as beans, legumes, cabbage, broccoli, and cauliflower. 4. Suggest foods with high-complex carbohydrates and a high-fiber diet.
Jaundice	1. Multivitamins and minerals daily. 2. Lipoic acid, 100 mg daily helps to improve liver function. 3. Colostrum, 500 mg qid has been shown to strengthen immune function and improve digestion. 4. Vitamin C and bioflavonoids, 500 mg five to six times daily have anti-inflammatory properties and can reduce duration of jaundice. 5. Vitamin E, 400 IU daily.	1. Eat raw vegetables and fruits for one week, then 75 percent raw, then take fresh lemon enemas daily. 2. Drink the following juices: lemon juice and water, beet and beet greens, black radish extract to cleanse the liver. 3. Do not consume any alcohol. 4. Oregano, celandine, chaparral and dandelion aids cleansing the liver. 5. Silymarin, an active flavonoid is known to repair liver damage.

Condition	Supplements / Vitamins	Nutrition
Knee pain	1. Glucosamine sulfate and chondroitin sulfate are well recognized for their nutritional support, as they are important for the formation of bones, tendons, ligaments, and cartilage. 2. Sulfur helps the absorption of calcium. Adequate intake and absorption of calcium is essential for the repair and the rebuilding of bones, tendons, cartilage, and connective tissues.	1. It is important to consume an adequate amount of various vitamins and minerals in foods, as they are essential to prevent bone loss and promote bone growth. 2. Consume foods high in sulfur such as asparagus, eggs, fresh garlic, and onions. 3. Sea cucumber is very beneficial, as it contains a rich source of compounds that are needed in all connective tissues, especially synovial joints and joint fluids. 4. Consume foods high in histidine such as rice, wheat, and rye. 5. Fresh pineapples are recommended as they contain bromelain, an enzyme that is excellent in reducing inflammation.
Libido	1. Ginseng is a primary tonic for male's sexual virility. 2. Consider Yohimbe caps, 750 to 1,000 mg to stimulate testosterone and revitalize male virility. 3. Royal Jelly, 60,000 to 120,000 mg daily helps boost healthy seminal fluids. 4. Vitamin E, 800 IU helps promote vaginal fluids. 5. Niacin, 100 mg, 30 minutes before sex to enhance sexual flush, mucus membrane tingling and intensity of the orgasm.	Women: 1. Increase soy foods for mild estrogenic effect. 2. Eat food rich in EFAs, such as seafoods, green vegetables, sea greens, whole grains, nuts, legumes, and seeds. 3. Vitamin-E-rich foods include soy foods, wheat germ, seeds, nuts and vegetable oils and beta-carotene foods like apricots, mangos and carrots. 4. Boost adrenal energy with brown rice. 5. Magnesium rich foods, like almonds, avocados, carrots, citrus fruits, lentils, and salmon counteract depression and anxiety.
Masses	1. Multivitamins and minerals daily. 2. Vitamin C, 500 to 1,000 mg tid. 3. Vitamin E, 400 to 800 IU daily. 4. EFAs, Flaxseed oil or evening primrose oil, 1 to 2 tablespoons daily help the body process estrogen. 5. Phosphatidylcholine, 500 mg tid. 6. Pancreatin, 350 to 700 mg tid between meals. 7. Magnesium, 1,000 to 1,500 mg daily aids in the stagnation of the uterus.	1. Eat certified organic foods as much as possible. 2. Base your diet around whole grains, unprocessed foods, vegetables, fruits, sea vegetables, beans, beets, carrots, artichokes, dandelion greens, onions, garlic, and soy products. 3. Increase consumption of soy foods and iodine from seaweeds. 4. Vitamin K will encourage proper blood clotting and reduce excessive flow. 5. Flaxseeds have been shown to help balance estrogen levels.
Memory	1. Choline, 500 to 100 mg daily. 2. DMAE, 75 mg bid boosts neurotransmitters, elevates mood, and increases energy. 3. Folic acid, 400 to 800 mg daily. 4. L-Carnitine. 50 to 500 mg daily. 5. Pantothenic acid, 30 to 100 mg daily. 6. High potency multivitamins and minerals that include: Vitamin B, B12, and Zinc for daily nutrients and enhanced memory function.	1. Make sure the diet contains an adequate amount of lecithin, which is essential for transmission of nerve impulses that control memory. Good sources of lecithin include flaxseed oil, walnut oil, sesame oil, egg yolk, soybean, and raw wheat germ. 2. The B vitamins are also important for energy and proper brain function. 3. Avoid smoking and alcohol.
Menopausal Syndrome	1. Vitamin C, 500 to 1,000 mg tid. 2. Vitamin E, 400 to 1,000 IU daily reduces symptoms, also applied topically for vaginal dryness. 3. EFAs, Flaxseed oil, 1 to 2 tablespoons daily. 4. Hesperidin, 900 mg daily. 5. Gamma-oryzanol, 300 mg daily relieves hot flashes. 6. Boron, 3 mg daily increases estrogen blood levels. 7. Vitamin D, 400 to 600 IU daily. 8. Vitamin B-complex, 50 to 100 mg helps stabilize estrogen levels.	1. Encourage a diet with a high content of raw foods, fruits and vegetables to stabilize blood-sugar. Wild yam is very helpful to nourish yin and reduce menopause symptoms. 2. Discourage dairy products and red meats, as they promote hot flashes. 3. Avoid alcohol, sugar, spicy foods, and caffeine as they trigger hot flashes and aggravate mood swings. 4. Increase the intake of soy products such as tofu, soymilk, and soy nuts. Soy products regulate the estrogen levels and are beneficial for menopause.
Menorrhagia	1. Vitamin A, 50,000 IU daily normalizes blood loss. 2. Vitamin E, 800 IU daily relieves menstrual symptoms and reduces excessive blood loss. 3. Vitamin C and bioflavonoids protect capillaries from damage. 4. Adding cayenne to any herbal tea can regulate bleeding internally and externally. 5. Drinking diluted lemon juice throughout the menstrual period will help reduce the flow.	1. Increase the intake of vegetable oil and fish oil. 2. Soy products are also beneficial as they help to regulate hormone imbalance. 3. Avoid cold or raw foods as they impair the Spleen function and create more dampness and stagnation.
Menstrual Irregularity	1. Multivitamins and minerals daily. 2. Vitamin C, 500 to 1,000 mg tid. 3. Vitamin E, 400 to 800 IU daily is beneficial for cramps and reduces breast tenderness. 4. EFAs, Flaxseed oil, 1 to 2 tablespoons daily aids in the production of prostaglandin and reduces breast tenderness. 5. Calcium, 500 to 1,000 mg daily prevents mood swings and reduces symptoms. 6. EFA capsules, 250 mg 1 to 3 daily. 7. Iron 10 to 15 mg daily. 8. Magnesium, 250 to 500 mg daily soothes the nervous system and reduces irritability. 9. Zinc, 15 mg bid. 10. Melatonin and Pregnenolone, 100 mg daily, or DHEA 10 mg daily.	1. Adequate intake of calcium is important to prevent menstrual cramps. Calcium level in the body is decreased about 10 days before a period. 2. Increase the intake of vegetable oil and fish. They are rich resources of prostaglandin, which relieves cramping and pain associated with painful menstruation. 3. Soy products are also beneficial as they help to regulate hormone imbalance. 4. Increase the intake of foods that are warm in nature, such as onions, garlic, mutton, chili, or chives. 5. Avoid cold or raw foods as they impair the Spleen function and create more dampness and stagnation.
Muscle Tension	1. Vitamin B6, 25 to 50 mg daily. 2. Vitamin B12, 100 to 1,000 mcg daily. 3. Vitamin C, 500 to 1,000 mg daily.	
Multiple Sclerosis	1. Multivitamins and minerals daily. 2. Vitamin C, 500 to 1,000 mg tid. 3. Vitamin E, 400 to 800 IU daily. 4. EFAs, Flaxseed oil, 1 or 2 tablespoons daily may lessen the harshness and duration of MS attacks. 4. Methylcobalamin (active vitamin B12), 1,000 mcg tid. 5. Pancreatin, 350 to 700 mg tid between meals. 6. Niacin, 200 to 500 mg tid. 7. Vitamin B6, 100 to 500 mg daily. 8. Vitamin B12, 1,000 mg daily. 9. L-cysteine, 500 mg daily. 10. Inositol, 1,000 mg daily. 11. DMG, 100 to 400 mg daily contributes to remyelinization of the sheath protecting the spinal column.	1. Eat organically grown foods with no chemical treatments or additives, including eggs, fruits, gluten-free grains, seeds, and vegetables. 2. Eat plenty of dark leafy greens with a normal allowance of protein. 2. Daily intake of 40 to 50 grams of polyunsaturated oils is recommended. At least 1 teaspoon of cod liver oil daily. 3. Consumption of fish three or more times a week is highly recommended. 4. Take a fiber supplement daily. 5. Avoid alcohol, chocolate, coffee, dairy products, meat, refined foods, sugar, wheat, and processed foods.

VITAMINS

Condition	Supplements / Vitamins	Nutrition
Neck Pain	1. Multivitamins and minerals daily. 2. Calcium, 1,500 to 2,000 mg daily. 3. MSM, 500 to 1,000 mg tid. 4. DLPA (dl-phenylalanine), 375 mg capsule pm 4/24 for discomfort. 5. Glucosamine sulfate, 700 to 1,000 mg daily. 6. Magnesium, 700 to 1,000 mg daily. 7. Zinc, 50 mg daily. 8. Bromelain, 400 mg tid, or curcumin, 600 mg tid, and grape seed extract for inflammation. 9. Manganese and free form amino acid complexes are good for ligaments and connective tissues. 10. Consider chondroitin sulfate, bovine cartilage, and shark cartilage.	1. Eat plenty of whole grains, seafood, dark-green vegetables, and nuts. These foods are rich in vitamin B complex and magnesium, which are essential for nerve health and relaxation of tense muscles. 2. Adequate intake of minerals, such as calcium and potassium, are essential for pain management. Deficiency of these minerals will lead to spasms, cramps, and tense muscles.
Nosebleed	1. Multivitamins and minerals daily. 2. Vitamin K, 25 mcg bid helps the blood clot more efficiently. 3. Vitamin C and bioflavonoids, 500 to 1,000 mg qid for two days after a nosebleed.	1. Eat organically grown foods with no chemical treatments or additives, including raw and cooked foods with good sources of vitamin K. 2. Avoid refined sugars which slow the healing process.
Obesity /Weight Control	1. 5-HTP, 50 to 100 mg, before meals for the first two weeks, then double the dosage if weight loss is less than one pound per week. Higher dosages are associated with nausea; both symptoms will disappear after six weeks. 2. Chromium, 200 to 400 mcg daily helps stabilize blood-sugar levels and reduce cravings for sweets. 3. Coenzyme Q10, 100 to 300 mg daily. 4. Hydrocitrate, 500 mg tid. 5. Colorad from Enhanced fitness, a liquid food supplement designed to help body lose fat without losing lean muscle. 6. L-carnitine, 500 to 1,000 mg daily helps fatty acids inside cells produce energy burning mitochondria. 7. Lecithin, one tablespoon daily at breakfast helps emulsify fat.	1. Increase the daily intake of cholesterol-lowering foods such as apples, bananas, carrots, cold-water fish, dried beans, garlic, grapefruit, olive oil, and fibers such as bran and oat. 2. Advise the patient to consume large quantities of fresh fruits and vegetables. 3. Decrease the intake of food that will raise cholesterol levels, including but not limited to beer, wine, cheese, tobacco products, aged and cured meats, sugar, and greasy or fried foods. 4. Eat small, frequent meals throughout the day instead of a few large ones. Eat slowly and chew thoroughly.
Obsessive-Compulsive	1. Calcium, 600 mg bid helps strengthen the nervous system. 2. Taurine, 500 mg tid assists in improving brain function and reducing anxiety. 3. Magnesium, 300 mg bid helps strengthen the nervous system. 4. St. Johns wort is useful in mild cases of OCD.	1. Maintaining a stable blood-sugar level is very important. Avoid sugar, caffeine, and stimulants that cause rapid fluctuation in blood-sugar. 2. Consider food allergies as the culprit for symptoms.
Osteo-arthritis	1. Multivitamins and minerals daily. 2. Vitamin C, 500 to 1,000 mg tid. 3. Vitamin E, 400 to 800 IU daily. 4. EFAs, Flaxseed oil, 1 or 2 tablespoons daily. 5. Vitamin A, 5000 IU daily. 6. Vitamin B6, 50 mg daily. 7. Pantothenic acid, 13 mg daily. 8. Zinc, 30 to 45 mg daily. 9. Glucosamine sulfate, 500 mg tid. 10. Boron (as sodium tetrahydraborate), 6 to 9 mg daily. 11. Topically applied capsaicin preparation can help reduce pain of osteoarthritis.	1. Raw carrot, beet, celery, parsley or alfalfa juices, 1 to 2 glasses daily can reduce arthritic conditions. 2. Consume iron in foods that include broccoli, Brussels sprouts, cauliflower, fish, lima beans, and peas. 3. Eat more sulfur-containing foods, such as asparagus, eggs, garlic, and onions as they help repair bone, cartilage and connective tissue. 4. Eat fresh pineapple, which contains bromelain, an enzyme that reduces inflammation. 5. Avoid nightshade vegetables, greasy foods, and NSAIDs.
Osteo-porosis	1. Multivitamins and minerals daily. 2. Vitamin C, 500 to 1,000 mg tid. 3. Vitamin E, 200 to 400 IU daily. 4. EFAs, Flaxseed oil, 1 or 2 tablespoons daily. 5. Boron (as sodium tetrahydraborate), 6 to 9 mg daily. 6. Vitamin D, 400 IU daily with calcium is necessary for absorption. 7. Magnesium, 400 to 800 mg daily can improve bone density.	1. Consume a sufficient amount of calcium and vitamin D, including broccoli, chestnuts, clams, dark-green vegetables, flounder, salmon, sardines, shrimp and soybeans. Eat whole grain and calcium-rich foods at different times of the day to prevent grains from binding to calcium, impeding its absorption in the body. 2. Consumption of foods rich in plant estrogen is beneficial, including soybeans and yams. 3. Eat sulfur-rich foods, like garlic and onions, to make bones healthy. 4. Avoid soft drinks, alcoholic beverages, smoking, yeast products, sugar and salt.
Pain	1. Calcium and magnesium, 500 mg of each tid can be effective for pain associated with muscle spasms. 2. Glucosamine sulfate, 500 mg tid is a natural alternative to aspirin and other NSAIDs. 3. Bromelain, 300 to 500 mg tid is a natural enzyme that reduces inflammation.	1. Eat organically grown foods with no chemical treatments or additives, including pineapple, soups made with garlic, onions, green leafy vegetables, ginger root, and turmeric root. 2. Avoid food containing saturated, hydrogenated fats including butter, red meat, shellfish, margarine, shortenings, and all fried foods.
Palpitations	1. B-complex, 50 mg tid calms and stabilizes your system. 2. Vitamin E, 200 to 800 IU daily is a powerful antioxidant and reduces clotting. 3. Selenium, 200 mcg daily keeps tissue elastic. 4. Multivitamins and minerals daily that include vitamin A, C, and E. 5. Pycnogenol, 400 mg daily keeps collagen elastic and softens platelets. 6. Vitamin C with bioflavonoids, 3,000 to 20,000 strengthens arterial walls. 7. CoQ10, 60 bid prevents free-radical damage. 7. CoQ10, 60 tid strengthens heart disease. 8. Magnesium, 500 to 1,000 mg daily helps reverse heart disease. 9. Bromelain, 1,500 mg daily.	1. A diet which is magnesium and potassium rich includes: fresh leafy green vegetables, sea food, and sea greens are essential in heart disease prevention. 2. Avoid MSG, baking soda, meat, fat, aged foods, alcohol, diet soft drinks, preservatives, sugar substitutes, and soy sauce since they can aggravate palpitations and arrhythmias. 3. Increase the intake of fresh, raw vegetables, nuts, sunflower, and sesame seeds.
Paralysis	1. Multivitamins and minerals daily. 2. Vitamin C, 500 to 1,000 mg tid. 3. Vitamin E, 400 to 800 IU daily. 4. EFAs, Flaxseed oil, 1 or 2 tablespoons daily may lessen the harshness of paralysis. 5. DMG, 100 to 400 mg daily contributes to remyelinization of the sheath protecting the spinal column. 6. Calcium, 2,000 mg daily. 7. Magnesium, 1,000 mg daily.	1. Eat soured milk products like yogurt and kefir, including beet greens, chard, eggs, green leafy vegetables, raw cheese, and raw milk. 2. Drink fresh "live" juices made from beets, carrots, green beans, green leafy vegetables, peas, red grapes, and seaweed. 3. Avoid dairy products, meat, sugar and white flour products.

VITAMINS

Condition	Supplements / Vitamins	Nutrition
Parkinson's Disease	1. Multivitamins and minerals daily. 2. Vitamin C, 500 to 1,000 mg daily. 3. Vitamin E, 400 to 800 IU daily. 4. Ginkgo biloba, 40 to 80 mg tid increases blood flow to the brain. 5. Phosphatidylserine, 100 mg tid helps boost energy level to the brain. 6. Consider Thiodox from Allergy Research, 200 mg which contains the essential glutathione to support the body. 7. Vitamin B thiamin, 3,000 to 8,000 mg daily and tyrosine, 500 to 1,000 mg daily helps boost dopamine levels for the brain. 8. CoQ10, 200 mg daily is crucial for cellular energy. 9. DHEA, 10 mg for women, 25 mg for men daily is a helpful hormone.	1. Eat a diet consisting of raw foods, with seeds, grains, nuts and raw milk. 2. Include diet foods containing amino acid, such as almonds, fish, pecans, sesame seeds, lentils. 3. Reduce intake of animal protein.
Pelvic Inflammatory Disease		1. Natural, plain yogurt with live cultures helps to minimize yeast infections by establishing a normal environment in the genital tract. 2. Eat plenty of fruits and vegetables, which provide the nutrients needed to resist infection and facilitate healing. 3. Regular consumption of unsweetened cranberry juice will help to prevent and treat urinary tract infections.
PMS	1. Multivitamins and minerals daily. 2. Vitamin C, 500 to 1,000 mg tid. 3. Vitamin E, 400 to 800 IU daily is beneficial for cramps and reduces breast tenderness. 4. EFAs, Flaxseed oil, 1 to 2 tablespoons daily aids in the production of prostaglandin and reduces breast tenderness. 5. Calcium, 500 to 1,000 mg daily prevents mood swings and reduces symptoms. 6. EFA capsules, 250 mg 1 to 3 daily. 7. Iron 10 to 15 mg daily. 8. Magnesium, 250 to 500 mg daily soothes the nervous system and reduces irritability. 9. Zinc, 15 mg bid. 10. Melatonin and Pregnenolone, 100 mg daily, or DHEA 10 mg daily.	1. A diet high in calcium, magnesium, phosphorus, potassium, and vitamins B and E is recommended. These nutrients are easily depleted by stress. 2. Encourage the consumption of fruits and vegetables such as apricots, wintermelon, asparagus, avocados, bananas, and broccoli in addition to brown rice, dried fruit, figs, salmon, garlic, green leafy vegetables, soy products, and yogurt. 3. Avoid caffeine (coffee, tea, soda, chocolate), tobacco, alcohol, and sugar. 4. Reduce exposure to environmental estrogens in foods.
Polycystic Ovarian	1. Multivitamins and minerals daily. 2. Vitamin C, 500 to 1,000 mg tid. 3. Vitamin E, 400 to 800 IU daily is an estrogen antagonist. 4. EFAs, Flaxseed oil or evening primrose oil, 1 to 2 tablespoons daily helps the body process estrogen and reduce inflammation. 5. Pancreatin, 350 to 700 mg tid between meals helps with fat metabolism. 6. Magnesium, 1,000 to 1,500 mg daily aids in the stagnation of the uterus. 7. Quercitin and bromelain are effective anti-inflammatory.	1. Eat certified organic foods as much as possible. 2. Base your diet around whole grains, unprocessed foods, vegetables, fruits, fish, sea vegetables, beans, beets, carrots, artichokes, dandelion greens, onions, garlic, and soy products. 3. Increase consumption of soy foods. 4. Flaxseeds have been shown to help balance estrogen levels. 5. Include green drinks to support detoxification. 6. Avoid red meat, dairy products, sugar, caffeine, alcohol, processed foods, fried foods, and refined sugars.
Rheumatoid Arthritis	1. Multivitamins and minerals daily. 2. Vitamin C, 500 to 1,000 mg tid. 3. Vitamin E, 400 to 800 IU daily. 4. EFAs, Flaxseed oil, 1 to 2 tablespoons daily. 5. Pancreatin, 350 to 700 mg tid between meals.	1. Fasting can bring temporary relief for RA. 2. Consume foods high in an iron which include broccoli, Brussels sprouts, cauliflower, fish, lima beans, and peas. 3. Eat more sulfur-containing foods, such as asparagus, eggs, garlic, and onions. 4. Eat fresh pineapple, which contains bromelain, an enzyme that reduces inflammation. 5. Avoid nightshade vegetables, greasy foods, and NSAIDs. 6. Avoid iron supplements because they are suspected of being involved in pain, swelling, and joint destruction.
Sciatica	1. Multivitamins and minerals daily. 2. Quercitin, 1,000 mg daily, bromelain, 1,500 mg daily to relieve nerve inflammation. 3. Niacin, 500 to 1,500 daily to stimulate circulation. 4. MSM, 3,000 to 8,000 mg daily in divided dosages for inflammation. 5. Consider horsetail, alfalfa, burdock, oat straw, slippery elm, white willow bark in capsules, extract, or tea form to reduce inflammation. 6. EFAs, in the form of flaxseed oil, fish oil, and evening primrose oil which are rich in fatty acids nourish the nervous system. 7. Consider bovine cartilage and shark cartilage as added support for back pain with sciatica.	1. Eat a diet with a wide variety of raw vegetables and fruits, and whole grain cereals to ensure a complete supply of nutrients for the bones, nerves, and muscles. 2. Fresh pineapples are recommended as they contain bromelain, an enzyme that is excellent in reducing inflammation. If the consumption of fresh pineapples causes stomach upset, eat it after meals. 3. Avoid red meat and seafood in the diet as they contain high levels of uric acid, which puts added strain on the kidneys. 4. Avoid cold beverages, ice cream, caffeine, sugar, tomatoes, milk, and dairy products.
Sinusitis	1. Vitamin C, 500 to 1,000 mg every waking hour reduces histamine levels. 2. Thymus extract, 750 mg once or bid. 3. Beta-carotene, 50,000 IU tid.	1. Avoid spicy, fried, or greasy foods. 2. Food or beverages that are cool or cold in nature should be consumed. Among these are watermelon, lotus nodes, melon, seaweed, cranberries, celery, cucumber, cactus and winter melon. 3. Drink plenty of water in order to urinate often. 4. Increase supplementation with vitamin C and B complex.
Smoking	1. Consider Smoking withdrawal from Natra-Bio Homeopathic. 2. Glutamine, 1,000 mg daily. Cysteine, 1,000 mg daily and Vitamin C, 1,000 mg daily for nicotine toxicity. 3. Magnesium, 800 mg daily to calm nerves. 4. Ginseng and licorice help normalize and control cravings. 5. Lycopene, 10 mg daily, germanium, 150 mg daily, CoQ10, 60 mg tid, aid oxygen flow to the brain and protect heart tissue. 6. Beta-carotene, 200,000 IU daily are great antioxidants and lung protectors. 7. Maitake 1,000 to 4,000 mg daily, inhibits carcinogenesis and protects against metastasis through the lungs.	1. Consume more asparagus, broccoli, cauliflower, spinach, sweet potatoes, nuts, seeds, yellow and deep-orange vegetables, pumpkin, squash, yams, apples, cantaloupe, grapes, legumes, and plums. 2. Drink fresh carrot juice daily as a preventative measure against lung cancer. 3. Avoid junk foods, processed refined foods, sugar, white flour or any animal protein, except for broiled fish.

Condition	Supplements / Vitamins	Nutrition
Sore Throat	1. Vitamin C chewable, 500 mg every hour during acute stages. 2. Consider Emergen-C every few hours. 3. Vitamin C, 5,000 mg daily to fight infection. 4. Zinc lozenges or colloidal silver as needed. 5. Lysine, 500 mg daily. 6. Echinacea to flush lymph glands for at least 7 days. 7. Garlic capsules, 8 daily.	1. Avoid spicy, fried, or greasy foods. 2. Food or beverages that are cool or cold in nature should be consumed. Among these are watermelon, lotus nodes, melon, seaweed, cranberries, celery, cucumber, cactus and winter melon. 3. Drink plenty of water in order to urinate often. 4. Increase supplementation with vitamin C and B complex. 5. Lemon juice and honey in hot water with a pinch of cayenne pepper each morning is helpful.
Stress	1. Calcium 500 to 1,000 mg daily. 2. DHEA, 25 to 50 daily. 3. Magnesium, 250 to 500 mg daily is a muscle relaxant. 4. Vitamin B Complex, 25 to 50 mg daily regulates nerves. 5. Siberian ginseng, astragalus, schisandra, and kava are great adaptogens which strengthen resistance to stress. 6. CoQ10, 100 mg qid helps fight fatigue and is a powerful antioxidant. 7. SAMe, 400 mg daily. glutamine, 1,000 mg daily, tyrosine, 500 mg daily and DLPA, 1,000 mg daily are good amino acids that boost your brain energy. 8. Ginseng, gotu kola, and ginkgo biloba provide excellent support to the nerves. 9. Licorice root extract helps support adrenal functions.	1. A diet high in calcium, magnesium, phosphorus, potassium, and vitamins B and E is recommended. These vitamins and minerals are easily depleted by stress. 2. Consider a raw diet. 3. Encourage the consumption of fruits and vegetables such as apricots, wintermelon, asparagus, avocados, bananas, and broccoli in addition to brown rice, dried fruit, figs, salmon, garlic, green leafy vegetables, soy products, and yogurt. 4. Avoid caffeine (coffee, tea, soda, chocolate), tobacco, alcohol, and sugar whenever possible.
Stroke	1. B-complex, 50 mg tid nourishes the brain and reduces homocysteine levels. 2. Beta-carotene has been shown to reduce the risk of ischemic stroke. 3. Vitamin E, 200 to 800 IU daily is a powerful antioxidant and reduces clotting. 4. Selenium, 200 mcg daily keeps tissue elastic. 5. Multivitamins and minerals daily that include vitamin A, C, and E. 6. Pycnogenol, 400 mg daily keeps collagen elastic and softens platelets. 7. Vitamin C with bioflavonoids, 3,000 to 20,000 strengthens arterial walls. 8. Melatonin, 500 to 3,000 mcg prevents free-radical damage.	1. Eliminate salt and fats from the diet and reduce blood pressure. 2. Avoid MSG, baking soda, meat, fat, aged foods, alcohol, diet soft drinks, preservatives, sugar substitutes, meat tenderizers, and soy sauce. 3. Increase the intake of fresh, raw vegetables and fruits to control blood pressure. Nuts and seeds should be consumed daily for a source of protein. 4. Vitamin C and bioflavonoids help to reduce blood pressure by stabilizing the blood vessel walls. 5. Garlic is effective to lower blood pressure and thin the blood.
Tendonitis	1. Vitamin E, 200 to 400 IU daily reduces trauma and torn cartilage. 2. Vitamin C with bioflavonoids tid is important in the production of collagen and helps speed repair of tissue. 3. Manganese, 3 to 5 mg tid. 4. Bromelain, 400 mg tid is a natural anti-inflammatory. 5. Pine bark and grape seed extract, 50 mg tid. 6. Zinc, 15 mg daily supports the immune system. 7. Flaxseed and fish oil rich in omega-3 fatty acid, 1,000 mg bid. 8. Bromelain, 400 mg tid has natural anti-inflammatory properties. 9. Glucosamine sulfate, 1,500 mg daily or Chondroitin sulfate, 1,200 mg daily to reduce trauma. 10. Creatine, 1,000 mg daily for muscles and joint injuries also help speed up recovery time.	1. Eat organically grown foods with no chemical treatments or additives, including fresh vegetables, especially dark-green vegetables, fruits, lean chicken, fish and tofu. 2. Avoid saturated, hydrogenated, processed foods, sugars, red meat, dairy products, caffeine, and alcohol.
Tinnitus	1. Vitamin A, 25,000 IU daily. 2. Vitamin B1, 100 to 500 mg daily. 3. Vitamin B12, 1 to 5 mg daily in lozenge form. 4. B-complex, 50 mg bid. 5. Vitamin E, 400 to 800 IU daily helps repair nerves. 6. Vitamin D, 500 to 1,000 daily. 7. Magnesium, 500 mg daily. 8. Potassium, 500 mg daily. 9. Silica helps strengthen vascular walls.	1. Encourage a diet with a high content of raw foods, fruits and vegetables to stabilize blood-sugar. 2. Discourage dairy products and red meats, as they promote hot flashes. 3. Avoid spicy or greasy foods, or anything else that may trigger a recurrent bacterial or viral attack.
TMJ	1. Vitamin B complex daily to relieve anxiety and improve sleep. 2. Vitamin C, 2,000 to 5,000 tid.	1. Eat a diet including lightly steamed vegetables, fresh fruit, whole-grain products, and white fish. Eat more sulfur-containing foods, such as asparagus, eggs, garlic and onions. Sulfur is needed for repair and rebuilding of bones, cartilage and connective tissue. 2. Eat fresh pineapple frequently. 3. Avoid high stress foods: all forms of sugar, all junk foods, alcohol, candy, colas, fast foods, and foods containing caffeine.
Toothache	1. Multivitamins and minerals daily. 2. Calcium, 1,000 mg daily. 3. Magnesium, 600 mg daily for healthy teeth. 4. Hydrogen peroxide, 3 percent, floss and swish in your mouth for few seconds helps kill infection in the gum or nerve of a tooth.	1. A diet consisting of lean protein, good concentration of calcium, phosphorous, and vitamin D. 2. Calcium rich foods include: green leafy vegetables, broccoli, cabbage and Brussels sprouts, figs, kelp, oats, prunes, sesame seeds, and tofu. 3. Phosphorous can be obtained from bananas, whole grain breads and cereals, eggs, fish and poultry. Foods rich in calcium include: eggs, dairy products, and saltwater fish.

Condition	Supplements / Vitamins	Nutrition
Ulcer	1. Vitamin C, 500 to 1,000 mg tid. 2. Vitamin E, 200 to 400 IU daily. 3. EFAs, Flaxseed oil, 1 tablespoon daily. 4. Vitamin A, 20,000 IU daily heals mucosal tissue of the stomach. 5. Zinc, 25 to 30 mg daily speeds the healing process. 6. Chewing tablets containing a special licorice extract, DGL (for deglycyrrhizinated licorice), 380 to 760 mg twenty minutes before meals is very effective in healing ulcers. In fact, clinical studies have shown DGL is more effective than standard anti-ulcer drugs. 7. Fish oil and corn oil can keep ulcers from coming back.	1. Increase the intake of papayas and pineapples as they contain bromelain, a digestive enzyme that helps with indigestion. 2. Acidophilus is also helpful for digestion. 3. For ulcers, intake of vitamin K, found in green leafy vegetables, should be increased as it helps with the healing process. 4. Avoid lentils, peanuts and soybeans because they contain enzyme inhibitors. 5. Avoid fried, spicy or greasy foods, refined sugar, tea, coffee, caffeine, salt, chocolate, strong spices, and carbonated drinks.
UTI	1. Consider Probiotics which can help improve digestive function and eliminate bacterial buildup. 2. Drink unsweetened cranberry juice (16 ounces daily) or take a cranberry extract to acidify the urine and inhibit bacterial growth. 3. Vitamin C, 2,000 to 6,000 mg daily expels infectious bacteria and is an effective preventative agent. 4. Zinc, 50 mg daily assists in WBC production and eliminates bacteria. 5. Vitamin A prevents irritation and improves function of WBC. 6. Colloidal silver is a natural antibiotic. 7. Calcium, 1,500 mg daily and magnesium 750 to 1,000 mg daily reduces bladder irritability.	1. Natural, plain yogurt with live cultures helps to minimize yeast infections by establishing a normal environment in the genital tract. 2. Eat plenty of fruits and vegetables, which provide the nutrients needed to resist infection and facilitate healing. 3. Regular consumption of unsweetened cranberry juice will help to prevent and treat urinary tract infection. 4. Drink watermelon and pear juice tid. 5. Drink carrot and celery juice tid. 6. Drink cornsilk tea freely. 7. Eat squash soup for at least seven days. 8. Eat steamed lotus root and water chestnuts bid.
Varicose Veins	1. Multivitamins and minerals daily. 2. Vitamin C, 500 to 1,000 mg to strengthen vein walls. 3. Vitamin E, 200 to 400 IU daily. 4. EFAs, Flaxseed oil, 1 tablespoon daily. 5. PCO extracts or flavonoids are excellent at strengthening vein walls. 6. Aorta glycosaminoglycans, 50 mg bid. 7. DMSO has been used to relieve the swelling and pain of severe varicose veins. 8. Bromelain, 1,500 mg daily, quercitin, 1,000 mg daily boost flavonoids for vein tone and reduce inflammation.	1. Eat a diet that is low in fat and refined carbohydrates and includes plenty of fish and fresh fruits and vegetables. 2. Eat as many blackberries and cherries as you wish. 3. Include garlic, onion, and pineapple in your diet. 4. Avoid animal protein, processed and refined foods, sugar, junk foods, tobacco, alcohol, and salt.
Warts Common	1. Adequate vitamin C intake is more important in managing effective immunity against the viruses that cause warts. 2. High potency multivitamin and mineral supplements. 3. Zinc, 75 mg daily, increases immunity against viruses. 4. N-acetyl cysteine, 2,000 mg daily helps boost immune response. 5. Vitamin E, 800 IU daily or apply the oil on the surrounding skin. 6. Vitamin A 100,000 IU daily for one month, then 50,000 IU daily for second month, then reduce to 25,000 IU daily for third month or until warts disappear.	1. Increase the amount of sulfur-containing amino acids in your diet by eating more asparagus, citrus fruits, eggs, onions, and garlic.
Weakened immune system	1. High potency multivitamin and mineral supplements. 2. Vitamin A, 10,000 IU daily. 3. Vitamin C with flavonoids, 5,000 to 20,000 mg daily. 4. Vitamin E, 400 IU daily. 5. Zinc, 50 to 80 mg daily. 6. Coenzyme Q10, 25 to 50 mg daily. 7. DHEA, 25 to 50 mg daily. 8. Pregnenolone, 10 mg daily. 9. Selenium, 100 to 200 mcg daily.	1. Begin diet of fresh fruits, vegetables, seeds, grains, and other foods that are high in fiber. 2. Include in your diet: chlorella, garlic, and pearl barley. 3. Consume green drinks daily. 4. Avoid animal products, processed foods, alcohol, smoking, and soda. 5. Follow a fasting program; consider the use of spirulina, especially after fasting.

ESSENTIAL OILS

There are many different essential oils available, each with its own special properties. The table lists some of the more commonly used oils for common conditions.

Conditions	Oils
Allergies	Roman Chamomile, Lavender, Myrrh
Arthritis	Birch, Ginger, Juniper, Lavender, Marjoram
Asthma	Cypress, Frankincense, Lavender, Peppermint, Eucalyptus
Bacterial & Fungal Infections	Oregano, Tea Tree, Lemon, Eucalyptus, Niaouli, Lavender
Bone Breaks, Dislocation & Damage	Eucalyptus, Chamomile, Lavender
Bronchitis	Eucalyptus, Fir, Pine, Tea Tree, Niaouli, White Thyme, Myrtle
Burns & Sunburns	Lavender, Chamomile, Niaouli
Bruising	Lavender, Roman Chamomile, Myrtle
Candida	Tea Tree, Lemongrass, Marjoram, Myrrh, Niaouli
Cellulite	Fennel, Juniper, Lemon
Circulation (Poor)	Cypress, Lemongrass, Ginger
Colds, Flu	Eucalyptus, Lavender, Pine, Fir, Myrtle
Cold Sores	Lemon, Chamomile, Tea Tree, Lavender
Cystitis	Birch, Cedarwood, Juniper, Cypress, Lavender
Digestion (Poor)	Anise, Fennel, Ginger, Lemongrasss, Nutmeg, Pepper
Ear Problems	Chamomile, Lavender, Tea Tree, Niaouli, Marjoram, Juniper
Fatigue	Caraway Seed, Clove Bud, Cypress, Peppermint
Hair Loss	Cedarwood, Sage
Hair (Oily)	Sage, Lemon, Neroli, Cedarwood
Headaches	German Chamomile, Lavender, Peppermint, Cedarwood
Hemorrhoids	Cypress, Myrtle, Juniper, Myrrh
Immune System (Low)	Lemon, Tea Tree, Angelica, Niaouli
Inflammation	Blue and German Chamomile, Patchouli, Myrrh, Frankincense
Insomnia	Neroli, Marjoram, Tangerine, Lavender, Chamomile
Jet Lag	Melissa, Angelica, Peppermint, Ginger, Lemon
Laryngitis	Chamomile, Lavender, Lemon, Cypress, Lemongrass, Myrrh
Menopause	Clary, Chamomile, Fennel, Sage, Rose, Jasmine
Menstrual Pain (Light Periods)	Chamomile, Lavender, Marjoram, Clary Sage, Cypress
Menstrual Pain (Heavy Periods)	Chamomile, Lavender, Cypress, Marjoram
Migraine	Peppermint, Chamomile, Lavender, Marjoram, Angelica
Muscle & Tendon Damage	Eucalyptus, Peppermint, Ginger, Lavender, Chamomile
Nausea	Peppermint, Spearmint, Ginger
Obesity	Fennel, Lemon, Ginger, Peppermint, Cardamon
Pain (Muscular)	Birch, Chamomile, Clove, Ginger, Pepper, Lavender, Nutmeg
Post Operative Care	Chamomile, Lavender, Niaouli,
Rheumatism	Birch, Juniper, Chamomile, Lavender, Pine
Sinusitis	Lavender, Eucalyptus, Peppermint, Angelica, Myrtle, Tea Tree
Snoring	Myrtle, Marjoram, Lavender
Soft Tissue Damage	Chamomile, Lavender, Eucalyptus, Ginger
Sore Throat	Ginger, Myrrh, Pine, Eucalyptus, Tea Tree, Lemongrass
Sprains	Ginger, Nutmeg, Clove, Peppermint
Stretch Marks	Rose, Lavender, Tangerine, Neroli
Urinary Infections	Cedarwood, Juniper, Tea Tree, Myrtle
Varicose Veins	Cypress, Lemon, Peppermint, Lavender
Water Retention	Cypress, Orange, Juniper, Lemon
Wounds	Lavender, Fir, Tea Tree, Myrrh

ESSENTIAL OILS

The table lists some of the more commonly used oils and their properties.

Oils	Properties
Basil	Aids concentration, clarity and helps fight colds, influenza and headaches.
Bergamot	A balancing and uplifting stress-relieving oil. Lifts depression and melancholy.
Cedarwood	An antiseptic, expectorant, astringent, and sedative. Normalizes sweat gland function. Good for bronchial problems and useful for controlling mildew and molds.
Chamomile	An analgesic, anti-inflammatory, and antispasmodic. Relieves muscular pain, as a sedative, which calms the mind and eases fear, eases anxiety, emotional stress, nervous tension, and insomnia. Excellent for headaches. A good remedy for gastrointestinal problems.
Cinnamon Bark	A useful scent enhancement in the home or office which makes a good air freshener and has antifungal properties.
Clary Sage	An aromatic oil that is used for healing eye problems. An antidepressant, anti-inflammatory, antispasmodic, and aphrodisiac. Helps relieve insomnia, menopause, PMS, and nervous exhaustion. Caution: Should not be used in the first months of pregnancy.
Cypress	An astringent, antiseptic, antispasmodic oil which is soothing and eases aches and pains and coughs. Used to increase circulation, relieve muscular cramps, bronchitis, whooping cough, painful periods, reduce nervous tension and other stress-related problems. Acts as an immune stimulant. Reduces coughing and excessive perspiration.
Eucalyptus	An antiseptic, antiviral chest rub, decongestant, and expectorant. Reduces fever, relieves congestion, muscle aches and asthma. Has a normalizing and balancing effect.
Frankincense	An anti-inflammatory, antiseptic, sedative and expectorant. Promotes cellular regeneration and elevates mind and spirit. Good to calm by slowing down breathing and controlling tension, it helps to focus the mind, enhance meditation, help breathing, and psychic cleansing. Also excellent for toning and caring for mature/aging skin.
Ginger	A fiery and fortifying oil used for massaging on the muscles and for nausea and sickness.
Geranium	An antidepressant, anti-diabetic, antiseptic, hormone balancer and insect repellant. A normalizing and balancing, flowery aroma which is both uplifting and calming oil good for PMS, hormone balancing, nervous tension, skin concerns, and neuralgia. Good as bath additive and in skin-care products for both its fragrance and cleansing properties.
Grapefruit	A citrus smell which is energizing and helps to elevate the spirits, reduces appetite and useful in treating obesity. Balances mood, relieves muscle fatigue, lifts depression, cleanses the body of toxins, reduces water retention, and detoxifies the skin.
Hyssop	An antiseptic, antidepressant, and sedative which promotes alertness and clarity of thought. Useful for anxiety, emotional imbalances, frigidity, and impotence. Benefits scalp and skin.
Jasmine	An antidepressant, aphrodisiac, antiseptic, and sedative which is emotionally warming, relaxing, soothing, uplifting and helps self confidence. Useful for anxiety, emotional imbalances, frigidity, and impotence. Benefits scalp and skin.
Juniper	An antiseptic, detoxifier, diuretic and internal cleanser which exerts a cleansing effect on the mental and spiritual planes as well as on the physical. Helps rid body of toxins, reduces spasms, improve arthritis and reduces cellulite. Caution: Do not use during pregnancies. Do not use if you have kidney problems.
Lavender	An overall first aid oil, antiviral and antibacterial, boosts immunity, antidepressant, anti-inflammatory, and antispasmodic which is relaxing and refreshing, uplifts the spirits, and helps to relieve the distress of muscle pain. Useful for improving immune system function, calming and normalizing the body fighting bacterial and fungal infect, easing depression and reducing inflammation. Good for acne, burns, eczema, skin healing, sleep disorders, and stress.
Lemon	An antiseptic, antibacterial, and astringent. Helps to increase the body's defenses against infections. Refreshing and uplifting for purification of the body. Good for varicose veins, stomach ulcers, anxiety depression and digestive disorders. Emulsifies and disperses grease and oil. Helpful in cleaning product and hair rinses and wound cleansing.
Lemongrass	An antiseptic and astringent oil which is refreshing, cleansing and stimulating body tonic. Serves as a good refreshing and deodorizing room fragrance.
Linden	A calming, sedating and soothing tonic. Moisturizes the skin.
Marjoram, sweet	A calming, soothing and warming effect on mind, body and spirit. It helps relieve common colds, including congestion and muscle aches and pains, and is also comforting in times of stress. Used to regulate the nervous system and treat insomnia.
Orange	Balances and uplifts emotions. Has an antispasmodic and regenerative property. Useful in skin-care products. Caution: This oil increases sensitivity to the sun. Do not use if you are spending considerable time outdoors.
Patchouli	An aphrodisiac used in personal fragrances to relieve stress and nervous exhaustion. Good for dry skin and athlete's foot. Has antidepressant, anti-inflammatory, antiseptic, aphrodisiac and anti-fungal properties.
Peppermint	An antiseptic, antispasmodic, mental stimulant and has regenerative properties which is energizing, penetrating, minty, and aromatic oil helpful for brightening moods, reduces pain, improves mental clarity, and memory. Good for headaches, congestion, fatigue, fever, indigestion, muscle soreness, sinus problems and stomach problems.
Pine	A refreshing and cleansing immune system stimulant which acts as an antiseptic, antiviral, expectorant, restorative, and stimulate. Helps to clear the mind. Repels lice and fleas.
Rose	An antidepressant, antiseptic, and tonic astringent which is soothing and cleansing oil which uplifts the spirit. Acts as a mild sedative. Good for female complaints, impotence, insomnia, and nervousness.
Rosemary	The ideal "pick you up" oil which is an antiseptic, antispasmodic, astringent, and mental stimulant. Enhances circulation. Energizing for muscle pains, cramps or sprains, brightens mood, for improving mental clarity and memory. Helpful for cellulite, dandruff, hair loss, memory problems, headache, and sore muscles. Caution: if irritation occurs, discontinue use. Do not use directly on the skin without diluting. Use caution if inhaling it if you have asthma or bronchitis. Do not use if you have epilepsy.
Rosewood	An antiseptic and regenerative. Helps relieve stress and balance the central nervous system. Calms and helps restore emotional balance. Good for jet lag, anxiety, cellular regeneration, depression headaches, nausea, PMS, and tension.
Sandalwood	An antidepressant, antiseptic, expectorant, aphrodisiac, and skin moisturizer. Lifts melancholy, enhances meditation, heals the skin, calms and reduces stress. Good for bronchitis and nervousness; it is soothing for both mind and body.
Tea Trea	A powerful, anti-infective, anti-inflammatory, antiseptic, antiviral, expectorant, antifungal, and anti-parasitic used as a cleansing agent. Powerful immuno-stimulant properties especially against bacteria and viruses. Good for athletes, foot, bronchial congestion, dandruff, ringworm, and yeast infection.
Thyme	An antiseptic, antispasmodic, and expectorant. Calming.
Yarrow	An anti-inflammatory and antispasmodic. Improves digestion and lowers blood pressure. Similar in function to chamomile
Ylang yiang	Antidepressant, antiseptic, aphrodisiac, and calming sedatives. Lifts mood, relieves anger, eases anxiety, relaxes muscles, reduces stress, normalizes the heartbeat, and lowers blood pressure. Good for frigidity, high blood pressure and impotence.

VITAMINS

Chief Complaint History (LOC-Q-SMAT)

1. (L) Location / radiation
- Where? Have patient point to the location.
- Write description of location that is as specific as possible (" thoracic or mid-thoracic" is more specific than "low back, "anterior & lateral right shoulder" is preferable to "shoulder")
- Indicate right, left or both sides.
- Does it radiate? If so, where and how far? (ankle, elbow, wrist, hand, fingertips?)
- What surface or aspect? (lateral/medial/anterior/posterior/dorsal)

2. (O) Onset (what happened & when did it occur?)
- When did you first notice this problem? Was it gradual or sudden? What was the cause?
- Look for specific actions, modifications in activities, posture, occupation, exercise.

3. (C) Chronology/Timing (symptom patterns)
- Constant or intermittent patterns (episodic).
- If persistent, is it actually 24 hours a day? Does it affect sleep?
- If irregular, is it associated with specific conditions? (e.g. consuming certain foods? particular activities? time of day?)
- Rate of recurrence & length of the episodes.
- Diurnal patterns (worse in morning or end of day?)
- Is there night pain that wakes you or prevents you from falling asleep?
- Worsening, improving, or staying the same?
- Prior history: Have you ever experienced this type of problem? When? For how long? How did you address it?

4. (Q) Quality
- Have patient describe pain or symptoms (sharp, dull, etc.).
- If description is uncommon, use patient's words in quotations or open-ended question.

5. (S) Severity/ADL affected (activities daily living)
- Is pain slight, moderate, or intense?
- How would you rate pain on scale from 1 to 10?
- ADL: Can patient perform regular daily activity such as work? Is performance affected? Hobbies? Sexual activity? Everyday activities such as putting on a jacket? Get specific actions & how the patient is affected (great source of functional outcome markers).

6. (M) Modifying factors
- Does anything make symptoms or pain worse? Be specific.
- Does anything make symptoms better? Avoiding certain things? Changing posture? Rest? Medication (how much relief & how often?)

7. (A) Associated symptoms
- Do you have any other symptoms or problems that you feel are related or relevant to this issue?
- Further detailed questions are asked based on what the patient presents with & what the examiner thinks it could be; for example:
  - Is there numbness, tingling, or lack of strength in an extremity?
  - Neck: Any cracking? Headaches? Numbness in the arms?
  - Knees: Any popping, clicking, or snapping? Knees ever lock? Swell? Give way?
  - Low back: Does your back ever catch or get locked? Any changes in bladder or bowel habits? Change in sexual performance?

8. (T) Treatment previous
- Have you been treated by other health care providers? Who did you see? When? What tests were performed?
- What diagnosis? What treatment? Did it help?

9. Relevant injuries
- When? What happened? (Include falls, broken bones, or motor vehicle accidents)
- Were you hospitalized? Did you have any relevant surgeries?
- What was the ultimate outcome? Were there any residual effects?

10. Goal (optional)
- What is the treatment goal of the patient?
- If it has been a long-term problem, why is s/he seeking treatment now?

Is there any more information you can provide regarding your condition?

Using appropriate terms, explain why you are inquiring & be compassionate towards patient.

Create a differential diagnosis list.

Family & Personal History / Past Health History

Family Health Problems
- Are there any conditions that run in your family, such as cancer, depression, diabetes, high blood pressure, stroke or heart disease?
- I'd like to start with your father. Is he still living? If so, describe any health problems he has
- How about your father's father?
- Your mother? Your siblings?
- If there is a deceased relative, what was their age at time of death? What was the cause of death?
- Are there any other health issues in the family?

1. Living Environment
- How would you describe your living environment? Is it a house/condo/apartment? What are the relationships of dwellers? Are there children?

2. Occupation
- What is your profession?
- Describe the nature of your work? What is involved? What are the hours you work?
- Do you enjoy your work?

3. Exercise
- Do you partake in regular exercise? (What type? How intense? How often?)

4. Interests/Avocations/ Activities
- Are there any other interests, avocations or activities you enjoy?

5. Diet/Nutrition
- Rate the quality of your overall diet (scale 1 to 10)
- What do you eat for breakfast? Lunch? Dinner? Between meals?
- What do you drink during the day?
- How often do you eat meat? Vegetables? Fruit? Sweets? Fast food?
- How much water a day do you consume?

6. Sleep Pattern
- How much sleep do you get each night?
- Any changes in your sleep lately?
- Do you think you get enough rest?

7. Bowel Habits
- How frequently do you have bowel movements? Any changes recently?
- Any rectal bleeding?

8. Urinary Habits
- Do you have any problems with urinating? Any recent changes? Problems starting or stopping?

9. Habits
- Do you drink alcohol? What type?
- Frequency and amount of alcohol?
- Smoke or use any tobacco products? What kind and how much?
- How long did you smoke? When did you stop?
- Use any recreational drugs? What and for how long? (reiterate patient confidentiality if needed)

10. Domestic Violence
- Are you now or have you ever been in a relationship in which you were physically injured or threatened?

11. Stress factors/Depression/Support system
- Any significant stresses in your life lately?
- Noticed a change in your ability to handle stress?
- Feel depressed?
- What resources do you have for support?

Assessing Pain and Symptoms (OPQRST)

O = Onset. When did pain first start? Over days or within hours. Acute vs. chronic.

P = Provoke. What causes the pain? What intensifies or lessens it?

Q = Quality. What does pain feel like? Sharp? Dull? Burning? Stabbing? Crushing? Throbbing?

R = Radiation. Does the pain travel to different places in the body?

S = Severity. Do you think the pain is mild, moderate, or severe?

T = Time. Is pain continuous or sporadic? Has it occurred before? Does it change (get better or worse)? When does it start?

PRACTICE

Past Health History

1. Serious Illness
- Ever had one or more serious illnesses?
- Other problems?

2. Hospitalizations/Surgeries
- Ever been hospitalized?
- Ever had surgery of any kind?

3. General Trauma, Accidents, Injury
- Have you experienced any physical trauma that was treated or that you think should have been treated?
- Ever had any accidents? MVA?
- Suffer any residual problems or long-lasting side effects?

4. Menses, Menopause
- What was the first day of your last menstrual period?
- Any problems with your menstrual cycle?
- Any changes in your menstrual cycle? Any abnormal bleeding?

Patients over 50:
- Do you continue to have menstrual periods? If yes, do you remember the first day of your last menstrual period?

Physiologic menopause:
- How old when you first experienced menopause?
- Taken hormone replacements in the past? Currently taking them?
- If yes, which one? How administered?

Surgical menopause:
- Why did you have a hysterectomy? For cancer?
- Were your ovaries removed?
- Taking hormone replacements?
- If yes, which one? How administered?

5. Contraceptives, Pregnancies
Contraceptives:
- Using any type of hormonal contraceptive or an IUD? If yes, have there been any problems?

Pregnancies:
- Ever been pregnant? If is yes, were there any complications?

6. Medications
- Take any prescribed medications?
- Any over-the-counter medications?
- Any vitamins?
- Ever taken any medication such as steroids, antidepressants, NSAIDs, antibiotics, hormones for an extended period of time?

7. Allergies
- Allergic to any foods or medications? If so, are they seasonal?

8. X-rays
- Have you ever had any x-rays? If so, why?
- Any problems identified on the x-ray?

9. Prior Care
- Have you ever received prior care?
- If so, what for? Describe the care. Did it help?
- This will tell what has and hasn't worked prior

10. Last Physical Exam
- When was your last physical exam? Were you experiencing your chief complaint when you had it?
- What was it for?
- Any problems identified?

Females:
- When was your last GYN exam and PAP smear?
- What were the results?

Females over 50:
- Have you had a mammogram? How often?
- Results?

Males 15-35:
- Do you perform self-testicular exams?
- Have you ever been taught how to?

Males over 40:
- Ever had a rectal exam or lab tests to evaluate your prostate?
- If so, do you remember the results?

10 Asking Diagnosis

1. Chills and fever
- Do you get chills, fever, or both?
- Is it made worse or better with heat or cold?
- Are there alternating chills and fever?

2. Sweat
- Is there profuse or scanty sweat?
- Indicate the area or times of the day when you sweat?
- What is the quality of the sweat?

3. Head and body
- Do you have headaches, dizziness, whole body pain, joint pain, backaches, or numbness and tingling in the body?
- If so, please indicate the onset, times, location, character, and condition of each pain?

4. Thorax and abdomen
- Do you have chest pain, epigastric pain, lower abdominal pain, hypogastric pain and/or abdominal distention?
- If so, please indicate the onset, times, location, character, and condition of each pain?
- Indicate if conditions are made worse or better with bowel movements or with food.

5. Food and taste
- Indicate if conditions are made worse or better with food?
- Indicate the preference for food quality?
- Describe taste in your mouth?
- Is there vomiting? If so, indicate quality and if conditions are made worse or better?

6. Sleep
- How many hours do you sleep each night?
- Describe the quality of the sleep, dreams, waking up, falling asleep, or lack of sleep, etc.?
- Have there been any recent changes in sleep?
- Do you feel you get enough sleep?
- Is there a feeling of lethargy involved? Describe the quality and character?

7. Stools and urine
- Describe the consistency, character, smell, and sensations of your stool sample?
- How often do you have a bowel movement? Any recent changes?
- Is there constipation, diarrhea, or both? Include the consistency, character, smell, and sensations of your stool.
- Do you ever notice any rectal bleeding or discoloration?
- Do you have any problems with urination? Any recent changes? (stopping or starting)
- Describe the frequency and color of your urine? Is there pain involved in urination?

8. Ears and eyes
- Do you have tinnitus? If so describe the onset, pressure, and character of the noise?
- Is there sudden or gradual deafness in the ear?
- Is there pain or dryness in the eye? If so, describe the character, location, and quality?

9. Thirst and drink
- How often and what is the amount of water you consume in a day?
- Is there absence or desire to drink water?

10. Pain
- Please indicate if there is any pain involved throughout the body and describe the following: type, temperature, onset, character, location, posture, made better or worse with pressure, bowel movements, rest and movement.

PRACTICE

Review of Findings (ROF)

Review of findings (ROF) is a significant aspect of acupuncture treatment and gives you the chance to determine benefits from your treatment and be an expert in its execution. It also is an excellent outline for acupuncture success by educating patient on how you will treat his or her complaints.

PRACTICE

Greeting
1. Greet patient by name
2. Ask about current status
3. Orient patient to ROF
    a. Review of findings and their meanings
    b. Make treatment suggestions
    c. Provide opportunity for questions
    d. Inform patient of anticipated duration of each treatment (30 min to 60 min)

Overview
1. Summarize the problem(s)
2. Establish your ability to help
3. Reassure patient about his/her condition

Describe condition(s)
1. Explain diagnosis in simple terms
2. The cause (mechanism of injury)
3. Review exam findings how they relate to diagnosis
4. How it manifests
5. How the treatment will address cause

Describe treatment
1. Type of therapy
2. Frequency and duration of treatments

Establish goals
1. Describe goals of acupuncture treatment
2. Relate goals to problem(s) and outcome measures

Describe importance of compliance
1. Relate to cause of problem and complaint
2. Stress patient's role in her/his own care
3. Determine and address obstacles to compliance

Describe expectations
1. Outcome measures
2. When to re-evaluate

PAR (Procedures, Alternatives, Risks)
1. Legally required for every new procedure
2. Describe procedures, alternatives to treatment and risks
3. Obtain written informed consent with patient's signature to proceed with treatment
4. Address any questions (legally required)

Conclusion
1. Educational materials
2. Answer any of patient's questions

Practice Building Tips
1. Be professional, prepared and competent
2. Ensure patient's comfort
3. Use appropriate language for patient's level of understanding
4. Communication between clinician and patient should flow naturally
5. Use clear explanations that make sense
6. Be a good listener
7. Adjust eye contact to patient's comfort
8. Have empathy for patient's concerns
9. Give patient opportunities to ask questions/verbalize concerns

SOAP NOTES

The purpose of the SOAP note is to be a brief report using abbreviations rather than complete sentences. Keep in mind that abbreviations differ for each specialty. SOAP notes can also be used as documentation on the necessity for continued treatment (especially when dealing with third-party payers or litigation).

S = SUBJECTIVE - Symptoms the patient verbally expresses or that are stated by a significant other. Include the patient's descriptions of pain or discomfort, the presence of nausea or dizziness and a multitude of other descriptions of dysfunction, discomfort or illness the patient describes.

- Record subjective information provided by the patient, using quotes if possible
- How has patient responded since last treatment
- Address each condition separately
- Keep this section brief unless patient has much new information
- If patient presents with a new condition, then a new chief complaint history is required

O = OBJECTIVE - Include symptoms that can actually be measured, seen, heard, touched, felt, or smelled. Vital signs such as temperature, pulse, respiration, skin color, swelling and the results of diagnostic tests.

- Record objective information observed about the patient
- General observations of the patient physical presentation are applicable
- Physical exam parameters are monitored

A = ASSESSMENT - The diagnosis of the patient's condition. In some cases the diagnosis may be clear, such as a low back pain, but an assessment might not be clear and could include several diagnosis possibilities.

- Record assessment as to the current status of condition
- Indicate whether improving or not
- For the action, record treatment that was administered during the visit
- Record patient response to treatment ask the patient how they felt afterwards
- Home care exercises, etc. provided

P = PLAN - May include laboratory and/or radiological tests ordered for the patient, medications ordered, treatments performed, patient referrals (sending patient to a specialist), patient disposition (e.g., home care, bed rest, short-term, long-term disability, days excused from work, admission to hospital), patient directions and follow-up directions for the patient.

- Patient to return (PTR), record the date you want patient to return for treatment
- Record any patient self-care instructions
- Record any future plans to examine or test

Soap Note Example:
Patient Name: KY DOB: 12/31/1961
Record No. XXX-XXX-XXXX
Date: 09/09/07

S: "Pt. says she has neck pain that cricks upon movement." Had a headache for last 2 weeks, unable to sleep because of pain. PMS symptoms with cramps. Current 7/10 pain.
O: Tight and tender, both sides at occipital ridge, temporal headaches > right side
A: Neck pain, heat to posterior cervical, manual neck stretches.
P: Acupuncture, Change habits to lessen workload and avoid being on computer long time. Short Term Goal: Client to begin stretching exercise for every 2 hours of work. Told patient to be aware of body and posture while working. Follow-up in one week.

SOAP

Subjective: M / F _____   Age_____
Chief
Complaint: _____
_____
_____
_____

Last Visit's _____
Symptom _____
Progress: _____

New _____
Symptoms: _____

(can check: energy level, sleep, sweats, thirst, urination, appetite, digestion, stools, head, eyes, ears, nose, lungs, heart, limbs, emotions, etc.)

Women:	LMP:	Color:	Interval:	Duration:	Flow:	Clots:

For Patients with Pain: Pain Scale: None   0   1   2   3   4   5   6   7   8   9   10   Severe

Objective Signs: Blood Pressure:_____   Temperature:_____   Pulse Rate:_____
Pulses: 1st   L:_____   R:_____
2nd
3rd
Overall _____
Tongue: _____

Other physical/emotional signs and orthopedic examinations:_____

Assessment/Diagnosis: <u>with</u> western dx, write "per doctor" or "per patient" or "per records"
or "NA" as is applicable
Western
Diagnosis: _____
TCM
Diagnosis: _____

Plan of Treatment:
Treatment
Principle: _____

Acupuncture: _____
Bilateral: _____
Right: _____
Left: _____

Herbs/
Recommendations: _____

Mark the" following" where patient feels pain:

X X X   Sharp/stabbing
P P P   Pins & Needles
D D D   Dull/Aching
N N N   Numbness

Ear Seed ☐		Infrared ☐
Exercise ☐		Ear Acp ☐
Patch ☐		Tuina ☐
Massage ☐		Other

ICD-9 Code: _____   _____
CPT Code: _____   _____
Acupuncturist: John Doe, LAc   Signature:
Patient Name: Date:

PRACTICE

Source: ADR; The following general health forms can be downloaded and customized for your usage at
www.acupuncturedeskreference.com

374

PATIENT INFORMATION FORM

Please Note: This is a confidential record of your medical history and will be kept in this office. Information contained here will not be released to any person except when you have authorized us to do so.

Name _____ M.I. _____ Last Name _____

Address _____ City _____ State _____ Zip _____

Home Phone ( ) _____ Cell ( ) _____ Work ( ) _____

SS# _____ Age _____ DOB _____

Drivers License # _____ Male ☐ Female ☐

Employer _____ Occupation _____

Married ☐ Single ☐ Divorced ☐ Name of Spouse _____

Emergency Contact _____ Telephone ( ) _____

Referred by _____ Friend ☐ Relative ☐ Insurance ☐ Other ☐

PRIMARY INSURANCE Cash ☐ Group ☐ Work/Comp ☐ Auto ☐ Other ☐

Name of Insurance Co. _____ ID#. _____ Group# _____

Name of Insured _____ Relationship to Patient: Self ☐ Spouse ☐ Parent ☐

Secondary Insurance _____ Name of Insured _____

I understand that this is a quotation of benefits and is NOT a guarantee of payment, and the agreement is between the Insurance Carrier and me. I authorize any and all payment from my insurance carrier directly to this office with the understand that all monies be credit to my account upon receipt. Any denial of payment becomes my responsibility (patient).

Patient Name (print) _____ Patient Signature _____ Date _____

24 HOUR CANCELLATION POLICY & CREDIT AUTHORIZATION RELEASE

_____ takes pride in the quality of care he offers his patients. In order to do this he has a strict cancellation policy. Dr. _____ requires a 24-hour cancellation notice prior to your appointment time. If sufficient time is not given, the full fee will be charged to the credit card we have on file.

I, _____ authorize Dr. _____ to charge the credit card given below, for cancellation fees, insurance co-payments and related charges.

_____-_____-_____-_____ Ex_____/_____ Visa ☐ / MC ☐

Patient Name (print) _____ Patient Signature _____ Date _____

PRACTICE

Source: ADR; The following general health forms can be downloaded and customized for your usage at www.acupuncturedeskreference.com

ACUPUNCTURE DESK REFERENCE ▮▮▮ 375

OUR CLINIC PROTECTS YOUR HEALTH INFORMATION AND PRIVACY

Dear Valued Patient,

This notice describes our office's policy for how medical information about you may be used and disclosed, how you can get access to this information, and how your privacy is being protected.

In order to maintain the level of service that you expect from our office, we may need to share limited personal medical and financial information with your insurance company and with Worker's Compensation (and your employer as well in this instance), or with other medical practitioners. We will obtain your authorization before disclosing any information.

Safeguards in place at our office include:

- Limited access to facilities where information is stored.
- Policies and procedures for handling information.
- Requirements for third parties to contractually comply with privacy laws.
- All medical files and records (including email, regular mail, telephone, and faxes sent) are kept on permanent file.

Types of information that we gather and use:

In administering your health care, we gather and maintain information that may include non-public personal information:

- About your financial transactions with us (billing transactions).
- From your medical history, treatment notes, all test results, and any letters, faxes, emails or telephone conversations to or from other health care practitioners.

- From health care providers, insurance companies, worker's comp and your employer, and other third party administrators (*e.g.* requests for medical records, claim payment information).

In certain states, you may be able to access and correct personal information we have collected about you, (information that can identify you -*e.g.* your name, address, Social Security number, etc.).

We value our relationship with you, and respect your right to privacy. If you have questions about our privacy guidelines, please call us during regular business hours at _____

Yours sincerely,

_____, L.Ac,
Your Office

PRACTICE

NAME_____   DATE_____

I. Goals: What would you most like to achieve through your work at the ABC Acupuncture Center?
1. _____
2. _____
3. _____
4. _____
5. _____

II. Major Symptoms: Please list in order of importance what symptoms are of concern to you.
(most concerning to least, along with the duration of the symptom)
1. _____
2. _____
3. _____
4. _____

Use the following illustration to indicate painful or distressed areas:

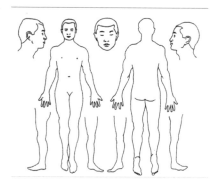

Are you experiencing pain/discomfort in any area of your body? **Y / N**

If yes, using the models to the left, please indicate the location of the discomfort by using the symbol that best describes the feeling:

X X X   Sharp/stabbing
P P P   Pins & Needles
D D D   Dull/Aching
N N N   Numbness

For Women:
1. Are you pregnant now? [ ]Yes   [ ]No   [ ]Unsure

2. Indicate number of occurrences:
Live Births _____ Pregnancies_____ Miscarriages _____ Abortions _____

3. Age: First period _____ Menopause (if applicable) _____

4. Date: Last Pap Smear _____ /_____ Last Mammogram _____ / _____

5. Any History of an Abnormal Pap Smear? [ ] Yes   [ ] No If so, what / when? _____

PRACTICE

Source: ADR; The following general health forms can be downloaded and customized for your usage at www.acupuncturedeskreference.com

ACUPUNCTURE DESK REFERENCE   377

6. Is your menses cycle regular? [ ] Yes [ ] No
a) Average number of days of flow _____
b) The flow is: [ ] Normal [ ] Heavy [ ] Light
c) The color is: [ ] Normal [ ] Dark [ ] Purple [ ] Light Brown [ ] Brown

7. Do you have the following menstruation related signs/symptoms?

[ ] Difficulty with Orgasm   [ ] Cramps   [ ] PMS   [ ] Heavy Vaginal discharge
                                                                                             between periods
[ ] Pain with Intercourse   [ ] Nausea   [ ] Bleeding between Periods

[ ] Blood Clots   [ ] Breast Distention   [ ] Vaginal Discharge

For Men:
1. Do you have any bothersome urinary symptoms? [ ] Yes   [ ] No

Describe:_____

2. Check all that apply:

[ ] Erectile dysfunction   [ ] Difficulty with orgasm   [ ] Pain or swelling of the   [ ] Frequent need to urinate
                                                                 testicles   at night
[ ] Impotence/erectile   [ ] Premature ejaculation   [ ] Feeling of coldness or
    dysfunction   numbness in genitalia
                               [ ] Pain/Subtly of testicles

3. Do you get up at night to urinate? [ ] Yes   [ ] No   How often? _____

4. To what extent do these conditions interfere with your daily activities (work, sleep, socializing, sex, etc.)?
_____

5. Have you sought Medical intervention for these problems? If so, when? _____
_____

6. What treatments have you tried for these problems and how successful have they been?
_____

III. Medical History

Please check all that apply	Date Diagnosed		Date Diagnosed
Diabetes	___ / ___ / ___	High Cholesterol	___ / ___ / ___
High Blood Pressure	___ / ___ / ___	High Blood Pressure	___ / ___ / ___
Thyroid Disease	___ / ___ / ___	Seizures	___ / ___ / ___
Cancer	___ / ___ / ___	Hepatitis	___ / ___ / ___
HIV	___ / ___ / ___	Others	___ / ___ / ___

IV. Surgical History

_____ Date _____
_____ Date _____
_____ Date _____

V. Family History

Please check all that apply and state how you are related to the family member with that condition.

Condition	Mother	Father	Sibling	Maternal Grandparent	Paternal Grandparent
Heart disease					
Cancer					
Hypertension					
Stroke					
Asthma					
Allergies					
Migraines					
Depression					
Other mental illness					
Substance abuse					
Osteoporosis					
Diabetes					
Glaucoma					

VI. Medications / Supplements

Medications you are currently taking (please include prescription medicine, supplement, herbal supplements and over the counter medicines you take on a regular basis, along with dosages and brands if known)

_____   _____   _____
_____   _____   _____
_____   _____   _____
_____   _____   _____
_____   _____   _____

Allergies (to medications, chemicals or foods):

_____   _____   _____
_____   _____   _____
_____   _____   _____
_____   _____   _____

VIII. Nutrition

1. Do you follow a special diet? [ ] Yes   [ ] No If yes, how would you describe the diet?
   (ie Vegetarian, Vegan, Low Carb, etc.)
   _____

2. What do you eat on a "typical" day? _____
a) Breakfast _____
b) Lunch _____
c) Dinner _____
d) Snacks _____
e) Foods you tend to crave: _____
f) Foods you dislike: _____

PRACTICE

Source: ADR; The following general health forms can be downloaded and customized for your usage at
www.acupuncturedeskreference.com

ACUPUNCTURE DESK REFERENCE   379

PRACTICE

IX. Social History

1. How much per day do you use of the following?
a) Coffee, tea, soft drinks: _____
b) Alcohol: _____
c) Cigarettes, cigars, other tobacco: _____
d) Other drugs: _____

2. Have you ever had a problem with *alcohol* or *alcoholism*? [ ] Yes   [ ] No

3. Have you ever had a problem with *dependency* on other drugs? [ ] Yes   [ ] No

4. If yes which and when?
_____

5. Do you have a known history of any exposure to *toxic* substances? [ ] Yes   [ ] No

6. If so, please list which and when you first noticed symptoms?
_____
_____

7. In the past year, how many days have been significantly affected by your health? _____

8. How many days did you feel generally poor? _____

9. How many times were you in the hospital? _____

10. Please describe your current exercise regimen:
Hours per week: _____ Activities: _____ [ ] No Exercise

11. How many hours of sleep do you usually get per night during the week? _____

12. Do you awake feeling rested? [ ] Yes   [ ] No   Do you feel you sleep well at night? [ ] Yes   [ ] No

13. Who would you describe as your source of primary social support? (relationship to you)

X. Other Information
Please list and briefly describe the most significant events in your life:
1. _____
2. _____
3. _____
4. _____
Have you been treated for emotional issues? [ ] Yes   [ ] No

Have you ever considered or attempted suicide? [ ] Yes   [ ] No

Do you have any other neurological or psychological problem? [ ] Yes   [ ] No

Please provide us with any other information that you think is relevant for us to know:
_____
_____
_____
_____
_____

HEALTH: **CHECK ALL THAT APPLY**

GENERAL

Past	Current	Condition
[ ]	[ ]	Poor appetite
[ ]	[ ]	Excessive appetite
[ ]	[ ]	Insomnia
[ ]	[ ]	Fatigue
[ ]	[ ]	Fevers
[ ]	[ ]	Night sweats
[ ]	[ ]	Sweat easily
[ ]	[ ]	Chills
[ ]	[ ]	Localized weakness
[ ]	[ ]	Poor coordination
[ ]	[ ]	Bleed or bruise easily
[ ]	[ ]	Catch cold easily
[ ]	[ ]	Change in appetite
[ ]	[ ]	Strong thirst
[ ]	[ ]	Other: _____

SKIN & HAIR

Past	Current	Condition
[ ]	[ ]	Rashes
[ ]	[ ]	Hives
[ ]	[ ]	Itching
[ ]	[ ]	Eczema
[ ]	[ ]	Pimples
[ ]	[ ]	Dryness
[ ]	[ ]	Tumors, lumps

HECK & NECK

Past	Current	Condition
[ ]	[ ]	Dizziness
[ ]	[ ]	Fainting
[ ]	[ ]	Neck stiffness
[ ]	[ ]	Enlarged lymph glands
[ ]	[ ]	Headaches
[ ]	[ ]	Concussions
[ ]	[ ]	Other: _____

EARS

Past	Current	Condition
[ ]	[ ]	Infection
[ ]	[ ]	Ringing
[ ]	[ ]	Decreased hearing
[ ]	[ ]	Other: _____

EYES

Past	Current	Condition
[ ]	[ ]	Blurred vision
[ ]	[ ]	Visual changes
[ ]	[ ]	Poor night vision
[ ]	[ ]	Spots
[ ]	[ ]	Cataracts
[ ]	[ ]	Glasses / contacts
[ ]	[ ]	Eye inflammation
[ ]	[ ]	Other: _____

NOSE, THROAT, MOUTH

Past	Current	Condition
[ ]	[ ]	Nose bleeds
[ ]	[ ]	Sinus infections
[ ]	[ ]	Hay fever or allergies
[ ]	[ ]	Recurring sore throats
[ ]	[ ]	Grinding teeth
[ ]	[ ]	Difficulty swallowing

CARDIOVASCULAR

Past	Current	Condition
[ ]	[ ]	High blood pressure
[ ]	[ ]	Low blood pressure
[ ]	[ ]	Blood clots
[ ]	[ ]	Palpitations
[ ]	[ ]	Phlebitis
[ ]	[ ]	Chest pain
[ ]	[ ]	Irregular heart beat
[ ]	[ ]	Cold hands / feet
[ ]	[ ]	Fainting
[ ]	[ ]	Difficult breathing
[ ]	[ ]	Swelling of hands / feet
[ ]	[ ]	Other: _____

RESPIRATORY

Past	Current	Condition
[ ]	[ ]	Asthma
[ ]	[ ]	Bronchitis
[ ]	[ ]	Frequent colds
[ ]	[ ]	Chronic obstructive
[ ]	[ ]	Pulmonary disease
[ ]	[ ]	Pneumonia
[ ]	[ ]	Cough
[ ]	[ ]	Coughing blood
[ ]	[ ]	Production of phlegm
[ ]	[ ]	Other: _____

GASTRO-INTESTINAL

Past	Current	Condition
[ ]	[ ]	Nausea
[ ]	[ ]	Vomiting
[ ]	[ ]	Diarrhea
[ ]	[ ]	Belching
[ ]	[ ]	Blood in stools/black
[ ]	[ ]	Stools
[ ]	[ ]	Bad breath
[ ]	[ ]	Rectal pain
[ ]	[ ]	Hemorrhoids
[ ]	[ ]	Constipation
[ ]	[ ]	Pain or cramps
[ ]	[ ]	Indigestion
[ ]	[ ]	Gall bladder disorder
[ ]	[ ]	Gas
[ ]	[ ]	Other: _____

GENITO-URINARY

Past	Current	Condition
[ ]	[ ]	Kidney stones
[ ]	[ ]	Pain or urination
[ ]	[ ]	Frequent urination
[ ]	[ ]	Blood in urine
[ ]	[ ]	Urgency to urinate
[ ]	[ ]	Unable to hold urine
[ ]	[ ]	Other: _____

MALE

Past	Current	Condition
[ ]	[ ]	Pain / itching genitalia
[ ]	[ ]	Genital lesions/ discharge
[ ]	[ ]	Impotence
[ ]	[ ]	Weak urinary stream
[ ]	[ ]	Lumps in testicles
[ ]	[ ]	Other: _____

FEMALE

Past	Current	Condition
[ ]	[ ]	Frequent urinary tract infections
[ ]	[ ]	Frequent vaginal infections
[ ]	[ ]	Pain / itching of genitalia
[ ]	[ ]	Genital lesions / discharge
[ ]	[ ]	Pelvic inflammatory disease
[ ]	[ ]	Abnormal pap smear
[ ]	[ ]	Irregular menstrual periods
[ ]	[ ]	Painful menstrual periods
[ ]	[ ]	Premenstrual syndrome
[ ]	[ ]	Abnormal bleeding
[ ]	[ ]	Menopausal syndrome
[ ]	[ ]	Breast lumps
[ ]	[ ]	Hot flashes
[ ]	[ ]	Menopausal syndrome
[ ]	[ ]	Other: _____

NEUROLOGICAL

Past	Current	Condition
[ ]	[ ]	Seizures
[ ]	[ ]	Tremors
[ ]	[ ]	Numbness/tingling of limbs
[ ]	[ ]	Concussion
[ ]	[ ]	Pain
[ ]	[ ]	Paralysis
[ ]	[ ]	Other: _____

PSYCHOLOGICAL

Past	Current	Condition
[ ]	[ ]	Depression
[ ]	[ ]	Anxiety / stress
[ ]	[ ]	Irritability
[ ]	[ ]	Treated for emotional or
[ ]	[ ]	Psychological problems
[ ]	[ ]	Other: _____

INFECTION SCREENING

Past	Current	Condition
[ ]	[ ]	HIV
[ ]	[ ]	TB
[ ]	[ ]	Hepatitis
[ ]	[ ]	Gonorrhea
[ ]	[ ]	Chlamydia
[ ]	[ ]	Syphilis
[ ]	[ ]	Genital warts
[ ]	[ ]	Herpes: oral
[ ]	[ ]	Herpes: genital

MUSCULAR-SKELETAL

Past	Current	Condition
[ ]	[ ]	Stiff neck / shoulders
[ ]	[ ]	Low back pain
[ ]	[ ]	Back pain
[ ]	[ ]	Muscle spasm, twitching, cramps
[ ]	[ ]	Sore, cold or weak knees
[ ]	[ ]	Joint pain

PRACTICE

© 2007 Acupuncture Desk Reference, Permission to Use Granted; www.acupuncturedeskreference.com

Source: ADR; The following general health forms can be downloaded and customized for your usage at www.acupuncturedeskreference.com

COMMON ICD-9 CODES

Condition	Codes	Condition	Codes	Condition	Codes
Abdominal pain	789.00	Gout	274.9	Sore throat, acute	462
Acid reflux	536.8	Hair loss, alopecia	704.0	Sore throat, chronic	472.1
Acne	706.1	**Headache**	784.0	**Stress, acute reaction**	308.9
Adrenal insufficiency	255.5	Headache, migraine	346.90	Stress, emotions	308.0
Alcohol abuse	305.00	Headache, tension	707.81	Stress, gross	308.9
Allergic rhinitis	477.9	Hearing loss, unspecified	389.9	Tendonitis	726.90
Allergy, unspecified	995.3	Hemorrhoids	455.6	Tennis elbow	726.32
Amenorrhea	626.0	Hepatitis	573.3	Thoracic outlet syndrome	353.0
Angina pectoris	413.9	Herpes zoster	053.9	Thyroiditis	245.1
Ankle sprain/strain	845.00	Herpes, genital	054.10	Tinnitus	388.30
Anxiety disorders	300.00	High blood pressure	796.2	TMJ	524.60
Arm/leg pain	729.5	Hip/thigh sprain/stain	843.9	Tonsillitis, acute	463
Arthritis	716.90	Hypertension	401.9	Trigeminal neuralgia	3501
Arthritis - osteoarthritis, hand	715.4	**Hyperthyroidism**	424.9	Trigger finger	727.03
Arthritis - osteoarthritis, lower leg	715.6	Hypotension	458.1	Ulcerative colitis	556.9
		Hypothyroidism	244.9	URI	465.9
Arthritis, gout	274.0	Hypothyroidism	244.9	Urinary incontinence	788.30
Asthma, unspecified	493.90	Impotence	302.71	Urticaria, allergic	708.0
Back pain	724.2	Indigestion, dyspepsia	536.8	Uterine fibroid	218.9
Bells palsy	351.0	Infertility, female	628.9	UTI	599.0
Bloating	787.3	Infertility, male	606.9	Vertigo, dizziness	780.4
Brachial radiculitis	723.1	Influenza	487.1	Voice loss - aphonia	784.41
Breast disorders	610.1	**Insomnia**	780.52	Vomiting	787.03
Bronchitis, acute	466.0	Insomnia, w/ sleep apnea	780.51	Wart, unspecified	078.10
Bronchitis, chronic	491.9	Irregular menstrual cycle	626.4	Weakness	780.79
Carbuncle or furnacle	680.0	Irritable bowel syndrome	564.1	Weight loss	783.2
Carpal tunnel syndrome	354.0	Jaundice	782.4	Wrist sprain/strain	842.00
Chest pain	786.5	**Joint pain**	719.4	Yeast infection	112.0
Choleycystis, acute	575.0	**Knee pain/strain**	844.9		
Chrohn's disease	555.9	Lumbar sprain/strain	847.2	**JOINT PAIN**	
Chronic fatigue syndrome	780.71	Mastitis	611.0	Ankle, foot	719.47
Colitis, gastroenteritis	558.9	Menopause	627.2	**Cervical, neck**	723.1
Common cold	460	Menorrhagia, excess	626.2	Coccyx	724.7
Constipation	564.00	Migraine	346.1	Forearm	719.43
Cough	786.2	MS pain/fibromyalgia	729.1	Hand	719.44
Cystitis, acute	595.0	Nausea, no vomiting	787.02	**Knee**	719.46
Depression	311.0	**Neck pain**	723.1	Lower leg	719.46
Depressive reaction, prolonged	309.1	Neuralgia, neuritis radiculitis	729.2	**Lumbar, Low back**	724.2
		Night sweats	780.8	Pelvic, thigh	719.45
Dermatitis, unspecified	564.00	Numbness	782.0	Sacrum	724.6
Diabetes	250.0	Obesity	278.0	**Sciatica**	724.3
Diarrhea	787.91	**Osteoarthritis**	715.00	Shoulder	719.41
Diarrhea, colitis	558.9	Osteoporosis	733.00	Thoracic	724.1
Diverticulitis	562.11	Painful limbs	729.5	Thoracic or lumbar	724.4
Dizziness/vertigo	780.4	Palpitations	785.1	Upper arm	719.42
Drug abuse	505.90	Paresthesias, numbness	782.0		
Drug dependence	304.00	Pelvic pain	625.9	**STRAINS**	
Dysmenorrhea	625.3	Pharyngitis, chronic	472.1	Ankle, foot, unspecified	845.00
Earache	388.70	**PMS**	625.4	Bursitis/ankle	726.70
Eczema	692.9	Polycystic ovarian syndrome	256.1	Bursitis/elbow	726.33
Elbow/forearm spr/str	841.9	Prostatitis	601.9	Bursitis/knee	726.60
Endometriosis	617.0	Psoriasis	696.1	Bursitis/shoulder	726.10
Fatigue, general	780.79	Radiculopathy	729.2	Coccyx	847.4
Fatigue/malaise	780.71	Respiratory difficulty, SOB	786.05	Elbow, forearm	841.9
Fever	780.6	**Rheumatoid arthritis**	714.0	Hip, thigh, unspecified	843.9
Fibromyalgia	729.1	Rotator cuff sprain/strain	840.4	Knee, leg, unspecified	844.9
Food poisoning	005.9	**Sciatica**	724.3	**Lumbar, Low back**	847.2
Foot sprain/strain	845.10	Shingles	053.9	**Neck**	547.0
Gastritis, w/ hemmorhage	535.01	**Shoulder pain**	719.41	Rotator cuff	840.4
Gastritis, w/o hemmorhage	535.00	Shoulder strain	840.9	Sacrum	847.3
GERD/reflux	530.81	Sinusitis, acute	461.9	**Shoulder, arm**	840.9
Gingivitis, acute	523.0	Sinusitis, chronic	473.9	Thoracic	847.1
				Wrist, carpal (joint)	842.01
				Wrist, unspecified	842.00

INSURANCE, ARBITRATION & CONSENT

Acupuncture Insurance & Protection Strategy

It is increasingly clear that acupuncturists no longer have the luxury of complacent belief that a malpractice suit "Can't happen to me." There are significant financial and legal risks of treating patients without the proper protections and documentation. Unless you can afford to lose you license and/or afford a litigious civil suit, make sure you have proper malpractice insurance coverage, arbitration and informed consent forms signed and dated by your patents prior to any treatment. We have provided a sample of the arbitration and informed consent for your review. It is advisable to purchase similar forms through your malpractice carrier.

American Acupuncture Council
1851 East First Street, Suite 1160
Santa Ana, CA 92705
(800) 838-0383
www.acupuncturecouncil.com

Patient Name_____

ARBITRATION AGREEMENT

Article 1: Agreement to Arbitrate: It is understood that any dispute as to medical malpractice, that is as to whether any medical services rendered under this contract were unnecessary or unauthorized or we improperly, negligently or incompetently rendered, will be determined by submission to arbitration as provided by California law, and not by lawsuit or resort to court process except as state and federal law provided for judicial review of arbitration proceeding. Both parties to this contract by entering into, are giving up their constitutional right to have any such dispute decided in a court of law before a jury, and instead are accepting the use of arbitration.

Article 2: All Claims must be Arbitrated: It is also understood that any dispute that does not relate to medical malpractice, including disputes as to whether or not a dispute is subject to arbitration, will also be determined by submission to bring arbitration. It is the intention of the parties that this agreement binds all parties as to all claims including claims arising out of the relating to treatment or services provided by the health care provider including any heir or past, present or future spouse(s) of the patient in relation to all claims, including loss of consortium. This agreement is intended to bind the patient and the health care provider and/or other licensed health care providers or preceptorship interns who now or in the future that the patient while employed by, working or associated with or serving as a back-up for the health care provider, including those working at the health care providers clinic or other clinic or office whether signatories to this form or not.

All claims for monetary damages exceeding the jurisdictional limit of the small claims court against the health care provider, and/or the health care provider's associates, association, corporation, partnership, employees, agents and estate, must be arbitrated including, without limitation, claims for loss of consortium, wrongful death, emotional distress, injunctive relief, or punitive damages.

Article 3: Procedures and Applicable Law: A demand of arbitration must be communicated in writing to all parties. Each party shall select an arbitrator (party arbitrator) within thirty days and a third arbitrator (neutral arbitrator) shall be selected by the arbitrators appointed by the parties within thirty days thereafter. The neutral arbitrator shall then be the sole arbitrator and shall decide the arbitration. Each party to the arbitration shall pay such party's pro rata share of the expenses and fees of the neutral arbitrator, together with other expenses of the arbitration incurred or approved by the neutral arbitrator, not including counsel fees, witness fees, or other expense incurred by a party for each party's own benefit.
Either party shall have the absolute right to bifurcate the issues of liability and damage upon written request to the neutral arbitrator. The parties consent to the intervention a joinder in this arbitration of any person or entity that would otherwise be a proper additional party in a court action, and upon such intervention and joinder any existing court action against such additional person or entity shall be stayed pending arbitration.
The parties agrees that the provisions of the California Medical Injury Compensations Reform Act shall apply to disputes within this arbitration agreement, including, but not limited to, selection establishing the right to introduce evidence of any amount payable as a benefit to the patient allowed be law (Civil Code 3333.1) the limitation on recovery for non-economic losses (Civil Code 3333.2), and the right to have a judgment for future damages conformed to periodic payments (CCP 667.7). The parties further agree that the Commercial Arbitration Rules of the American Arbitration Association shall govern any arbitration conducted pursuant to this Arbitration Agreement.

Article 4: General Provision: All claims based upon the same incident, transaction or related circumstances shall be arbitrated in one proceeding. A claim shall be waived and forever if (1) on the date notice thereof is received, the claim, if asserted in a civil action, would be barred the applicable legal statue of limitations, or (2) the claimant fails to pursue the arbitration claim in accordance with the procedures prescribed herein with reasonable diligence.

INSURANCE, ARBITRATION & CONSENT

Article 5: Revocation: This agreement may be revoked by written notice delivered to the health care provider within 30 days of signature and if not revoked will govern all professional service received by the patient and all other disputes between the parties.

Article 6: Retroactive Effect: If patient intends this agreement to cover service rendered before the date it is signed (for example, emergency treatment) patient should initial here. _____. Effective as the date of first professional services.

If any provision of this Arbitration Agreement is held invalid or unenforceable, the remaining provisions shall remain in full force and shall not be affected by the invalidity of any other provisions. I understand that I have the right to receive a copy of this Arbitration Agreement. By my signature below, I acknowledge that I have received a copy.

NOTICE: BY SIGNING THIS CONTRACT YOU ARE AGREEING TO HAVE ANY ISSUE OF MEDICAL MALPRACTICE DECIDED BY NEUTRAL ARBITRATION AND YOU ARE GIVING UP YOUR RIGHT TO A JURY OR COURT TRIAL. SEE ARTICLE 1 OF THIS CONTRACT.

Patient Signature_____ Date_____
Office Signature_____ Date_____

ACUPUNCTURE INFORMED CONSENT TO TREAT

I hereby request and consent to the performance of acupuncture treatment and other procedure within the scope of the practice of acupuncture on me (or on the patient named below, for whom I am legally responsible) by the acupuncturist named below and/or other license acupuncturist who now or in the future treat me while employed by, working or associated with or serving as back-up for the acupuncturist name below, including those working at the clinic or office listed below or any other office or clinic, whether signatories to this form or not.

I understand that the methods of treatment may include, but are not limited to, acupuncture, moxibustion, cupping, electrical stimulation, Tui-Na (Chinese massage), Chinese herbal medicine, and nutritional counseling. I understand that the herbs may need to be prepared and the teas consumed according to the instruction provided orally in writing. These herbs may have an unpleasant smell or taste. I will immediately notify a member of the clinical staff of any unanticipated or unpleasant effects associated with the consumption of the herbs.

I have been informed that acupuncture is a generally safe method of treatment, but that I may have some side effects, including bruising, numbness or tingling near the needling sites that may last a few days, and dizziness or fainting. Bruising is a common side effect of cupping. Unusual risks of acupuncture include spontaneous miscarriage, nerve damage and organ puncture, including lung puncture (pneumothorax). Infection is another possible risk, although the clinic uses sterile disposable needles and maintains a clean and safe environment. Burns and/or scarring are a potential risk of moxibustion and cupping. I understand that while this document describes the major risks of treatment, other side effects and risks may occur. The herbs and nutritional supplements (which are from plant, animal and mineral sources) that have been recommended are traditionally consider safe in the practice of Chinese Medicine, although some may be toxic in large does. I understand that some herbs may be inappropriate during pregnancy. Some possible side effects of taking herbs are nausea, gas, stomachache, vomiting, headache, diarrhea, rashes, hives, and tingling of the tongue. I will notify a clinical staff member who is caring for me if am or become pregnant.

I do not expect the clinical staff to be able to anticipate and explain all possible risks and complications of treatment, and I wish to rely on the clinical staff to exercise judgment during the course of treatment which the clinical staff thinks at the time, based upon the facts then known is in my best interest. I understand that results are not guaranteed.

I understand the clinical and administrative staff may review my patient records and lab reports, but all my records will be kept confidential and will not be released without my written consent.

By voluntarily signing below, I show that I have read, or have had read to me, the above consent to treatment, have been told about the risks and benefits of acupuncture and other procedures and have had an opportunity to ask questions. I intend this consent form to cover the entire course of treatment for my present condition and for any future condition(s) for which I seek treatment.

Patient Signature_____ Date_____

Insurance Providers

The following is a listing of some health-care providers, some of which will provide some form of coverage for varying health plans. This information is provided to enable you to contact health-care providers directly in order to obtain benefit information for your patients. Be aware that telephone numbers reflect the current numbers at the printing of the book and are subject to change and will vary according to state and regional plans.

Company	Telephone	Notes
Aetna	(800) 624-0756	
Aetna (HMO)	(800) 323-9930	
Aftra	(800) 562-4690	
American Specialty Health Plan (ASHP)	(800) 972-4226	
Blue Cross / Anthem	(800) 333-0912	
Blue Cross / Anthem (HMO)	(800) 972-4226	
Blue Cross of California / Anthem	(800) 677-6669	
Blue Shield	(800) 351-2465	
Cigna	(800) 832-3211	
Directors Guild	(323) 866-2200	
Empire (Red Bluff)	(800) 676-2583	
Great West / One Health Plan	(800) 663-8081	
Guardian	(800) 685-4542	
Health Net	(800) 641-7761	
Medicare	(866) 931-3903	
Motion Pictures	(310) 769-0007	
Oxford / United Healthcare	(800) 666-1353	
PacifiCare	(866) 863-9776	
PacifiCare (HMO)	(800) 542-8789	
SAG	(818) 954-9400	
United Healthcare	(877) 842-3210	
Writers Guild	(818) 846-1015	

CPT Codes

Acupuncture

97810	Acupuncture
97811	Each additional 15 minutes

97010	Hot or Cold Packs (supervised)
97024	Diathermy (supervised)
97026	Infrared (supervised)
97028	Ultraviolet (supervised)
97035	Ultrasound
97140	Manual Therapy techniques (e.g. myofascial release, mobilization, manipulation, manual traction
97530	Therapeutic activities
99070	Supplies and materials
97124	Massage

Electro-Acupuncture

97813	Electro-acupuncture, one or more needles, with electrical stimulation
97814	Each additional 15 minutes

New patient office visit
99201-205 (not treatment)

Established patient office visit
99211-215 Review Office Consultation (not treatment)

Important Phone Numbers for Emergency, Local, National, and Health-care Referrals

Local Numbers

Agency	Telephone Number	Notes
Emergency	911	
Police		
Fire		
Poison Control		
Hospital 1		
Hospital 2		
Hospital 3		
County Health Department		
Mental Health Referral		
Domestic Abuse Hotline		
Alcoholic Anonymous		
Rape and Battering Hotline		
Alcoholic Anonymous		
Elder Abuse		
Child Abuse		
Suicide Prevention		
Other		

Many of the numbers can be found in your local telephone directory. We have also listed national directory information in this section that will provide you the number.

Other Acupuncturists & Their Specialties

The best practice management is to know when to refer out. Regardless of your specialty, building a referral network with other health-care professionals can be a great resource for your patients and compliment your practice. The following section offers a location where you refer your patients or specialties. Check with your colleagues or other physicians in the area.

Acupuncturist	Specialty/Area	Telephone	Address
John Doe, LAc	OBGYN	555-1212	123 ABC Street, Los Angeles

Referral to other Health-care Professionals

Acupuncturists who successfully work with other health-care professionals have found that one of the key ingredients in development of such relationships is the quality of referrals. MDs are more likely to work with L.Acs and OMDs who demonstrate a high level of professionalism with referrals. The following section provides a list of other health-care professionals that are essential to patient care. Talk to your patient as well as with your colleagues to find the out which MD's are open to building a referral network in your area.

Health-care Professional Referral Numbers

Specialty	Physician	Telephone	Address
Allergy			
Cardiologist			
Chiropractor			
Chiropractor			
Chiropractor			
Emergency Medicine			
Endocrinology			
Family Practice			
Family Practice			
Family Practice			
Family Practice			
Gastroenterology			
General Surgery			
General Surgery			
Infectious Diseases			
Internal Medicine			
Midwife			
Neurology			
OB/GYN			
OB/GYN			
Oncology			
Optometry			
Orthopaedic Surgery			
Orthopaedic Surgery			
Pediatrics			
Podiatry			
Psychiatry			
Psychologist			
Radiology			
Rheumatology			
Urology			

Acupuncture-Related Numbers

Acupuncture Agency	Telephone	Notes
National Provider Identifier (NPI)	(800) 465-3203	
National Acupuncture & OM Regulatory		
State Regulatory Agency		
National OSHA	(800) 232-4346	
State OSHA		
U.S. Food and Drug Administration	(888) 463-6332	
CDC	(800) 232-4636	
National Organizations		
State Acupuncture Organizations		
Sharps Injury Prevention		www.sharpslist.org

Many of the addresses and phone numbers can be found on the following pages. It is
advisable to have them on hand in case of emergencies or questions regarding your practice.

National Numbers

You can contact the following agencies to get more information on local or regional offices,
and many provide a wealth of information on their websites. The numbers are subject to
change.

	Agency	Telephone
Aging	National Council on Aging	(800) 424-9046
Aging	National Institute on Aging Information Center	(800) 222-2225
AIDS / HIV	AIDS Hotline	(800) 933-3413
AIDS / HIV	National AIDS Hotline	(800) 232-4636
AIDS / HIV	Sexually Transmitted Disease National Hotline	(800) 227-8922
AIDS/HIV	HIV/AIDS Treatment Hotline	(800) 822-7422
Alcohol	A1-Anon/Alateen Family Group Headquarters, Inc	(800) 344-2666
Alcohol	Alcohol and Drug Addictions/Trauma hotline	(800) 544-1177
Alcohol	Alcohol and Drug Information	(800) 729-6686
Alcohol	Alcohol Hotline	(800) 331-2900
Alcohol	Alcoholism and Drug Dependence Hopeline	(800) 622-2255
Alcohol	National Drug and Alcohol Treatment Referral Service	(800) 662-HELP
Child Abuse	Child Abuse Hotline	(800) 4-A-CHILD
Child Abuse	Child Abuse Hotline	(800) 792-5200
Child Abuse	Child Abuse prevention	(800) 257-3223
Child Abuse	Information Services for Child Support	(800) 537-7072
Child Abuse	National Child Abuse Hotline	(800) 422-4453
Depression	National Depressive & Manic-Depressive Association	(800) 826-3632
Disease	Center for Disease Control	(800) 232-4636
Domestic Abuse	Domestic Abuse Hotline	(800) 799-7233
Drug Abuse	Alcohol and Drug Abuse Hotline	(800) 237-6237
Drug Abuse	American Council for Drug Education	(800) 488-3784

Drug Abuse	Center for Substance Abuse Treatment	(800) 662-HELP
Drug Abuse	Cocaine Hotline	(800) 992-9239
Drug Abuse	Drug and Alcohol Treatment Routing Service	(800) 662-4357
Drug Abuse	Marijuana Anonymous	(800) 766-6779
Eating Disorder	Eating Disorders - Bulimia, Anorexia Self Help	(800) 931-2237
Eating Disorder	Eating Disorders Hotline	(800) 445-1900
Elder Abuse	Elder Abuse Hotline	(800) 752-6200
Family Violence	National Domestic Violence/Abuse Hotline	(800) 799-7233
Family Violence	Parent Helpline	(800) 942-4357
Family Violence	Parents' Stress Hotline	(800) 632-8188
Health - Alzheimer's	Alzheimer's Association	(800) 272-3900
Health - Cancer	Cancer Information Service	(800) 422-6237
Health - Cystic	Cystic Fibrosis Foundation	(800) 344-4823
Health - Diabetes	Juvenile Diabetes Foundation	(800) 223-1138
Health - Down	National Down Syndrome Congress	(800) 232-6372
Health - Dyslexia	Dyslexia Society	(800) 222-3123
Health - Epilepsy	Epilepsy Foundation	(800) 332-1000
Health - Hearing	Better Hearing Institute	(800) 327-9355
Health - Heart	American Heart Association	(800) 242-8721
Health - Info	National Health Information Center	(800) 336-4797
Health - Info	National OCD Information Hotline	(800) NEWS-4-OCD
Health - Kidney	American Kidney Fund	(800) 638-8299
Health - Liver	American Liver Foundation	(800) 223-0179
Health - Lupus	Lupus Foundation of America	(800) 558-0121
Health - MS	National Multiple Sclerosis Society	(800) 532-7667
Health - Nutrition	National Center for Nutrition	(800) 366-1655
Health - Panic	Panic Disorder Information Hotline	(800) 64-PANIC
Health - Parkinson	National Parkinson Foundation	(800) 327-4545
Health - Reyes	National Reyes Syndrome Foundation	(800) 233-7393
Health - SID	Sudden Infant Death Syndrome Alliance	(800) 221-7437
Health - Spina	Spina Bifida Association	(800) 621-3141
Health - STD	Center for Disease Control-National STD Hotline	(800) 227-8922
Mental Health	Anxiety and Panic	(800) 64-PANIC
Mental Health	Depression Awareness	(800) 421-4211
Mental Health	Mental Health Referral	(800) 950-6264
Mental Health	National Council on Compulsive Gambling	(800) 522-4700
Mental Health	National Foundation for Depressive Illness	(800) 826-3232
Mental Health	National Mental Health Association	(800) 969-6642
Poison	Poison Information Center	(800) 222-1222
Pregnancy	Planned Parenthood	(800) 230-7526
Pregnancy	Pregnancy Hotline	(800) 848-5683
Rape	Crisis Help Line -For Any Kind of Crisis	(800) 233-4357
Rape	Crisis Line	(800) 999-9999
Rape	National Victims Center (for rape or assault)	(800) FYI-CALL

RESOURCE

Rape	Rape, Abuse, Incest National Network (RAINN)	(800) 656-HOPE
Rape	Sexual Assault Crisis Line -Hotlines & Information	(800) 643-6250
Runaways	Boys Town National Hotline	(800) 448-3000
Runaways	Center For Missing and Exploited Children	(800) 843-5678
Runaways	Missing and Exploited Children Hotline	(800) 843-5678
Runaways	Missing Children Hotline	(800) THE-LOST
Runaways	National Child Safety Council	(800) 327-5107
Runaways	National Hotline for Missing & Exploited Children	(800) 843-5678
Runaways	National Runaway Hotline	(800) RUNAWAY
Runaways	National Runaway Hotline	(800) 621-4000
Runaways	National Youth Crisis Hotline	(800) 442-HOPE
Spousal Abuse	National Domestic Violence/Abuse Hotline	(800) 799-7233
Substance Abuse	Cocaine Anonymous (CA)	(800) 347-8998
Substance Abuse	National Treatment Hotline	(800) 662-HELP
Suicide	National Adolescent Suicide Hotline	(800) RUNAWAY
Suicide	National Cocaine and Suicide Prevention Hotline	(800) 288-1022
Suicide	National Suicide Referral	(202) 237-2280
Suicide	Suicide Crisis Intervention Center	(800) 784-2433

RESOURCE

Manufacturer and Distributor Information

Below are the manufacturers and distributors of some of the brand name formulas and single herbs mentioned in this book, plus their addresses and phone numbers and website. This information is provided to enable you to contact these companies to order or to obtain further information about their products. None of the manufacturers or distributors mentioned has had any connection with the production of this book. Rather, we list these companies because we believe their products to be effective and of high quality. Be aware that addresses, numbers, and URLs are subject to change.

BioEssence
1030 Ohio Ave
Richmond, CA 94804
(510) 215-5588
www.bioessence.com

Blue Poppy Enterprises
5441 Western Ave, #2
Boulder, CO 80301
(800) 487-9296
www.bluepoppy.com

Brion Herbs Corporation
Distributes Sun Ten Formulas
9200 Jeronimo Road,
Irvine, CA 92618
(949) 587-1238
www.sunten.com

Chinese Herbs Direct
2421 W. 205th St, Suite D103
Torrance, CA 90501
(800) 608-9056
www.chineseherbsdirect.com

Crane Herb Company
745 Falmouth Road
Mashpee, MA 02649
(508) 539-1700
www.craneherb.com

Evergreen Herbs
17431 East Gale Ave
City of Industry, CA 91748
(866) 473-3697
www.evherb.com

Far East Summit
P.O. Box 2486
Culver City, CA 90231
(888) 441-0489
www.fareastsummit.com

Golden Flower Chinese Herbs
2724 Vassar Place NE
Albuquerque, NM 87107
(800) 729-8509
www.gfcherbs.com

Health Concerns
8001 Capwell Drive
Oakland, CA 94621
(800) 233-9355
www.healthconcerns.com

Herbmax Inc.
12155 Mora Dr. Unit 13
Santa Fe Springs, California 90670
(562) 941-8881
www.herbmaxinc.com

Honso USA, Inc.
4602 E Elwood Street, Suite 6
Phoenix, AZ 85040
(888) 461-5808
www.honsousa.com

Jen-On Herbal Science International
1015 S. Nogales Street, Suite 120
Rowland Heights CA 91748
(800) 828-6618
www.hsusa.net

Kan Herb Company
6001 Butler Lane
Scotts Valley, CA 95066
(831) 438.9450
www.kanherb.com

KPC Products, Inc.
16 Goddard
Irvine, CA 92618
(800) KPC-8188
www.kpc.com

Mayway Corporation
1338 Mandela Parkway
Oakland, California 94607
(800) 2MAYWAY
www.mayway.com

Nuherbs Co
3820 Penniman Ave.
Oakland, Ca, 94619
(800) 233-4307
www.nuherbs.com

Oriental Pharmacy.com
P.O. Box 255.
Northvale, NJ 07647
(201)264-0888
www.orientalpharmacy.com

Qualiherb
119-40 Metropolitan Avenue
Kew Gardens, NY 11415
(877) 776-4372
www.qualiherb.com

Secara Herbs
2342 Shattuck Ave. #410
Berkeley, CA 94704
(888) SECARA-1
www.secara.com

Acupuncture Supplies Companies

Below are the acupuncture supply companies with their appropriate web site contact. This information is provided to enable you to contact these companies to order or to obtain further information about their products. Be aware that web addresses are subject to change.

Acu International Supplies, Inc. – Acupuncture supplies
http://acuinternational.com

Acu-Market – Acupuncture supplies & herbal remedies
www.acu-market.com

Acu-Mart International, Inc. – Acupuncture supplies
www.acu-mart.com

AcuExpress.com – Acupuncture supplies
www.AcuExpress.com

CAI Industries Corp – Acupuncture & Medical supplies
http://caicorporation.com/

Coastal Medical Supplies, Inc. – Acupuncture & Medical supplies
http://coastalmedicalsupplies.com

GoldenNeedle Acupuncture, Acupuncture, Herbal, & Medical supplies
http://goldenneedleonline.com

Health Point Products – Acupuncture & Medical supplies
www.1hpi.com

K.S. Choi Corp – Acupuncture & Medical supplies
www.goacuzone.net

Lhasa OMS – Acupuncture & Medical supplies
www.LhasaMedical.com/

Massage Chairs from Massage Unlimited – Massage supplies
www.massageunlimited.com

Mayway Corporation – Acupuncture supplies, herbs & formulas
www.mayway.com

Pantheon Research – Pantheon e-stim units in the USA
www.PantheonResearch.com/

Quality Medical Supplies – Medical supplies
www.qualitymedicalsupplies.com

Seirin Brand Needles – SEIRIN-America products
www.SeirinAmerica.com/

Sinic Avenue Online – Acupuncture, books, and medical supplies
www.sinicave.com

UPC Medical Supplies, Inc. – Acupuncture & medical supplies
www.goacupuncture.com

Resources You Can Use

There are many reliable resources and information in alternative health. We have listed the following professional associations and health organizations. Besides brochures, booklets and hotlines, many provide valuable information online in their respective fields as well as referrals to other health-care professionals.

Acupuncture & Oriental Medicine

Accreditation Commission for Acupuncture and Oriental Medicine (ACAOM)
Maryland Trade Center #3, 7501 Greenway Center Drive,
Suite 760, Greenbelt, MD 20770
(301) 313-0855
www.acaom.org

American Association of Acupuncture & Oriental Medicine (AAAOM) AKA AOM Alliance
PO Box 162340
Sacramento, CA 95816
(916) 443-4770
www.aaom.org or www.aaaomonline.org

Council of Acupuncture and Oriental Medicine Associations
1217 Washington Street
Calistoga, CA 94515
(707) 942-9380
www.acucouncil.org

National Acupuncture Detoxification Association (NADA)
PO Box 1927
Vancouver WA 98668-1927
(360) 254 0186
http://acudetox.com

National Certification Commission for Acupuncture and Oriental Medicine (NCCAOM)
76 South Laura Street, Suite 1290
Jacksonville, FL 32202
(904) 598-1005
www.nccaom.org

Aromatherapy

The National Association for Holistic Aromatherapy
3327 W. Indian Trail Road PMB 144
Spokane, WA 99208
(509) 325-3419
www.naha.org

Ayurvedic Medicine

American Academy of Ayurvedic Medicine, Inc.
100 Jersey Avenue
Building B, Suite 300
New Brunswick, N.J. 08901
(732) 247-3301
www.ayurvedicacademy.com

National Institute of Ayurvedic Medicine
584 Milltown Road Brewster,
New York 10509
(845) 278-8700
www.niam.com

Biofeedback

Association for Applied Psychophysiology and Biofeedback
10200 W 44th Ave #304
Wheat Ridge, CO 80033
(303) 422-8436
www.aapb.org

Chelation Therapy

American Association of Naturopathic Physicians
4435 Wisconsin Ave NW Ste 403
Washington DC 20016
(866) 538-2267
www.naturopathic.org

Chiropractic

American Chiropractic Association
1701 Clarendon Boulevard
Arlington, VA 22209
(703) 276-8800
www.amerchiro.org

Craniosacral Therapy

The Upledger Institute, Inc
11211 Prosperity Farms Road, Suite D-325
Palm Beach Gardens, FL 33410
(800) 233-5880
www.upledger.com

Herbal Medicine

American Botanical Council
6200 Manor Road
Austin, TX 78723
(512) 926-4900
www.herbalgram.org

Herb Research Foundation
4140 15th St.
Boulder, CO 80304
(303) 449-2265
www.herbs.org

Homeopathy

National Center for Homeopathy
801 North Fairfax Street Suite 306
Alexandria, VA 22314
(703) 548-7790
http://nationalcenterforhomeopathy.org

North American Society of Homeopaths
PO BOX 450039
Sunrise, FL 33345-0039
(206) 720-7000
www.homeopathy.org

Massage

American Massage Therapy Association
500 Davis Street, Suite 900
Evanston, IL 60201
(877) 905-2700
www.amtamassage.org

Naturopathic Medicine

American Association of Naturopathic Physicians
4435 Wisconsin Ave NW Ste 403
Washington DC 20016
(866) 538-2267
www.naturopathic.org

Nutrition

National Association of Nutrition Professionals
P.O. Box 1172
Danville, CA 94526
(800) 342-8037
www.nanp.org

American Dietetic Association
120 South Riverside Plaza, Suite 2000
Chicago, Illinois 60606-6995
(800) 877-1600
www.eatright.org

Council for Responsible Nutrition
1828 L Street, NW, Suite 900
Washington, DC, 20036-5114
(202) 776-7929
www.crnusa.org

Osteopathic Medicine

American Osteopathic Association
142 East Ontario Street
Chicago, IL 60611
(800) 621-1773
www.osteopathic.org

Reflexology

Reflexology Association of America
4012 Rainbow Ste. K-PMB#585
Las Vegas, NV 89103
(740) 657-1695
www.reflexology-usa.org

Yoga

American Yoga Association
P.O. Box 19986
Sarasota, FL 34276
(941) 927-4977
www.americanyogaassociation.org

Acupuncture & Oriental Medicine Regulatory State Agencies

We have listed the following state regulatory agencies for information on licensing and acupuncture laws and regulation. Codes and laws can be found through your repective agencies. Due to the changing nature of laws, the information, regulations, and regulatory agencies are subject to change.

NCCAOM Certification Examination
National Certification Commission for Acupuncture
and Oriental Medicine (NCCAOM)
76 South Laura Street, Suite 1290
Jacksonville, FL 32202
(904) 598-1005
(904) 598-5001 Fax

For information on laws/statutes:
http://www.nccaom.org

Alabama
Alabama Association of Oriental Medicine
Hidden Creek Professional Park
28311 N. Main St. Ste B-101
Daphne, AL 36526
(866) 606-6866
(251) 626-5066 Fax

According to AOM Alliance, Alabama is a state in which there is no legislation or rules authorizing the practice by licensed acupuncturists. However, a statute has been introduced.

Alaska
Department of Commerce and Economic
Development
Division of Occupational Licensing - Acupuncture
P.O. Box 110806
Juneau, Alaska 99811-0806
(907) 465-2695
(907) 465-2974 Fax

For information on laws/statutes:
http://www.commerce.state.ak.us/occ/pacu.htm

Arizona
Arizona Board of Acupuncture Examiners
1400 W. Washington #230
Phoenix, AZ 85007
(602) 542-3095
(602) 542-3093 Fax

For information on laws/statutes:
http://www.azacuboard.az.gov/statutes.htm

Arkansas
Arkansas State Board of Acupuncture & Related
Techniques
1401 West 6th Street
Little Rock, AR 72201
(501) 683-3583
(501) 244-2333 Fax

For information on laws/statutes:
http://www.asbart.org/rules.htm

California
The Acupuncture Board
444 N. 3rd Street, Suite 260
Sacramento, CA 95814
(916) 445-3021
(916) 445-3015 Fax

For information on laws/statutes:
http:// www.acupuncture.ca.gov/

Colorado
Department of Regulatory Agencies
Office of Acupuncturists Registration
1560 Broadway, Suite 1340
Denver, CO 80202 - 5140
(303) 894-7429
(303) 894-7764 Fax

For information on laws/statutes:
http:// www.dora.state.co.us/acupuncturists/

Connecticut
Department of Public Health, Acupuncturist
Licensure
410 Capitol Ave.
MS # 12 APP
P.O. Box 34308
Hartford, CT 06134-0308
(860) 509-7603

Delaware
According to AOM Alliance, Delaware is a state in which there is no legislation or rules authorizing the practice by licensed acupuncturists.

District of Columbia
Department of Health Advisory Committee on
Acupuncture
717 14th Street, NW
Suite 600
Washington, DC 20005
(877) 672-2174
(202) 727-8471 Fax

For information on laws/statutes:
http://hpla.doh.dc.gov/hpla/cwp/view,A,1195,Q,488827,h plaNav,|30661|,.asp

Florida
Division of Medical Quality Assurance (MQA)
Board of Acupuncture
4052 Bald Cypress Way Bin #C06
Tallahassee, Florida 32399
(850) 245-4161

For information on laws/statutes:
http://www.doh.state.fl.us/mqa/acupunct/acu_statutes. html

Georgia
Composite State Board of Medical Examiners
2 Peachtree Street, N.W., 36th Floor
Atlanta, Georgia 30303-3465
(404) 656-3913
(404) 656-9723 Fax

For information on laws/statutes:
http://www.ganet.org/meb/licensure_rr.html#acu

Hawaii
Department of Commerce and Consumer Affairs
Professional and Vocational Licensing Division
Board of Acupuncture
P.O. Box 3469
Honolulu, Hawaii 96801
(808) 586-2698 or 3000

For information on laws/statutes:
http://www.hawaii.gov/dcca/areas/pvl/boards/acupuncture/statute_rules/

Idaho
Idaho State Board of Acupuncture
Bureau of Occupational Licenses
1109 Main Street, Suite 220
Boise, Idaho 83702-5642
(208) 334-3233
(208) 334-3945 Fax
http://ibol.idaho.gov/acu.htm

For information on laws/statutes:
http://www3.state.id.us/idstat/TOC/54047KTOC.html

Illinois
Technical Assistance Unit
Illinois Department of Professional Regulation
320 W. Washington Street, 3rd Floor
Springfield, IL 62786
(217) 782-8556
(217) 524-2169 Fax
http://www.idfpr.com/dpr/WHO/acupnt.asp

For information on laws/statutes:
http://www.ilga.gov/commission/jcar/admincode/068/
06801140sections.html

Indiana
Professional Licensing Agency
(Attn: Indiana Acupuncture Advisory Committee)
402 W. Washington St., Room W072
Indianapolis, IN 46204
(317) 234-2060
http://www.in.gov/pla/acupuncture.htm

For information on laws/statutes:
http://www.in.gov/pla/2347.htm

Iowa
Iowa Board of Medical Examiners
400 SW 8th Street, Suite C
Des Moines, Iowa 50309-4686
(515) 281-5171
(515) 242-5908 Fax
http://www.docboard.org/ia/Acupuncture.htm

For information on laws/statutes:
http://www.legis.state.ia.us/IACODE/1999SUPPLEMENT/
148E/

Kansas
**Kansas State Board of Healing Arts (Regulatory
Agency)**
234 SW Topeka Blvd.
Topeka, KS 66603-3068
(785) 296-7413
(888) 886-7205
(785) 296-0852 Fax

For information on laws/statutes:
http://www.ksbha.org/

Kentucky
Kentucky Board of Medical Licensure
310 Whittington Parkway, Ste. 1B
Louisville, KY 40222
(502) 429-7150
(502) 429-7158 Fax

For information on laws/statutes:
http://kbml.ky.gov/ah/ac.htm

Louisiana
Louisiana State Board of Medical Examiners
630 Camp Street
New Orleans, Louisiana 70130
(504) 568-6820

For information on laws/statutes:
http:// www.lsbme.louisiana.gov/

Maine
Maine Dept. of Professional and Financial Regulation
Office of Licensing and Enforcement
35 State House Station
Augusta, Maine 04333-0035
(207) 624-8600
(207) 624-8637 Fax

Maryland
State Board of Acupuncture
4201 Patterson Avenue, Room 320
Baltimore, MD 21215
(410) 764-4766
(410) 358-7258 Fax
http://dhmh.state.md.us/bacc/

For information on laws/statutes:
http://dhmh.state.md.us/bacc/

Massachusetts
Commonwealth of Massachusetts
Board of Registration in Medicine
Committee on Acupuncture
560 Harrison Avenue, Suite G-4
Boston, MA 02118
(617) 654-9810
(617) 426-9358 Fax
http://www.massmedboard.org/acupuncture/

For information on laws/statutes:
http://www.mass.gov/legis/laws/mgl/112-148.htm

Michigan
**Michigan Association of Acupuncture and Oriental
Medicine**
P.O. Box 4404
East Lansing MI 48826-4404
(517) 381-0299
(517) 381-9950 Fax

For information on standards and training:
http://www.michiganacupuncture.org/

Minnesota
Minnesota Board of Medical Practice
University Park Plaza
2829 University Ave. SE - Suite 500
Minneapolis, MN 55414-3246
(612) 617-2130
(612) 617-2166 Fax
http://www.state.mn.us/portal/mn/jsp/home.
do?agency=BMP

For information on laws/statutes:
http://www.revisor.leg.state.mn.us/stats/147B/

Mississippi
According to AOM Alliance, Mississippi is a state in which
there is no legislation or rules authorizing the practice by
licensed acupuncturists.

Missouri
Missouri State Acupuncturist Advisory Committee
3605 Missouri Boulevard
P.O. Box 1335
Jefferson City, MO 65102-1335
(573) 526-1555
(573) 751-0735 Fax
http://pr.mo.gov/acupuncturist.asp

For information on laws/statutes:
http://pr.mo.gov/acupuncturist-statutes.asp

Montana
Montana Board of Medical Examiners
301 South Park, 4th Floor
P.O. Box 200513
Helena, MT 59620-0513
(406) 841-2360
(406) 841-2305 Fax

For information on laws/statutes:
http://mt.gov/dli/bsd/license/bsd_boards/med_board/
licenses/med/lic_acup.asp

Nebraska
Nebraska Health and Human Services
PO Box 94986
Lincoln, NE 68509-4986
(402) 471-2118

For information on laws/statutes:
http://www.hhs.state.ne.us/crl/profindex1.htm
http://www.sos.state.ne.us/business/regsearch/Rules/
Health_and_Human_Services_System/Title-172/Chapter-
89.pdf

Nevada
Nevada State Board of Oriental Medicine
9775 S. Maryland Pkwy., Ste. F-280
Las Vegas, NV 89123
(702) 837-8921
(702) 914-8921 Fax

For information on laws/statutes:
http://oriental_medicine.state.nv.us/

New Hampshire
New Hampshire Board of Acupuncture Licensing
NH DHHS Office of Program Support
Licensing & Regulative Services
129 Pleasant Street
Concord, NH 03301-3857
(603) 271-4814
(603) 271-5590 Fax

For information on laws/statutes:
http://www.nh.gov/acupuncture/

New Jersey
State of New Jersey
Acupuncture Examining Board
PO Box 46019
Newark, NJ 07101
(973) 273-8092
(973) 273-8075 Fax
http://www.state.nj.us/lps/ca/medical.htm#bme5

For more information:
http://www.state.nj.us/lps/ca/medical/acupuncture.htm

New Mexico
Board of Acupuncture and Oriental Medicine
2550 Cerrillos Road
Santa Fe, NM 87505
(505) 476-4630
(505) 476-4545 Fax
http://www.rld.state.nm.us/acupuncture/index.html

For information on laws/statutes:
http://www.rld.state.nm.us/acupuncture/ruleslaw.html

New York
NY State Education Department
Office of the Professions
Division of Professional Licensing Services
Acupuncture Unit
89 Washington Avenue
Albany, New York 12234-1000
(518) 474-3817 , ext. 270
(518) 402-5354 Fax

For information on laws and legislation:
http://www.op.nysed.gov/acupun.htm

North Carolina
North Carolina Acupuncture Licensing Board
P.O. Box 10686
Raleigh, NC 27605
(919) 821-3008
(919) 833-5743 Fax

For information on laws and legislation:
http://www.ncalb.state.nc.us/

North Dakota
According to AOM Alliance, North Dakota is a state in
which there is no legislation or rules authorizing the
practice by licensed acupuncturists. However, a statute
has been introduced.

Ohio
Ohio State Medical Board
77 South High Street, 17th Floor
Columbus, Ohio 43215-6127
(614) 466-3934
(614) 728-5946 Fax
http://med.ohio.gov/ACUsubwebindex.htm

For information on laws/statutes:
http://med.ohio.gov/4762index.htm

Oklahoma
Contact: State Board of Medical Licensure.

MDs and DOs alone are allowed to practice acupuncture.
No training is required. Supervision of an acupuncturist
by an MD is not allowed. Chiropractors can practice
acupuncture with additional training.

Oregon
Oregon Board of Medical Examiners
1500 SW First Avenue, Suite 620
Portland, Oregon 97201
(971) 673-2700
(971) 673-2670 Fax
http://egov.oregon.gov/BME/

For information on laws/statutes:
http://landru.leg.state.or.us/ors/677.html
http://arcweb.sos.state.or.us/rules/OARS_800/OAR_
847/847_070.html

Pennsylvania
Board of Osteopathic Examiners/Board of Medical Examiners
P.O. Box 2649
Harrisburg, Pennsylvania 17105
(717) 787-8503
http://www.dos.state.pa.us/bpoa/site/default.asp

Rhode Island
State of Rhode Island & Providence Plantations
Department of Health, Cannon Building
Three Capitol Hill, Room 104
Providence, Rhode Island 02908
(401) 222-2827
(401) 222-1272 Fax
http://www.health.state.ri.us/hsr/professions/acup.php

For information on laws/statutes:
http://www.rules.state.ri.us/dar/regdocs/released/pdf/
DOH/DOH_191_.pdf

South Carolina
Department of Labor, Licensing and Regulation
P.O. Box 11289
Columbia, SC 29211
(803) 896-4500
(803) 896-4515
For information:
http://www.llr.state.sc.us/POL/Medical/

South Dakota
According to AOM Alliance, South Dakota is a state in
which there is no legislation or rules authorizing the
practice by licensed acupuncturists.

Tennessee
Tennessee Department of Health
425 Fifth Avenue, North
Cordell Hull Building, 3rd Floor
Nashville, TN 37247
(615) 532-4384
(615) 253-4484 Fax
http://www.state.tn.us/health/

For information on rules/regulations:
http://tennessee.gov/sos/rules/0880/0880-12.pdf

Texas
Texas State Board of Medical Examiners
P.O. Box 2018 MC - 231
Austin, TX 78768-2018
(512) 305-7030
(512) 305-9416 Fax
http://www.tmb.state.tx.us/professionals/acupuncturists/
acupuncturists.php

For information on statutes/rules:
http://www.tmb.state.tx.us/rules/acu/acurandr.php

Utah
Division of Occupational and Professional Licensing
160 East 300 South
Salt Lake City, UT 84114
(801) 530-6628
(801) 530-6511
http://www.dopl.utah.gov/licensing/acupuncture.html

For information on rules/regulations:
http://www.dopl.utah.gov/licensing/acupuncture_sub_
page.html#acupustatutes

Vermont
Office of Professional Regulation
26 Terrace Street, Drawer 09
Montpelier, VT 05609-1106
(802) 828-2191
(802) 828-2465 Fax
http://vtprofessionals.org/opr1/acupuncturists/

For information on statutes/laws:
http://www.leg.state.vt.us/statutes/fullchapter.
cfm?Title=26&Chapter=075

Virginia
Virginia Board of Medicine
6603 West Broad St., 5th Fl.
Richmond, VA 23230-1712
(804) 662-9900
http://www.dhp.state.va.us/medicine/advisory/lac/default.
asp

For information on statutes/laws:
http://www.dhp.state.va.us/medicine/leg/
LicensedAcupuncture2-8-06.doc

Washington
Washington Department of Health
Health Professions Quality Assurance
310 Israel Road
Tumwater, WA 98501
(360) 236-4700
Fax: (360) 236-4818
https://fortress.wa.gov/doh/hpqa1/hps3/Acupuncture/
default.htm

For information on statutes/laws:
https://fortress.wa.gov/doh/hpqa1/hps3/Acupuncture/
laws.htm

West Virginia
West Virginia Acupuncture Board
P.O. Box 252
Huntington, WV 25707-0252
(304) 529-4558
http://www.wvs.state.wv.us/acupuncture/

For information on rules/regulations:
http://www.wvs.state.wv.us/acupuncture/rules.html

Wisconsin
State of Wisconsin
Dept. of Regulation and Licensure
Bureau of Health Service Professions
Acupuncture Certification
PO Box 8935
Madison, Wisconsin 53708
(608) 266-2811
http://drl.wi.gov/prof/acup/def.htm
http://drl.wi.gov/boards/rla/index.htm

Wyoming

According to AOM Alliance, Wyoming is a state in which
there is no legislation or rules authorizing the practice by
licensed acupuncturists. However, a statute has been
introduced

Diagnostic Laboratories

The following diagnostic laboratories offer innovative tests for integrative health professionals, including female and male hormone screenings, adrenal stress hormone tests, thyroid panels, platelet or urine catecholamine panels, digestive stool analysis, candida antibody tests, Chronic Fatigue Immune Dysfunction Syndrome evaluation, ELISA food allergy testing, hair analysis for toxic and essential elements, nutritional assays, amino acid assays, essential fatty acids profile, vitamin and mineral analysis. Many of the laboratories are physician-friendly and can be obtained by blood, saliva or urine. The range of tests will vary according to specialties and will require TCM practioners to setup an account. We have listed some specialties, however many labs offer a broad spectrum of tests.

Accu-Chem Laboratories
990 N. Bowser Rd., Suite 800
Richardson, TX 75081
(214) 234-5412
(800) 451-0116
www.accuchem.com

Specialists in toxicology tests, environmental and occupational chemical exposures, including pesticide and herbicides. Also specialize in substance-of-abuse screenings.

Aeron Lifecycles Clinical Laboratory
1933 Davis St., Suite 310
San Leandro, CA 94577
(800) 631-7900
www.aeron.com

Aeron LifeCycles is a clinical laboratory with research interests in linking hormonal changes with many of the diseases and symptoms of aging including osteoporosis, cardiovascular disease and cancer. Accurate salivary hormone tests are currently available for: estradiol, progesterone, testosterone, DHEA, and melatonin.

AAL Reference Laboratories, Inc.
1715 E. Wilshire #715
Santa Ana, CA 92705
(714) 972-9979
(800) 522-2611
www.antibodyassay.com

Provides a wide range of services including immunology, infectious diseases, nutrition, and oxidative medicine tests.

Biochemical Laboratories
P.O.Box 157
Edgewood, NM 87015
(505) 832-4100

Specializes in hair trace mineral analysis tests.

Doctors Data, Inc.
3755 Illinois Avenue
St. Charles, IL 60174-2420
(800) 323-2784
(708) 231-3649
www.doctorsdata.com

Doctor's Data, Inc. is an independent reference laboratory that provides tests in the following area: toxic and hair analysis, amino acids, and metabolites in blood and urine tests.

ELISA/ACT Biotechnologies
14 Pidgeon Hill #300
Sterling, VA 22181
(800) 553-5472
703.450.2980
www.elisaact.com

Provides a range of comprehensive allergy and hypersensitivity tests.

Genova Diagnostics (Formerly Great Smokies Laboratories)
63 Zillicoa Street
Asheville, N.C. 28801-1074
(704) 253-0621
(800) 522-4762
www.gsdl.com

Specializes in tests of physiological function. All tests use samples of stool, urine, saliva, blood, and hair. Results focus on how well the body is doing its job in six important areas: digestion, nutrition, detoxification/oxidative stress, immunology/allergy, production and regulation of hormones, and heart and cardiovascular systems.

Immuno Laboratories, Inc.
1620 W. Oakland Park Blvd.
Ft. Lauderdale, FL 33311
(305) 486-4500
(800) 231-9197
www.immunolabs.com

Offers ELISA delayed food allergy testing, a highly sensitive candida assay, as well as an ELISA gluten/gliadin assay.

Immunosciences Lab, Inc.
8730 Wilshire Blvd., Suite 305
Beverly Hills, CA 90211
(310) 657-1077
(800) 950-4686
www.immuno-sci-lab.com

A diagnostic and research facility that specializes in innovative microbiology and immunology laboratory testing. Tests in the following categories: allergy, autoimmune diseases, cancer and its early diagnosis, chronic fatigue syndrome, immunology and serology, immunotoxicology and intestinal health.

King James Medical Laboratory/Omegatech
24700 Center Ridge Rd., #113
Cleveland, OH 44145
(216) 835-2150
(800) 437-1404
www.kingjamesomegatech-lab.com

The King James Medical Laboratory, Inc. provides
the analysis of metals in hair and water samples to
both the general public and healthcare practitioners.

Meridian Valley Lab
801 SW 16th Street Suite 126
Renton, WA 98055
425.271.8689
www.meridianvalleylab.com

A clinical reference lab and nutritional testing for
practioners. The lab offers the following tests: Allergy
(Elisa), amino acids, bone density, complete stool
and digestive analysis, essential fatty acids profile,
mineral analysis, steroid, hormone panels, thyroid
panels.

Metametrix Clinical Laboratory
4855 Peachtree Industrial Blvd Suite 201
Norcross GA, 30092
770-446-5483
800-221-4640
www.metametrix.com

Metametrix Clinical Laboratory provides a wide
range of test in nutritional insufficiencies, metabolic
dysfunction, and toxicity and detoxification.

Optimum Health Resource Laboratories, Inc.
2700 North 29th Avenue, Suite # 205
Hollywood, Florida 33020
(888) 751-3388
www.yorkallergyusa.com

Optimum Health Resource provides food intolerance
testing.

Pantox Laboratories
4622 Santa Fe Street
San Diego, CA 92109
(619) 272-3885
(800) 726-8696
www.pantox.com

Pantox Laboratories analyzes and interprets the
biochemical defense system that prevents aging and
degenerative diseases.

Spectracell Laboratories, Inc.
515 Post Oak Blvd., Suite 830
Houston, TX 77027
(800) 227-5227
(713) 621-3101
www.spectracell.com

SpectraCell Laboratories Inc. specializes in
functional intracellular testing. Their tests offer
application for assessing many clinical conditions
including cardiovascular risk, immunological
disorders, metabolism measurements and nutritional
analysis.

U.S. BioTek Laboratories
13758 Lake City Way NE
Seattle, WA 98125
(877) 318-8728
(206) 365-1256
www.usbiotek.com

US BioTek Laboratories provides a range of tests
including: antibody, amino acids, bone density,
complete stool and digestive analysis, urinary
metabolic tests, hormone panels, thyroid panels.

**Vitamin Diagnostics/European Laboratories of
Nutrients**
Industrial Drive & Route 35
Cliffwood Beach, N.J. 07735
(732) 583-7773
www.europeanlaboratory.com

Offers specialized nutritional testing for nutrient
status.

RESOURCE

RESOURCES FOR THE STUDY OF CHINESE MEDICINE

The following pages detail the resources for the study of Chinese medicine, providing for each the name of the book and its author(s), the publication date, publisher, and principal city for the publisher's distribution.

1. **MATERIA MEDICA & GUIDES TO INDIVIDUAL HERBS** - Materia Medica and other books that provide information about the traditional uses of individual medicinal materials.
2. **CHINESE FORMULA & GUIDES TO FORMULATION** - Traditional Chinese formula books that provide information about the content and applications of numerous traditional formulas, sometimes with modern formulas included.
3. **CLINICAL EXPERIENCE & TREATMENT RECOMMENDATIONS** - Clinical experience reports (herbal medicine), which represent suggestions for treatments of a large number of different diseases based on the experience of an individual practitioner or a group of practitioners who collaborated in writing about clinical efforts.
4. **ACUPUNCTURE & MOXIBUSTION** - Acupuncture and moxibustion texts. There are dozens of books available on this subject, but many present essentially the same information.
5. **CHINESE NUTRITION** - Food as medicine books, depicting Oriental efforts to understand the health impact of foods and Chinese nutrition. Some of these books review the historical developments of food use in China, with only passing reference to medicine.
6. **GENERAL SUBJECT** - General subjects, including overviews of Oriental medicine, special topics within the field of Chinese medicine (including physiology and diagnosis), and general analysis of the application of herbs based on the theoretical framework applied mainly to traditional prescriptions, rather than direct clinical experience of the author(s).
7. **HISTORICAL RECORDS** - Translations of traditional texts, analysis of archeological and historical records, and discussions of the development of traditional Chinese medicine and its cultural context.
8. **MEDICAL SPECIALTIES** - Books on TCM focused on cancer, ophthalmology, pediatric disorders, gynecology, and dermatology.
9. **WESTERN MEDICINE** - Books that are used primarily for the purpose of brief description of disease characteristics and associated therapeutics, or studies of nutrients and herbal active ingredients that do not focus on Chinese herbs.
10. **ALTERNATIVE MEDICINE** - These are books that present information about alternative medicine not specific to Chinese medicine and provide alternative perspective to healing.
11. **LISTING OF PUBLISHERS & BOOKSELLERS**
12. **BOARD EXAMINATION PREPERATIONS & STUDY RESOURCES**

Clearly, there will be substantial differences in opinion about the quality of each book; in fact, it was not always easy to place the books within one of the categories based on the criteria established here since many books overlap categories and many provide broad discussions on wide ranging topics of TCM and acupuncture. Emphasis is placed on such features as: inclusion of quality of work; comprehensiveness in dealing with the subject at hand; apparent reliability of the information presented; and readability.

An acupuncturist that prescribes Chinese herbs should develop an extensive library that includes books from each category (at least from those that correspond to their scope of practice). A minimum library of about 35-40 such books in these categories would likely provide the resource information that is essential to conduct a successful acupuncture practice.

1. MATERIA MEDICA & GUIDES TO INDIVIDUAL HERBS

Hong-Yen Hsu, *Oriental Materia Medica: A Concise Guide*, 1986, Oriental Healing Arts Institute, Long Beach, CA.

John Chen & Tina Chen, *Chinese Medical Herbology and Pharmacology*, 2001, Art of Medicine Press, Industry, CA.

Dan Bensky & Andrew Gamble, *Chinese Herbal Medicine: Materia Medica*, 1993, Eastland Press, Seattle, WA.

Bingshan Huang & Yuxia Wang, *Thousand Formulas and Thousand Herbs of Traditional Chinese Medicine, vol. 1*, 1993, Heilongjiang Education Press, Harbin China.

Yifan Yang, *Chinese Herbal Medicines*, 2002, Churchill Livingstone, London.

Charles Belanger, *The Chinese Herb Selection Guide*, 1997, Phytotech Publishing, Richmond, CA.

Dafang Zheng, *Essentials of Chinese Medicine Materia Medica*, 2003, Bridge Publishing Group, Walnut, CA.

Ming Ou, *Chinese-English Manual of Common-Used Herbs in Traditional Chinese Medicine*, 1989, Joint Publishing Co., Hong Kong.

Pharmacopoeia Commission of PRC, *Pharmacopoeia of the PRC*, 1988, People's Medical Publishing House, Beijing.

Philippe Sionneau, *Pao Zhi: An Introduction to the Use of Processed Chinese Medicinals*, 1995, Blue Poppy Press, Boulder, CO.

Kun-ying Yen, *Illustrated Chinese Materia Medica*, 1986, Southern Materials Center, Inc., Taipei.

Enquin Zhang, *Chinese Materia Medica*, 1990, Publishing House of Shanghai College of Traditional Chinese Medicine, Shanghai.

Junying Geng, *Practical Traditional Chinese Medicine and Pharmacology: Medicinal Herbs*, 1991, New World Press, Beijing.

Him-che Yeung, *Handbook of Chinese Herbs*, 1998, Institute of Chinese Medicine, Los Angeles, CA.

2. CHINESE FORMULA & GUIDES TO FORMULATION

Dan Bensky & Randall Barolet, *Chinese Herbal Medicine: Formulas and Strategies*, 1990, Eastland Press, Seattle, WA.

Him-che Yeung, *Handbook of Chinese Herbal Formulas*, 1998, Institute of Chinese Medicine, Los Angeles, CA.

Jake Paul Fratkin, *Chinese Herbal Patent Medicines: The Clinical Desk Reference*, 2001, Shya Publications, Boulder, CO.

Will Maclean & Jane Lyttleton, *The Clinical Manual of Chinese Herbal Patent Medicines*, 2000, Pargolin Press, Campleton Australia.

Junying Geng, *Practical Traditional Chinese Medicine and Pharmacology: Herbal Formulas*, 1991, New World Press, Beijing.

HY Hsu & CS Hsu, *Commonly Used Chinese Herb Formulas Companion Handbook*, 1997, Oriental Healing Arts Institute, Long Beach, CA.

Nigel Wiseman & Craig Mitchell, *Ten Lecturers on the Use of Formulas from the Personal Experience of Jiao Shu De*, 2005, Paradigm Publications, Taos, NM.

Ou Ming, *Chinese-English Manual of Common-Used Prescriptions in Traditional Chinese Medicine*, 1989, Joint Publishing Co., Hong Kong.

Bob Flaws, *160 Essential Patent Formulas*, 1999, Blue Poppy Press, Boulder, CO.

Margaret Naeser, *Outline Guide to Chinese Herbal Patent Medicines in Pill Form*, 1990, Boston Chinese Medicine, Boston, MA.

CH Zhu, *Clinical Handbook of Chinese Prepared Medicines*, 1989, Paradigm Publications, Brookline, MA.

Linda Morse, *Examination Workbook for Oriental Medicine,* 2004, Linda Morse, Los Angeles, CA,

3. CLINICAL EXPERIENCE & TREATMENT RECOMMENDATIONS

Xianmin Shang, *Practical Traditional Chinese Medicine and Pharmacology: Clinical Experiences*, 1990, New World Press, Beijing.

Tietao Deng, *Practical Diagnosis in Traditional Chinese Medicine*, 1999, Churchill Livingstone, London.

John Chen, *Clinical Manual of Oriental Medicine 2nd Edition*, 2006, Lotus Institute of Integrative Medicine, Industry, CA.

Sun Peilin, *The Treatment of Pain with Chinese Herbs and Acupuncture*, 2002, Churchill Livingstone, London.

Yan Wu & Warren Fischer, *Practical Therapeutics of Traditional Chinese Medicine*, 1997, Paradigm Publications, Brookline, MA.

Enquin Zhang, *Clinic of Traditional Chinese Medicine*, 1990, Publishing House of Shanghai College of Traditional Chinese Medicine, Shanghai.

Liu Chongyun & Deng Yong, *Encyclopedia of Chinese and US Patent Herbal Medicines*, 1999, Keats Publishing, Lincolnwood, IL.

Giovanni Maciocia, *The Practice of Chinese Medicine*, 1994, Churchill Livingstone, London.

Giovanni Maciocia, *Diagnosis in Chinese Medicine, A Comprehensive Guide*, 2004, Churchill Livingstone, London.

Will Maclean & Jane Lyttleton, *Clinical Handbook of Internal Medicine, Volume 1 & 2*, 2002, University of Western Sydney, Campleton Australia.

Nianfang Shao, *The Treatment of Knotty Diseases with Chinese Acupuncture and Chinese Herbal Medicine*, 1990, Shandong Science and Technology Press, Jinan.

Richard Tan, *Twenty-Four More in Acupuncture*, 1991, Richard Tan, San Diego, CA.

Richard Tan, *Dr. Tan's Strategy of Twelve Magical Points, Advanced Principles and Techniques in Acupuncture,* 1991, Richard Tan, San Diego, CA.

Richard Tan, *Twelve and Twelve*, 1991, Richard Tan, San Diego, CA.

Richard Tan, *Acupuncture 1, 2, 3*, 2006, Richard Tan, San Diego, CA.

Qi Wang & Zhilin Dong, *Modern Clinical Necessities for Traditional Chinese Medicine*, 1990, China Ocean Press, Beijing.

Anshen Shi, *Essentials of Chinese Medicine: Internal Medicine*, 2003, Bridge Publishing Group, Walnut, CA.

Junwen Zhang, *Integrating Chinese and Western Medicine: A Handbook for Practitioners*, 1993 Foreign Languages Press, Beijing.

Zhou Zhong Ying & Jin Hui De, *Clinical Manual of Chinese Herbal Medicine and Acupuncture*, 1997, Churchill Livingstone, London.

Kiiko Matsumoto & Steven Birch, *Extraordinary Vessels*, 1986, Paradigm Publications, Brookline, MA.

Barbara Kirschbaum, *Atlas of Chinese Tongue Diagnosis Volume 2*, 2002, Eastland Press, Seattle, WA.

4. ACUPUNCTURE & MOXIBUSTION

Andrew Ellis, Nigel Wiseman, & Ken Boss, *Fundamentals of Chinese Acupuncture*, 1988, Paradigm Publications, Brookline, MA.

Maoliang Qiu, *Chinese Acupuncture and Moxibustion*, 1993, Churchill Livingstone, London.

Ken Chen & Yonquiang Cui, *Handbook to Chinese Auricular Therapy*, 1990, Foreign Language Press, Beijing.

Alon Lotan, *Acupoint Location Guide*, 2000, Estem, Yodfat, Isreal.

Xinnong Cheng, *Chinese Acupuncture and Moxibustion*, 1987, Foreign Languages Press, Beijing.

Peter Deadmean & Mazin Al-Khafaji, *A Manual of Acupuncture*, 1998, Journal of Chinese Medicine Publications, East Sussex, England.

Terry Oleson, *Auriculotherapy Manual 3rd Edition*, 2003, Churchill Livingston, London England.

Andrew Ellis, Nigel Wiseman, & Ken Boss, *Grasping the Wind*, 1989, Paradigm Publications, Brookline, MA.

Zhu Ming Ching, *Zhu's Scalp Acupuncture*, 1992, Eight Dragons Publishing, Hong Kong.

John & Dan Bensky, *Acupuncture: A Comprehensive Text*, 1981, Eastland Press, Seattle, WA.

Yu Hui Chan & Han Fu Ru, *Golden Needle Wang Leting*, 1996, Blue Poppy Press, Boulder, CO.

Zhang Enquin, *Chinese Acupuncture and Moxibustion*, 1990, Publishing House of Shanghai College of Traditional Chinese Medicine, Shanghai.

Jeremy Ross, *Acupuncture Point Combinations: The Key to Clinical Success,* 1995, Churchill Livingstone, London.

Zhang Ruifu, Wu Xifen, & Wang NS, *Illustrated Dictionary of Chinese Acupuncture*, 1986, Sheep's Publication, U.S.A., San Francisco, CA.

Zhu Ming Ching, *A Handbook for Treatment of Acute Syndromes by Using Acupuncture and Moxibustion*, 1992, Eight Dragons Publishing, Hong Kong.

Robert Johns, *The Art of Acupuncture Techniques*, 1996, North Atlantic Books, Berkeley, CA.

Miriam Lee, *Insights of a Senior Acupuncturist,* 1992, Blue Poppy Press, Boulder, CO.

Angela Hicks, Five Element Constitutional Acupuncture, 2004, Churchill Livingstone, London.

Zhang Denbu, *Acupuncture Cases from China, 1994*, Churchill Livingstone, London.

Zhong Meiquan, *The Chinese Plum-Blossom Needle Therapy*, 1984, The People's Medical Publishing House, Beijing.

5. CHINESE NUTRITION

Henry Lu, *Chinese System of Food Cures*, 1986, Sterling Publishing Co. Inc., New York, NY.

Paul Pitchford, *Healing with Whole Foods*, 2002, North Atlantic Books, Berkeley, CA.

Maoshing Ni & Cathy NcNease, *The Tao of Nutrition*, 1987, College of Tao & Traditional Chinese Healing, Los Angeles, CA.

Rosa LoSan & Suzanne LeVert, *Chinese Healing Foods*, 1998, Pocket Books, New York, NY.

E.N. Anderson, *The Food of China*, 1988, Yale University Press, New Haven, CT.

Zhang Enquin, *Chinese Medicated Diet*, 1988, Publishing House of Shanghai College of Traditional Chinese Medicine, Shanghai.

6. GENERAL SUBJECT

Giovanni Maciocia, *The Foundations of Chinese Medicine*, 1989, Churchill Livingstone, London.

Ted Katpchuk, *The Web That Has No Weaver: Understanding Chinese Medicine*, 1983, St. Martins Press, New York, NY.

Claude Larre C & Elisabeth De La Vallée ER, *Rooted in Spirit: The Heart of Chinese Medicine,* 1995 Station Hill Press, Barrytown, NY.

Harriet Beinfield & Efrem Korngold, *Between Heaven and Earth*, 1992, Ballantine Books, London.

Philippe Sionneau, *Dui Yao: The Art of Combining Chinese Medicinals*, 1997, Blue Poppy Press, Boulder, CO.

Jeremy Ross, *Zang Fu: The Organ Systems of Traditional Chinese Medicine*, 1989, Churchill Livingstone, London.

Paul Unschuld, *Chinese Medicine*, 1998, Paradigm Publications, Brookline, MA.

Nigel Wiseman & Andrew Elli' *ndamentals of Chinese Medicine*, 1985, Pa   ., Brookline, MA.

Miriam Lee, *Master Tor Alternative Style in Mr* Blue Poppy Press, P

David Legge, *Clc* College Press, \

7. HISTORICAL RECORDS

Maoshing Ni, *The Yellow Emperor's Classic of Medicine: A New Translation of the Neijing Suwen with Commentary*, 1995, Shambhala, Boston, MA.

Paul Unschuld, *Forgotten Traditions of Ancient Chinese Medicine*, 1990, Paradigm Publications, Brookline, MA.

Ping Chen, *History and Development of Traditional Chinese Medicine*, 1999, Science Press, Beijing.

HY Hsu & Peacher, *Shang Han Lun: The Great Classic of Chinese Medicine*, 1981, Oriental Healing Arts Institute, Long Beach, CA.

HY Hsu & SY Wang, *The Theory of Feverish Diseases and Its Clinical Applications*, 1985, Oriental Healing Arts Institute, Long Beach, CA.

Paul Unschuld, *Medicine in China: History of Pharmaceutics*, 1986, University of California Press, Berkeley, CA.

Paul Unschuld, *Medicine in China: A History of Ideas*, 1985, University of California Press, Berkeley, CA.

Yang Shou Zhong & Li Jianyong, Li Dongyuan's, *Treatise on the Spleen and Stomach*, 1993, Blue Poppy Press, Boulder, CO.

Ming Zhu, *The Medical Classic of the Yellow Emperor*, 2001, Foreign Languages Press, Beijing.

Yang Shou Zhong, *Extra Treatises based on Investigation and Inquiry*, 1994, Blue Poppy Press, Boulder, CO.

Yang Shou Zhong, *Master Hua's Classic of the Central Viscera*, 1993, Blue Poppy Press, Boulder, CO.

Yang Shou Zhong, *The Divine Farmer's Materia Medica*, 1997, Blue Poppy Press, Boulder, CO.

Yang Shou Zhong & Charles Chace, *The Systematic Classic of Acupuncture and Moxibustion*, 1994, Blue Poppy Press, Boulder, CO.

Zhang Zhong Jing, *Treatise on Febrile Diseases Caused by Cold with 500 Cases*, 1993, New World Press, Beijing.

8. MEDICAL SPECIALTIES

CANCER

Minyi Chang, *Anticancer Medicinal Herbs*, 1992, Hunan Science and Technology Publishing House, Changsha.

HY Hsu, *Treating Cancer with Chinese Herbs*, 1990, Oriental Healing Arts Institute, Long Beach, CA.

Ming Ou, *An Illustrated Guide to Antineoplastic Chinese Herbal Medicine*, 1990, The Commercial Press, Hong Kong.

Lanling Shi & Peiquan Shi, *Experience in Treating Carcinomas with Traditional Chinese Medicine*, 1992, Shandong Science and Technology Press, Shandong.

E Lien & L Wen, *Structure Activity Relationship Analysis of Chinese Anti-Cancer Drugs and Related Plants*, 1985, Oriental Healing Arts Institute, Long Beach, CA.

Mingji Pan, *How to Discover Cancer Through Self-Examination*, 1992, Fujian Science and Technology Publishing House, Fujian.

Chiyuan Sun, *A Probing into the Treatment of Leukemia with Traditional Chinese Medicine*, 1990, Hai Feng Publishing Company, Hong Kong.

Daizhao Zhang, *The Treatment of Cancer by Integrated Chinese-Western Medicine*, 1989, Blue Poppy Press, Boulder, CO.

...wen, Management of Cancer with Chinese ...2003, Donica Publishing, London,

DERMATOLOGY

Lin Li, *Practical Traditional Chinese Dermatology*, 1995, Hai Feng Publishing Company, Hong Kong.

Xu Yihou, *Dermatology in Traditional Chinese Medicine*, 2004, Donica Publishing, London England.

Jian Hui Liang, *A Handbook of Traditional Chinese Dermatology*, 1988, Blue Poppy Press, Boulder, CO.

De-hui Shen, Hsiu-Fen Wu, & Wang N, *Manual of Dermatology in Chinese Medicine*, 1995, Eastland Press, Seattle, WA.

Xu Xiangcai, *The English-Chinese Encyclopedia of Practical Traditional Chinese Medicine, vol. 16: Dermatology*, 1991, Higher Education Press, Beijing.

INFECTIONS & FEVERISH DISEASES

Jinglun Hou, *Traditional Chinese Treatment of Infectious Diseases*, 1997, Academy Press, Beijing.

Gary Seifert & JM Wen, *Warm Disease Theory*, 2000, Paradigm Publications, Brookline, MA.

GuoHui Liu, *Warm Pathogen Diseases*, 2002, Eastland Press, Seattle, WA.

PEDIATRICS

Cao Jiming, Su Xinming, *Essentials of Traditional Chinese Pediatrics*, 1990, Foreign Language Press, Beijing.

Xiao Shuqin, Zhang Xiwen, *Pediatric Bronchitis: Its TCM Cause, Diagnosis, and Treatment*, 1991, Blue Poppy Press, Boulder, CO.

GYNECOLOGY/UROLOGY

Charlotte Furth, *A Flourishing Yin: Gender in China's Medical History, 960-1665*, 1999, University of California Press, Berkeley, CA.

Giovanni Maciocia, *Obstetrics & Gynecology in Chinese Medicine*, 1998, Churchill Livingstone, London.

Anna Lin, *A Handbook of TCM Urology & Male Sexual Dysfunction*, 1992, Blue Poppy Press, Boulder, CO.

Zita West, *Acupuncture in Pregnancy and Childbirth*, 1998, Churchill Livingstone, London.

Yoshiharu Shibata & Jean Wu, *Kampo Treatment for Climacteric Disorders*, 1997, Paradigm Publications, Brookline, MA.

Ye Heng-Yyin, *Guide to Gynecology*, 2001, Blue Poppy Press, Boulder, CO.

NEUROLOGY

Cheung CS, Lai YK, & Kaw UA, *Mental Dysfunction as Treated by Traditional Chinese Medicine*, 1981, Traditional Chinese Medicine Publisher, San Francisco, CA.

OPHTHALMOLOGY

Xu Xiangcai, *The English-Chinese Encyclopedia of Practical Traditional Chinese Medicine, vol. 17: Ophthalmology*, 1994, Higher Education Press, Beijing.

Paul Unschuld & J Kovacs, *Essential Subtleties on the Silver Sea*, 1998, University of California Press, Berkeley, CA.

ORTHOPEDICS, TRAUMATOLOGY, & RHEUMATOLOGY

Xu Xiangcai, *The English-Chinese Encyclopedia of Practical Traditional Chinese Medicine, vol. 14: Orthopedics and Traumatology*, 1992, Higher Education Press, Beijing.

C. Vangermeersch & Sun Peilin, *Bi-Syndromes*, 1994, SATAS, Belgium.

9. WESTERN MEDICINE

Mark Beers & Robert Porter, *The Merck Manual (18th ed.)*, 2007, Merck & Co., Rahway, NJ.

John Boik, *Natural Compounds in Cancer Therapy*, 2001, Oregon Medical Press, Princeton, MN.

AMA, *AMA Encyclopedia of Medicine*, 2003, Random House, New York.

Winter Griffith and Stephen Moore, *Complete Guide to Prescription and Nonprescription Drugs 2007 (Complete Guide to Prescription and Nonprescription Drugs), 2007*, Harper Collins, New York, NY.

James J. Rybacki, *The Essential Guide to Prescription Drugs*, 2006, Harper Perennial, New York.

Melvyn R. Werbach, *Foundations of Nutritional Medicine*, 1997, Third Line Press, Tarzana, CA

Melvyn R. Werbach, *Healing Through Nutrition*, 1993, Harper Collins, New York, NY.

Melvyn R. Werbach, *Nutritional Influences on Illness, Second Edition*, 1993, Third Line Press, Tarzana, CA.

Melvyn R. Werbach, *Nutritional Influences on Mental Illness, Second Edition*, 1999, Third Line Press, Tarzana, CA.

Kathleen Mahan and Sylvia Escott-Stump, *Krause's Food, Nutrition, & Diet Therapy, 10th Edition*, 2000, Saunders Company, New York, NY.

Stanley Hoppenfeld, *Physical Examination of the Spine Extremities*, 1976, Prentice Hall, Saddle River, NJ.

Lawrence M. Tierney, *Current Medical Diagnosis & Treatment, 2006*, 2006, McGraw Hill, New York, NY.

Fred Ferri, *Practical Guide to the Care of Medical Patient, 4th Edition*, 1998, Mosby, Inc. St. Louis. MO.

10. ALTERNATIVE MEDICINE

James Balch & Mark Stengler, *Prescription for Natural Cures : A Self-Care Guide for Treating Health Problems with Natural Remedies Including Diet and Nutrition, Nutritional Supplements, Bodywork, and More*, 2004, John Wiley & Sons, Hoboken, NJ.

Vance Ferrell & Edgar Archbold, *Natural Remedies Encyclopedia*, 2004, Harvestime Books, Altamount, TN.

Larry Trivieri & John Anderson, *Alternative Medicine: The Definitive Guide (2nd Edition)*, 2002, Celestial Arts, Berkeley, CA.

Michael Murray & Joseph E. Pizzorno, *Encyclopedia of Natural Medicine*, 1998, Prima Publishing, Rocklin, CA.

Phyllis Balch, *Prescription for Nutritional Healing, 4th Edition: A Practical A-to-Z Reference to Drug-Free Remedies Using Vitamins, Minerals, Herbs & Food Supplements ... A-To-Z Reference to Drug-Free Remedies)*, 2004, Penguin Putnam, New York, NY.

Hazel Courtney, *500 of the Most Important Health Tips You'll Ever Need*, 2001, Cico Books, London, England.

Phyllis Balch, *Prescription for Herbal Healing: An Easy-to-Use A-Z Reference to Hundreds of Common Disorders and Their Herbal Remedies*, 2002, Penguin Putnam, New York, NY.

Phyllis Balch, *Prescription for Nutritional Healing: The A-to-Z Guide to Supplements: The A-to-Z Guide to Supplements,* 2002, Penguin Putnam, New York, NY.

Daniel Krinsky & James LaValle, *Lexi-Comp's Natural Therapeutics Pocket Guide, 2nd Edition,* 2003, Lexi-Comp, Inc., Hudson, OH.

Gary Null, *The Complete Encyclopedia of Natural Healing,* 2005, Kensington Books, New York, NY.

Michael Murray & Joseph Pizzorno, *Encyclopedia of Natural Medicine, Revised Second Edition,* 1997, Three Rivers Press, New York, NY.

Michael Murray & Joseph Pizzorno, *Encyclopedia of Nutritional Supplements: The Essential Guide for Improving Your Health Naturally,* 1996, Three Rivers Press, New York, NY.

Bill Gottlieb, *Alternative Cures: The Most Effective Natural Home Remedies for 160 Health Problems,* 2002, Rodale Publishing.

Winter Griffith, *Vitamins, Herbs, Minerals, & Supplements: The Complete Guide,* 1998, Da Capo Press, Cambridge, MA.

Linda Skidmore-Roth, *Mosby's Handbook of Herbs & Natural Supplements,* 2001, Mosby, St. Louis, MO.

Steven Brantman & Andrea Girman, *Mosby's Handbook of Herbs and Supplements and Their Therapeutic Use,* 2003, Mosby, St. Louis, MO.

Charles Fetrow, *The Complete Guide to Herbal Medicines,* 2000, Pocketbooks, New York, NY.

Linda Page, *Healthy Healing: A Guide to Self-Healing for Everyone,* 12th Edition, 2004, Traditional Wisdom, Inc.

Michael Van Straten, *Organic Super Foods,* 2003, Octopus Publishing, London, England.

Earl Mindell & Virginia Hopkins, *Prescription Alternatives, Third Edition: Hundreds of Safe, Natural Prescription-Free Remedies to Restore and Maintain Your Health,* 2003, McGraw Hill, New York, NY

11. PUBLISHERS & BOOKSELLERS

Blue Poppy Press
www.bluepoppy.com

Churchill Livingstone
www.harcourt-international.com/acupuncture

Eastland Press
www.eastlandpress.com

Eastwind Books
www.ewbb.com

Great Wall Bookstore
www.gwbooks.com

National Acupuncture Foundation
http://nationalacupuncturefoundation.org

Paradigm Publications
www.paradigm-pubs.com

Redwing Books
www.redwingbooks.com

Snow Lotus Press
www.snowlotus.org

12. BOARD EXAMINATION PREPARATIONS & STUDY RESOURCES

Linda Morse Acupuncture Board Preparation Review - National & California State Board preparations workshop - Linda Morse, *(Linda's nationally acclaimed workshop has the highest passing ratio for national and California state board preparations for the last 4 years. Her preparation workshop and workbook is essential to your success. The best investment for your boards)* - www.lindamorselac.com

Creative Memory Tools - Audio cds & software for students & practitioners of TCM, acupuncture - www.creativememorytools.com

Chinese Herb Flash Cards - Chinese Herb Flash Cards, effective way to learn Chinese herbs - www.chineseherbcards.com

Musical Formula Study Guide - Double-CD musical study guide to the functions and ingredients of the most popular Chinese herbal formulas. All California State Board required formulas are included - www.cdbaby.com/cd/curcio

TCMtests.com is the largest online test preparation site for Oriental Medicine practitioners who wish to pass professional licensing examinations - www.tcmtests.com

INTERNET RESEARCH SITES

National Library of Medicine (NIH) - http://www.nlm.nih.gov/

National Institutes of Health - http://www.ncbi.nlm.nih.gov/

National Center for Complimentary and Alternative Medicine - http://nccam.nih.gov/

Medscape - http://www.medscape.com

World Health Organization - http://www.who.int/en/

British Medical Journal - http://www.bmj.com/

The Office of Dietary Supplements (NIH) - http://ods.od.nih.gov/index.aspx

BIBLIOGRAPHY

AMA, AMA *Encyclopedia of Medicine*, Random House, New York, 2003.

Bakerman, Seymour, *ABCs of Interpretative Laboratory Data 4th Edition*, Interpretative Laboratory Data, Phoenix, AZ, 2002.

Balch, James & Stengler, Mark, *Prescription for Natural Cures: A Self-Care Guide for Treating Health Problems with Natural Remedies Including Diet and Nutrition, Nutritional Supplements, Bodywork, and More*, John Wiley & Sons, Hoboken, NJ, 2004.

Balch, Phyllis, *Prescription for Herbal Healing: An Easy-to-Use A-Z Reference to Hundreds of Common Disorders and Their Herbal Remedies*, Penguin Putnam, New York, NY, 2002.

Balch, Phyllis, *Prescription for Nutritional Healing, 4th Edition: A Practical A-to-Z Reference to Drug-Free Remedies Using Vitamins, Minerals, Herbs & Food Supplements ... A-To-Z Reference to Drug-Free Remedies*, Penguin Putnam, New York, NY, 2004.

Balch, Phyllis, *Prescription for Nutritional Healing: The A-to-Z Guide to Supplements: The A-to-Z Guide to Supplements*, Penguin Putnam, New York, NY, 2002.

Beers, Mark & Porter, Robert, *The Merck Manual (18th ed.)*, Merck & Co., Rahway, NJ, 2007.

Belanger, Charles, *The Chinese Herb Selection Guide*, Phytotech Publishing, Richmond, CA, 1997.

Bensky, Dan & Barolet, Randall, *Chinese Herbal Medicine: Formulas and Strategies*, Eastland Press, Seattle, WA, 1990.

Bensky, Dan & Gamble, Andrew, *Chinese Herbal Medicine: Materia Medica*, Eastland Press, Seattle, WA, 1993.

Bensky, John & Bensky, Dan, *Acupuncture: A Comprehensive Text*, Eastland Press, Seattle, WA, 1981.

Boik, John, *Natural Compounds in Cancer Therapy*, Oregon Medical Press, Princeton, MN, 2001.

Brantman, Steven & Girman, Andrea, *Mosby's Handbook of Herbs and Supplements and Their Therapeutic Use*, Mosby, St. Louis, MO, 2003.

Chen, John & Chen, Tina, *Chinese Medical Herbology and Pharmacology*, Art of Medicine Press, Industry, CA, 2001.

Chen, John, *Clinical Manual of Oriental Medicine 2nd Edition*, Lotus Institute of Integrative Medicine, Industry, CA, 2006.

Chen, Ken & Cui, Yonquiang, *Handbook to Chinese Auricular Therapy*, Foreign Language Press, Beijing, 1990.

Chongyun, Liu & Yong, Deng, *Encyclopedia of Chinese and US Patent Herbal Medicines*, Keats Publishing, Lincolnwood, IL, 1999.

Cline, David & Ma, John, *A Comprehensive Study Guide Emergency Medicine 5th Edition*, McGraw-Hill, New York, NY, 2000.

Courtney, Hazel, *500 of the Most Important Health Tips You'll Ever Need*, Cico Books, London, England, 2001.

Deadman, Peter & Al-Khafaji, Mazin, *A Manual of Acupuncture*, Journal of Chinese Medicine Publications, East Sussex, England, 1998.

Deng, Tietao, *Practical Diagnosis in Traditional Chinese Medicine*, Churchill Livingstone, London, 1999.

Ellis, Andrew, Wiseman, Nigel, & Boss, Ken, *Fundamentals of Chinese Acupuncture*, Paradigm Publications, Brookline, MA, 1988.

Ferrell, Vance & Archbold, Edgar, *Natural Remedies Encyclopedia*, Harvestime Books, Altamount, TN, 2004.

Ferri, Fred, *Practical Guide to the Care of Medical Patients, 4th Edition*, Mosby, Inc. St. Louis. MO, 1998.

Fetrow, Charles, *The Complete Guide to Herbal Medicines*, Pocketbooks, New York, NY, 2000.

Flaws, Bob, *160 Essential Patent Formulas*, Blue Poppy Press, Boulder, CO, 1999.

Fratkin, Jake Paul, *Chinese Herbal Patent Medicines: The Clinical Desk Reference*, Shya Publications, Boulder, CO, 2001.

Gottlieb, Bill, *Alternative Cures: The Most Effective Natural Home Remedies for 160 Health Problems*, Rodale Publishing, 2002.

Griffith, Winter & Moore, Stephen, *Complete Guide to Prescription and Nonprescription Drugs 2007 (Complete Guide to Prescription and Nonprescription Drugs)*, Harper Collins, New York, NY, 2007.

Griffith, Winter, *Vitamins, Herbs, Minerals, & Supplements: The Complete Guide*, Da Capo Press, Cambridge, MA, 1998.

Hoppenfeld, Stanley, *Physical Examination of the Spine Extremities*, Prentice Hall, Saddle River, NJ, 1976.

Hsu, HY & Hsu, CS, *Commonly Used Chinese Herbal Formula Companion Book*, Ohai Press, Long Beach, CA, 1997.

Katpchuk, Ted, *The Web That Has No Weaver: Understanding Chinese Medicine*, St. Martins Press, New York, NY, 1983.

Kim, HB, *California State Board Tutorial Workbook*, HB Kim, Los Angeles, CA.

Krinsky, Daniel & LaValle, James, *Lexi-Comp's Natural Therapeutics Pocket Guide*, 2nd Edition, Lexi-Comp, Inc., Hudson, OH, 2003.

LoSan, Rosa & LeVert, Suzanne, *Chinese Healing Foods*, Pocket Books, New York, NY, 1998.

Lotan, Alon, *Acupoint Location Guide*, Estem, Yodfat, Isreal, 2000.

Lu, Henry, *Chinese System of Food Cures*, Sterling Publishing Co. Inc., New York, NY, 1986.

Maciocia, Giovanni, *Obstetrics & Gynecology in Chinese Medicine*, Churchill Livingstone, London, 1998.

Maciocia, Giovanni, *The Foundations of Chinese Medicine*, Churchill Livingstone, London, 1989.

Maciocia, Giovanni, *The Practice of Chinese Medicine*, Churchill Livingstone, London, 1994.

BIBLIOGRAPHY

Maciocia, Giovanni, *Diagnosis in Chinese Medicine, A Comprehensive Guide*, Churchill Livingstone, London, 2004.

Maclean, Will & Lyttleton, Jane, *The Clinical Manual of Chinese Herbal Patent Medicines*, Pargolin Press, Campleton Australia, 2000.

Maclean, Will & Lyttleton, Jane, *Clinical Handbook of Internal Medicine, Volume 1 & 2*, University of Western Sydney, Campleton Australia, 2002.

Magee, David, *Orthopedic Physical Assessment Enhanced Edition, 4th Edition*, 2006, W.B. Saunders Company, New York, NY.

Mahan, Kathleen & Escott-Stump, Sylvia, *Krause's Food, Nutrition, & Diet Therapy, 10th Edition*, Saunders Company, New York, NY, 2000.

Matsumoto, Kiiko & Birch, Steven, *Extraordinary Vessels*, Paradigm Publications, Brookline, MA, 1986.

Mindell, Earl & Hopkins, Virginia, *Prescription Alternatives, Third Edition: Hundreds of Safe, Natural Prescription-Free Remedies to Restore and Maintain Your Health*, McGraw Hill, New York, NY, 2003.

Miriam Lee, *Master Tong's Acupuncture: An Ancient Alternative Style in Modern Clinical Practice*, Blue Poppy Press, Boulder, CO, 1992.

Morse, Linda, *Examination Workbook for Oriental Medicine*, Linda Morse, Los Angeles, CA, 2004.

Murray, Michael & Pizzorno, Joseph, *Encyclopedia of Natural Medicine, Revised Second Edition*, Three Rivers Press, New York, NY, 1997.

Murray, Michael & Pizzorno, Joseph, *Encyclopedia of Nutritional Supplements: The Essential Guide for Improving Your Health Naturally*, Three Rivers Press, New York, NY, 1996.

Ni, Maoshing & NcNease, Cathy, *The Tao of Nutrition*, College of Tao & Traditional Chinese Healing, Los Angeles, CA, 1987.

Null, Gary, *The Complete Encyclopedia of Natural Healing*, Kensington Books, New York, NY, 2005.

Oleson, Terry, *Auriculotherapy Manual 3rd Edition*, Churchill Livingston, London England, 2003.

Page, Linda, *Healthy Healing: A Guide to Self-Healing for Everyone, 12th Edition*, Traditional Wisdom, Inc. 2004.

Peilin, Sun, *The Treatment of Pain with Chinese Herbs and Acupuncture*, Churchill Livingstone, London, 2002.

Pharmacopoeia Commission of PRC, *Pharmacopoeia of the PRC*, People's Medical Publishing House, Beijing, 1988.

Qiu, Maoliang, *Chinese Acupuncture and Moxibustion*, Churchill Livingstone, London, 1993.

Ross, Jeremy, *Acupuncture Point Combinations: The Key to Clinical Success*, Churchill Livingstone, London, 1995.

Ross, Jeremy, *Zang Fu: The Organ Systems of Traditional Chinese Medicine*, Churchill Livingstone, London, 1989.

Shi, Anshen, *Essentials of Chinese Medicine: Internal Medicine*, Bridge Publishing Group, Walnut, CA, 2003.

Skidmore-Roth, Linda, *Mosby's Handbook of Herbs & Natural Supplements*, Mosby, St. Louis, MO, 2001.

Tan, Richard, *Acupuncture 1, 2, 3*, Richard Tan, San Diego, CA, 2006.

Tan, Richard, *Dr. Tan's Strategy of Twelve Magical Points, Advanced Principles and Techniques in Acupuncture*, Richard Tan, San Diego, CA, 1991.

Tan, Richard, *Twelve and Twelve*, Richard Tan, San Diego, CA, 1991.

Tan, Richard, *Twenty-Four More in Acupuncture*, Richard Tan, San Diego, CA, 1991.

Tierney, Lawrence M., *Current Medical Diagnosis & Treatment*, 2006, McGraw Hill, New York, NY, 2006.

Trivieri, Larry & Anderson, John, *Alternative Medicine: The Definitive Guide (2nd Edition)*, Celestial Arts, Berkeley, CA, 2002.

Van Straten, Michael, *Organic Super Foods*, Octopus Publishing, London, England, 2003.

Vizniak, Nikita, *Quick Reference Clinical Consultant Physical Assessment Manual*, Professional Health Systems Inc., Canada, 2006.

Werbach, Melvyn R., *Foundations of Nutritional Medicine*, Third Line Press, Tarzana, CA, 1997.

Werbach, Melvyn R., *Healing Through Nutrition*, Harper Collins, New York, NY, 1993.

Werbach, Melvyn R., *Nutritional Influences on Illness*, Second Edition, Third Line Press, Tarzana, CA, 1993.

Werbach, Melvyn R., *Nutritional Influences on Mental Illness*, Second Edition, Third Line Press, Tarzana, CA, 1999.

Wiseman, Nigel & Ellis, Andrew, *Fundamentals of Chinese Medicine*, Paradigm Pub., Brookline, MA, 1985.

Wiseman, Nigel & Mitchell, Craig, *Ten Lecturers on the Use of Formulas from the Personal Experience of Jiao Shu De*, Paradigm Publications, Taos, NM, 2005.

Wu, Yan & Fischer, Warren, *Practical Therapeutics of Traditional Chinese Medicine*, Paradigm Publications, Brookline, MA, 1997.

Yang, Yifan, *Chinese Herbal Medicines*, Churchill Livingstone, London, 2002.

Yeung, Him-che, *Handbook of Chinese Herbs*, Institute of Chinese Medicine, Los Angeles, CA, 1998.

Yeung, Him-che, *Handbook of Chinese Herbal Formulas*, Institute of Chinese Medicine, Los Angeles, CA, 1998.

Zheng, Dafang, *Essentials of Chinese Medicine Materia Medica*, Bridge Publishing Group, Walnut, CA, 2003.

Zhou Zhong Ying & Jin Hui De, *Clinical Manual of Chinese Herbal Medicine and Acupuncture*, Churchill Livingstone, London, 1997.

Zhu, CH, *Clinical Handbook of Chinese Prepared Medicines*, Paradigm Publications, Brookline, MA, 1989.

Zhu, Ming Ching, *Zhu's Scalp Acupuncture*, Eight Dragons Publishing, Hong Kong, 1992.

NOTES

Tell the Editors

The information is constantly evolving. We view ADR similar to a clearing house of information for the acupuncture community. Our research and editorial team analyzes information periodically. If you spot information that needs to be changed or updated, you can use this form, or a copy of it, to communicate directly with the editors. You can email or snail-mail the information. We appreciate your help!

We are constantly looking for feedback to improve future versions of Acupuncture Desk Reference.

1. What part of ADR are you commenting about?	Page Number

2. What wording should be added?	
(Please specific about exact wording that you propose adding)	

3. What wording should be deleted?	

4. What reference citations support this change?	
(Please give us specific reference citations.) We base on reliable studies published in peer-reviewed professional literature. Please give us enough information so that we can find the reference.	

5. What would you like to see in future versions of ADR?	

Name..

Address ....

City, State, Zip ....

Phone..

Email ....

Acumedwest Inc.
P.O. Box 14068
San Francisco, CA 94114
(310) 395-9573

www.acupuncturedeskreference.com
Email: adrguide@yahoo.com

About the author

David J Kuoch, LAc, (D.J.). began his early training in Traditional Chinese Medicine in China. He is a graduate of UCLA as well as a graduate of Emperors College of Traditional Chinese Medicine. He was an acupuncture fellow at Guang Xi Traditional Chinese Medical University in Nanning, China in the department of Orthopaedics and Integrative Medicine. Soon after finishing his training, he received advanced hospital training in the Acupuncture and Internal Medicine Departments at Guangzhou Chinese Traditional Medicine in Guangzhou, China. He is a licensed acupuncturist with a practice in San Francisco, CA specializing in pain management and orthopaedic acupuncture. DJ's work is derived from his passion for the promotion of Acupuncture and clinical excellence. When he is not actively involved in clinical practice or software development he enjoys, yoga, hiking, classic car restoration, riding vintage Ducati's & Moto Guzzi's, NPR, Bruins basketball, running, Chinese food, independent films, and great coffee.

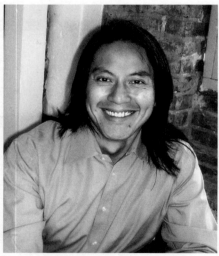

天佑中医
发揚光大
仁心仁术
救死扶伤

母親勉

David J. Kuoch, (D.J.) L.Ac.

To acquire knowledge, one must study;
but to acquire wisdom, one must observe.
~ *Marilyn vos Savant*

ORDER FORM

ACUPUNCTURE DESK REFERENCE ™
ACUPUNCTURE DESK REFERENCE VOLUME 2 ™

David J Kuoch, LAc

A Clinical Guide for the Modern Acupuncturist

Please Print Clearly

Name...
Address ....
City, State, Zip ....
Phone..

Books		Quantity	Price	Total
Acupuncture Desk Reference	$44.95			
Acupuncture Desk Reference Volume 2	$44.95			
(please indicate volumes)				
Subtotal				
California Residents, add 8.25% sales tax				
Shipping & Handling			5.00	
Shipping & Handling (2 books)			7.00	
Total				$

Make checks or money order or purchase orders payable to **Acumedwest.** We do not accept credit cards, however credit cards payments are available through paypal. Visit us at www.acupuncturedeskreference.com to order your copy today. International shipping is available. Please call for wholesale pricing or institutional orders.

Acumedwest Inc.
P.O. Box 14068
San Francisco, CA 94114
(310) 395-9573

www.acupuncturedeskreference.com
Email: adrguide@yahoo.com

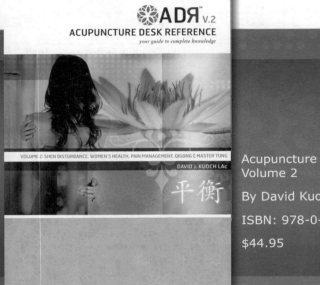